T0187745

PEDIATRIC NASAL
AND SINUS DISORDERS

LUNG BIOLOGY IN HEALTH AND DISEASE

Executive Editor

Claude Lenfant

Former Director, National Heart, Lung, and Blood Institute
National Institutes of Health
Bethesda, Maryland

The opinions expressed in these volumes do not necessarily represent the views of the National Institutes of Health.

PEDIATRIC NASAL AND SINUS DISORDERS

Edited by

Tania Sih
University of São Paulo
São Paulo, Brazil

Peter A. R. Clement
Free University of Brussels
Brussels, Belgium

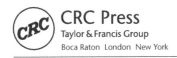

CRC Press
Taylor & Francis Group
Boca Raton London New York

CRC Press is an imprint of the
Taylor & Francis Group, an **informa** business
A TAYLOR & FRANCIS BOOK

CRC Press
Taylor & Francis Group
6000 Broken Sound Parkway NW, Suite 300
Boca Raton, FL 33487-2742

First issued in paperback 2019

© 2005 by Taylor & Francis Group, LLC
CRC Press is an imprint of Taylor & Francis Group, an Informa business

No claim to original U.S. Government works

ISBN-13: 978-0-8247-5448-8 (hbk)
ISBN-13: 978-0-367-39304-5 (pbk)

Library of Congress Cataloging-in-Publication Data

Catalog record is available from the Library of Congress

Introduction

Nose, nose, jolly red nose,
And who gave thee this jolly red nose? . . .
The Knight of the Burning Pestle
Francis Beaumont (1584–1616)

No one ever denied the importance of the nose, but it was really the December 1897 debut of *Cyrano de Bergerac*, a play by the French poet-dramatist Edmond Rostand, that made the nose famous. Cyrano, a poet and swordsman, was cursed with an enormous beak-like nose that, he believed, constituted an insurmountable impediment to attracting the love of a woman.

Today we still recognize the esthetic significance of the nose, but also—and perhaps more important—we now acknowledge and appreciate the functional significance of the interaction of the nasal airways with the lower airways. In fact, because of the similarities between the nasal and bronchial mucosa, the concept of "one airway, one disease" has been introduced. This concept is strongly supported by the relationship between rhinitis and asthma.

Over the years, the series of monographs *Lung Biology in Health and Disease* has presented many volumes and chapters in which the biology and pathology of the nose and the paranasal sinuses were discussed. However, never before has a volume like *Pediatric Nasal and Sinus Disorders*, edited by Drs. T. M. Sih and P. A. R. Clement, been included in the series. This work not only presents a comprehensive review of the physiology of the nose, and of its disorders, but also established the relationship between the nasal and the bronchial airways in health and disease.

The data presented in this volume come from well-recognized investigators and clinicians working in as many as 14 countries distributed in all continents. Thus, the readership is given a detailed and panoramic view of the subject area. As the editor of this series of monographs, I am grateful to the editors and contributors for the opportunity to present this new volume.

Claude Lenfant, M.D.
Gaithersburg, Maryland

Foreword

This is the first compendium dealing exclusively with rhinologic and sinus disorders *in children*, where differentiation of a "harmless" from a severe problem can be extremely difficult, and where under- and overtreatment are very close neighbors.

The list of authors reads like a "who's who" of today's specialists in rhinologic and sinus disorders worldwide, many of whom have dedicated their work exclusively to the pediatric age group. Tania Sih and Peter Clement have to be congratulated for achieving an outstanding task, first by stimulating the experts mentioned to contribute their outstanding knowledge and skills and second, by succeeding in making the book easy and interesting to read, as if it were written by one person.

The editors have left room for controversy and individual approaches: a solution in one country need not necessarily be applicable to another one, and depends on regional, even medico-social differences. This book, therefore, is very honest, not dogmatic, and reflects the state of the art of our knowledge in the new millenium. It is designed to help physicians and surgeons and clinical and basic researchers devoted to rhinologic and sinus problems—but most of all to help those children in the world suffering from the latter.

Dr. Heinz Stammberger
Professor and Chair
Department of General ENT,
Head, and Neck Surgery
University Medical School
Graz, Austria

Preface

Over the last two decades, significant progress has been made in the field of rhinology—some even feel they have been the two most exciting decades for rhinology so far. Basic research increased our knowledge of the pathophysiology of rhinosinusitis, of allergy and immunology, environmental and developmental problems, as well as of smell, taste, and genetic features. Imaging technologies with reduced or even no radiation, CT and MRI, allowed for pictures of anatomical structures and pathological processes, for three-dimensional visualization unheard of before. Microscopes and endoscopes gave insight on the nose and its sinuses with unprecedented clarity, resulting in new diagnostic and surgical procedures, all aiming to avoid unnecessary trauma to the delicate structures or, even better, to avoid surgery at all, based on better diagnosis and prevention.

This book has been written for every physician who deals with children with upper respiratory infections (URIs), allergy, and related diseases (i.e., asthma and allergic rhinitis/sinus infection, cystic fibrosis, choanal atresia, HIV infection, gastroesophageal reflux, obstructive sleep apnea). As URIs are very common in childhood, it is mandatory to make a correct diagnosis followed by an appropriate therapy. There exist, however, a lot of controversies about the "appropriate therapy." Some authors are very conservative, others are very surgically minded. It is the editors' opinion that in the future, on the one hand, one has to be very conservative, especially in our use of antibiotics, and on the other, one also has to be firm in performing the necessary surgery for the right indications in order to prevent complications that can sometimes jeopardize the life of a child. More emphasis, however, has to be put on prevention. In the long run, prevention is the cheapest mode of treatment with the best benefit/cost ratio, which is not only the right way to keep the national health budget in balance, but also the only way to create an environment where the quality of life is good for the generations to come. This book discusses all such aspects of health care.

The chapters in the book are written by authors from 14 different countries all over the world (i.e., Australia, Austria, Brazil, Belgium, Canada, France, Italy, Mexico, Norway, Singapore, Spain, The Netherlands, United Kingdom, and United States). This worldwide approach is necessary because the problems in highly industrialized countries are not similar to those in developing countries. We have tried to give a balanced coverage to the more commonly encountered problems as well as the more complex infections. Similarly, both concepts and advanced techniques are discussed and therefore this book will be beneficial to specialists as well as students and residents in pediatrics, infectious disease, ENT, immunology, and pneumonology.

The book is organized into four complementary sections: basic sciences/epidemiology, diagnosis, medical management, and surgery. The first section delves into the basic science of URIs and allergies as well as the latest research findings regarding epidemiology and pathophysiology. The second and third sections covering diagnosis and medical management discuss the most current methods in diagnosing and treating URIs and allergies. The chapters on antimicrobial agents will be especially relevant to practitioners who encounter these cases on a daily basis and need guidance on dosage and follow-up. The fourth section on surgery details the surgical options available and will be useful in determining the most optimal treatment plan. Chapter 23, Allergic Rhinitis and Its Impact on Asthma (ARIA document), summarizes the guidelines under which definitions were determined, and the management of rhinosinusitis in children is discussed. We are confident that the book gives a complete review of the field and will find wide readership as the most practical and accessible reference on the market for pediatric nasal/sinus infections, allergies, and related diseases.

T. M. SIH and P. A. R. CLEMENT
Editors

List of Contributors

Dayse Carneiro Alt, M.D. *Department of Pulmonology, Federal University of Rio Grande do Sul, Porto Alegre, Brazil.*

Marco Anselmi, M.D. *Department of Otorhinolaryngology, University of Siena, Siena, Italy.*

Elizabeth Araújo, M.D. *Brazilian Society of Rhinology, Porto Alegre, Brazil.*

Claus Bachert, M.D. *Department of Otorhinolaryngology, University Hospital Ghent, Ghent, Belgium.*

Luisa Bellussi, M.D. *Department of Otorhinolaryngology, University of Siena, Siena, Italy.*

Joel M. Bernstein, M.D., Ph.D., P.C. *Department of Otolaryngology, State University of New York, Buffalo, New York, USA.*

William E. Bolger, M.D. *Department of Otorhinolaryngology, Head and Neck Surgery, University of Pennsylvania Health System, Philadelphia, Pennsylvania, USA.*

Marcella Bothwell, M.D. *Department of Pediatric Otolaryngology, University of Missouri, Columbia, Missouri, and Department of Pediatric Otolaryngology, Washington University, St. Louis, Missouri, USA.*

Jean Bousquet, M.D. *Department of Respiratory Disease, University of Montpellier, Montpellier, France.*

Lucia Ferro Bricks, M.D., Ph.D. *Department of Pediatrics & Otolaryngology, University of São Paulo, São Paulo, Brazil.*

Pierre Brihaye, M.D. *Department of Otorhinolaryngology, Free University of Brussels, Brussels, Belgium.*

Itzhak Brook, M.D., M.Sc. *Georgetown University, Washington, D.C., USA.*

Paul van Cauwenberge, M.D. *Department of Otolaryngology, University Hospital Ghent, Ghent, Belgium.*

Peter A. R. Clement, M.D., Ph.D. *Department of Otolaryngology, Free University of Brussels, Brussels, Belgium.*

Harvey Coates, M.D., F.A.C.S. *Princess Margaret Hospital for Children, Perth, Australia.*

Philip Cole, M.D., F.R.C.S.C. *Department of Otolaryngology, University of Toronto, Toronto, Ontario, Canada.*

Valerio Damiani *Department of Otolaryngology, University of Siena, Siena, Italy.*

Ellen Deutsch, M.D. *Division of Pediatric Otolaryngology, Alfred I. Dupont Hospital for Children, Wilmington, Delaware, USA.*

Javier Dibildox, M.D. *Department of Pediatrics & Otorhinolaryngology, Autonomous University of San Luis Potosí, San Luis Potosí, Mexico.*

Per Djupesland, M.D., Ph.D. *Department of Otorhinolaryngology, Head and Neck Surgery, Ullevål University Hospital, Oslo, Norway.*

Amy Doherty, M.D. *Clinical Neuroscience Branch, NIMH, National Institutes of Health (NIH), Bethesda, Maryland, USA.*

Scott F. Dowell, M.D. *Centers for Disease Control and Prevention, Atlanta, Georgia, USA.*

Bernardo Ejzemberg, M.D., Ph.D. *Division of Pediatrics and Department of Otolaryngology, University of São Paulo, São Paulo, Brazil.*

Patrick Froehlich, M.D., Ph.D. *Department of Otorhinolaryngology, Head and Neck Surgery, E. Herriot Hospital, Lyon, France.*

Frans Gordts, M.D., Ph.D. *Pediatric ENT Department, Free University of Brussels, Brussels, Belgium.*

Rainer Haetinger, M.D. *Head and Neck Radiology, Hospital Beneficência Portuguesa, São Paulo, Brazil.*

Helen van Hcecke *Department of Otorhinolaryngology, University Hospital Ghent, Ghent, Belgium.*

Robert I. Henkin, M.D. *Center for Molecular Nutrition and Sensory Disorders, Washington, D.C., USA.*

Muriel van Kempen, M.D. *Department of Otorhinolaryngology, University Hospital Ghent, Ghent, Belgium.*

David W. Kennedy, M.D. *Department of Otorhinolaryngology, Head and Neck Surgery, University of Pennsylvania, Philadelphia, Pennsylvania, USA.*

Bernd Kremer, M.D., Ph.D. *Department of Otorhinolaryngology, Head and Neck Surgery, Maastricht University, Maastricht, The Netherlands.*

Paola Marchisio, M.D. *Department of Pediatrics, University of Milan, Milan, Italy.*

Brian M. Martin, M.D. *Clinical Neuroscience Branch, NIMH, National Institutes of Health (NIH), Bethesda, Maryland, USA.*

Maria Carolina Gouveia Miorim, M.D. *Department of Pulmonology, Federal University of Rio Grande do Sul, Porto Alegre, Brazil.*

Bruno Carlos Palombini, M.D., Ph.D. *Federal University of Rio Grande do Sul, Porto Alegre, Brazil.*

Carlos Oliveira Palombini, M.D. *Department of Pulmonology, Federal University of Rio Grande do Sul, Porto Alegre, Brazil.*

Yoke Teen Pang, M.D. *Department of Otorhinolaryngology, The National University of Singapore, Singapore, Republic of Singapore.*

David S. Parsons, M.D., F.A.A.P., F.A.C.S. *Pediatric Otolaryngology and Sinus Care, Greenville, South Carolina, USA.*

Desiderio Passàli, M.D. *Department of Otorhinolaryngology, University of Siena, Siena, Italy.*

Francesco Maria Passàli, M.D. *Department of Otorhinolaryngology, University of Genova, Genova, Italy.*

Giulio Cesare Passàli, M.D.   *Department of Otorhinolaryngology, University of Genova, Genova, Italy.*

Nicola Principi, M.D.   *Department of Pediatrics, University of Milan, Milan, Italy.*

Tania Quintella, M.D., Ph.D.   *Department of Pediatrics, Pediatric Society of São Paulo, São Paulo, Brazil.*

Molakala Reddy, Ph.D.   *Department of Oral Biology, State University of New York, Buffalo, New York, USA.*

James S. Reilly, M.D.   *Jefferson Medical College, Philadelphia, Pennsylvania, USA.*

Renato Roithmann, M.D., Ph.D.   *Department of Otorhinolaryngology, Head and Neck Surgery, Universidade Luterana do Brasil, Canoas, Brazil.*

Francisco Giménez Sánchez, M.D., Ph.D.   *Unidad de Investigaciòn en Medicina, Tropical y Salud Internacional, Instituto de Salud Carlos III, Madrid, Spain and Centers for Disease Control and Prevention (CDC), Atlanta, Georgia, USA.*

Glenis K. Scadding, M.D.   *Royal National Throat, Nose and Ear Hospital, London, UK.*

Lalitha Shankar, M.D.   *Department of Medical Imaging and Otolaryngology, University of Toronto, Toronto, Canada.*

Isaac Shubich, M.D.   *Department of Pediatric Otorhinolaryngology, Miami Children's Hospital, Miami, Florida, USA.*

Tania Maria Sih, M.D., Ph.D.   *Professor of Medical School, Laboratory of Medical Investigation, University of São Paulo, São Paulo, Brazil.*

Carel D. A. Verwoerd, M.D.   *Department of Otorhinolaryngology, Erasmus University Medical Center, Rotterdam, The Netherlands.*

Henriette L. Verwoerd-Verhoef, M.D.   *Department of Otorhinolaryngology, Erasmus University Medical Center, Rotterdam, The Netherlands.*

Ellen R. Wald, M.D.   *Department of Pediatrics & Otorhinolaryngology, University of Pittsburgh, Pittsburgh, Pennsylvania, USA.*

De-Yun Wang, M.D., Ph.D.   *Department of Otolaryngology, The National University of Singapore, Singapore, Republic of Singapore.*

Erin D. Wright, M.D., C.M., F.R.C.S.(C).   *Department of Otolaryngology, University of Western Ontario, Ontario, Canada.*

Contents

A. Basic Sciences/Epidemiology

1

Immune Defense Mechanisms in Viral Upper Respiratory Tract Infections

PAUL VAN CAUWENBERGE, MURIEL VAN KEMPEN, and CLAUS BACHERT

University Hospital Ghent,
Ghent, Belgium

I. Introduction

An upper respiratory tract infection or common cold is characterized by rhino-rrhea, nasal congestion, and sneezing, sometimes accompanied by fever, sore throat, and malaise. It is one of the most frequent infectious diseases in man (1). Throughout our lifetime, we spend between 1 and 2 years suffering from a cold (2). Especially, preschool children often (approximately 6 up to 12 times a year) suffer from an upper respiratory tract infection, while the incidence decreases with age and averages two to three common colds a year in adolescents and adults (3). Although these infections are generally mild and self-limiting, they account for a big economical burden due to high medical costs and high morbidity. Each year, US physicians are consulted for an upper respiratory tract infection about 27 million times and almost $2 billion are spent on over-the-counter medications for treatment of common cold symptoms (4). In addition, approximately 26 million days of school absence annually have been attributed to an upper respiratory tract infection (3).

In some cases, however, a bacterial invasion may follow the initial infection and it is these invaders that may produce complications like otitis media, acute sinusitis, or even pneumonia (5). Besides, several epidemiological studies have demonstrated a relationship between upper respiratory tract infections and increased lower airway reactivity and asthma (6,7).

Approximately 80% of the acute upper respiratory tract infections are caused by viruses (8). Rhinoviruses are responsible for about half of these viral colds in adults while coronaviruses account for about 15% (9,10). Although rhinoviruses can also cause an acute upper respiratory tract infection in children, other viral agents like respiratory syncytial virus (RSV) and para-influenza more frequently induce viral upper respiratory tract illnesses (11). However, since most people associate viral colds with rhinoviruses we will focus on this virus while discussing the host immune defense mechanisms to an acute viral upper respiratory tract infection.

II. Rhinovirus

A rhinovirus is a nonenveloped 30 nm RNA virus with over 100 serotypes (10). It belongs to the Picornaviridae family, consisting of small RNA viruses (Pico RNA viruses) and only replicates in primates (5). The viral capsid has an icosahedral symmetry and is characterized by deep canyons, with a receptor-binding domain (12).

The rhinovirus is spread from person to person by virus contaminated respiratory secretions, partially through inhalation of small- or large-particle aerosols, but mainly via direct or indirect contact with infected secretions (3). In 40–90% of common cold patients, the rhinovirus could be detected on the hands, presumably due to frequent contact with the virus-shedding nose (13). Hendley and Gwaltney (14) supported the importance of hand-to-hand transmission by demonstrating that treatment of the hands with a virucidal compound significantly reduced transmission of rhinovirus infection. Since rhinoviruses retain their virulence for up to 3 days on plastic surfaces, transmission is very easy. Once the hands are contaminated, introduction of a finger in the eyes or nose will initiate infection.

III. Host Defense Against Rhinovirus Infection

The host defense against acute upper respiratory tract infections generally consists of three mechanisms, namely, the nonspecific passive and active mechanisms and the specific, active immune responses.

A. Nonspecific, Passive Defense Mechanisms

Nonspecific, passive defense mechanisms are innate mechanical or chemical barriers that prevent colonization and penetration of the epithelium by pathogens. A true mechanical barrier in the upper respiratory tract is formed by the vibrissae in the nasal vestibule filtering the inhaled air. However, due to the small size of a rhinovirus this first line of defense does not inhibit rhinovirus entry into the nasal cavity.

Once the rhinovirus has entered the nasal cavity, it is exposed to the second nonspecific mechanical as well as chemical barrier: the epithelium and the mucociliary clearing system.

Nasal mucus covering the epithelium consists of various locally produced or serum derived substances (15). These substances can be divided into specific immunoglobulins that will be discussed later in this chapter and nonspecific substances like lactoferrin and lysozyme that inhibit the growth and spread of microorganisms. The former is an iron-chelating protein with bacteriostatic effects while lysozyme has bactericidal properties by breaking down the bacterial core (15,16). However, both of these proteins, produced by submucosal glands, do not exert an influence on the spread of viruses. Therefore nasal secretions also contain antiviral interferons and complement components (15,17). These complement proteins can be activated on the one hand via the classical pathway by interaction between the complement component C1 and antigen–antibody complexes (18). The alternative pathway, on the other hand, is activated by lipopolysaccharides present on gram-negative bacterial cell surfaces. The various complement components interact with each other and with other elements of the immune system. Once activated, the complement system exerts various functions like opsonization of antigen thus facilitating subsequent phagocytosis. It furthermore induces chemotaxis and activation of leucocytes, the release of various enzymes like bacterial proteases, and an increased vascular permeability.

Not only the nasal mucus but also the ciliary transport inhibits pathogen adhesion to the nasal epithelium. Synchronized wavelike motion of the cilia at a frequency of 700 beats per minute conveys the mucus toward the nasopharynx where it is swallowed and finally digested by the gastrointestinal tract (19). However, instead of blocking infection, rhinoviruses benefit from this clearing system as rhinovirus infection starts in the nasopharynx (20).

Thus, in spite of the various nonspecific defense mechanisms a rhinovirus can easily arrive at the site of infection, the adenoid or the lymphoid tissue in the nasopharynx. In this area we have a lympho-epithelium rich in the intercellular adhesion receptor molecule-1 (ICAM-1), a member of the immunoglobulin superfamily and a major ligand binding site for rhinoviruses (21). Approximately 90% of the rhinoviruses infect their host by binding to this receptor (22,23). Once bound to the epithelial cell surface the rhinovirus penetrates the cell. After intracellular invasion and replication, the infection spreads to the nasal mucosa and to the pharynx (20). Typical for rhinovirus infections are the isolated scattered foci of infected epithelium between large areas of normal epithelium (24,25). In contrast to other common cold viruses like influenza and adenoviruses, the epithelium does not show any striking damage or cytopathic alterations during a rhinovirus infection (26,27).

B. Nonspecific Active Defense Mechanisms

Once the epithelium is invaded and viral replication has started, inflammatory responses are evoked by the host. These nonspecific inflammatory responses are generated within hours after rhinovirus infection. Vasodilatation and increased vascular permeability, cellular infiltration, and the release of various mediators characterize this response. In addition, increased mucus production by seromucous glands and irritation of the sensible nerve receptors in the subepithelium and epithelium are observed. The ultimate goal of this response is phagocytosis and lysis of the invading microorganism.

The Plasma Exudate

Largely contributing to our current understanding of the common cold was the work of Naclerio and Proud (28), who challenged healthy volunteers with two strains of rhinoviruses (T 39 and HH) and performed nasal washes every 4 h around the clock for 5 days. They found significantly increased levels of albumin in nasal secretions of infected symptomatic subjects compared to controls, indicating increased permeability of the nasal vessels.

Various inflammatory mediators may induce vasodilatation of local blood vessels and increased capillary permeability. Reversibly, the resulting increased blood supply and plasma exudation provides additional mediators and substrates for the inflammatory and immune response. This plasma exudate may also be of sufficient volume to contribute to the rhinorrhea associated with a common cold.

The Cellular Inflammatory Response

Several studies have demonstrated increased neutrophil counts in the nasal mucosa and nasal secretions as well as in the peripheral blood of symptomatic subjects during both natural and experimental common colds (28–31). A nasal biopsy study demonstrated increased neutrophil numbers on the first and second days of infection while others failed to show an alteration in neutrophil number in the biopsies performed on day 4 of illness (29,32). Naclerio and Proud (28) also observed an early but transient increase in neutrophil count in nasal washes within 24 h after rhinovirus inoculation.

Since neutrophils express Fc and complement receptors on their surface which recognize opsonizing IgG and activated complement components (C3b, C3d), they are able to effectively phagocytose antigenic material. However, even though they limit the spread of rhinoviruses, the extracellular release of their cytotoxic proteins like myeloperoxidase (MPO), lysozyme, and elastase, the generation of superoxide radicals on their surface, and the release of mediators (e.g., LTB4) also enhance tissue damage and continuation of the inflammatory response.

Some days after the start of the inflammatory response, recruitment of monocytes crossing the endothelium and becoming tissue macrophages has been observed (33). These macrophages are activated by complement components and cytokines, which results in phagocytosis of the debris left over from the attack of the neutrophils. Furthermore, macrophages present antigen together with major histocompatibility complex (MHC) class I or II molecules to T-lymphocytes and produce cytokines like IL-1β, a T-cell activating cytokine (18). Thus, macrophages do not only play an important role in the inflammatory response but are also of critical importance for the initiation of the specific active immune defense mechanisms.

Inflammatory Mediators

Bradykinin

In the previously mentioned study by Naclerio and Proud (28) a 10-fold increase in kinin concentrations in nasal lavage fluids of infected symptomatic subjects was observed compared to baseline values. These alterations contrasted with the relatively unchanged kinin concentrations in infected asymptomatic and control subjects. In addition, the increased kinin levels were shown to correlate with the severity of common cold symptoms.

Bradykin is a well-known potent inflammatory mediator, which causes vasodilatation and increased vascular permeability and stimulates pain and glandular secretion via neuronal reflexes. When administered intranasally in normal subjects, symptoms of nasal obstruction, rhinorrhea, and a sore throat appear, suggesting that this mediator may indeed contribute to the typical common cold symptoms (34).

Histamine

In an experimentally induced rhinovirus infection no significant alterations in histamine concentrations were observed in nasal secretions of infected symptomatic subjects compared to controls (28). This observation, together with nasal biopsy studies showing no change either in mast cell number or in mast cell degranulation, suggests that mast cells do not exert a major role in the patho-physiology of a rhinovirus infection (26).

Cytokines

The observed migration of inflammatory cells and their subsequent acti-vation is orchestrated by cytokines (35). These proteins regulate chemotaxis, and cellular differentiation and activation by the induction of adhesion molecule expression and the release of additive, synergistic, or antagonistic cytokines. A rhinovirus infection is supposed to trigger synthesis and release of these mediators and cytokines resulting in a cascade of inflammatory reactions.

In Vitro Experiments

In vitro studies of cell cultures have demonstrated the production of IL-8 in response to rhinovirus stimulation in both fibroblasts as well as respiratory epi-thelial cells (36–38).

Not only IL-8 but also IL-6 were found to be released in human rhino-virus infected epithelial cell lines (39). The same cytokines were produced after RSV challenge, indicating that the cytokine production is not specific to a certain virus (40,41).

Especially IL-8 is of great importance in rhinovirus colds, as it is a strong chemoattractant for neutrophils (42,43). It belongs to the C–X–C family of che-mokines and induces the expression of $\beta2$-integrins, namely, LFA-1 and Mac-1, on neutrophils, which bind to the endothelium via adhesion receptor molecules that mediate their transendothelial migration (44). In addition, IL-8 is capable of activating the recruited neutrophils (45).

Another cytokine found to be released is IL-6. Zhu et al. (39) demonstrated in an *in vitro* model significantly elevated IL-6 protein production 24–72 h after a rhinovirus infection. IL-6 is a pleiotropic cytokine. It has activating and prolifera-tive effects on lymphocytes (43,46). Indeed, under the influence of IL-6, B-lymphocytes mature and differentiate into plasma cells and the subsequent production of immunoglobulins is stimulated (47,48). In addition, IL-6 mediates T-cell activation, growth, and differentiation (49). The critical role of IL-6 in initiating humoral responses is confirmed by IL-6 knockout mice with deficient immunoglobulin responses after viral challenge (50). Furthermore, IL-6 plays an important role in the host response to trauma by inducing "acute phase proteins" such as C-reactive protein (43,46). Finally, it could participate in common cold symptoms, as it induces pyrexia (49). In fact, a direct correlation between IL-6 and symptom severity has been shown in experimentally induced rhinovirus colds (39).

The rhinoviruses do not only induce the local production of cytokines, they also influence *per se* the expression of their receptor molecule—ICAM-1—on epithelial cells (51). *In vitro* studies have shown that nasal epithelial cells infected by rhinoviruses display a significant upregulation of ICAM-1 expression (52). This direct effect of rhinovirus infection on ICAM-1 expression facilitates further viral spread by increasing cell attachment and entry. In addition, rhino-viruses also exert indirect ICAM-1 upregulating effects via the induction of cyto-kine production (53,54). For instance, *in vitro* pretreatment of uninfected nasal epithelial cells with IL-8 increases ICAM-1 expression, while IL-8 pretreatment followed by rhinovirus inoculation additionally upregulates epithelial ICAM-1 expression (55). However, it has been shown that epithelial ICAM-1 expression depends on the kind of mediator released, and ICAM-1 downregulating cytokines have also been found.

Studies on Experimentally Induced Common Cold

Mediator and cytokine production was not only studied in *in vitro* experi-ments but also in experimentally induced rhinovirus upper respiratory tract infections in humans. Proud et al. (56) recently reported increased IL-1β concen-trations in nasal lavage fluids of infected symptomatic subjects compared to infected asymptomatic and noninfected volunteers during an experimental rhinovirus cold.

IL-1β has important proinflammatory properties. It enhances the expression of adhesion molecules such as E-selectin and ICAM-1 on endothelial cells (49,57). These endothelial receptor molecules induce the recruitment and migration of granulocytes and lymphocytes to the site of inflammation by inter-acting with their cognate receptor. However, IL-1β also upregulates ICAM-1 expression on epithelial cells (54). Therefore, by upregulating ICAM-1 expression, IL-1β possibly exerts a dual effect on rhinovirus infections. First, it initiates the host response to infection by enhancing the recruitment of immune effector cells into the inflammatory site, and second, it could increase rhinoviral spread via upregulation of its receptor. Besides, IL-1β also exerts important activating and proliferative effects on lymphocytes via IL-2 receptor induction, thus stimulating the specific cellular host response as well (57). In addition, IL-1β increases vascular permeability and induces the release of other proinflammatory mediators like platelet-activating factor as well as the cytokine IL-8 from epithelial cells (58,59).

Because viruses, unlike bacteria, remain intracellular, a cell-mediated immune response is essential to eradicate a rhinovirus infection. The most important cytokine for macrophage activation and thereby for cell-mediated immunity is IFN-γ (60). It upregulates MHC expression, and stimulates macro-phage accumulation and activation and cytokine production (42,60). In addition, it stimulates natural killer cell function and antigen-specific B-cell proliferation (49,61). In fact, in experimentally induced upper respiratory tract infections increased concentrations of IFN-γ were observed in nasal secretions of sympto-matic subjects (62). Interestingly, *in vitro* experiments have shown an additional antiviral function of IFN-γ, as it persistently downregulates ICAM-1 expression on rhinovirus infected epithelial cells (55).

Studies on naturally acquired upper respiratory tract infections have confirmed the increased concentrations of IL-1β, IL-6, IL-8, and IFN-γ in nasal washes of symptomatic subjects compared to baseline values (8,63,64). Noah et al. (63) also observed significantly elevated TNF-α levels, which gradually returned to normal values, in nasal lavage fluids of children during acute upper respiratory tract infections. Like IL-1β, TNF-α has strong proinflammatory properties, as it costimulates T- and B-lymphocytes and activates endothelial cells to express adhesion molecules and to release further cytokines (49,65). In addition, it is a potent activator of neutrophils, mediating adherence, chemotaxis, and degranulation (9). Furthermore, it induces vascular leakage and regulates MHC expression on various cells (42,65). Finally, it activates macrophages and augments their capacity to release inflammatory mediators and cytokines such as IL-6 and IL-8 (42).

Recently, we have focused on the time course of release of various cytokines and chemokines in nasal lavages of subjects during a naturally acquired upper respiratory tract infection (66). Compared to baseline, we found transient, significantly elevated concentrations of IL-1β, IL-6, TNF-α, IL-8, MPO, IFN-γ, and monocyte chemotactic protein-1 (MCP-1) in nasal secretions, which all returned to baseline levels 3 weeks after the symptomatic cold. In addition, we measured the concentrations of IL-1ra, a naturally occurring IL-1 receptor antagonist; its levels were found to be unaltered during the overall study period. Since IL-1ra binds to the IL-1 receptors without effecting a biological response, constant IL-1ra concentrations and increased levels of IL-1β would result in favoring the proinflammatory process. Interestingly, we observed a rapid increase in IL-8 levels, which is held responsible for the early neutrophil recruitment observed in nasal biopsy studies. A subsequent decrease in IL-8 concentrations from study day 3 is also in agreement with the previously mentioned nasal biopsy and lavage studies, showing no significant alterations in neutrophil numbers on day 4 of a rhinovirus cold (32). Furthermore, a strong correlation was found between IL-8 and neutrophil MPO levels, a cytoplasmic granule constituent, which is set free by activated neutrophils. This observation demonstrates the major role of IL-8 in neutrophil recruitment and activation with subsequent degranulation in rhinovirus colds. MPO and other neutrophilic enzymes like elastase and also superoxide radicals on their surface have been shown to cause severe tissue damage. In fact, Teran et al. (64) found a direct relation between MPO concentrations and the severity of common cold symptoms in children with virus induced asthma. These correlations between IL-8, MPO, and common cold symptoms were very recently confirmed by Turner et al. (67) who observed a direct relation between the magnitude of the rise in IL-8 and the severity of common cold symptoms in volunteers after rhinovirus type 23 inoculation.

In contrast to the early increase in IL-8 levels, we found gradually increasing concentrations of MCP-1 during the study period. MCP-1 is a member of the

C–C chemokine family, which preferentially attracts and stimulates monocytes (68). The slow increase in MCP-1 levels is in accordance with the delayed monocyte mucosal infiltration observed in other studies (33).

Finally, besides cytokines and chemokine, we also focused on the soluble form of the adhesion molecule ICAM-1—sICAM-1—which was found to be elevated in nasal secretions of patients with naturally acquired common cold (66). This increase is likely to be secondary to the upregulated epithelial ICAM-1 expression by cytokines, followed by shedding of the molecule from the cell surface into nasal secretions (69). In contrast to cell-bound ICAM-1, the exact function of sICAM-1 is not clarified yet. It could inhibit rhinovirus infection, block the recruitment of inflammatory cells, or just serve as a marker of infection (70,71).

C. Specific, Active Immune Defense Mechanisms

Upon stimulation with proinflammatory cytokines the host-specific active immune defense consisting of cellular and humoral immunity is initiated.

The Cellular Immune Response

Since rhinoviruses remain intracellular, the major mechanism to terminate infection is by cell-mediated immunity. In this process antigens are either recognized by MHC class I restricted CD8+ cytotoxic T-lymphocytes or processed and expressed in association with class II MHC molecules on the cell surface of antigen presenting cells in a way that they are recognized by CD4+ helper T-lymphocytes. Antigenic stimulation in the presence of macrophage derived IL-1β induces T-lymphocytes to differentiate into IL-2 producing cells. The subsequent binding of secreted IL-2 to high-affinity IL-2 receptors on activated T-lymphocytes induces clonal T-cell proliferation.

In contrast to the clear increase in neutrophils, the involvement of lymphocytes in rhinovirus colds is still a matter of debate. Winther et al. (72) studied lymphocyte populations in the nasal mucosa during an experimentally induced viral rhinitis by immunohistochemistry and found no striking alterations in the number or subset distribution of T- and B-lymphocytes in comparison to normal nasal mucosa. Nevertheless, Lewandowski et al. (30) demonstrated an increased number of T-lymphocytes in nasal secretions, a reduced number of circulating lymphocytes, and a decreased serum T-helper/T-suppressor ratio during an experimentally induced rhinovirus infection. They assumed that the reduced number of circulating T-lymphocytes was related to the recruitment of T-lymphocytes in the nasal mucosa. It is not clear whether these discrepant findings on lymphocyte count are based on different viral serotypes, alterations in symptom severity, or differences in methodology.

However, unanimity exists on T-helper cell polarization. As mentioned previously, following a rhinovirus infection, significantly increased concentrations of IFN-γ and IL-2 were observed in nasal secretions indicating the development of T-helper-1 cells (63,66). Generally upon antigenic stimulation T-helper-0 cells, producing an unrestricted cytokine profile, may differentiate into either T-helper-1 lymphocytes inducing cellular immune responses or T-helper-2 lymphocytes inducing a humoral response (73). Intracellular antigenic stimulation, as in rhinovirus infection, promotes a T-cell cytokine polarization toward T-helper-1 cells with their specific cytokine profile of IL-2 and IFN-γ (33). In addition, it has recently been shown that CD8+ cytotoxic T-lymphocytes synthesize a T-helper-1 pattern of lymphokines like IFN-γ, also influencing the differentiation of uncommitted T-helper cells in favor of T-helper-1 cells (61). This propagation of the immune response toward a T-helper-1 lymphocyte pathway induces several effector functions like macrophage accumulation and activation, thus enhancing the cell-mediated immunity necessary to eradicate the viral infection.

The Humoral Immune Response

Humoral immunity is mediated by immunoglobulins produced by plasma cells. This type of immune response is principally important against extracellular pathogens (18). In the case of intracellular viruses its function is restricted to antigen opsonization facilitating phagocytosis. In addition, antibodies in association with complement can cause a lysis of the virus-bearing cells. Immunoglobulins, furthermore, activate the classical complement pathway and play a key role in the immune exclusion at the nasal epithelium.

During the early course of a rhinovirus infection, an increase in IgG concentrations in nasal secretions can be observed (74). This IgG is partially produced locally but is predominantly serum derived (74,75). However, as it is not virus specific, it only amplifies the inflammatory process by activating the classical complement pathway and contributes to the host immune response by antigen opsonization. Local and systemic neutralizing antibodies are usually not detectable until 2–3 weeks after rhinovirus infection, indicating that alternate cell-mediated defense mechanisms combat the acute symptomatic infection (76). Therefore, the role of neutralizing antibodies in rhinovirus infections seems limited to rhinovirus serotype-specific protection. Following the first viral contact, an immunologic memory is built up. This memory consists of "memory" T- and B-lymphocytes. During repeated antigen contact this memory enables T-lymphocytes to react on lower antigen concentrations and B-lymphocytes to produce immunoglobulins more rapidly and more abundantly. This secondary response facilitates rapid elimination at lower antigen concentrations.

In an earlier study, we investigated the protective serum antibody level in subjects experimentally infected by rhinovirus type 2 (77). A seroconversion, defined as a fourfold increase of specific neutralizing antibodies, could be observed in 41 out of 50 volunteers (82%) 3 weeks after inoculation (Table 1.1).

Table 1.1 Seroconversion of Neutralizing Antibodies after Intranasal Challenge of 50 Volunteers with Rhinovirus Type 2 in Relation to the Prechallenge Serum Antibody Titer (77)

Initial antibody titer	Seroconversion (n)	No seroconversion (n)
<2	11	1
2	9	1
4	14	1
8	6	1
16	1	0
32	0	4
>128	0	1
Total	41	9

Note: n = number of subjects.

Subjects with an initial antibody titer greater than 16 did not show seroconversion, indicating the protective serum level of specific neutralizing antibodies. Six months after inoculation, only 41% of the subjects still demonstrated a seroconversion. After 9 months, this percentage dropped to 10% indicating only a transient increase in specific neutralizing antibodies. This results in susceptibility to a rhinovirus infection even with the same serotype as early as 9 months after primary infection. Furthermore, it has been suggested recently that the protection against upper respiratory tract infection results rather from a transient production of secretory IgA (sIgA) by mucosal plasma cells than from increased serum neutralizing antibodies, indicating that even a high serum level of specific neutralizing antibodies does not always protect against reinfection (17).

Indeed, the pioneering work of Brandzaeg and colleagues strongly indicates that immunoglobulin polymers, especially dimeric sIgA, play a key role in epithelial surface protection. Exported through secretory epithelial cells by binding to a constitutively expressed epithelial receptor protein complex—called the transmembrane secretory component—sIgA performs immune exclusion. By binding to microorganisms in the airways forming an insoluble complex, it prevents epithelial attachment and further rhinovirus spread.

IV. Conclusion

A rhinovirus infection represents a neutrophilic inflammatory reaction with relatively mild symptoms. *In vitro* and *in vivo* data have demonstrated a time-limited, rhinovirus induced release of epithelial derived proinflammatory cytokines and an increase in bradykinin, chemokine, and sICAM-1 concentrations. The epithelial derived proinflammatory cytokines initiate an adhesion cascade and activate the recruited inflammatory cells. These cells produce in their turn cytokines, resulting in an amplification of the inflammatory process. The typical selective neutrophil recruitment seems linked to the increased concentrations of IL-8 and common cold symptoms. In addition, T-lymphocytes are activated to create a T-helper-1-type cytokine environment, necessary to eradicate the virus infection. The cytokine-regulated production of specific neutralizing immunoglobulins only contributes to a temporary protection against rhinovirus reinfection.

These observations confirm the crucial role that cytokines and mediators play in the pathogenesis of a rhinovirus infection.

References

1. Kirkpatrick GL. The common cold. Primary Care 1996; 23:657–675.
2. Rowlands DJ. Rhinoviruses and cells: molecular aspects. Am J Respir Crit Care Med 1995; 152:S31–S35.
3. Turner RB. Epidemiology, pathogenesis and treatment of the common cold. Ann Allergy Asthma Immunol 1997; 78:531–540.
4. Rosenthal I. Expense of physician care spurs OTC, self-care market. Drug Top 1988; 132:62–63.
5. Brooks GF, Butel JS, Ornston LN. Medical Microbiology. 19th ed. Appleton & Lange Publishers, 1991.
6. Busse WW, Lemanske RF, Dick EC. The relationship of viral respiratory infections and asthma. Chest 1992; 101(6):S385–S388.
7. Gern JE, Busse WW. The effects of rhinovirus infections on allergic airway responses. Am J Respir Crit Care Med 1995; 152:S40–S45.
8. Röseler S, Holtappels G, Wagenmann M et al. Elevated levels of interleukins IL-1beta, IL-6, IL-8 in naturally acquired viral rhinitis. Eur Arch Otorhinolaryngol 1995; 252(suppl):S61–S66.
9. Klebanoff SJ, Vadas MA, Harlan JM et al. Stimulation of neutrophils by tumor necrosis factor. J Immunol 1986; 136:4220–4225.
10. Winther B. Pathogenesis of viral induced rhinitis. In: van Cauwenberge P, Wang D-Y, Ingels K et al. eds. The Nose, Kugler Publications, Amsterdam. 1997:135–140.
11. Dolin R. Common viral respiratory infections. In: Wilson JD, Braunwald E, Isselbacher KJ et al. eds. Principles of Internal Medicine. New York: McGraw-Hill, 1991:700–705.
12. Johnston SL, Bardin PG, Pattemore PK. Viruses as precipitants of asthma symptoms III. Rhinoviruses: molecular biology and prospects for future intervention. Clin Exp Allergy 1993; 23:237–246.
13. Gwaltney JM Jr, Hendley JO. Transmission of experimental rhinovirus infection by contaminated surfaces. Am J Epidemiol 1982; 116:828–833.
14. Hendley JO, Gwaltney JM Jr. Mechanisms of transmission of rhinovirus infections. Epidemiol Rev 1988; 10:243–258.
15. van Cauwenberge P, Ingels K. Effects of viral and bacterial infection on nasal and sinus mucosa. Acta Otolaryngol (Stockh) 1996; 116:316–321.
16. Bernstein JM. Mucosal immunology of the upper respiratory tract. Respiration 1992; 59(suppl):3–13.
17. Brandtzaeg P. Immunocompetent cells of the upper airway: functions in normal and diseased mucosa. Eur Arch Otorhinolaryngol 1995; 252(suppl):S8–S21.

18. Roitt I. Innate immunity. In: Roitt I. Essential Immunology. 8th ed. Oxford: Blackwell Scientific Publications, 1994:3–20.
19. Maltinski G. Nasal disorders and sinusitis. Prim Care 1998; 25(3):663–683.
20. Winther B, Gwaltney JM Jr, Mygind N et al. Sites of recovery after point inoculation of the upper airway. J Am Med Assoc 1986; 256:1763–1767.
21. Rossman MG, Palmenberg AC. Conservation of the putative receptor attachment site in picornaviruses. Virology 1988; 164:373–382.
22. Staunton DE, Merluzzi VS. A cell adhesion molecule, ICAM-1, is the major surface receptor for rhinoviruses. Cell 1989; 56:849–853.
23. Greve JM, Davis G, Mayer AM. The major human rhinovirus receptor is ICAM-1. Cell 1989; 56:839.
24. Arrunda E, Boyle TR, Winther B et al. Localisation of human rhinovirus replication in the upper respiratory tract by in situ hybridisation. J Infect Dis 1995; 171:1329–1333.
25. Turner RB, Winther B, Henley JO et al. Sites of virus recovery and antigen detection in epithelial cells during experimental rhinovirus infection. Acta Otolaryngol 1984; 413(suppl):9–14.
26. Winther B, Brofeldt S, Christensen B et al. Light and scanning electron microscopy of nasal biopsy material from patients with naturally acquired common colds. Acta Otolaryngol (Stockh) 1984; 97:309–318.
27. Winther B, Gwaltney JM Jr, Hendley JO. Respiratory virus infection of monolayer cultures of human nasal epithelial cells. Am Rev Respir Dis 1990; 141:839–845.
28. Naclerio RM, Proud D. Kinins are generated during experimental rhinovirus colds. J Infect Dis 1988; 157:133–142.
29. Winther B, Farr B, Turner RB et al. Histopathologic examination of polymorphonuclear leukocytes in the nasal mucosa during experimental rhinovirus colds. Acta Otolaryngol (Stockh). 1984; 413(suppl):19–24.
30. Levandowski RA, David W, Jackson GG. Acute-phase decrease of T lymphocyte subsets in rhinovirus infection. J Infect Dis 1986; 153:743–748.
31. Cheung D, Dick EC, Timmers MC et al. Rhinovirus inhalation causes long-lasting excessive airway narrowing in response to metacholine in asthmatic subjects in vivo. Am J Respir Crit Care Med 1995; 151:879–886.
32. Fraenkel DJ, Bardin PG, Sanderson G et al. Immunohistochemical analysis of nasal biopsies during rhinovirus experimental colds. Am J Respir Crit Care Med 1994; 150:1130–1136.
33. Gaur S, Kesarwala H, Gavai M et al. Clinical immunology and infectious diseases. Pediatr Clin North Am 1994; 41:745–779.
34. Proud D, Reynolds CJ. Nasal provocation with bradykinin induced symptoms of rhinitis and a sore throat. Am Rev Respir Dis 1988; 137:613–616.
35. Bachert C, Wagenmann M, Holtappels G. Cytokines and adhesion molecules in allergic rhinitis. Am J Rhinol 1998; 12(1):3–8.
36. Turner RB. Rhinovirus infection of human embryonic lung fibroblast induces the production of a chemoattractant for polymorphonuclear leucocytes. J Infect Dis 1988; 157:346–350.
37. Subauste MC, Jacoby DB, Richards SM et al. Infection of a human respiratory epithelial cell line with rhinovirus. J Clin Invest 1995; 96:549–557.
38. Johnston SL, Papi A, Bates PJ et al. Low grade rhinovirus infection induces aprolonged release of IL-8 in pulmonary epithelium. J Immunol 1998; 160:6172–6181.

39. Zhu Z, Tang W, Ray A et al. Rhinovirus stimulation of interleukin-6 in vivo and in vitro. J Clin Invest 1996; 97:421–430.
40. Arnold R, Humbert B, Werchau H et al. Interleukin 8, interleukin 6, and soluble tumor necrosis factor receptor type I release from a human pulmonary epithelial cell line (A549) exposed to respiratory syncytial virus. Immunology 1994; 82:126–133.
41. Noah TL, Becker S. Respiratory syncytial virus-induced cytokine production by a human bronchial epithelial cell line. Am J Physiol 1993; 265:L472–L478.
42. Baggiolini M, Dewald B, Moser B. Interleukin-8 and related chemotactic cytokines—CXC and CC chemokines. Adv Immunol 1994; 55:97–179.
43. Borish L, Rosenwasser LJ. Update on cytokines. J Allergy Clin Immunol 1996; 97:719–734.
44. Paccaud JP, Schifferli JA, Baggiolini M. NAP-1/IL-8 induces up-regulation of CR1 receptors on human neutrophil leucocytes. Biochem Biophys Res Commun 1990; 166:187–192.
45. Bazzoni F, Cassatella MA, Rossi F et al. Phagocytosing neutrophils produce and release high amounts of the neutrophil activating peptide 1/interleukin-8. J Exp Med 1991; 173:771–774.
46. Akira S, Taga T, Kishimoto T. Interleukin-6 in biology and medicine. Adv Immunol 1993; 54:1–78.
47. Muraguchi A, Hirano T, Tang B et al. The essential role of B cell stimulatory factor 2 (BSF/IL-6) for the terminal differentiation of B cells. J Exp Med 1988; 167:332–344.
48. Ramsay AJ, Husband AJ, Ramshaw AI et al. The role of interleukin-6 in mucosal IgA antibody responses in vivo. Science 1994; 264:561–563.
49. Luger TA, Schwarz T. The role of cytokines and neuroendocrine hormones in cutaneous immunity and inflammation. Allergy 1995; 50:292–302.
50. Kopf M, Baumann H, Freer G et al. Impaired immune and acute-phase responses in interleukin-6-deficient mice. Nature 1994; 368:339–342.
51. Terajima M, Yamaya M, Sekizawa K et al. Rhinovirus infection of primary cultures of human tracheal epithelium: role of ICAM-1 and IL-1β. Am J Physiol 1997; 273:L749–L759.
52. Bianco A, Sethi SK, Allen JT, Knight RA et al. Th2 cytokines exert a dominant influence on epithelial cell expression of the major group human rhinovirus receptor, ICAM-1. Eur Respir J 1998; 12:619–626.
53. Bloemen PGM, van den Tweel MC, Hendricks PAJ et al. Expression and modulation of adhesion molecules on human bronchial epithelial cells. Am J Respir Cell Mol Biol 1993; 9:586–593.
54. Paolieri F, Battifora M, Riccio AM et al. Intercellular adhesion molecule-1 on cultured human epithelial cell lines: influence of proinflammatory cytokines. Allergy 1997; 52:521–531.
55. Sethi SK, Bianco A, Allen JT et al. Interferon-gamma (IFN-γ) down-regulates the rhinovirus-induced expression of intercellular adhesion molecule-1 (ICAM-1) on human airway epithelial cells. Clin Exp Immunol 1997; 110:362–369.
56. Proud D, Gwaltney JM, Hendley JO et al. Increased levels of interleukin-1 are detected in nasal secretions of volunteers during experimental rhinovirus colds. J Infect Dis 1994; 169:1007–1013.
57. Dinarello CA. Biology of interleukin-1. FASEB J 1988; 2:108–115.
58. Becker S, Koren HS, Henke DC et al. Interleukin-8 expression in normal nasal epithelium and its modulation by infection with respiratory syncytial virus and

cytokines tumor necrosis factor, interleukin-1 and interleukin-6. Am J Respir Cell Mol Biol 1993; 8:20–27.

59. Bussolino F, Brevario F, Tetta C et al. Interleukin-1 stimulates platelet activating factor production in cultured human endothelial cells. J Clin Invest 1986; 77:2027–2033.

60. Farrar MA, Schreiber RD. The molecular cell biology of interferon-γ and its receptor. Ann Rev Immunol 1993; 11:571–611.

61. Biron C. Cytokines in the generation of immune responses to, and resolution of, virus infection. Curr Opin Immunol 1994; 6:530–538.

62. Linden M, Greiff L, Andersson M et al. Nasal cytokines in common cold and allergic rhinitis. Clin Exp Allergy 1995; 25:166–172.

63. Noah TL, Henderson FW, Wortman IA et al. Nasal cytokine production in viral acute respiratory infection of childhood. J Infect Dis 1995; 171:582–584.

64. Teran LM, Johnston SL, Schroder JM et al. Role of nasal interleukin-8 in neutrophil recruitment and activation in children with virus-induced asthma. Am J Respir Crit Care Med 1997; 115:1362–1366.

65. Akira S, Hirano T, Taga T et al. Biology of multifunctional cytokine: IL-6 and related molecules (IL-1 and TNF). FASEB J 1990; 4:2860–2867.

66. Bachert C, van Kempen M, Höpken K et al. Elevated levels of mediators, cytokines and sICAM-1 in naturally acquired viral rhinitis. Eur Arch ORL 2001; 258:406–412.

67. Turner RB, Weingand KW, Yeh C-H et al. Association between interleukin-8 concentration in nasal secretions and severity of symptoms of experimental rhinovirus colds. Clin Infect Dis 1998; 26:840–846.

68. Becker S, Quay J, Koren H et al. Constitutive and stimulated MCP-1, GROα,β, and γ expression in human airway epithelium and bronchoalveolar macrophages. Am J Physiol. 1994; 266:L278–L286.

69. Rothlein R, Mainolfi EA, Czajkowski M et al. A form of circulating ICAM-1 in human serum. J Immunol 1991; 147:3788–3793.

70. Becker N, Abel U, Stiepak C et al. Frequency of common colds and serum levels of sICAM-1 (CD 54), sLFA-3 (CD58) and sIL-2r (CD25). Eur Cytokine Netw. 1992; 3(6):545–551.

71. Marlin SD, Stauton DE, Springer TA et al. A soluble form of ICAM-1 inhibits rhinovirus infection. Nature 1990; 344:70–72.

72. Winther B, Innes DJ, Bratsch J et al. Lymphocyte subsets in the nasal mucosa and peripheral blood during experimental rhinovirus infection. Am J Rhinol 1992; 6:149–156.

73. Romagnani S. Induction of Th1 and Th2 responses: a key role for the 'natural' immune response? Immunol Today 1992; 13:379–381.

74. Igarishi Y, Skoner DP, Doyle WJ et al. Analysis of nasal secretions during experimental rhinovirus upper respiratory infections. J Allergy Clin Immunol 1993; 92:731–733.

75. Remington JS, Vosti KL, Lietze A et al. Serum proteins and antibody activity in human nasal secretions. J Clin Invest 1964; 43:1613–1624.

76. Butler WT, Waldmann TA, Rossen RD et al. Changes in IgA and IgG concentrations in nasal secretions prior to the appearance of antibody during viral respiratory infection in man. J Immunol 1970; 105:584–591.

77. van Cauwenberge PB, Ectors L. Antibodies against rhinoviruses. In: Mogi G, Veldman JE, Kawauchi H. Immunobiology in Otolaryngology: Progress of a Decade. Amsterdam: Kugler Publications, 1994:539–542.

2

The Role of Nasal Mucus in Upper Airways Function

ROBERT I. HENKIN

Center for Molecular Nutrition and
  Sensory Disorders,
Washington, D.C., USA

AMY DOHERTY* and
BRIAN M. MARTIN

National Institutes of Health (NIH),
Bethesda, Maryland, USA

I. Introduction

It is commonly assumed that the role of nasal mucus is to bathe mucous membranes of the upper airways, supplying moisture, electrolytes, and mucinous substances to moisten their surface, warm, filter, and humidify incoming air, trap inhaled particles

---

**Current affiliation*: Wyeth Nutrition, Collegeville, Pennsylvania, USA.

and pollutant gases, and thereby condition incoming air. Although much scientific effort has been expended by many previous investigators to analyze these secretions their roles in nasal function have not been clearly defined.

In reality, nasal mucus is a complex mixture of substances, in part secreted from glands in the nasal mucosa, in part absorbed from internal and external sources by the mucosa and secreted, in part secreted by various cell types in nasal mucus following their recruitment from the systemic and local vasculature and in part by substances trapped in nasal mucus from inhalation of outside air or from inhaled pharmaceuticals. This complex mixture of substances from these multiple sources plays multiple roles in nasal function of which we know little. Inherent in the presence of this complex mixture is a story of the physiology and pathology of the nasal milieu. By use of tools of modern biochemistry this story can be told and functions of these substances can be investigated.

It is useful in understanding the function of nasal mucus to recognize that the nasal airways can be defined as a complex homeostatic system in which the structures present in this anatomical area are supported and maintained by nasal mucus. It is the nasal mucus, which acts as one of the primary nutritive source for these structures, as a source of growth factors, and a source of other substances upon which these various structures depend for health and development.

This concept is important since many and varied processes take place in the nasal cavity. Some of these processes are mechanical in nature, some are biochemical, and some are a mixture of several different processes. However, each of these processes depends upon the presence and function of nasal mucus and its various components for these processes to take place. Since several of the processes in the nasal cavity do not depend upon blood borne nutrition or support, it falls upon nasal mucus to provide the substance which supports these processes. Without nasal mucus these processes develop pathological patterns of behavior.

Hyposecretion of nasal mucus occurs in response to several clinical events. For example, following irradiation to the nasal cavity for nasal or sinus tumors, nasal mucus glands exhibit a reactive fibrotic process and mucus secretion either diminishes or stops. This results in a continuum of nasal pathology including propensity for recurrent rhinitis and sinusitis, propensity for lower airways infection, loss of smell and flavor perception, difficulty in nasal breathing, and propensity for enhanced allergic reactions and other pathological events. In the past, a clinical condition termed ozena was used to describe a dry, fibrotic, crusted nasal mucosa with the presence of mucosal atrophy and nasal eschars. In this condition, difficulty in nasal breathing and recurrent infections were common symptoms and clinical management was difficult due to the anatomical and functional changes resulting from the loss of nasal mucus. Patients with Sjögren's syndrome exhibit xerorhinia due to infiltration of mucosal glands with chronic inflammatory cells; this infiltration causes glandular destruction with development of nasal eschars and mucous membrane fibrosis.

Hypersecretion of nasal mucus occurs in other clinical conditions. For example, in patients with chronic obstructive pulmonary disease and in chronic bronchitis, mucus hypersecretion occurs not only in lower airways but also in upper airways due primarily to the presence of both acute and chronic inflammation. Thus, nasal mucus plays a variety of roles in maintaining the function of the upper airways.

Nasal mucus also plays a specific role in supporting the nasal mucosa. For example, the normal nasal mucosa absorbs a wide variety of substances. Hydrophilic molecules up to 1 kDa were reported to be readily absorbed by nasal respiratory mucosa of animals (1) although larger molecules were not absorbed. Absorption has been hypothesized to occur by free intracellular diffusion through functional aqueous pores in the mucosal membrane (2). Studies in rabbits suggested that polypeptides found in nasal respiratory tissues of rabbit were dependent upon active transport of receptor-mediated endocytosis (3). Mechanisms underlying this activity were related to the physiological process of antigen sampling (4). Through these and other mechanisms, xenobiotics from the external environment impinge directly upon the nasal mucosa and secretions from the mucosa alter the components of nasal mucus.

The first step in understanding this complex system is to begin with the initial event in nasal function, intake of air from the external environment. The nose is involved with the fate of the air sample which enters it. At rest, approximately 10,000–15,000 L of air move over the upper airways daily (5). From the nose, air goes through the upper airway, the trachea, the larynx, and the bronchi to reach the lungs where gas exchange takes place and respiration occurs. All air which enters the nose is required to remain in the body to reach the lungs, to be exchanged at the alveolar-capillary membrane; there is no possibility for escape from the body once air has entered the lower airways although sneezing and coughing represent physiological attempts to deal with air samples which may be considered noxious prior to entry into the lower airways. Air continually entering the nose may dry underlying tissues; however, because external air must be passed directly into the lungs other critical functions were added to this moisturizing effect and these additional functions need to be examined critically.

These additional functions resulted teleologically in the development of a complex fluid, which we know as nasal mucus and more specifically relate to the proteins in nasal mucus. It is our hypothesis that these nasal mucus proteins act not only to condition incoming air but also to protect and maintain integrity of nasal mucous membranes and the structures they subserve and to inhibit potential pathological effects of inhaled xenobiotics of all types—they perform these functions by specific and concerted biological actions. In so doing they maintain the homeostasis of the upper airways and play both general and specific roles in nasal disease processes.

II. The Nose

The nose is the normal anatomical entry port into the lungs. It is equipped with two passages filled with hair cells and cilia, which filter some portion of external air, particularly particulate matter, and turbinates or baffles that warm, humidify, and deflect incoming air, thereby conditioning it prior to its passage into the lungs. Nasal airflow must be turbulent in order to project incoming particles against the nasal mucosa (6). Sinus cavities in the head are present and their secretions normally empty into the nose. The nose acts as a resonator for speech and sound. As in the mouth, a specific sensory control mechanism, smell receptors, at the nasal vault, control and judge content of air taken into the nose on its voyage into the lungs. Air containing noxious substances is rejected by various maneuvers (forced expiration, sneezing, coughing, etc.) at its point of entry, as in the mouth; air containing agreeable substances is accepted. These receptors monitor intake of outside air to assist in controlling intake of food and fluids, (flavor perception) and, in males of lower species, recognize the presence of ovulatory signals in the environment to initiate mating behavior. Females of lower species also utilize these receptors, both before and after copulation, to accept a male of an appropriate species and to inhibit further male contact following copulation. Receptors in the nose associated with the vomeronasal organ, particularly in lower organisms, play a significant role in this complex reproductive behavior. Other receptors perceive pain, pressure, touch, and temperature and act with other structures in the nose to respond to these sensations and assist in control and judgment of passage of outside air into the lower airways. Thus, the nose is not simply a conduit or a simple tubular system whereby air enters the body. Rather the nose is a complex organ in which homeostatic mechanisms maintain structures within it, as in the mouth, and act on xenobiotics presented to it. It is a complex, epithelial lined structure through which air normally passes continuously and *involuntarily* into the lungs. It is different from the mouth since intake of air is essentially continuous and there is no physiological mechanism to turn off this air intake without seriously compromising the required presentation of oxygen to the lungs. Because of this continuous, reflexive, nonvolitional process of acceptance of outside air and the lack of any obvious chemical filtering mechanism, teleologically, defense mechanisms developed in the upper airways to protect both structures of the upper airways and the lungs from potentially noxious effects of inhaled air, particularly those not associated with any noxious sensory quality. Sensory receptors in the nose, despite their greater sensitivity than those in the mouth, are not equipped to deal with the host of potentially noxious, xenobiotic, and nonvolatile substances which they cannot perceive (due to their lack of specific sensitivity) and which can easily gain entry into the pulmonary system. Thus, protective mechanisms were developed in the nose in the form of nasal mucus due to this lack of sensory recognition.

III. Nasal Mucous Membranes

Nasal mucous membranes are continuous with skin outside the nares, the mucous membranes of the pharynx, the conjunctiva through the nasolacrimal and lacrimal ducts, and the frontal, ethmoidal, sphenoidal, and maxillary sinuses through several openings in the meatae, and with the middle ear (7). All surface linings are moist due to nasal secretions (5). Mucous membranes covering the surface are composed of three distinct types: (a) stratified, keratinized squamous epithelium in the nasal vestibule and nasopharynx, which covers the entrance of the nasal cavity; (b) respiratory epithelium, which covers the posterior two-thirds of the nasal cavity; and (c) specialized ciliated epithelium (olfactory epithelium), which covers two very small areas at the nasal vault (8). The respiratory portion is a pseudostratified ciliated columnar epithelium containing several distinct secretory cell types including goblet, mucous, and serous glands (9). Goblet cells are the major nonciliated cell type found and secrete high molecular weight mucins (10). Several other glands are present in this epithelium (9).

A mucosal basal cell layer normally initiates replacement cells for both ciliated and nonciliated cells of this columnar epithelium (11,12). Basal cells play a role in attachment of columnar cells to airways basement membrane (13). They act as a bridge to columnar cells and to the cellular basement membrane (13). They secrete factors which enhance their ability to migrate (14). They also gradually decrease in number distally in lower airways until there are none in terminal and respiratory bronchioles (14a). *Clara cells* have been suggested as forming the stem cell (basal cell?) compartment (15) and play a role in cellular renewal.

The basement membrane acts as an extracellular scaffold upon which the basal cell layer rests (8). It is a structural boundary below which is a layer of areolar connective tissue infiltrated with lymphocytes and a lamina propria, a relatively thin elastofibrous tissue layer, containing a layer of glands toward its surface and a layer of blood vessels and lymphatics next to the periosteum. In deeper layers of the lamina propria are both veins and blood spaces which form a rich plexus and bear a resemblance to erectile tissue which becomes engorged following a variety of physiological and pathological events causing the mucosa to swell. This deeper submucosal zone consists of an admixture of seromucous glands and vasoerectile structures (16).

The olfactory epithelium is defined by two olive-sized slightly pigmented areas, located bilaterally at the nasal vault composed mainly of sustentacular (supporting) and mitral (receptor) cell types. Other cell types are also found, including two types of basal cells, dark/horizontal and light globose (17,18); mitoses are present only in these basal cells, particularly those of the light globose basal cells (17,19) which renew the other cell types. There are no blood vessels or lymphatics in olfactory mucosa in contrast to respiratory mucosa. While both respiratory and olfactory epithelial cells are renewed by the same general scheme of stem cell or basal cell differentiation, respiratory epithelial cells are replaced slowly (1% of cells are in division at any one time) (20), whereas olfactory epithelial cells are replaced rapidly (some cells turn over every 24 h but do so by apoptosis with only basal cells exhibiting mitosis).

IV. Nasal Secretions

The nose is bathed with a film of fluid from 5 to 100 μm in depth secreted from several major cellular sources (21). Volume of upper airways secretion has been estimated to be 10–100 mL/day. Secretions cover all nasal surfaces but they differ in character due to specific requirements of growth and development of cells of underlying structures in specific areas. The mucus layer is continually propelled posteriorly by epithelial cell cilia and is disposed of by swallowing. The mucus layer has been estimated to be replaced rapidly, every 15–20 min (22). Mucus secretions, as noted previously, are comprised of a mixture of glandular secretions, vascular transudates, cellular debris of many cellular types, including leukocytes, bacteria, etc., mucosal cells and many other elements. This airway lining fluid consists of two layers, a relatively thick mucous blanket lying on top of a thinner watery layer adhering to cilia (23). The periciliary fluid is of constant depth, related to ciliary length and is a watery sol of low viscosity (24); the upper layer is of variable thickness and is of much higher viscosity (25). This two-layer system also overlies the olfactory epithelium but constituents of this system may differ from that overlying respiratory epithelium.

Glandular secretions of respiratory epithelium contain 95% water, 1% protein, 0.9% carbohydrate, 0.8% lipid (26), various combinations of these substances, and multiple other small molecular weight moeities. Goblet, serous, mucous, and other cells of the respiratory mucosa secrete specific substances. Mucous glands secrete mucins and other carbohydrate containing glycans. Serous glands secrete proteins and proteoglycans and are the major protein-secreting glands in the nose. Almost all proteins in nasal secretions are also found in external secretions from most other glandular tissues, including lacrimal, bronchial, cervical, seminal, mammary gland secretions, and hepatic bile and pancreatic juice. The proteins in these secretions are similar in their composition and concentration and in their functions in the various entities in which they serve. However, these protein secretions differ significantly in composition and concentration from those found in saliva which developed in a different manner and perform many different physiological functions. Blood plasma derived secretions are also found and contain similar substances to those found in blood plasma albeit their concentrations in nasal mucus are quite different, some greater than in blood plasma, many lower.

A. Nasal Mucus

We have attempted to determine the composition of nasal mucus after collection from seven normal volunteers without upper or lower airways disease and from 11 patients with various diseases involving the upper airways. It was collected directly from the nose without any external lavage in plastic containers in the morning hours from spontaneous discharge from the nares without external stimulation (27). Using this technique, this secretion reflects the basic secretory products of nasal glands with no exogenous stimulated contribution from plasma filtrates that might be expected following nasal lavage, the most common technique used to collect nasal secretions. In this manner, we analyzed nasal secretions directly without contamination from bronchial, pulmonary, or other lower airway sources. Patients included two with smell loss (hyposmia) who had no inflammatory upper or lower airways disease, five with active acute and chronic sinusitis, three with inactive chronic sinusitis and in one with acute and chronic sinusitis before and after successful therapy with antibiotics for this infectious disorder.

Mucus was centrifuged at 20,000 rpm for 20–90 min, the supernatant protein removed from the underlying precipitate and a sample chromatographed on HPLC using an UpChurch C-18 reverse phase column (2.1 mm × 15 cm). A linear gradient from 95% solvent A (0.12% TFA in water) to 60% solvent B (0.1% TFA in acetonitrile) was developed over 60 min at 0.200 mL/min flow rate. Elutes from peaks of chromatograms were subjected to protein sequence analysis. Elutes which were not sequenceable were subjected to digestion with Asp-N proteinase, trypsin, V8 proteinase, and peptides and separated by HPLC prior to resubmission for sequence analysis. Identity of digests were confirmed by a computer search of the Swiss Protein Database (28) which detected greater than 98% identity between proteins eluted from the column and comparative database standards. Peaks demonstrated on HPLC chromatograms reflect the seroproteins present in nasal mucus, their concentration demonstrated by their area, their presence identified by elution time, in minutes, from the origin.

These same nasal mucus samples were subjected to metal analysis and results compared to similar analyses performed in parotid saliva and in serum. Analysis was performed by flame aspiration atomic absorption spectrophotometry on an IL (Instrumentation Laboratory, Wilmington, MA) Model 951 dual beam spectrophotometer by methods previously described (29).

Major seroproteins measured in normal subjects (Fig. 2.1) were albumin, eluted at 51 min; lysozyme, eluted at 49 min; β_2 microglobulin, eluted at 46 min; and lumicarmine, eluted at 28 min. Many other proteins were also eluted including histones, statherin, α-trypsin protease inhibitor, and the Clara cell phospholipid binding protein.

Metals identified in nasal mucus include zinc, copper, magnesium, and calcium (Table 2.1). Results indicate that calcium is the major metal present both in parotid saliva and in nasal mucus; in parotid saliva its concentration is 100 times that of magnesium, 1000 times that of copper, and 500 times that of zinc. In nasal mucus its concentration is over three times that of magnesium, over 300 times that of copper, and over 350 times that of zinc. Zinc concentration in nasal mucus is about 1.7 times greater than in parotid saliva, copper concentration about 4.5 times greater than in parotid saliva and magnesium about 46 times greater than in parotid saliva. On the other hand, zinc and copper in nasal mucus are 15% their concentration in serum, magnesium is 72% its concentration in serum and calcium is about 50% its concentration in serum. These

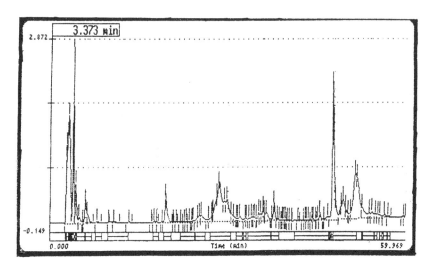

Figure 2.1 HPLC of seroproteins from whole human nasal mucus from a normal subject (66-year-old Caucasian male) without any disease of upper or lower airways with normal smell function. See text for details of methodology. Absorbance at 225 nm is plotted on the ordinate, time in minutes on the abscissa. This chromatogram is representative of results obtained in normal subjects. The proteins, identified by peak elution times from the reversed phase column (left to right) are as follows: 18 min, histone H_2B_1; 28 min, lumicarmine; 36 min, statherin; 38 min, α-trypsin proteinase inhibitor; 46 min, β_2 microglobulin precursor; 49 min, lysozyme; 51 min, albumin; 63 min, Clara cell phospholipid binding protein.

results raise the question of the role of calcium and magnesium in nasal mucus and of calcium in parotid saliva. Since both calcium and magnesium are active chemical elements they are usually found in their major form bound to protein. In parotid saliva, calcium is bound to amylase which represents 5–10% of

Table 2.1 Metals in Nasal Mucus and in Parotid Saliva in Normal Volunteers

METAL	Serum (20) ($\mu g/dL$)	Nasal mucus (7) ($\mu g/L$)	Parotid saliva (18) ($\mu g/L$)
Zn	92 ± 4	14.0 ± 2.2[a]	8.3 ± 1.3
Cu	106 ± 4	16.3 ± 1.4[b]	3.6 ± 1.0
Mg	2150 ± 80	1554 ± 188[b]	33.9 ± 3.7
Ca	9820 ± 148	5303 ± 334	3885 ± 215

Note: Number in parentheses in column head indicates number of subjects.
Values represent mean ± SEM.
[a]$p < 0.05$ with respect to parotid saliva.
[b]$p < 0.001$ with respect to parotid saliva.

total protein and magnesium is bound to the a specific magnesium containing protein, magnesin, which represents about 1% of total protein. Presently known calcium-binding proteins in nasal mucus consist of statherin, amylase, and several others including visinin-like protein (30), calbindin (31,32), calmodulin (31,33), calcimycin (33), calretinin (31), and neurocalcin (34). No specific magnesium binding proteins have been found in nasal mucus. The role of these calcium-binding proteins in nasal mucus has not been established.

Because zinc in both nasal mucus and parotid saliva is a cofactor in gustin/carbonic anhydrase (CA VI), a major growth factor which supports growth and development of both taste buds and olfactory epithelial cells (see following text), CA VI was measured in both secretions in normal subjects and in patients with loss of smell following a viral illness (Table 2.2) by a variation of the method of Richli et al. (35). Results (Table 2.2) indicate that CA VI is significantly lower than normal in both nasal mucus and parotid saliva in patients with smell loss.

B. Nasal Seroproteins

Results of HPLC analysis shown in Fig. 2.1 and from studies of many previous investigators indicate that nasal mucus contains five major proteins which comprise about half its total protein (Table 2.3).

The most prevalent protein in nasal mucus, comprising between 10% and 15% of the total, is albumin (36). Lysozyme (37), and lactoferrin (37,38) each represent about 10% of mucus protein (38). Immunoglobulin G represents about 5% of the total protein and the α-trypsin proteinase inhibitor represents about 3% of the total protein. Other proteins, each of which represents $<3\%$ of the total protein, are the Clara cell phospholipid binding protein, and in still smaller amounts, histones, statherin, β_2 microglobulin, lumicarmine, gustin (CA VI), secretory IgA, and various phase reactants including other immunoglobulins, cytokines, including several interleukins, eosinophilic cationic protein, transferrin, haptoglobin, C_3, C_4, kallikrein and other secreted proteins (39), several serum proteins including fibrinogen, prothrombin, plasminogen, antithrombin (40) and many other substances, including uric acid (40) and nitrous

Table 2.2 Gustin/Carbonic Anhydrase CA VI in Nasal Mucus and Parotid Saliva in Normal Subjects and in Patients with Loss of Smell

Subjects	Nasal mucus (μg/mL)	Parotid saliva (μg/mL)
Normals (12)	0.08 ± 0.008[a]	0.24 ± 0.01
Patients (150)	0.06 ± 0.004[a,c]	0.13 ± 0.006[b]

Note: Values represent mean $\pm$ SEM. Number in parentheses indicates number of subjects.
[a]$p < 0.001$ with respect to parotid saliva.
[b]$p < 0.001$ with respect to normals.
[c]$p < 0.025$ with respect to normals.

Table 2.3 Protein Constituents

Nasalmucus relative total protein (%) or presence	Protein	MW (kDa)	Composition characteristics	Function	Saliva relative total protein (%)
+	Lumicarmine	36	Phosphoglycoprotein 80% Pro, Gly, Glu 10% Val, Arg No aromatic amino acids	Structural protein covering all surfaces	75
+	Amylase	58	Ca Metalloprotein two isoforms (a) Glycoprotein (b) Asialoprotein	Digest starch Antimicrobial agent	8
+	Carbonic anhydrase VI (gustin)	33	Zn Metalloprotein 8% His Glycoprotein (3 sites)	Taste bud/olfactory epithelial cell growth factor	3
?	Magnisin	30	Mg Metalloprotein binds Cu, Zn	?	1
+?	$Zn\text{-}x_2$ Glycoprotein	38	Zn Metalloprotein x (Heavy) chain Class I MHC molecule	Immune response	<1
15	Albumin	69	Water soluble Heat coagulable	Binds Fe, Zn ? Antimicrobial agent	<1
10	Lysozyme	17.5	Mucolytic protein Single chain Four Intra CysCross-links	Antimicrobial agent	<1
10	Lactoferrin	78	Fe Metalloprotein	Antimicrobial agent	<1

	Protein				
5	Immunoglobulin G (Ig G)	150	Two "Heavy chains" / Two "Light chains" / Two Antigen binding sites	Binds foreign proteins (antigens)	<1
5	x-Trypsin proteinase inhibitor	12	Acid stable / Four Disulfide core / Inhibits trypsin, chymotrypsin, elastase	Protects mucosal surface from toxic effects of PMN, microbial breakdown products	<1
+	β₂ Microglobulin	12	β (Light) chain-monomorphic / Class I MHC molecule	Immune response	<1
3	Clara cell phospholipid binding protein	15.8	Homodimer joined by 2 disulfide bonds / Secreted by clara cells	Binds potentially toxic xenobiotics by cytochrome P-450 activity	<1
+	Histones	8–26	10–20% Lysine / Found in cell chromatin	? Reflects nuclear breakdown products of mucosal, microbial cells	—
+	Statherin	5.4	Phosphoprotein pro rich	Adsords onto OH-apatite / Inhibits Ca precipitation / Inhibits crystal growth / Formally found only in saliva	<1
+	Phase reactant proteins		Cytokines (interleukins) / Eosinophilic cationic protein / Immunoglobulins A,M,E / Many other proteins	Reactive products to infection / Other effects?	<1

oxide (NO) (41). It seems reasonable to assume that those proteins which comprise the majority of the total protein in nasal mucus play important roles in the nose and in nasal function.

Albumin is the most abundant protein in nasal mucus. It is a simple, water-soluble, ellipsoidal protein with molecular weight of 69 kDa. It contains multiple reversible binding sites for various substances, especially those carrying negative charges, but also those containing iron and zinc, such that it may have antimicrobial properties similar to lactoferrin.

Lactoferrin is a 78 kDa iron binding protein which is capable of binding two atoms of iron and the major iron binding protein found in all external secretions. It is the major iron binding protein found in these secretions. This contrasts with transferrin, which is the major iron binding protein found in serum. Concentrations of lactroferrin from secretory glands are much greater than its concentration in blood. In plasma, its concentration is $0.02-0.2$ µg/mL protein, in serum, $0.18-1.0$ µg/mL protein in human tears, $1-3$ mg/mL or $15-30\%$ of total protein, and in human milk it represents about 12% of total protein (42). It is synthesized by both nasal serous glands and neutrophils and has been shown to exhibit both bacteriostatic and bactericidal activity. This action has been attributed to its ability to bind iron and thus render this essential nutrient unavailable to invading microorganisms which require it for their growth and development. In this sense, apolactoferrin is a more potent antimicrobial agent than lactoferrin which may contain some iron. Lactoferrin trimer, since it can bind three times as much iron as lactoferrin monomer, has enhanced antimicrobial activity. Lactoferrin in leukocytes may also play a role in their antimicrobial activity. If lactoferrin is iron saturated it is without antimicrobial activity. The iron-containing protein siderophilin was previously reported to represent $2-2.5\%$ of nasal serous protein (43).

Lysozyme is a 17.5 kDa mucolytic enzyme that catalyzes hydrolysis of glycosidic linkages in complex polysaccharides found in cell walls of many Gram-positive and Gram-negative bacteria. It has 129 residues in a single chain with four intrachain cysteine cross-links; its bactericidal activity occurs by dissolving bacterial cell walls by catalyzing hydrolysis of the $1-4$ glycosidic linkages of the polysaccharide backbone of mureins, yielding dissacharides of N-acetyl-D glucosamine and N-acetyl muramic acid to which muropeptides are attached. Gram-positive bacteria in the presence of lysozyme yield protoplasts, essentially a naked Gram-positive bacterial cell, surrounded only by its membrane, which is then susceptible to swelling and rupture of its membrane with subsequent bacterial cell death. Lysozyme has also been shown to be bactericidal in the absence of cell lysis since it can initiate microorganism aggregation and thereby inhibit colonization of mucosal surfaces. It can act also with other proteins to initiate bacteriolysis; in combination with complement and secretory IgA it has been shown to be bactericidal for *Escherichia coli*. Its bacteriolytic properties were initially reported by Fleming in 1922 (44). Its specific distribution in secretory proteins has been previously reported with a serum concentration of $1-1.5$ $\mu g/mL$ of protein, in tears, $1-3$ mg/mL of protein, and in lung secretions reflecting $5-6\%$ of total protein (45).

Immunoglobulin G (IgG) is the fourth most abundant protein in nasal mucus with a molecular weight of 150 kDa. It has four peptide chains characterized as two identical "heavy" chains (molecular weight 50 kDa) and two identical "light" (molecular weight 25 kDa) chains linked together by disulfide bonds; it has two binding sites for antigens. Each heavy chain contains a covalently bound oligosaccharide component. Its function in nasal mucus, presumably, is to bind foreign proteins (antigens) and thereby inhibit their activity in the nose.

The α-trypsin proteinase inhibitor is a 12 kDa acid stable protein consisting of a four-disulfide core with two homologous consecutive domains of equal length, each containing eight cysteine residues similar to several snake neurotoxins and neurophysin. It is structurally similar to whey protein of rat and mouse, Red Sea turtle proteinase inhibitor and ragweed pollen allergen Ra 5 (46). It has strong affinity and strong inhibitory effects on trypsin, chymotrypsin, and neutrophil lysosomal elastase. When polymorphonuclear cells (PMNs) disintegrate they liberate lysosomal proteins which are potentially harmful to cells which line the nasal mucosal surface. The inhibitor's function may be to protect the mucosal surface by inhibiting these proteinases and their proteolytic activity upon their release from PMNs. These proteins thus act to protect the mucosal surface from release of enzymes and proteins from PMNs and other sources which have been designed to be antimicrobial (47) and represent part of the homeostatic mechanisms by which integrity of the nasal mucosa in maintained during acute and chronic infection. This protein has also been found in the human parotid gland (48).

The Clara cell phospholipid binding protein is a water-soluble, 15.8 kDa homodimer of 8.5 kDa monomers joined by two disulfide bonds (49). It is the predominant protein secreted by Clara cells which comprise part of the repertoire of protein-secreting cells that line mucous membranes of both nose and lung (50). These cells may act by thwarting unnecessary and potentially destructive immune responses against inhaled allergens to which the nose is constantly exposed (49). These cells have been found predominantly in the lung and only in our research has secretion of this protein been found in human nasal mucus. These cells are nonciliated and have been considered instrumental in repair of epithelium of both nasal mucosa and distal airways of the lung (50). The secreted protein specifically binds methylsulfonyl-polychlorated biphenyls (PCBs) and inhibits phospholipase A_2 (46). It has been considered a site of metabolism of xenobiotics by activity of cytochrome P-450-dependent mixed function oxidases (51) indicating that it acts to bind, inhibit, and inactivate substances entering the nose which may be toxic, allergenic, or both. In this sense it can play a detoxifying role acting against xenobiotics entering the nose. It has 61% homology with uteroglobin found in cervical secretions, which acts as a natural immunosuppressant protecting the female genital tract from unwanted immune response (52). It also has homology with Fel dI which is secreted from cat salivary glands and has been found to be a factor in initiation of human allergic reactions to cat dander since it is also found in cat hair and skin (53). It also has some homology with the annexin family, a series of lipid-binding proteins. Clara cells have been previously observed in the respiratory epithelium of various species, including the mouse, where it is found in submucosal glands which are both serous and seromucous in nature (54). It also has been considered as antiproteinase and can act with antitrypsin, antichymotrypsin, and macroglobulins associated with leukocytes as an antibacterial agent and may act along with the α-trypsin-proteinase inhibitor as part of the homeostatic activity of nasal mucus proteins to protect the nasal mucosa from substances released from PMNs and other sources which are antibacterial and could harm the integrity of the nasal mucosa.

Histones are basic proteins ranging from 8 to 26 kDa found in cell chromatin with 10–20% of their amino acid residues as lysine. These proteins are characterized by regularly spaced positive changes contributed by R groups of lysine and arginine residues through which they combine with negatively charged groups on the periphery of the DNA double helix to form complexes. These nuclear proteins function by interacting with cellular DNA to form nucleasomes, which are essential for both regulation of transcription and packaging of DNA within chromosomes. Histones are architectural proteins and their action on transcriptional cellular machinery is essential in nuclear function. These proteins in nasal mucus may reflect the nuclear breakdown products of cells shed from nasal mucous membranes or from viral, bacterial or other microbial breakdown products. We have identified this protein in nasal mucus for the first time.

Statherin is a 43-residue, 5.4 kDa phosphopeptide with one-quarter of its residues derived from aromatic amino acids, one-quarter derived from acidic amino acids, and the remainder containing a relatively large amount of proline (55). It was originally described in parotid saliva where it was characterized as having two unusual inhibitory properties: the first, its selective adsorption onto hydroxyapatite which may explain, through its inhibitory properties, that mineral deposits do not form spontaneously on teeth (56); the second, its action to inhibit precipitation of supersaturated calcium phosphate salts from solution and its presence has been considered the reason why human saliva can be supersaturated with these salts with respect to dental enamel yet lack properties which normally characterize the supersaturated state (57). It also inhibits crystal growth in seeded systems through its binding onto the tooth surface and blocks crystal formation. While these properties may explain its function in saliva with respect to tooth formation, its presence in nasal mucus has not been previously described prior to the present study. We report its presence in nasal mucus for the first time. While its function in nasal mucus is unexplained, it seems reasonable that it possesses properties other than the ones attributed to it in saliva.

β_2 Microglobulin (β_2m) is a monomorphic single peptide chain of 12 kDa devoid of carbohydrate, encoded on chromosome 15 (58,59) which we identify in nasal mucus for the first time. It is uniquely characterized by three di-prolyl sequences in the first one-third of the molecule (60). It is a cell-membrane component closely associated with HLA antigens (60). It is a member of the immunoglobulin superfamily required for proper expression and function of class I major histocompatibility complex (MHC) antigens (61,59). It is the light chain which appears to provide the conformation of the human class I MHC molecule (62,61). In this molecule, comprised of two polypeptides, a polymorphic heavy chain encoded in the MHC on chromosome 6, depends upon a noncovalent interaction with a light chain molecule, β_2m protein. Its X-ray crystal structure has been determined and it has a common evolutionary origin with immunoglobulin (59). In nasal mucus, the heavy chain portion of this molecule could be supplied by the Zn-α_2 glycoprotein (63), although identification of this latter polypeptide was initially blocked in nasal mucus in our amino acid sequence assay. However, this latter protein has been found by us and by other investigators before us in normal human parotid saliva and we suspect that it is also present in human nasal mucus.

Functions of the β_2m proteins are multiple consisting of (a) stabilizing tertiary structure of class I MHC antigens, (b) processing and intracellular transport of antigen after synthesis, and (c) interacting with the complement-like killing structure on T cells to initiate cell destruction in a manner similar to interaction of the Fc portion of IgG and complement (62,61). It has been proposed that class I molecules mediate cell destruction by T cell activation (64) and that histocompability antigens play a complement-like role (65). It is water soluble and binds to cell surface proteins of plasma membranes. It is found in trace amounts in most body fluids including saliva (66) although the present work is the first study identifying its presence in nasal mucus. Although considered a nonspecific clinical marker its concentration is increased in several diseases including myeloproliferative and lymphoproliferative disorders, rheumatoid arthritis, systemic lupus erythematosus, Sjögren's syndrome, and primary biliary cirrhosis (60,67). In patients with lymphoma or acute leukemia, its level in cerebral spinal fluid exceded that in plasma in 10–20% of patients with these disorders and its level decreased following intrathecal chemotherapy (60). Increased β_2m in saliva in patients with Sjögren's syndrome has occurred with development of lymphoproferative complications and has been considered related to changes in cellular turnover. In these disease states it was hypothesized that it either stabilized the tertiary structure of histocompatability antigens or that the β_2m-histocompatability antigen complex was necessary for subsequent processing and intracellular transport of antigen after synthesis (59,68).

Discovery of β_2m in nasal mucus raises the question of whether all three main classes of loci of the major histocompatability complex (69) are present in nasal mucus. Class I loci code for polypeptides of 45 kDa and are expressed on the surface of virtually all nucleated cells (70). Class II loci code for a family of cell surface proteins of 30 kDa and are present on B lymphocytes, macrophages and some T lymphocytes. Several cells (71) express class II MHC complex molecules which serve to process and present antigen to T-cell lymphocytes via appropriate receptors (72). Class III loci code for molecules that are components of the complement system. Class I products are attached to the plasma membrane by a hydrophobic segment and their extracellular portion is noncovalently associated with β_2m (70) which shows significant homology to the C_H3 domain of immuno-globulin-γ chains (73). Because of the presence of this protein it seems reasonable to predict that other components of the major histocompatibility complex are also present in nasal mucus either as a direct or indirect result of activity of B and T lymphocytes. HLA class II antigens have been found by histochemical techniques and by tissue culture in epithelial cells of nasal polyps; interferon-γ (IFN-γ) regulates its expression in upper airways epithelial cells from nasal polyps at a transcriptional level (74) and class I MHC alleles also appear to play a role in this system (75). These results suggest that a complex immunological system is present in nasal mucus which operates on xenobiotics through well known protective systems to inhibit foreign invaders.

Many other proteins are present in nasal mucus and play roles in various aspects of nasal function. These proteins include phase reactant proteins, immuno-globulins, cytokines, including the interleukins IL-1β, IL-2, and IL-6 (76), tumor necrosis factor-α (TNF-α) (77), kallikrein (78), substance P (79), calcito-nin gene-related peptide (78), vasoactive intestinal protein (79), IgE (79), trans-ferrin (80), haptoglobin (80) and other proteins whose function is not clear at this time.

Cytokines found in several human tissues (81) are also found in nasal mucus. IL-1, IL-6, and TNF-α are glycoproteins produced by a variety of cells in nasal and lower airways when exposed to bacteria and viruses (82). These substances mediate a broad spectrum of biological activities including triggering acute phase responses and T and B lymphocyte proliferation and differentiation. IL-1β has been shown to be increased 12–24 h after experimental rhinovirus infection in lavaged nasal secretions in normal volunteers but not in noninfected subjects (82). Increased mRNA for IL-2, IL-4, IL-5, IL-6, IL-10, IL-13, and IFN-γ was found in lavaged nasal mucus from subjects exposed to a challenge of particulates from diesel exhaust whereas only mRNA from IL-2, IL-13, and IFN-δ was found in lavaged samples prior to this challenge (83). IL-1α, IL-6, and IL-8 have been synthesized following *in vitro* tissue culture of nasal epithilial cells (84).

Gustin is a protein found in nasal mucus whose function we hypothesize is to enhance growth and development of olfactory cells (27) similar to its action on taste buds (85,86). It is the third most prevalent protein in parotid saliva where it comprises about 3% of the total protein (85); it is a minor protein in nasal mucus. It is a zinc metalloprotein also known as carbonic anhydrase (CA) VI (87–90) and is an oligomer of 36 kDa molecular weight with two glycosylation sites (89). It is comprised of five isomers with varying amounts of sialic acid residues as termini on these carbohydrate chains (90). Its major function in saliva is to act as a growth factor which supports growth and development of the cellular reper-toire of taste buds (87–90). It may play a similar role in nasal mucus to support growth and development of olfactory epithelial cells (27) but not in cells of the vomeronasal organ. It has some enzymatic activity similar to nerve growth factor (NGF) (91,92) and specifically activates calmodulin-dependent brain cAMP phosphodiesterase (93), an enzymatic action that is inhibited by removal of zinc from the protein (92). Removal of zinc from the protein also inhibits growth and development of taste buds, *per se*; hence it has been considered a taste bud growth factor (88,90). In some patients with loss of smell it has also been found to be decreased in nasal mucus (27) and some of these patients also exhibit zinc deficiency (89). Zinc treatment has been useful to restore taste and/or smell function in these patients (94–97), but some are resistent to this therapy (98). This may relate, in part, to the di-, tri-, and tetrasiaylated isoforms of CA VI (90) since it is well known that siaylated TSH is inactive as a thyroid hormone stimulator whereas its activity increases with progressive desiaylation (99). Both taste buds and some olfactory epithelial cells are renewed every 24–48 h based upon activity of taste bud and olfactory epithelial stem cells, respectively. These cells are the only cells of the taste bud or olfactory epithelium to exhibit mitosis and are dependent upon gustin/CA VI, which acts as growth factor for at least part of this activity.

Lumicarmine is a phosphoglycoprotein containing six moles of phosphate per mole protein, is 80% pro, gly, glu, 10% val, and arg and belongs to the family of proline-rich proteins. It constitutes 70–80% of parotid saliva protein but is a minor component of nasal mucus. It is devoid of aromatic amino acids, has a molecular weight of 36 kDa, has very little molecular structure with a circular dichroism (CD) peak at 202 nm and has little inherent structure, assuming the shape of a random coil (100). It is the major constituent of salivary pellicle and covers every surface in the oral cavity as a thin biofilm. It is the protein which forms the structural foundation for rapid healing of wounds in the oral cavity and is the protein which, when applied to wounds by animals through licking, initiates a rapid healing process (101). A small proline-rich protein has been found to be upregulated in nasal epithelial cells of rats exposed to tobacco smoke (102); this small protein may be a breakdown product of lumicarmine.

We identify the presence of lumicarmine in nasal mucus for the first time in this work. Its role in nasal mucus is unclear. While its concentration in nasal mucus is much lower than in saliva, it could act as the biofilm layer in the nose as it does in the mouth. In this sense it may be the thin periciliary mucus layer which coapts to all nasal mucosal surfaces to which bacteria, viruses, inflammatory cells, and cellular debris and other substances bind.

Amylase, a calcium-containing glycoprotein of 58 kDa, has been found in nasal mucus as a secretory product from nasal serous glands (103). In saliva it has two isoforms, a glycoprotein and an asioloprotein. It is an important component of saliva, comprising between 5% and 10% of its total protein (104). Its function in saliva may be as an antibacterial agent although it is commonly considered to act as a digestive agent since it actively hydrolyzes starch. Its antibacterial properties in the oral cavity have been well defined (105–107) and in this antibacterial action, it is inhibitory to *Streptococcus sanguis*, one of the more important oral bacteria, binding to its cellular surface through a heat stable protein receptor (107). It inhibited the growth of *Neisseria gonorrhoeae* grown in starch (106,107) but not in saliva. Removal of calcium from the protein inhibits all its activity, including starch digestion. It has a proclivity to bind copper and zinc (108) and this could play a role in its antibacterial action since zinc enhances bacterial and viral growth and copper inhibits this growth.

We found copper ion in nasal mucus (see Table 2.1) and previous investigators have found evidence of ceruloplasm in these secretions (109). Its function in nasal mucus may be as an antibacterial and antiviral growth factor although it may have other functions as well.

Magnesin is a 30 kDa Mg-containing metalloprotein found in parotid saliva which binds both copper and zinc (110); it may act, as does amylase, as an antibacterial agent. However, it has not been isolated in nasal mucus although there is a significant amount of magnesium in nasal mucus and it would be expected that magnesium is associated with this protein.

Calmodulin is an 18 kDa calcium-containing protein found both in parotid saliva and in the nasal area (31,33). Its concentration is decreased in patients with both taste and smell loss (111) but its concentration in nasal mucus has not been determined. Its presence, similar to that of gustin/CA VI, may be an index of growth and development of both taste bud and olfactory epithelial stem cell turnover.

Among other proteins whose functions are unclear, and there are many, is the odorant-binding protein found in bovine olfactory and respiratory mucosa and in nasal mucus and tears but not in saliva (112,113). It may act by binding to and inactivating xenobiotic substances which are potentially harmful to the pulmonary tract (112,113).

Among other substances found in nasal mucus is NO, which is composed of two species, constitutive, found in endothelial cells, and inducible, found after activation in macrophages, neutrophils and may other cells. Its synthesis is catalyzed by NO synthase with L-arginine as substrate. It has been found in exhaled air from humans (41), found to be increased in air exhaled by asthmatics (113), and decreased in air exhaled by patients with Kartagener's syndrome (114). Although originally considered to be mainly of nasal origin (114) studies in asthmatics suggest contributions from lower airways (115). Uric acid has been reported to be a major antioxidant in nasal mucus (40) and to act as a protective agent against potential oxidant stress due to ozone exposure (116) or to nasal action of inflammatory cells (117). Large, nonsulfated glycosaminoglycans such as hyaluronan and similar proteoglycans are also found among the nasal seroproteins (118).

Seroproteins secreted from nasal serous glands may serve an analogous function in nasal mucus as do proteins secreted from oral parotid glands in saliva. However, while both glands serve their respective organs by secreting proteins, and while most proteins secreted are similar in both sets of glands, those proteins found in high concentrations in nasal mucus are in relatively low concentration in parotid saliva and vice versa (see Table 2.3).

Many other substances including those which play roles in cellular signaling are present in nasal mucus. Indeed, we have recently discovered that cAMP is present in nasal mucus and plays a role as a growth factor interacting with olfactory stem cells to promote growth and maturation of olfactory epithelial cells (100). These results mark the first demonstration of cAMP in nasal mucus and correlate with its previous finding in saliva. While absolute concentrations of cAMP in nasal mucus is approximately one-third that of saliva, expressed as per milligram protein, its concentration is about 30% greater than in saliva (Table 2.4).

C. Changes in Nasal Seroproteins with Disease and Other Conditions

Following nasal xenobiotic challenge there is usually a hypersecretion of nasal mucus. Changes in secretion of nasal seroproteins following nasal exposure to xenobiotics take two forms, increases and decreases. These changes are important to understand the pathophysiology of nasal seroproteins during infection and after exposure to various xenobiotics. In general, proteins which increase in concentration are those which combat infection, bind allergens or protect integrity of the nasal surface epithelium. Proteins which decrease in concentration are those which are destroyed by xenobiotic invasion, metabolized due to increased utilization, inhibited by direct action of invading bacteria, virus, fungi, etc., or whose cofactors are made unavailable to their appropriate substrate by a variety of pathological factors.

Following infectious, allergic, or other xenobiotic invasion, significant changes occur in nasal secretions derived from a variety of sources. Changes occur in (a) secretion of nasal seroproteins, (b) secretion from other glands of respiratory epithelium, (c) proteins derived from recruitment of acute and chronic inflammatory cells which enter areas of invasion to assist in combatting xenobiotics, and (d) secretions from cells of respiratory epithelium which themselves respond to invasion by undergoing hyperplasia (80). Lymphocytes are the major

Table 2.4 cAMP in Human Nasal Mucus and Parotid Saliva

Nasal mucus[a]			Parotid saliva[b]		
cAMP (pmol/mL)	Protein (mg/mL)	cAMP/Protein (pmol/mg)	cAMP (pmol/mL)	Protein (mg/mL)	cAMP/Protein (pmol/mg)
2.7 ± 2.7	16.3 ± 9.0^c	2.87 ± 1.52	7.39 ± 1.9^c	3.48 ± 0.40	2.21 ± 0.60

Note: Values are mean $\pm$ SEM.
[a]6 subjects.
[b]17 subjects.
[c]$p < 0.001$.

recruited inflammatory cells (119) with T cells more numerous than B cells by a ratio of 3:1 (120). Mast cells and macrophages are also heavily recruited (121). These cells generate and release specific inflammatory mediators and cytokines and express inflammatory cell-adhesion molecules and major MHC class I and II antigens (122,123).

Following acute viral or bacterial rhinitis (124–128), following acute or chronic sinusitis, or following exposure to allergens which affect upper airways and nasal mucosa (129), major proteins of nasal mucus, albumin, lysozyme, immunoglobulin, other glandular proteins, other phase reactant proteins, proteins from recruited cells, serum-derived proteins, etc., increase in both absolute and relative terms with albumin increasing disproportionately more than any other protein (125,126). Immunoglobulins and phase reactant proteins also increase over levels measured in the noninfected state (80). In addition, mediators of and products of inflammatory cells such as cytokines, GM-CSF (granulocyte calony-stimulating factor) and GCSF, are recruited to and are found in nasal mucus and include products of amino acid metabolism, prostaglandins, leukotrienes, and cell-specific products including neutrophil elastase, cathepsin G, mast-cell chymase, monocyte-macrophage secretogogue, eosinophil granule derived proteins, and oxygen metabolites (80). Mucosal secretory cells undergo hyperplasia (129) during acute and chronic infection and after exposure to other xenobiotics and express increased amounts of secretory products. Patients with nasal disease of several types have been reported to synthesize different cytokines from those without nasal disease (121).

In patients with viral rhinitis, lysozyme and lactoferrin have been reported to *increase* in nasal mucus by a factor of 2 to reflect an 100% increase to reach 10–20% of total nasal serous protein concentration. There appears to be a timed pattern of change in these proteins following infection (125–128). In one study, albumin and what has been considered to be plasma proteins, (IgG), increased on days 2 and 3 after experimental viral infection whereas there was little concomitant increase in so called glandular proteins (126). These investigators appear to have assumed that all albumin in nasal mucus was a transudate from plasma. However, careful analysis of these data indicate that all nasal seroproteins increased after experimental viral infection with albumin increasing from 10–20 to 300 $\mu g/mL$ in both controls and infected subjects (126). Since these samples of nasal mucus were obtained after nasal lavage and since changes were observed in both patients and controls, these results question both the results obtained and the validity of use of nasal lavage to obtain nasal mucus. Indeed, several investigators have criticized nasal lavage as having inherent disadvantages (130).

Several investigators suggested that plasma and plasma derived mediators represent the major respiratory defense mechanism (131). These investigators considered plasma exudation as a first line of respiratory mucosal defense (132). These investigators indicated that the more pronounced was the airways inflammation the greater was the plasma exudative response at the nasal airways (133). They contend that all nasal mucus albumin results from "airways exudation" resulting from increased submucosal microvascular and mucosal permeability secondary to rhinitis or asthma (130–132). However, these same investigators note that albumin was not a good index of inflammatory response (134) and that plasma proteins may stimulate glandular secretions (135); for example, albumin may prevent normal hydration of secreted mucins (135). These suggestions indicate the difficulty in identifying the origin of proteins secreted in nasal mucus since some, due to their concentration, are obviously secreted from glands in the mucosa, some may be derived from plasma and some may be derived from recruited inflammatory cells. Present data do not offer definitive information about the source of these proteins.

In our studies, in one patient with acute sinusitis, albumin *increased* not by 100% but by over 900-fold to account for about 90% of the total protein in nasal serous fluid (Fig. 2.2). Our studies suggest that albumin may not only be a plasma-derived protein, as suggested by other investigators (130–132), but may also be a direct secretion from nasal serous glands. The reason for the great increase in albumin is unclear for its function in nasal mucus is uncertain. Whether it can bind and thereby inhibit invading xenobiotics and inactivate them due to its structural characteristics or putative antibacterial function is unclear.

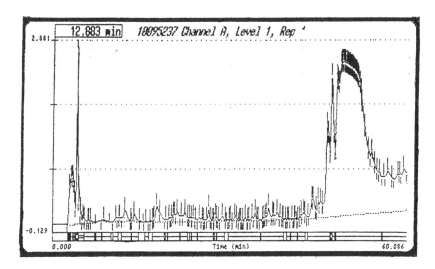

Figure 2.2 HPLC of seroproteins from whole nasal mucus of a patient (23-year-old Caucasian female) with acute sinusitis. Albumin, eluted at 51 min, is increased to reflect about 90% of the total eluted protein. β_2-m, eluted at 46 min and lysozyme, eluted at 49 min, are also significantly elevated above concentrations found in normal subjects (cf. Fig. 2.1). Lumicarmine, eluted at 28 min, is decreased in concentration compared to that measured in normal subjects and may reflect either increased destruction or utilization (see text for details).

Other proteins were also *increased* in the nasal mucus in this patient, including lysozyme and β_2m. As noted previously, lysozyme plays a well-known active role as an antibacterial, antiviral agent, and β_2m may be a manifestation of activation of the immune system complex to combat xenobiotic invasion.

Other proteins, including lumicarmine and histones, were *decreased* in this patient (Fig. 2.2). Decreased lumicarmine may be a manifestation of its activity in wound or epithelial structure healing. Since we hypothesize that it is the major scaffold maintainance protein of the epithelial surface, if xenobiotic invasion disrupted the epithelial surface, then lumicarmine, the biofilm which coapts the surface epithelium of the nose, would be functionally inactivated. In order to maintain epithelial surface integrity, a rapid repair process would be required. Since lumicarmine could be the major functional component of this process its concentration in mucus may decrease as it laid down over the nasal surface due either to increased utilization and/or an accompanying increased destruction due to xenobiotic activity. After mechanical disruption of respiratory epithelium both *in vivo* (136–138) and *in vitro* (139), a specific repair process has been demonstrated within hours after injury which can be blocked by inhibitors of protein synthesis (139). This scenario raises the hypothesis that lumicarmine itself may be the substance which has been described as the "thin" periciliary mucus layer which underlies the "thick" viscous mucus layer of both respiratory and olfactory epithelial mucus.

In a normal subject after recovery from and during an acute coryza, *increased* secretion of albumin, lactoferrin, lysozyme, and phase reactants was observed during the acute infectious process but after spontaneous recovery from the acute process these proteins, particularly albumin, decreased in concentration toward normal (Fig. 2.3). During the acute inflammatory phase, lumicarmine and histones were decreased in concentration, as previously shown, but after recovery, they increased in concentration.

In another example of this complex, reactive system, following a viral infection, gustin/CA VI has been shown to *decrease* in concentration with, presumably, a concomitant decrease in growth and development of olfactory epithelial cells and induction of smell loss (27). With treatment of the infection, gustin may *increase* in concentration, consistent with return of smell function to normal.

Thus, seroproteins in nasal mucus may increase or decrease following a variety of pathological events. Upregulation appears to be a function of protective nature of these proteins. Downregulation may indicate active destruction, decreased protein synthesis or increased utilization. Several disease processes such as nasal polyposis (84), natural (140,141) or iatrogenic allergic diatheses (142), acute infectious processes of the nose (126), recurrent middle ear infections (77), or exposure to particulates from diesel fuel (83) can induce upregulation of various components of nasal mucus proteins not only including albumin, lysozyme, and lactoferrin, but also cytokines, chemokines and other substances (Fig. 2.4).

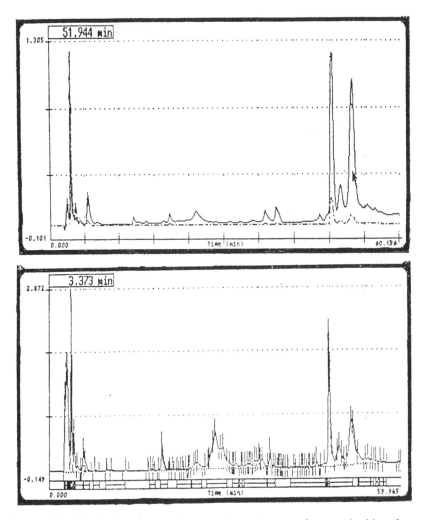

Figure 2.3 HPLC of seroproteins from whole nasal mucus of a normal subject (lower panel) (66-year-old Caucasian male) without upper or lower airways disease and from this same subject during an acute coryza (upper panel). Note *increased* concentrations of β_2m precursor, 46 min; lysozyme, 49 min; and albumin, 51 min during the acute coryza (upper panel). Also note decreased histones, 18 min and lumicarmine, 28 min (upper panel).

During allergy season mRNA of IL-4 and IL-5 has been shown to increase (142). After an antigen challenge in late phase allergic reactions associated with antigen-induced rhinitis, IL-1β, IL-5, IL-6, and GM-CSF reportedly increased associated with modulated activation of basophils, initiating histamine release (142). TNF-α has been reported to be released in nasal mucus in acute allergic rhinitis (82). Bradykinin has been reported to increase in nasal secretion after

NORMAL

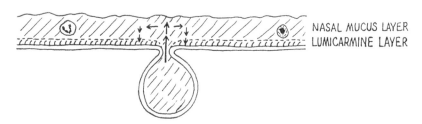

ACUTE INFLAMMATION

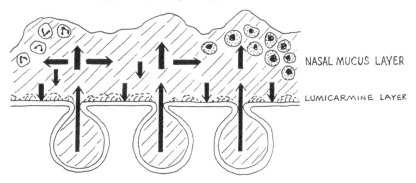

Figure 2.4   Representational illustration of nasal mucosa under normal conditions (top) and during acute inflammation (bottom) showing nasal serous glands and nasal mucus. Under *normal conditions* nasal serous glands secrete many proteins which form both the basal, thin, pericilliary mucus layer comprised predominantly of lumicarmine and the thick mucus layer comprised of major proteins (albumin, lysozyme, lactoferrin, IgG, etc.) which lies on top of the thin layer (see text for details). Small numbers of neutrophils and lymphocytes are present in the thick nasal mucus layer. Proteins present in the thick mucus layer derived from serous glands and recruited cells control homeostasis of the nasal mucosal membrane. During *acute inflammation*, nasal serous glands become hyperplastic. They increase protein secretion which causes an increase in thickness of the nasal mucus layer. Lymphocytes, mast cells, and macrophages which are recruited to the thick mucus layer increase in number and increase their secretion of cytokines, leukotrienes, etc. The thin mucus lumicarmine layer is decreased by xenobiotic activity, which acts to partially denude this thin layer.

experimental viral infection (124). Occupational exposure to methyl tetra-hydrophthalic anhydride induces an asthmatic condition and alters concentrations of many nasal proteins (39).

However, *differential changes* in concentration of these cytokines have been observed. For example, children with recurrent otitis media have been reported to have significantly lower levels of IL-1β, IL-6, and TNF-α in their nasopharyngeal secretions than do healthy children (77). While nasal secretions generally contained measureable levels of IL-1β, IL-6, and TNF-α, these substances were undetected in serum (67). Differential levels of these cytokines were also found with some subjects demonstrating high levels of IL-1β with lower undetectable levels of IL-6 or TNF-α or vice versa with low levels of IL-1β (77).

Protein upregulation also occurs in secretions from analogous glandular structures in epithelia of other tissues, such as in bovine mammary gland secretions. In response to experimental infection with *E. coli*, lactoferrin trimer synthesis is upregulated with respect to monomer and this change has been demonstrated to enhance the inhibitory effect of lactoferrin by increasing its iron-binding capacity threefold and thereby enhancing its antibacterial capacity.

There is analogous upregulation and downregulation of some of these proteins in parotid gland secretion in the mouth following infection. However, since most of these proteins (i.e., albumin, lysozyme, lactoferrin, etc.) comprise such a small percentage of total parotid saliva protein they do not alter significantly the total protein concentration or protein distribution in parotid saliva as they do in nasal mucus. Lumicarmine represents about 80% of total saliva protein, amylase about 5–10% and gustin/CA VI about 3%. Changes in these latter proteins are relatively small following infection, whereas upregulation of salivary proteins considered to be protective in nasal mucus are limited on an absolute scale. Following acute or chronic parotitis, albumin was reported to increase significantly in parotid saliva proteins and large relative increases in lactoferrin, lysozyme, immunoglobulins (IgA, IgG, IgM) and transferrin were measured (143–145). However, since these proteins represent <1–2% of total parotid protein, although the relative changes in protein concentration may increase by 50–100%, these changes are small relative to their absolute concentration in saliva. In addition, the observed changes were unduly influenced by significantly decreased saliva flow of over 10-fold, which exaggerates these relative changes by changes in total protein concentration (143,145). Thus, while major salivary proteins which comprise about 90% of the total parotid protein do not change significantly with infection, phase reactive proteins in saliva such as albumin, lysozyme, lactoferrin, etc., may be upregulated percentage wise but still reflect only a small change in total protein concentration.

Differences between protein secretion following infection in nose and mouth may also be observed following stimulation by other factors. Saliva is uniformly stimulated by a variety of physiological factors including the sight and smell of food, oral placement of food or sweet or sour substances (candies, lemon drops, etc.). Nasal mucus is occasionally stimulated by food, usually warm beverages, but is commonly physiologically stimulated by vigorous exercise, extremely cold or hot external temperatures, or sneezing. Nasal mucus is also stimulated by oral ingestion of noxious or intensely overpowering substances such as chilli peppers or extremely spicy foods and these substances, while they also induce an excessive production of saliva, may not do so to the extent noted in nasal mucus. These results suggest that capsaicin, through its action on substance P and similar neurotransmitters, may stimulate nasal secretion to protect nasal mucous membranes from harmful substances.

V. Discussion

Teleological functional differences between nose and mouth help explain development of nasal secretions. Phylogenetically, because external air entering the nose is delivered directly and without apparent modification to the lungs, an elaborate defense system developed to protect the lungs from potential toxic substances in incoming air. Air, if contaminated, and not perceived as such by sensory receptors in the nose, could induce serious pathological consequences if allowed direct, unhindered passage into the lungs, since they have been programmed to accept air without volition. Nasal sensory receptors may recognize some noxious substances but many substances which are potentially harmful, including bacteria, viruses, fungi, allergens, particulate matter, and other potential toxins, may not be recognized. For example, in some areas, airborne spores which have no odor, may be present in concentrations 1000 times those of pollens (146), but may go unrecognized by nasal sensory receptors yet cause severe disease. Indeed, systemic host defense mechanisms for fungi have not been clearly elucidated (147). Smell receptors in humans are adapted primarily to recognize very low concentrations of distant volatile substances in search for food in order to reduce energy required to obtain nourishment (usually sugars of various types (148)) or, in lower species, to recognize time of ovulation (usually, so called pheromones) and thereby conserve energy in performance of the reproductive process (148). The olfactory system, in spite of its exquisite sensitivity, *is not capable of recognizing* many pathologically important xenobiotic substances due to their lack of volatility; bacteria and viruses may not emit volatiles which olfactory receptors can detect or recognize. By contrast, samples entering the mouth *are recognized* since resident sensory receptors, albeit less sensitive than those in the nose can, more readily than those in the nose, deal with potentially noxious samples by easily and quickly identifying them by taste as noxious and eliciting rejection by spitting out the sample. Taste receptors in the mouth are specifically adapted to perform this task of identifying acceptable or rejectable substances (148). In this sense, sensory receptors in the mouth act as the guardian of the gastrointestinal tract (148). They are part of the program of the gastrointestinal tract designed to accept pleasant, sweet substances for food and reject noxious substances which may be poisonous. If acceptable, the sample is taken in and swallowed; if unacceptable the sample is rejected, spit out, or vomited. Even if, by error, the sample were disguised or unrecognized as toxic (e.g., sugar of lead) and taken into the gastrointestinal tract, only a portion would be absorbed, the majority passing out of gastrointestinal tract as waste. Of course, this does not infer that accidental or human-induced poisonings do not occur. If air is taken into the lungs from the mouth these oral sensory receptors are ill adapted to recognize potentially toxic substances as opposed to their ability to recognize toxic food or fluid and they cannot protect the lungs either by sensory means or by protein inactivation.

In a similar sense, sensory receptors of the nose were designed to act as the guardian of the respiratory system (148). However, their ability to do this is limited to recognition of noxious, volatile substances and thus, samples which do not have an obnoxious odor, do not initiate coughing or sneezing or are not highly volatile enter into the system without recognition. Teleologically, because of this sensory lack, other mechanisms developed, designed specifically to inhibit, bind, and inactivate xenobiotics in incoming air so that these substances could be inhibited before reaching their final destination in the lung.

But is examination of nasal seroproteins just an interesting teleological and biochemical exercise or does it have some clinical importance which relates to care of patients? Are there specific at-risk patient groups in whom examination of nasal seroproteins may offer diagnostic and therapeutic benefit? While answers to these questions are presently uncertain there are several patient groups in whom present treatment methods have not proven clinically effective. For example, patients with chronic sinusitis who are nonresponsive to repeated antibiotic trials may benefit from examination of nasal seroproteins to determine if some missing, decreased, or increased protein might assist in specifying an underlying disease process. Perhaps some lack of response of one or more proteins during an active infective process may identify mechanisms which inhibit therapeutic effectiveness. Examination of seroproteins in treatment refractory patients of many types may assist in determination of novel pathology and may assist in understanding the refractory nature of their treatment and thereby further understanding of their underlying disease process.

A. Clinical Effects of Xerorhinia

Decreased or altered secretion of proteins in nasal mucus may not only affect nasal mucosa but also the entire pulmonary system. As in the mouth decreased secretion of gustin/CA VI is associated with loss of smell function (27) and increased secretion of this protein following therapeutic intervention is associated with return of smell function to normal (27). As would be expected, in patients with xerorhinia with either Sjögren's syndrome (149) or following irradiation to the head and neck, smell loss was reported (150–154). In Sjögren's syndrome, pathological changes in nasal glands (155) similar to those observed in oral glands were observed secondary to dryness associated with this syndrome. However, in patients with Sjögren's syndrome and xerorhinia in whom secretion of these protective proteins is inhibited, reports have indicated that between 25% and 75% of patients exhibit severe bronchopulmonary disease of several types (156–160) and associated impairment of pulmonary function (161).

In one study in patients with primary Sjögren's syndrome, patients exhibited a variety of pulmonary pathology including bronchopneumonia, lymphocytic interstitial fibrosis, pseudolymphoma and malignant lymphoma (162). Patients found to have lymphocytic interstitial pneumonia have been observed to have Sjögren's syndrome as an etiological factor. Many patients with primary Sjögren's syndrome have associated sinopulmonary infections and bronchiectasis (162). Among these patients as many as 25% with pulmonary disease have diffuse interstitial lung disease (163,164) demonstrated by histological tissue examination (131,164). Alveolitis has been reported in 55% of patients with primary Sjögren's syndrome (165) and bronchiolitis obliterans has been reported in others (166,167).

While decreased nasal secretions may play an important role in decreased lung protection associated with the etiology of pulmonary disease in these patients it must be pointed out that Sjögren's syndrome can be a manifestation of a systemic collagen-vascular disease. In addition to xerorhinia decreased secretion from all glands associated with external secretions occur in Sjögren's syndrome. Thus, these patients not only exhibit xerorhinia but also xerotrachea and xerobronchia associated with a chronic dry, nonproductive cough. Decreased secretions from glands lining the mucosal surface of the upper and lower airways also contribute to pneumonia, bronchiectasis, and interstitial lung disease observed in these patients (163,165–167). However, as mentioned earlier, the same protective proteins secreted in nasal mucus are secreted from glands in these tissues and their decreased secretion may compound the lack of pulmonary protection.

In other diseases in which decreased nasal mucus occurs, the relationship to pulmonary disease onset is less clear. In the disorder labeled ozena, no clear cut association with pulmonary disease has been described although ozena is commonly associated with acute and chronic rhinitis and sinusitis which are associated with an increased incidence of respiratory infections. Similarly, whether or not there is an increased incidence of pulmonary disease among chronic mouth breathers, *per se*, is also unclear since many mouth breathers do so out of necessity due to nasal obstruction associated with either rhinitis, sinusitis, or other upper respiratory pathology. Pulmonary changes associated with sleep apnea have not been specifically described albeit changes in pO_2 have been associated with significant pathology related to several organ systems. Following therapeutic radiation to the nasopharynx for treatment of malignancies of various types there is an associated xerorhinia and, on occasion, mucositis, similar to that observed following therapeutic radiation to the oral cavity for oral or laryngeal tumors. However, little information is available about subsequent pulmonary disease in these former patients although if the present hypothesis were valid an increase in pulmonary dysfunction would be present. Patients with Wegener's granulomatosis or with midline granuloma in the early disease stages may exhibit nasal dryness with associated chronic inflammatory and giant cell infiltration of nasal glands and glands of the lower airways (10). One of the earliest symptoms in this disorder is loss of smell (R.I. Henkin, A.S. Fauci, S.M. Wolff, unpublished observations) in addition to their pulmonary and upper airways changes. Most of these patients exhibit chronic pulmonary disease as well as sinusitis and rhinitis. In the disorder labeled "limited" Wegener's granulomatosis (168), as many as 60% of patients may exhibit sinusitis at presentation (169,170) and one of the most practical and fruitful methods of diagnosis employs nasal mucosal, turbinate mucosal or sinus biopsy (168). As the disease progresses the necrotizing granulomatous character becomes more apparent.

B. Consequences of Treatment to Control Rhinorrhea and Other Nasal Usage

These results raise several questions about treatment used to control nasal secretion. While antihistamines, inhaled nasal decongestants, including α-adrenergic agonist and imidazolines, intranasal steroid sprays, and anticholinergic agents [ipratropium (171)] are used clinically to inhibit rhinorrhea and are socially useful, they act to decrease flow of nasal secretions; thus, their use inhibits secretions of those very proteins whose role it is to protect both nose and lungs from allergic or infectious agents which initiate rhinorrhea. In this sense, questions about their clinical use need to be raised since their application may initiate and aggravate rather than lessen the pathology for which they are prescribed. These drugs may also initiate "side effects" of nasal burning, drying, epistaxis, and systemic symptoms related to taste distortion, urinary retention, and prostate disorders. While these symptoms may occur in a relatively small number of patients, the underlying therapeutic concept of inhibiting nasal secretions designed to protect the nose needs to be reevaluated.

The role of these proteins in terms of their interactions with new nasal inhalation drug delivery systems for various agents, including insulin, etidronate, vaccines, nonabsorbable steroids, and other drugs, also needs further evaluation. Since nasal inhalation of many therapeutic agents is a growing pharmaceutical practice based upon the excellent and available vascular system in the nose, the manner in which these drugs and pharmaceuticals may alter nasal function is relatively unexplored "side effects" of these agents, considered relatively unimportant in relation to the beneficial pharmacological effects, need to be considered. However, novel techniques for drug delivery via nasal inhalation have been developed such that changes in particle size and density of inhalation aerosols can enhance delivery of inhaled therepeutics into the systemic circulation (172).

Finally, knowledge of these proteins and their secretion characteristics at rest and after xenobiotic invasion raise several questions related to function of both upper and lower airways reflecting both a challenge and an opportunity to otolaryngology in the 21st century:

1. Is any nasal seroprotein necessary or sufficient to protect upper airways from disease?
2. What role does each nasal seroprotein play individually or together as a group in initiation of or in protection from nasal–sino-pulmonary disease?

3. Does impaired secretion of any nasal seroprotein indicate a propensity for upper airways disease or aid in its diagnosis?

4. Does differential secretion of nasal seroproteins identify any patient group (e.g., children with recurrent, acute otitis media)?

5. Are the major seroproteins found in nasal mucus secreted from nasal glands (albumin, lysozyme, lactoferrin, IgG, α-trypsin proteinase inhibitor, the Clara cell phospholipid binding protein) more relevant clinically or more important as protectors of upper and lower airways structures than proteins secreted from cells recruited to the nasal mucus (cytokines, leukotrienes)?

6. Does failure to upregulate or downregulate any nasal seroprotein indicate a disease process and does it offer an opportunity for specific therapy?

7. What factors control upregulation and downregulation of nasal seroproteins and other substances in nasal mucus and by what mechanisms do these changes occur?

8. Is downregulation of lumicarmine during nasal infection an indication that the nasal lining requires immediate replacement in order to form a physiological nasal mucous membrane scaffold?

9. Would treatment with any nasal seroprotein improve nasal–sino-pulmonary disease?

10. Since these seroproteins and other substances contribute to a complex homeostatic system in the upper airways, how is this homeostasis regulated?

11. Does this putative regulation occur locally, are systemic factors involved or do both events occur simultaneously or in a timed pattern of change?

With answers to these and other more definitive questions, we should be better able to understand the function of nasal seroproteins and better able to diagnose and treat infectious, allergic and other processes which commonly affect the nose and interfere with nasal function, normal nasal breathing, sinus function, and to some extent, pulmonary function. While nasal seroproteins may play important roles in protecting nasal mucous membranes these roles are presently poorly defined. With a comprehensive understanding of these roles it will be possible to define more efficient therapy for disorders which afflict the nose and sinuses based upon sound biochemical and pathological principles inherent in our understanding of the function of the proteins and other substances present in nasal mucus.

References

1. McMartin CL, Hutchinson EF, Hyde R, Peters GE. Analysis of structural requirements for the absorption of drugs and macromolecules from the nasal cavity. J Pharm Sci 1987; 76:525–540.

2. Boucher RC. Chemical modulation of airway epithelial permeability. Environ Health Perspect 1980; 53:3–12.

3. Cremaschi D, Rosetti C, Draghetti MT, Manzoni C, Alberti V. Active transport of polypeptides in rabbit nasal mucosa: possible role in the sampling of potential antigens. Pflugers Arch 1991; 419:425–432.

4. Cremaschi D, Porta C, Ghirardelli R. Endocytosis of polypeptides in rabbit nasal respiratory mucosa. News Physiol Sci 1997; 12:219–225.

5. Jeffrey PK. Structural, immunologic and neural elements of the normal human airway wall. In: Busse WW, Holgate ST, eds. Asthma and Rhinitis. Cambridge, MA: Blackwell, 1995:80.

6. Cole P. Modification of inspired air. In: Mathew OP, Sant'Ambroglio G, eds. Lung Biology in Health and Disease. Vol. 35. New York: Marcel Dekker, 1988:415–445.

7. Gray H. Anatomy of the Human Body. Philadelphia, PA: Lea and Febriger, 1954:1198–1202.

8. Davies RJ, Devalia JL. Epithelial cell dysfunction in rhinitis. In: Busse WW, Holgate ST, eds. Asthma and Rhinitis. Cambridge, MA: Blackwell, 1995:612.

9. Jeffery PK. Morphologic features of airway surface epithelial cells and glands. Am Rev Respir Dis 1983; 128:514–520.

10. Verdugo P. Goblet cell secretion and mucogenesis. Am Rev Physiol 1990; 52:157–176.

11. Hyams VJ. Pathology of the nose and paranasal sinuses. In: English GM, ed. Otolaryngology. Vol. 2. Philadelphia, PA: Lippincott, 1986:1–95.

12. Blenkinsopp WK. Proliferation of respiratory tract epithelium in the rat. Exp Cell Res 1967; 46:114–154.

13. Evans MJ, Plopper CG. The role of basal cells in adhesion of columnar epithelium to airway basement membrane. Am Rev Respir Dis 1988; 138:481–483.

14. Takizawa H, Romberger D, Beckmann J et al. Separation of bovine bronchial epithelial cell subpopulations by density centrifugations: a method to isolate ciliated and non-ciliated cell fractions. Am J Respir Cell Mol Biol 1990; 3:553–562.

14a. Carson JL, Collier AM, Boucher RC. Ultrastructure of the respiratory epithelium in the human nose. In: Mygind N, Pitcorn U, eds. Allergic and Vasomotor Rhinitis: Pathophysiological Aspects. Copenhagen: Munksgaard, 1987:11–27.

15. Evans MJ, Cabral-Anderson LJ, Freeman G. Role of the Clara cell in renewal of bronchiolar epithelium. Lab Invest 1978; 38:648–655.

16. Ash JE, Raum M. An Atlas of Otolaryngic Pathology. Armed Forces Institute of Pathology. Washington, DC: US Government Printing Office, 1956.

17. Goldstein BJ, Fang H, Youngentob SL, Schwob JE. Transplantation of multipotent progenitors from the adult olfactory epithelium. Neuroreport 1998; 9:1611–1617.

18. Schwob JE, Huard JMT, Luskin MB, Youngentob SL. Retroviral lineage studies of the rat olfactory epithelium. Chem Senses 1994; 19:671–672.

19. Huard JMT, Schwob JE. Cell cycle of globose basal cells in rat olfactory epithelium. Dev Dyn 1995; 203:17–26.

20. Ayers M, Jeffrey PK. Proliferation and differentiation in adult mammalian airways epithelium: a review. Eur Respir J 1988; 1:58–80.

21. Widdicome JH. Structure and function of epithelial cells in controlling airway lining fluid. In: Busse WW, Holgate ST, eds. Asthma and Rhinitis. Cambridge, MA: Blackwell, 1995:565.

22. Baraniuk JN, Kaliner MA. Functional activity of upper airway nerves. In: Busse WW, Holgate ST, eds. Asthma and Rhinitis. Cambridge, MA: Blackwell, 1995:652.

23. Lucas AM, Douglas LC. Principles underlying ciliary activity in the respiratory tract. II. A comparison of nasal clearance in man, monkey and other mammals. Arch Otolaryngol 1934; 20:518–541.

24. Sanderson MJ, Sleigh MA. Ciliary activity of cultured rabbit tracheal epithelium: beat pattern and metachromy. J Cell Sci 1981; 47:331–347.

25. Yomeda K. Mucous blanket of rat bronchus: ultrastructural study. Am Rev Respir Dis 1976; 114:837–842.

26. Havez R, Rousel P. Bronchial mucus: physical and biochemical features. In: Weiss EB, Segal MS, eds. Bronchial Asthma: Mechanisms and Therepeutics. Boston, MA: Little Brown, 1976:409–422.

27. Doherty AE, Martin BM, Dai WL, Henkin RI. Carbonic anhydrase (CA) activity in nasal mucus appears to be a marker for loss of smell (hyposmia) in humans. J Invest Med 1997; 45:237A.

28. Swiss Protein Data Base-PC Gene (Release 14), 1999.

29. Meret S, Henkin RI. Simultaneous direct estimation by atomic absorption spectrophotometry of copper and zinc in serum, urine, and cerebrospinal fluid. Clin Chem 1971; 17:369–373.

30. Boekhoff I, Braunewell KH, Andreini I, Breer H, Gundelfinger E. The calcium-binding protein VILIP in olfactory neurons: regulation of secondary messenger signaling. Eur J Cell Biol 1997; 72:151–158.

31. Bastianelli E, Polans AS, Hidaka H, Pochet R. Differential distribution of six calcium-binding proteins in the rat olfactory epithelium during post natal development and adulthood. J Comp Neurol 1995; 354:395–409.

32. Fujiwara M, Nakamura H, Kawasaki M, Nakano Y, Kuwano R. Expressions of a calcium-binding protein (spot 35/calbindin-D28K) in mouse olfactory cells: possible relationship to neuronal differentiation. Eur Arch Otorhinolarygol 1997; 254:105–109.

33. Smith RP, Shellard R, Dhillon DP, Winter J, Mehta A. Asymmetric interactions between phosphorylation pathways regulating ciliary beat frequency in human nasal respiratory epithelium in vitro. J Physiol (Lond) 1996; 496:883–889.

34. Iino S, Kobayashi S, Okazaki K, Hidaka H. Neurocalcin-immunoreactive receptor cells in the rat olfactory epithelium and vomeronasal organ. Neurosci Lett 1995; 191:91–94.

35. Richli EE, Ghazanafar AS, Gibbons BH, Edsall JT. Carbonic anhydrases from human erythrocytes. J Biol Chem 1964; 239:1065–1078.

36. Raphael GD, Baraniuk JN, Kaliner MA. How and why the nose runs. J Allergy Clin Immunol 1991; 87:457–491.

37. Klockars M, Reitano S. Tissue distribution of lysozyme in man. J Histochem Cytochem 1975; 23:932–940.

38. Raphael GD, Jeney EV, Baraniuk JN, Kim I, Meredith SD, Kaliner MA. The pathophysiology of rhinitis: lactoferrin and lysozyme in nasal secretions. J Clin Invest 1989; 84:1528–1535.

39. Lindahl M, Ståhlbom Tagesson C. Two dimensional gel electrophoresis of nasal and bronchoalveolar lavage fluid after occupational exposure. Electrophoresis 1995; 16:1199–1204.

40. Peden DB, Hohman R, Brown ME, Mason RT, Berkebile C, Fales HM, Kaliner MA. Uric acid is a major antioxidant in human nasal airways secretions. Proc Natl Acad Sci USA 1990; 87:7638–7642.

41. Imada M, Iwamoto J, Nonaka S, Kobayashi Y, Unno T. Measurement of nitric oxide in human nasal airways. Eur Respir J 1996; 9:556–559.

42. Hegnhj Schaffalitsky de Muckadell OB. An enzyme-linked immunosorbent assay for measurement of lactoferrin in duodenal aspirates and other biological fluids. Scand J Clin Lab Invest 1985; 45:489–495.

43. Rossen RD, Schade AL, Butler WT, Kasel JA. The proteins in nasal secretion: a longitudinal study of the γA-globulin, γG-globulin, albumin, siderophilin and total protein in nasal washings from adult male volunteers. J Clin Invest 1966; 45:768–776.

44. Fleming A. On a remarkable bacteriolytic element found in tissues and secretions. Proc R Soc Lond B Biol Sci 1922; 93:306–317.

45. Raphael GD, Igarashi Y, White MV, Kaliner MA. The pathophysiology of rhinitis V. Sources of proteins in allergen-induced nasal secretions. J Allergy Clin Immunol 1991; 88:33–42.

46. Sümuller U, Arnhold M, Fritz H, Wiedenmann K, Machleidt W, Heinzel R, Appelhaus H, Gassen HG, Lottspeich F. The acid stable proteinase inhibitor of human mucous secretions (HUSI-1 antileukoprotease). FEBS Lett 1986; 199:43–48.

47. Lee CH, Igarash Y, Hohman RJ, Kaulbach H, White MV, Kaliner MA. Distribution of secretory leukoprotease inhibitor in the human nasal airway. Am Rev Respir Dis 1993; 147:710–716.

48. Stetler G, Brewer MT, Thompson RC. Isolation and sequence of a human gene encoding a potent inhibitor of leukocyte proteases. Nucleic Acids Res 1986; 14:7883–7896.

49. Umland TC, Swaminathan S, Singh G, Warty V, Furey W, Platcher J, Sax M. Structure of a human Clara cell phospholipid-binding protein–ligand complex at 1.9 Å resolution. Nat Struct Biol 1994; 1:538–549.

50. Singh G, Katyah SL, Brown WE, Phillips S, Kennedy AL, Anthony J, Squeglia N. Amino acid and cDNA nucleotide sequence of human Clara cell 10 kDa protein. Biochim Biophys Acta 1988; 950:329–337.

51. Boyd MR. Evidence for the Clara cell as a site of cytochrome P 450-dependent mixed-function oxidase in lung. Nature 1977; 269:713–715.

52. Mornon JP, Fridlansky F, Bally R, Milgrom E. X-ray crystallographic analyses of a progesterone-binding protein: the c222 crystal form of oxidized interoglobin at 2.2 Å resolution. J Mol Biol 1980; 137:415–429.

53. Morgenstern JP, Griffith IJ, Brauer AW, Rogers BL, Bond JF, Chapman MD, Kuo MC. Amino acid sequence of Fel dI, the major allergen of the domestic cat: protein sequence analysis and cDNA cloning. Proc Natl Acad Sci USA 1991; 88:9690–9694.

54. Matulionis DH, Parks HF. Ultrastructural morphology of the normal nasal respiratory epithelium of the mouse. Anat Rec 1973; 176:65–84.

55. Schlesinger DH, Hay DI. Complete covalent structure of statherin, a tyrosine-rich acidic peptide which inhibits phosphate precepitation from human parotid saliva. J Biol Chem 1977; 252:1689–1695.

56. Hay DI. The interaction of human parotid salivary proteins with hydroxyapatite. Arch Oral Biol 1973; 18:1517–1529.

57. Gron P. The demonstration of a dicalcium phosphate stabilizing factor in saliva. Arch Oral Biol 1973; 18:1379–1383.

58. Goodfellow PN, Jones EA, VanHeyningen V et al. The β_2-microglobulin gene is on chromosome 15 and not in the HL-A region. Nature (Lond) 1975; 254:267–269.

59. Lawlor DA, Warren E, Ward FE, Parham P. Comparison of class 1 MHC alleles in humans and apes. Part II. Immunol Rev 1990; 114:127–132.

60. Mavlight GM, Stuckey SE, Cabinillas FF et al. Diagnosis of leukemia or lymphoma in the central nervous system by beta$_2$-microglobulin determination. New Engl J Med 1980; 303:718–722.

61. Güssow D, Rein R, Ginjaar I, Hochstenback F, Seeman G, Kottman A, Ploegh HL. The human β_2-microglobulin gene. Primary structure and definition of the transcriptional unit. Part I. J Immunol 1987; 139:3132–3138.

62. Groves ML, Greenberg R. Complete amino acid sequence of bovine β_2-microglobulin. J Biol Chem 1982; 257:2619–2626.

63. Araki T, Gejyo F, Takagi K, Haupt H, Schwick HG, Bürge W, Marti T, Schaller J, Rickli E, Bussmer R, Atkinson PH, Putnan FW, Schmid K. Complete amino acid sequence of human plasma Zn-α_2-glycoprotein and its homology to histocompatability antigens. J Immunol 1988; 85:679–683.

64. Klein J. In: Quastel MR, ed. Cell Biology and Immunobiology of Leukocyte Function. New York: Academic Press, 1979:309–314.

65. Barnstable CJ, Jones EA, Bodmer WF, Bodmer JG, Arce-Gomez B, Smary D, Crompton M. Genetics and serology of HL-A linked human Ia antigens. Cold Spring Harbor Symp Quant Biol 1976; 41:443–455.

66. Plesner T. Immunochemical studies of human β_2-microglobulin. Allergy 1980; 35:627–637.

67. Michalski JP, Daniels TE, Talal N, Gray HM. Beta$_2$ microglobulin and lymphocytic infiltration in Sjögren's syndrome. New Engl J Med 1975; 293:1228–1231.

68. Gates FT, Coligan JE, Kindt TJ. Complete amino acid sequence of rabbit β_2-microglobulin. Biochemistry 1979; 18:2267–2272.

69. Klein J. The major histocompatability complex of the mouse. Science 1979; 203:516–521.

70. Goding JW, Walker ID. Allelic forms of β_2-microglobulin in the mouse. Proc Natl Acad Sci USA 1980; 77:7395–7399.

71. Unanue ER, Beller DI, Lu CY, Allen PM. Antigen presentation: comments on its regulation and mechanism. J Immunol 1984; 132:1–5.

72. Marrack P, Kappler J. The T cell receptor. Science 1987; 238:1073–1079.

73. Peterson PA, Cunningham BA, Berggard I, Edelman GM. β_2-microglobulin-a free immunoglobulin domain contains an intrachain disulfide loop of 57 residues similar in size to that found in IgG. Proc Natl Acad Sci USA 1972; 69:1697–1701.

74. Wang D, Levasseur-Acker GM, Janowski R, Kanny G, Moneret-Vantrin DA, Charron D, Lockhart A, Swierczeski E. HLA class II antigens and T lymphocytes in human nasal epithelial cells. Modulation of the HLA class II gene transcripts by gamma interferon. Clin Exp Allergy 1997; 27:306–314.

75. Lawler DA, Warren E, Ward FE, Parham P. Comparison of class I MHC alleles in humans and apes. Part I. Immunol Rev 1990; 113:147–185.

76. Alam R, Sim TS, Hilsmeier K, Grant JA. Development of a new technique for recovery of cytokines from inflammatory sites in situ. J Immunol Methods 1992; 155:25–29.

77. Lindberg K, Rynnel-Dagoo M, Sundquist KG. Cytokines in nasopharyngeal secretions: evidence for defective IL-1β production in children with recurrent episodes of acute otitis media. Clin Exp Immunol 1994; 97:396–402.

78. Baumgarten CR, Nichols RC, Naclerio RM, Lichtenstein LM, Norman PS, Proud D. Plasma kallikrein during experimentally induced allergic rhinitis: role to kinin formation and contribution to TAME-esterase activity in nasal secretions. J Immunol 1986; 137:977–982.

79. Mosimann BL, White MV, Hohman RJ, Goldrich MS, Kaulbach HC, Kaliner MS. Substance P, calcitonin gene-related peptide and vasoactive intestinal peptide increase in nasal secretions after allergen challenge in atopic patients. J Allergy Clin Immunol 1993; 92:95–104.

80. Johnson CW, Larivee P, Shelhamer JH. Epithelial cells: regulation of mucus secretion. In: Busse WW, Holgate ST, eds. Asthma and Rhinitis. Cambridge, MA: Blackwell, 1995:584–598.

81. Balkwill F, Burke F. The cytokine network. Immunol Today 1989; 10:299–304.

82. Proud D, Gwaltney JMJ, Hendley O, Dinorello CA, Gillis S, Schleiner RP. Increased levels of interleukin-1 are detected in nasal secretions of volunteers during experimental rhinovirus colds. J Infect Dis 1994; 169:1007–1013.

83. Diaz-Sanchez D, Tsien A, Casillos A, Dotson AR, Saxon A. Enhanced nasal cytokine production in human lungs after in-vivo challenge with diesel exhaust particulates. J Allergy Clin Immunol 1996; 98:114–123.

84. Kenny JS, Baker C, Welch MR, Altman LC. Synthesis of interleukin-1α, interleukin-6 and interleukin-8 by cultured human nasal epithelial cells. J Allergy Clin Immunol 1994; 93:1060–1070.

85. Henkin RI, Lippoldt RE, Bilstad J, Edelhoch H. A zinc protein isolated from human parotid saliva. Proc Natl Acad Sci USA 1975; 72:488–492.

86. Henkin RI, Lippoldt RE, Bilstad J, Wolf RO, Lum CKL, Edelhoch R. Fractionation of human parotid saliva. J Biol Chem 1978; 253:7556–7565.

87. Henkin RI, Martin BM, Agarwal RP. Carbonic anhydrase VI deficiency: a viral induced enzyme disorder amenable to treatment with exogenous zinc. J Invest Med 1995; 43:242A.

88. Henkin RI, Martin BM, Agarwal RP. Efficacy of exogenous zinc in treatment of patients with carbonic anhydrase VI deficiency. Am J Med Sci 1999; 318:392–404.

89. Henkin RI, Martin BM, Agarwal RP. Decreased parotid saliva gustin/carbonic anhydrase VI secretion: an enzyme disorder manifested by gustatory and olfactory dysfunction. Am J Med Sci 1999; 318:380–391.

90. Thatcher B, Doherty AE, Orvisky E, Martin BM, Henkin RI. Gustin from human parotid saliva is carbonic anhydrase (CA) VI. Biochem Biophys Res Commun 1998; 250:635–641.

91. Henkin RI. Zinc, saliva and taste: interrelationships of gustin, nerve growth factor, saliva and zinc. In: Hambidge KM, Nichols BL, eds. Zinc and Copper in Clinical Medicine. Jamaica, USA: Spectrum Publ Inc, 1978:35–48.

92. Henkin RI, Law JS, Nelson NR. The role of zinc on the trophic growth factors nerve growth factor and gustin. In: Hurley LS, Keen CL, Lonnerdal B, Rucker RB, eds. Trace Elements in Man and Animals. New York: Plenum Press, 1988:385–388.

93. Law JS, Nelson NR, Watanabe K, Henkin RI. Human salivary gustin is a potent activator of calmodulin-dependent brain phosphodiesterase. Proc Natl Acad Sci USA 1987; 84:1674–1678.

94. Henkin RI, Patten BM, Re P, Bronzert DA. A syndrome of acute zinc loss. Arch Neurol 1975; 32:745–751.
95. Henkin RI, Schechter PJ, Hoye RC. Idiopathic hypogeusia with dysgeusia, hyposmia and dysosmia: a new syndrome. J Am Med Assoc 1971; 217:434–440.
96. Shatzman AR, Henkin RI. Gustin concentration changes relative to salivary zinc and taste in humans. Proc Natl Acad Sci USA 1981; 78:3867–3871.
97. Yoshida S, Endo S, Tomita H. A double blind study of therapeutic efficacy of zinc gluconate on taste disorder. Auris Nasus Larynx 1991; 18:153–161.
98. Henkin RI, Schechter PJ, Friedemold WT, Demets DL, Raff MS. A double blind study of the effects of zinc sulfate on taste and smell dysfunction. Am J Med Sci 1976; 272:285–299.
99. Persani L, Borgato S, Ramoli R, Asteria C, Pizzocavo A, Beck-Piccoz P. Changes in the degree of sialylation of carbohydrate chains modify the biological properties of circulating thyrotropin isoforms in various physiological and pathological states. J Clin Endocrinol Metab 1998; 83:2486–2492.
100. Henkin RI, Papathanassiu A. cAMP is present in human nasal mucus and may act as a growth factor for cells of the olfactory epithelium. FASEB J 2002; 16:A1153.
101. Henkin RI. US Patent No. 5,384,308. Composition and method for enhancing wound healing. US Patent Office, 1995.
102. Tesfaigzi J, Th'ng J, Hotchkiss JA, Harkema JR, Wright PS. A small proline-rich proline, SPRR1, is upregulated early during tobacco smoke-induced squamous metaplasia in rat nasal epithelium. Am J Resp Cell Mol Biol 1996; 14:478–486.
103. Tachibana M, Mouska H, Machino M, Tamimura F, Mizukohi O. Amylase secretion by nasal glands. An immunocytochemical study. Ann Otol Rhinol Laryngol 1986; 95:284–287.
104. Agarwal RP, Henkin RI. Metal binding characteristics of human salivary and porcine pancreatic amylase. J Biol Chem 1987; 262:2568–2575.
105. Douglas CWI. The binding of human salivary α-amylase by oral strains of streptococcal bacteria. Arch Oral Biol 1983; 28:567–573.
106. Gregory MR, Gregory WW, Bruns DE, Zakowski JJ. Amylase inhibits *Neisseria gonorrhoeae* by degrading starch in the growth medium. J Clin Microbiol 1983; 18:1366–1369.
107. Mellersh A, Clark A, Hafiz S. Inhibition of *Neisseria gonorrhoeae* by normal human saliva. Br J Vener Dis 1979; 55:20–23.
108. Agarwal RP, Henkin RI. RIA of human salivary amylase: cross-reactivity with human and porcine pancreatic amylase and other salivary proteins. Metabolism 1984; 33:797–807.
109. Rossen RD, Butler WT, Cate TR, Szwed CF, Couch RB. Protein composition of nasal secretion during respiratory virus infection. Proc Soc Exp Biol Med 1965; 119:1169–1176.
110. Henkin RI, Martin BM. A magnesium protein found in human parotid saliva. FASEB J 1995; 9:452A.
111. Law JS, Henkin RI. Low parotid saliva calmodulin in patients with taste and smell dysfunction. Biochem Med Met Biol 1986; 36:118–124.
112. Pevsner J, Sklar PB, Snyder SH. Odorant-binding protein: localization to nasal glands and secretions. Proc Natl Acad Sci USA 1986; 83:4942–4946.
113. Pevsner J, Snyder SH. Odorant binding protein: odorant transport function in the vertibrate nasal epithelium. Chem Senses 1990; 15:217–222.

114. Lundberg JON, Weitzburg E, Nordvall SL, Kaydenstierna R, Lundberg JM, Alving K. Primarily nasal origin of exhaled nitric oxide and absence in Kartagener's syndrome. Eur Respir J 1994; 7:1501–1504.

115. Alving K, Weitzburg E, Lundberg JM. Increased amount of nitric oxide in exhaled air of asthmatics. Eur Respir J 1993; 6:1368–1370.

116. Kreit JW, Gross KB, Moore TB, Lorenzen TJ, D'Arcy J, Eschenbacher WL. Ozone-induced changes in pulmonary function and bronchial responsiveness in asthmatics. J Appl Physiol 1989; 66:217–222.

117. Molech HL, Gallin JI. Neutrophils in human disease. New Engl J Med 1987; 317:687–694.

118. Baraniuk JN, Shizari T, Sabol M, Ali M, Underhill CB. Hyaluronan is excytosed from serous, but not mucous cells of human nasal and trachiobronchial submucosal glands. J Invest Med 1996; 44:47–52.

119. Okuda M. Migrating cells in the epithelium of allergic nasal mucosa. Rhinology 1988; 26(suppl 1):136.

120. Mygind N, Bisgaard H. Applied anatomy of the airways. In: Mygind N, Pipkorn U, Dahl R, eds. Rhinitis and Asthma: Similarities and Differences. Copenhagen: Munskgaard, 1990:21–37.

121. Denburg JA, Dolovich J, Harnish D. Basophil, mast cell and eosinophil growth and differentiation factors in human allergic disease. Clin Exp Allergy 1989; 19:249–254.

122. Glanville AR, Tazelaar HD, Theodore J et al. The distribution of MHC class I and II antigens on bronchial epithelium. Am Rev Respir Dis 1989; 139:330–334.

123. Kalb TH, Chuang MT, Marom I, Mayer L. Evidence for accessory cell function by class I MHC antigen expressing airway epithelial cells. Am J Respir Cell Mol Biol 1991; 4:320–329.

124. Butler WT, Waldman TA, Rossen RD, Douglas RG Jr, Couch RB. Changes in IgA and IgG concentrations in nasal secretions prior to the appearance of antibody during viral respiratory infection in man. J Immunol 1970; 105:584–591.

125. Doyle WJ, Skoner DP, White M, Hayden F, Kaplan AP, Kaliner MA, Shibayama V, Fireman P. Pattern of nasal secretions during experimental virus infection. Rhinology 1996; 34:2–8.

126. Igarashi V, Skoner DP, Doyle WJ, White MV, Fireman P, Kaliner MA. Analysis of nasal secretions during experimental rhinovirus upper respiratory infections. J Allergy Clin Immunol 1993; 92:722–731.

127. Kaliner MA. Human nasal respiratory secretions and host defense. Am Rev Respir Dis 1991; 144(suppl):52–56.

128. Raphael GD, Jeney EV, Baranick JN, Kim I, Meredith SD, Kaliner MA. Pathophysiology of rhinitis: lactoferrin and lysozyme in nasal secretion. J Clin Invest 1989; 84:1528–1535.

129. Lundgren JD, Shelhamer JH. Pathogenesis of airway mucus hypersecretion. J Allergy Clin Immunol 1990; 85:399–419.

130. Naclerio RM, Kagey-Sobotka A, Togias A et al. Nasal lavage: a technique for elucidating the pathophysiology of allergic rhinitis. In: Mygind N, Pipkorn U, Dahl R, eds. Rhinitis and Asthma: Similarities and Differences. Copenhagen: Munksgaard, 1990:213–221.

131. Persson CGA. Role of plasma exudation in asthmatic airway. Am Rev Respir Dis 1986; 133:1126–1129.

132. Persson CGA, Erjefalt I, Alkner U et al. Plasma exudation as a first line respiratory mucosal defense. Clin Exp Allergy 1991; 21:17–21.

133. Erjefalt A, Persson CGA. Inflammatory passage of plasma macromolecules into airway tissue and lumen. Pulm Pharmacol 1989; 2:93–102.

134. Persson CGA. Mucosal exudation mechanisms. Allergy Clin Immunol News 1991; 3:142–149.

135. Aitken ML, Verdugo P. Donnan mechanism of mucin release and conditioning. In: Chantler FN, ed. Goblet Cells: The Role of Polions in Mucus and Related Topics. New York: Plenum, 1989:1–8.

136. Gordon RE, Lane BP. Regeneration of rat tracheal epithelium after mechanical injury. II. Restoration of surface integrity during the early hours after injury. Am Rev Respir Dis 1976; 113:799–807.

137. Keenan KD, Combs JW, McDowell EM. Regeneration of hamster tracheal epithelium after mechanical injury. I. Focal lesions: quantitative morphologic study of cell proliferation. Virchows Arch (Cell Pathol) 1982; 41:193–214.

138. Marin ML, Gordon RE, Lane BP. Development of tight junctions in rat tracheal epithelium during the early hours after mechanical injury. Am Rev Respir Dis 1979; 119:101–106.

139. Zahm JM, Chevillard M, Pachelle E. Wound repair of human surface respiratory epithelium. Am J Respir Cell Mol Biol 1991; 5:242–248.

140. Lee CH, Rhee CS, Min YG, Oh SH, Lee MS. Increase in expression of IL-4 and IL-5 mRNA in the nasal mucosa of patients with perennial allergic rhinitis during natural allergen exposure. Ann Otol Rhinol Laryngol 1997; 106:215–219.

141. Saito H, Asakura K, Kataura A. Study on the IL-5 expression is allergic nasal mucosa. Int Arch Allergy Immunol 1994; 104(suppl 1):39–40.

142. Sim TC, Grant A, Hilsmeier KA, Fukuda Y, Alam R. Proinflammatory cytokines in nasal secretions of allergic subjects after antigen challenge. Am J Respir Crit Care Med 1994; 149:339–344.

143. Mandel ID. Defense of the oral cavity. In: Kleinberg I, Ellison SA, Mandel ID, eds. Saliva and Dental Caries. London: Information Retrieval Ltd, 1978:473–491.

144. Tabak L, Mandel ID, Baurmash H. Alterations in lactoferrin in salivary gland disease. J Dent Res 1978; 57:43–53.

145. Tabak L, Mandel ID, Herreru M, Baurmash H. Changes in lactoferrin and other proteins in a case of chronic recurrent parotitis. J Oral Pathol 1978; 7:91–99.

146. Bush RK, Yunginger JW. Standardization of fungal allergens. Clin Rev Allergy 1987; 5:3–21.

147. Deshazo RD, Chapin K, Swain RE. Fungal sinusitis. New Engl J Med 1997; 337:254–259.

148. Henkin RI. Drug induced taste and smell disorders: incidence, mechanisms and management related primarily to treatment of sensory receptor dysfunction. Drug Safety 1994; 11:310–377.

149. Henkin RI, Talal N, Larson AL, Mattern CFT. Abnormalities of taste and smell in Sjögren's syndrome. Ann Intern Med 1972; 76:375–383.

150. Kalmus H, Farnsworth D. Impairment and recovery of taste following irradiation of the nasopharynx. J Laryngol Otol 1959; 73:180–182.

151. MacCarthy-Levinthal EM. Post-radiation month blindness. Lancet 1959; 2:1138–1139.

152. Mossman KL, Henkin RI. Radiation induced changes in taste acuity in cancer patients. Int J Radiat Oncol Biol Phys 1978; 4:663–670.
153. Mossman KL, Chencharick JD, Scheer AC, Walker WP, Ornitz RD, Rogers CC, Henkin RI. Radiation-induced changes in gustatory function: comparision of effects of neuron and photon irradiation. Int J Radat Oncol Biol Phys 1979; 5:521–528.
154. Rubin R, Casarett G. Clinical Radiation Pathology. Vol. 1. Philadelphia, PA: Saunders, 1968:260–261.
155. Powell RD, Larson AL, Henkin RI. Nasal mucous membrane biopsy in Sjögren's syndrome: a new diagnostic techinique. Ann Intern Med 1974; 81:25–31.
156. Bardana E, Montanero A. Sjögren's syndrome: a rheumatic disorder with prominent respiratory manifestations. Ann Allergy 1990; 64:3–10.
157. Constantopoulos SH, Papadimitirou CS, Moutsopoulos HM. Respiratory manifestations in primary Sjögren's syndrome: a clinical, functional and histologic study. Chest 1985; 88:226–229.
158. Fairfax AJ, Haslam PL, Pavia P, Sheahan NF, Bateman JRN, Agnew JE, Clarke SW, Turner-Warwick M. Pulmonary disorders associated with Sjögren's syndrome. Qu J Med 1981; 199:279–295.
159. Newball HH, Brahim SA. Chronic obstructive lung disease in patients with Sjögren's syndrome. Am Rev Respir Dis 1977; 115:295–304.
160. Strimlan CV, Rosenow EC III, Divertie MB, Harrison EG. Pulmonary manifestations of Sjögren's syndrome. Chest 1976; 70:354–361.
161. Shima H. Pulmonary function abnormalities and respiratory manifestations in Sjögren's syndrome. Nippon Rinsha 1995; 53:16–20 (in Japanese, English Abstract).
162. Robinson DA, Meyer CF. Primary Sjögren's syndrome associated with recurrent sinopulmonary infections and bronchiectasis. J Allergy Clin Immunol 1995; 94:263–264.
163. Deheinzelin D. Interstitial lung disease in primary Sjögren's syndrome: clinical–pathological evaluation and response to treatment. Am J Resp Crit Care Med 1996; 154:794–799.
164. Kadota J, Kusano S, Kawakami K, Morikawa T, Kohno S. Usual interstitial pneumonia associated with primary Sjögren's syndrome. Chest 1995; 98:1756–1758.
165. Hatron PY, Wallaert B, Gosset AB, Tonnel B, Gosselin B, Voisin C, Devulder B. Subclinical lung inflammation in primary Sjögren's syndrome: relationship between findings and characteristics of the disease. Arthritis Rheum 1987; 30:1226–1231.
166. Matterson EL, Ike RW. Bronchiolitis obliterans organizing pneumonia and Sjögren's syndrome. J Rheumatol 1990; 17:676–679.
167. Usui Y, Kimula Y, Miura H, Kodaira Y, Takayama S, Nakamura M, Kataoka N. A case of bronchiolitis obliterans organizing pneumonia associated with primary Sjögren's syndrome who died of superimposed diffuse alveolar damage. Respiration 1992; 59:122–124.
168. Simms RW, Kirby RE. A 64 year old man with cranial-nerve palsies and a positive test for antinuclear cytoplasmic antibodies. N Engl J Med 1998; 339:755–764.

169. Fauci AS, Haynes BF, Katz P, Wolff S. Wegener's granulomatosis: prospective clinical and therapeutic experience with 85 patients for 21 years. Ann Intern Med 1983; 98:76–85.
170. McDonald TJ, DeRemee RA. Head and neck involvement in Wegener's granulomatosis (WG). Adv Exp Med Biol 1993; 336:309–313.
171. BoehringerIngelheim. Atrovent (ipratropiun bromide) nasal spray. Physicians Desk Ref 1998; 52:708–709.
172. Edward DA, Hanes J, Caponetti G, Hrkach J, Ben-Jebria A, Eskew ML, Mintzer J, Deaner D, Lotan N, Langer R. Large porous paticles for pulmonary drug delivery. Science 1997; 276:1868–1871.

3

Mechanisms of Viral and Bacterial Infections of the Nose and Sinuses

PAUL VAN CAUWENBERGE, MURIEL VAN KEMPEN, and CLAUS BACHERT

University Hospital Ghent,
Ghent, Belgium

I. Introduction

Rhinorrhoea, mouth breathing, snoring, and hyponasal speech are very common problems in childhood. Children with these symptoms cannot be diagnosed as having either rhinitis or sinusitis. The more precise term for this symptom complex is "rhinosinusitis" since the mucous membranes of the nose and parana-sal sinuses are contiguous and one is rarely affected without the other. This was confirmed by Gwaltney et al. (1), who found CT abnormalities of the sinuses of 87% healthy adults suffering from a common cold for 48–96 h.

Besides allergy, the most common cause for inflammation of the nose and paranasal sinuses is an infection. Whereas viruses like rhinoviruses, respiratory syncytial virus (RSV), coronaviruses, and (para)-influenza viruses are the most frequently recovered microorganisms in nasal secretions, the bacteria *Streptococcus pneumoniae*, nontypable *Haemophilus influenzae*, and *Moraxella catarrhalis* are often cultured from sinus aspirates (Tables 3.1 and 3.2) (2).

For a long time it was believed that bacterial rhinosinusitis seldom occurred in infants and young children as their sinuses were not completely developed yet. Today, we know that rhinosinusitis is also a common pediatric disease. Approximately 5–10% of the upper respiratory tract infections in early childhood are complicated by an acute bacterial sinusitis (3). Since children present an average of six to eight upper respiratory tract infections per year, the potential for developing rhinosinusitis in childhood is therefore not rare (4).

II. The Local Host Defense

From the moment we are born, the mucosa of our respiratory tract is continuously exposed to potential harmful substances from the environment. In order to prevent infection or damage to the respiratory mucosa we have adequate local defense mechanisms including a continuous epithelial barrier and a mucociliary transport system. The epithelium lining the nasal cavity consists of pseudostratified, ciliated, columnar epithelial cells covering an area of $100–200 \ cm^2$ and extends into the sinuses (5). Epithelial goblet cells and submucosal seromucous glands contribute to a mucous layer that covers the epithelium. This mucous

Table 3.1 Bacterial Species Cultured from 79 Maxillary Sinus Aspirates in 50 Children with Acute Sinusitis

Species	Total
S. pneumoniae	22
M. catarrhalis	15
H. influenzae	15
Eikenella corrodens	1
Group A *Streptococcus*	1
Group C *Streptococcus*	1
α-*Streptococcus*	2
Moraxella sp.	1
Anaerobes	1

Source: Modified from Wald ER et al. J Allergy Clin Immunol 1992; 90:452–460.

Table 3.2 Bacterial Species Cultured from
Sinus Aspirates of 37 Children with Chronic
Sinusitis

Species	Total
Aerobic and facultative	
α-hemolytic *Streptococcus*	7
Group A *Streptococcus*	3
Group F *Streptococcus*	1
Staphylococcus aureus	7
Staphylococcus epidermis	1
Escherichia coli	1
Haemophilus influenzae	2
Haemophilus parainfluenzae	2
Total	24
Anaerobes	
Anaerobic cocci	34
Gram-positive bacilli	14
Gram-negative bacilli	13
Bacteroides sp.	36
Total	97

Source: Modified from Brook I. J Am Med Assoc
1981; 246:967–969.

layer, $\sim$10–15 μm thick, consists of a mixture of glandular products like lysozyme and sIgA, plasma proteins like albumin and IgG, and glycoproteins (6). In this secretory blanket inspired particles will be trapped and subsequently conveyed toward the nasopharynx by the coordinated wavelike motions of epithelial cilia. In physiologic conditions, this transport occurs continuously at a speed of $\sim$5 mm/min and is always directed toward the posterior pharynx where the particles are swallowed and digested finally in the gastrointestinal tract (7).

Although these local defense mechanisms prevent us from being ill with every breath we take, they do not completely prevent the adherence, colonization, and infection of certain pathogens. This is confirmed by the fact that we still spend between 1 and 2 years of our life suffering from rhinosinusitis (8).

The ability of microorganisms to infect the respiratory mucosa of their host depends first on the characteristics of the antigen and second on the accuracy of the host respiratory epithelium and mucociliary transport system.

A. The Antigen

Some bacteria are capable of forming structures on their surface such as pili that enhance their ability to adhere to the epithelium. *H. influenzae*, for example, expresses pili that adhere to human nasopharyngeal epithelial cells while

S. pneumoniae selectively binds to carbohydrate-containing protein receptors of the host epithelium through specific surface molecules (9). The viral shell of rhinoviruses is characterized by deep canyons with a receptor binding site for the intercellular adhesion receptor molecule-1 (ICAM-1), a receptor that is highly expressed on nasopharyngeal epithelial cells (10). Furthermore, it has been shown that some bacteria frequently colonizing the upper respiratory tract produce proteolytic enzymes that break down the immunoglobulins in nasal mucus like some *H. influenzae* and *S. pneumoniae* strains secreting IgA-proteases that degrade sIgA in the mucous layer (11).

B. The Host Respiratory Epithelium and Mucociliary Transport System

The integrity of the epithelium, the density and activity of the cilia, and the quality of the mucus all affect the ability of antigens to adhere to and infect the nasal mucosa.

First, a disruption of the epithelial lining, due to trauma, for example, is clearly associated with a greater potential for antigen adherence. In addition, Tsang et al. (12) have shown that *Pseudomonas aeruginosa* also preferentially adheres to extruded and damaged epithelial cells and not to normal cells.

Second, alterations in ciliary function, inherited (primary) ciliary dyskinesia as well as acquired (secondary) ciliary dyskinesia due to bacteria like *Pseudomonas* species, *H. influenzae*, and *S. pneumoniae* or viruses such as (para)-influenza or toxic gases like SO_2 or cigarette smoke, are associated with a disturbed mucociliary clearance, leaving more time for microorganisms to bind to the respiratory epithelium.

Third, increased mucus viscosity in children with cystic fibrosis or lower mucus concentrations of IgA or IgG subclasses have been reported with frequent upper respiratory tract infections.

Once one or more of the properties of the respiratory epithelium and mucociliary transport are impaired, microorganisms may easily adhere to and colonize the host epithelium.

III. Pathogenesis of Rhinosinusitis

Several nasal mucosal pathologies may predispose for bacterial colonization as they act on various levels of the local host defense. The two most common predisposing conditions for sinus disease are an upper respiratory tract infection and allergic rhinitis.

A. Viral Infection

As mentioned previously, colds are very common in younger children. This is presumably the result of, on the one hand, the physiologic immature immune system in young children significantly increasing their susceptibility to upper respiratory tract infections and, on the other, their frequent exposure to infectious agents from other children in day-care centers or in the family. Unlike in adults, where it is the rhinoviruses that mainly induce a common cold, the most common pathogens causing an upper respiratory tract infection in children are not only the rhinoviruses but also the RSV and the parainfluenza virus types 1 and 3 (13).

B. Respiratory Syncytial Virus

RSV is the most important respiratory pathogen in young children and is the major cause of lower respiratory disease in infants. Infection with RSV is seen in all parts of the world in annual epidemics occurring most frequently during the winter. The highest rates of illness occur in infants between 1 and 6 months of age with peak rates occurring between 2 and 3 months of age (13). RSV is transmitted primarily by close contact with contaminated hands and self-inoculation. Following an incubation period of 4–6 days a wide variety of upper as well as lower respiratory tract symptoms become manifest. In fact RSV accounts for 20–25% of the hospital admissions for pneumonia in childhood and up to 75% of cases of bronchiolitis in this age group. Interestingly, RSV infection has been shown to induce specific RSV-IgE antibodies. In a study with 79 infants with various forms of respiratory illness due to RSV, Welliver et al. (14) demonstrated a significant correlation between histamine concentrations in their nasal secretions and the degree of hypoxia. It was suggested that this IgE binds to mast cell and basophil surfaces. Re-exposure to antigen would lead to IgE binding with subsequent release of inflammatory mediators like histamine, adversely affecting the outcome of RSV infection.

C. Parainfluenza

Parainfluenza viruses are the second cause of respiratory illness in young children. There are four distinct serotypes of parainfluenza viruses; however, type 4 has been reported less widely. Generally, parainfluenza virus infection occurs in early childhood so that by their eighth birthday most children show antibodies to serotypes 1–3. Parainfluenza types 1 and 2 cause epidemics during the fall while type 3 has been detected during all seasons. They are spread through infected respiratory secretions, primarily by person-to-person contact or by large droplets. Parainfluenza types 1 and 2 are the most common causes of croup (laryngotracheobronchitis) in children, while serotype 3 frequently causes bronchiolitis and pneumonia in infants.

Influenza, adenoviruses, rhinoviruses, and coronaviruses cause upper respiratory tract infections less frequently in children than in adults. Mumps and measles are strictly speaking not respiratory viruses; however, at the onset of infection rhinitis can be observed and therefore these two viruses should be included in the differential diagnosis.

Even though viruses are not frequently recovered from sinus aspirates, they are clearly associated with sinusitis. Gable et al. (15) studied more than 1.5 million patients and found a significant correlation between upper respiratory tract infections and sinusitis in winter. In the 0- to 1-year age group 71% of the subjects had suffered from a cold within 90 days preceding the sinusitis episode. Saito et al. (16) documented high titers of neutralizing antibodies to parainfluenza virus type 3 in 18 out of 31 patients following an acute exacerbation of sinusitis.

An upper respiratory tract infection may indeed indirectly predispose to sinusitis by disturbing the local immune defense mechanisms as it

1. impairs ciliary function
2. changes viscosity of the mucous layer
3. creates edema
4. leads to damage of the epithelial surface.

D. Allergy

Allergy has long been associated with sinusitis. Savolainen (17) found ~25–30% of his acute sinusitis patients to be allergic, compared to ~19.5% in control subjects. Also, Furukawa (18) noted in a literature survey a coincidence of allergy and sinusitis between 25% and 70%. Shapiro (19) and Wald (20) described sinusitis to be a common complication of allergy in adults and children.

Indeed, allergic inflammation may indirectly act on the same levels to predispose to bacterial superinfection as the viral upper respiratory tract infections do. In addition, it impairs humoral and cellular defense mechanisms by inducing a T-helper-2 cytokine predominance.

Even though it has been demonstrated that allergens do not enter the sinus cavities, there are several studies suggesting a direct reaction of the sinus mucosa to allergen exposure. Pelikan et al. (21) demonstrated radiographic changes in the sinuses with increased mucosal edema or opacification up to 12 h after allergen challenge. In a study by Harlin et al. (22) paranasal tissue from allergic subjects was shown to be intensively infiltrated by eosinophils, which released major basic protein into the tissue, near the sites of epithelial damage. Georgitis et al. (23) recently investigated the level of mediators in sinuses with chronic infection and found increased concentrations of histamine, LTC4/D4/E4, and prostaglandin D2, which were comparable to those found in nasal secretions of allergic patients. Finally, we demonstrated a large amount of IgE-positive mast cells in the ethmoidal mucosa of chronic sinusitis patients (24).

Thus, it has been shown that upper respiratory tract infections and allergic rhinitis increase the potential for bacterial colonization by impairing mucociliary clearance, destructing the epithelial integrity, and inducing edema of the rhinosinusal mucosa.

Normally, the ventilation and drainage of the paranasal sinuses occur via the ostium. The ostia of the maxillary sinus and the anterior ethmoid and frontal sinus meet in the ostiomeatal complex. This is a 1.5–2.0 cm long area located between the inferior and middle turbinate. Under normal anatomic conditions the ostiomeatal complex is rather narrow. Alterations in ostiomeatal patency compromise sinus drainage, presenting a potential risk for developing sinus disease. Among those are anatomical variations such as septal deviations or spurs, Haller cells, and concha bullosa. There is, however, no consensus on this. In addition, exactly in this area the inspired nasal airflow changes direction from an upward to a more horizontal direction, which causes many inspired particles to impact here (5). As allergens or infectious or toxic agents reside here, an inflammatory process is initiated. But also, more general nasal mucosal inflammation due to adenoid hypertrophy or foreign bodies may cause an impairment of the ostiomeatal complex.

The subsequent mucosal edema compromises ostiomeatal drainage and produces stasis of sinus contents. Additionally, the impairment of the normal clearance mechanisms allows sinus secretions to further accumulate within the sinus. At this stage, the sealed-off sinus fails to drain and becomes susceptible to secondary bacterial infection. As the intrasinus hydrostatic pressure increases, the mean oxygen tension in the sinus cavity falls. Normally, when the ostium of the human maxillary sinus is patent, oxygen tension is about 16% but when the sinus ostium becomes obstructed it is reduced to $\sim11\%$ and lower (25). Interestingly, mucus synthesis and mucociliary activity are both oxygen dependent processes, for which mainly the absorption of the sinus oxygen content rather than oxygen supply by the mucosal blood flow is important. However, as the pO_2 decreases, aerobe glycolysis becomes insufficient resulting in an altered mucus secretion and further reduction in ciliary activity. In addition, anaerobic glycolysis is initiated leading to a lactate accumulation that contributes to local metabolic acidosis (drop in pH), which additionally aggravates the mucociliary transport. These changes favor the growth of microorganisms such as *S. pneumonia* and *H. influenzae* (Table 3.1). In fact, bacterial colony forming units in aspirates of acutely infected sinuses are $>10^5/mL$ and may exceed $10^8/mL$ (26). The subsequent bacterial overgrowth and infection of the sinus mucosa results in a purulent acute sinusitis.

In response to bacterial metabolites and mediators released by damaged tissue, an exudate develops within the sinus cavity containing polymorphonuclear leucocytes usually in excess of 5000 cells/mL. As the normal defense mechanisms come to the fore, sometimes aided by antibiotic therapy, the inflammatory process subsides, edema lessens, coordinated mucociliary flow returns, and mucus stagnation disappears.

However, in children with perennial allergic rhinitis, primary ciliary dyskinesia, or cystic fibrosis the ostia remain obstructed, ciliary activity impaired, and mucus stagnated and this results in the development of chronic rhinosinusitis. Under these conditions the oxygen tension within the sinuses is further reduced, favoring the growth of anaerobes (Table 3.2). In addition, repeated episodes of infection result in epithelial hyperplasia, squamous metaplasia, and accumulation of eosinophils, lymphocytes, and plasma cells. These mucosal changes further impair sinus drainage, and thus a vicious circle ensues (Fig. 3.1).

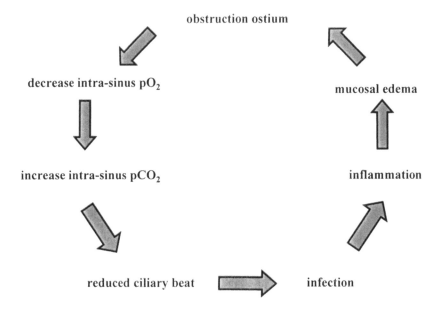

Figure 3.1 Vicious circle for chronic sinusitis due to ostial obstruction.

IV. Conclusion

Rhinosinusitis is the result of complex interactions between infectious and environmental factors. Altered ventilation and impaired drainage of the sinus cavities lead to abnormal secretion in the cavities, stagnation of fluids, and release of inflammatory mediators. The subsequent bacterial infection adds to the chronicity of the inflammatory and infectious process.

References

1. Gwaltney JM, Phillis CD, Miller RD et al. Computed tomographic study of common cold. N Engl J Med 1994; 330:25–30.
2. van Cauwenberge P, Ingels K. Effects of viral and bacterial infection on nasal and sinus mucosa. Acta Otolaryngol (Stockh) 1996; 116:316–321.
3. Wald ER. Rhinitis and acute and chronic sinusitis. In: Bluestone CD, Stool SE, Kenna MA, eds. Pediatric Otolaryngology. Philadelphia, PA: WB Saunders, 1996:843–858.
4. Turner RB. The epidemiology, pathogenesis and treatment of the common cold. Semin Pediatr Infect Dis 1995; 6:57–61.
5. Wagenmann M, Nacleiro RM. Anatomic and physiologic considerations in sinusitis. J Allergy Clin Immunol 1992; 90:419–423.
6. Kaliner MA. Human nasal host defense and sinusitis. J Allergy Clin Immunol 1992; 90:424–430.

7. Maltinski G. Nasal disorders and sinusitis. Prim Care 1998; 25(3):663–683.
8. Rowlands DJ. Rhinoviruses and cells: molecular aspects. Am J Respir Crit Care Med 1995; 152:S31–S35.
9. Cappelletty D. Microbiology of bacterial respiratory infections. Pediatr Infect Dis 1998; 17:S55–S61.
10. Rowlands DJ. Rhinoviruses and cells: molecular aspects. Am J Respir Crit Care Med 1995; 152:S31–S35.
11. Male CJ. Immunoglobulin A1 protease production by Haemophilus influenzae and Streptococcus pneumoniae. Infect Immunol 1979; 26:254–261.
12. Tsang KWT, Rutman A, Tanaka E et al. Interaction of Pseudomonas aeruginosa with human respiratory mucosa in vitro. Eur Respir J 1994; 7:1746–1753.
13. Dolin R. Common viral respiratory infections. In: Wilson JD, Braunwald E, Isselbacher KJ et al. eds. Principles of Internal Medicine. New York: McGraw-Hill, 1991:700–705.
14. Welliver RC, Wong DT, Sun M et al. The development of respiratory syncytial virus-specific IgE and the release of histamine in nasopharyngeal secretions after infection. N Engl J Med 1981; 301(15):841–846.
15. Gable C, Jones JK, Lian J et al. Temporal occurrence and relationship to medical claims for respiratory infections and allergic rhinitis. Pharmaco-epidemiol Drug Saf 1994; 3(6):337–349.
16. Saito H, Takenaka H, Hoshino A et al. Antiviral defense mechanisms of the nasal mucosa. Rhinology 1981; 19(suppl):19–27.
17. Savolainen S. Allergy in patients with acute maxillary sinusitis. Allergy 1989; 44:116–122.
18. Furukawa CT. The role of allergy in sinusitis in children. J Allergy Clin Immunol 1992; 90:515–517.
19. Shapiro GG. Sinusitis in children. J Allergy Clin Immunol 1988; 81:1025–1027.
20. Wald ER. Sinusitis in children. N Engl J Med 1992; 326:319–323.
21. Pelikan Z, Pelikan-Filipek M. Role of nasal allergy in chronic allergic sinusitis—diagnostic value of nasal challenge with allergen. J Allergy Clin Immunol 1990; 86:484–491.
22. Harlin SL, Ansel DG, Lane SR et al. A clinical and pathologic study of chronic sinusitis: the role of the eosinophil. J Allergy Clin Immunol 1988; 81:867–875.
23. Georgitis JW, Matthews BL, Stone B. Chronic sinusitis: characterization of cellular influx and inflammatory mediators in sinus lavage fluid. Int Arch Allergy Immunol 1995; 106:16–21.
24. Bachert C, Ganzer U. Die Darstellung der IgE-assoziierten Zellen in der atopischen Nasenschleimhaut mit Hilfe der Immunoperoxidase-Methode. Laryngol Rhinol Otol 1987; 66:573–576.
25. Ebenfelt A, Lundberg C, Otori N et al. Basic mechanisms of sinusitis. In: van Cauwenberge P, Wang DY, Ingels K et al. eds. The Nose. Amsterdam: Kugler Publications, 1998:143–153.
26. van Cauwenberge PB, Ingels KJ, Wang DY. Mechanisms of viral and bacterial infection of nose and sinuses. In: van Cauwenberge P, Wang DY, Ingels K et al. eds. The Nose. Amsterdam: Kugler Publications, 1998:155–163.

4

Bacteria-Mucin Interaction in the Upper Aerodigestive Tract Shows Striking Heterogeneity: Implications in Otitis Media, Sinusitis, and Pneumonia

JOEL M. BERNSTEIN and MOLAKALA REDDY

State University of New York,
Buffalo, New York, USA

I. Introduction

In an era of rapidly emerging bacterial resistance to antibiotics, other strategies of eliminating infectious diseases must be sought. Among the latter mechanisms are systemic vaccination with specific bacterial outer-membrane proteins (OMPs), bacterial interference, and mucosal vaccination with bacteria or bacterial products.

Bacterial colonization or adherence to epithelial cells is the hallmark of initiation of bacterial or viral inflammatory disease of the mucous membranes of the upper and lower respiratory tracts. This colonization requires the interaction of bacterial adhesins, which are usually proteins or glycoproteins, and receptors on the surface of epithelial cells, which are usually glycoproteins or glycolipids, the carbohydrate moiety probably in most instances being the critical specific receptor. Therefore, one of the strategies for preventing bacterial colonization could be the prevention of attachment of potentially pathogenic bacteria to the receptors on epithelial cells.

Several recent reports (1,2), however, suggest that most of the bacteria that cause infectious diseases of the upper respiratory tract, in particular nontypable *Haemophilus influenzae* (NTHI) and *Moraxella catarrhalis*, are found in the mucous layer of the nasopharynx in the normal healthy child and are rarely present on or in the epithelium, although recently a report suggests that NTHI may be found in the macrophages of the nasopharyngeal tonsil (3). Our laboratory, however, has found that most bacterial organisms are present in the mucous layer of the nasopharyngeal tonsil (4).

This report demonstrates the heterogeneity of bacterial-purified mucin interaction in various mucins of the upper and lower respiratory tracts including saliva (MG1, MG2), human nasopharyngeal mucin (HNM), human middle ear mucin (HMEM), and human tracheo-bronchial mucin (HTBM). The implications of this specific bacterial-mucin interaction is discussed in relation to the pathogenesis of otitis media, sinusitis, and lower respiratory tract infections.

II. Materials and Methods

The specific study design of this research is to identify the specific OMPs of four major bacterial pathogens that are associated with otitis media and sinusitis and to determine their interaction with purified mucins of saliva (MG1, MG2), HNM, HMEM, and HTBM.

A. Bacteria

NTHI strains were recovered from the nasopharynx of infants who were followed up from birth to 2 years of age. Twelve strains were utilized in the bacterial-mucin interaction assay. *H. influenzae* type b strains DL42 and DL42/2F4− were provided by Dr. Eric J. Hansen, University of Texas, Southwestern Medical Center. DL42/2F4− is a mutant that lacks the P2 protein and DL42 is the isogenic parent strain. Strain 1128 was isolated from the middle ear and was provided by Dr. Lauren Bakaletz, Department of Otolaryngology, Ohio State University. Strain 1128f− was constructed as detailed by Sirakova et al. (5) in 1994. The fimbrin gene was disrupted via insertion of a chloramphenicol resistance cassette; this strain, therefore, lacked the fimbrin P5 protein.

The OMPs were purified from NTHI strains using previously published methods (6). Polymodal antiserum to the P2 protein of *H. influenzae* 1479 was produced by immunizing rabbits with purified P2. Monoclonal antibody 2C7 (provided by Dr. Allen J. Lesse, State University of New York at Buffalo) recognizes an epitope on the P5 protein of *H. influenzae* and the OMP A-like protein of many Gram-negative bacteria (A.J. Lesse, unpublished data, June 1994).

Seven strains of *M. catarrhalis* were obtained from the nasopharynges of children undergoing adenoidectomy for either hypertrophy or persistent otitis media with effusion. The OMPs of *M. catarrhalis* were purified using the methods previously described (7).

A suspension of *Pseudomonas aeruginosa* 1244 isolated from the tracheo-bronchial tree of a patient with cystic fibrosis was suspended in phosphate buffered saline (PBS) and blended for 3 min in a Waring blender and centrifuged at $12,000 \times g$ for 30 min. Clear supernate was dialyzed and lyophilized. Isolation of 18 and 15 kDa adhesins from the PBS extract was achieved by a combination of filtration and electroelution.

Twenty-five isolates of *Streptococcus pneumoniae* were separated by sodium dodecylsulfate polyacrylamide gel electrophoresis (SDS-PAGE) and transferred by Western blotting to a polyvinyldifluoride (PVDF) membrane. Three groups of patients were used for this assay to ensure that the source of isolation did not have an effect on the specificity of adhesion between the organism and the purified mucins; 10 isolates were from the middle ear, 10 from the blood, and 5 from cerebrospinal fluid.

B. Purification of Mucins

The purification of mucins from MG1, HNM, HMEM, and HTBM has been previously described in various communications (1,2,6–9). Briefly, these secretions were lyophilized and fractionated in a column of Sepharose CL-2B with Tris–guanidine buffer. Chromatography of these secretions yields pools of proteins which consist of mucin and serum proteins. The mixtures were then reduced with dithiothreitol, alkylated with iodoacetamide, and then fractionated in a column of Sepharose CL-2B to obtain a very high molecular weight purified mucin glycoprotein. Only purified glycoproteins which have no protein contaminants are used in the overlay technique. The purification of the lower molecular weight salivary protein MG2 has been previously described (8).

C. Overlay Binding Assay

Outer membrane proteins of nontypable *H. influenzae*, *M. catarrhalis*, *P. aeruginosa*, and *S. pneumoniae* were separated by SDS-PAGE and transferred by Western blotting to a PVDF membrane (125 mA for 1 h) using a Semiphor TE 70 transfer unit (Hoefer Scientific Instruments, San Francisco, CA) and 0.1 M Tris with 0.192 M glycine in 20% methanol as transfer buffer. The membrane was blocked with bovine serum albumin (BSA) [2% w/v in 10 mM Tris–0.154 M NaCl, pH 7.5 (TBS) for 1 h at room temperature]. ^{125}I-mucins ($\sim 10^6$ cpm in 10–20 µL) were then added and incubated overnight at room temperature. Unbound radioactivity was removed by washing the membrane with TBS buffer. The membrane was gently blotted on a filter paper, air dried, and subjected to autoradiography.

D. Inhibition of Binding

To determine the mechanism of interaction between the various mucins and the adhesins of the bacteria, binding experiments have been performed in the presence of various monosaccharides. After incubation of the PVDF membrane with BSA, various monosaccharides and O-glycosidically linked oligosaccharides solubilized in $\sim$0.5 mL of TBS buffer were added and incubation continued for $\sim$16 h at room temperature. The monosaccharides used in this study were 10 mM galactose, 10 mM fucose, 10 mM N-acetylglucosamine, 10 mM N-acetylgalactosamine, and 5 mM N-acetylneuraminic acid. The oligosaccharides were derived from fetuin, a calf serum glycoprotein. The terminal sugar of fetuin is N-acetylneuraminic acid ^{125}I-HNM or HMEM was then added and binding was determined as above.

The overlay binding assay also was performed with asialo-^{125}I-mucins. To remove the sialic acid, ^{125}I-mucins ($\sim$10^6 cpm) in 150 μL of water were mixed with 50 μL of 0.1 M H_2SO_4 and heated for 90 min at 80°C in a water bath. The reaction mixture was then mixed with 50 μL of 0.2 M NaOH and used in the binding assay. As a control, ^{125}I-mucins in 150 μL of water were mixed with 50 μL of 0.1 M H_2SO_4 and 50 μL of 0.2 M NaOH, heated at 80°C, and used in the binding assay.

III. Results

Binding of radiolabeled mucins to OMPs of the four bacteria was examined by an overlay assay. In all the strains of NTHI examined ^{125}I-HNM and -HMEM bound to two OMPs migrating between 45 and 31 kDa. The binding patterns of representative strains to HNM are represented in Fig. 4.1(a).

On the basis of electrophoretic mobility and immunoblotting, these two proteins were identified as OMPs P2 and P5. Unequivocal identification of OMPs P2 and P5 was done by employing OMPs of bacterial strains and their respective isogenic mutants lacking the respective OMPs in the binding assay. Thus, OMPs of Hib DL42 and its isogenic mutant lacking OMP-2 and OMPs of NTHI 1128 and its isogenic mutant lacking OMP P5 were employed in the assay to confirm that OMPs P2 and P5 function as adhesins for HNM and HMEM. However, in addition, in some strains of NTHI, HNM and HMEM also bound to additional lower molecular weight OMPs migrating at $\sim$16 kDa [Fig. 4.1(a), lane 9]. These lower molecular weight OMPs have not yet been identified; however, the utilization of purified OMP P6 in a binding assay indicated that it was not one of the lower molecular weight adhesins.

From these observations, it can be concluded that only selected OMPs of NTHI bind HNM and HMEM and that the binding is not concentration dependent. In contrast to its ability to bind to HNM and HMEM, there are

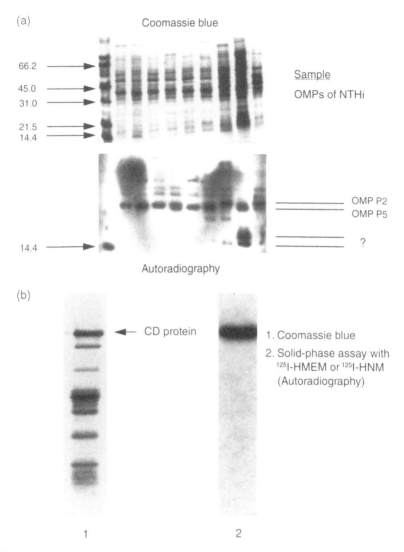

Figure 4.1 (a) Binding between human nasal mucin and OMPs of NTHI. Proteins were subjected to SDS-PAGE and transferred by Western blotting to a PVDF membrane (immobilon-P transfer membrane; Millipore Corp., Bedford, MA). Top: Membrane was stained with Coomassie blue to visualize the transferred proteins. Bottom: Membrane was subjected to overlay binding assay and iodinated human nasal mucin to locate the protein that binds mucin. Lane 1: Molecular weight markers (14.4, 21.5, 31, 45, 66.2, and 97.4 kDa); lanes 2–10: OMPs of NTHI. The autoradiography demonstrates P2 and P5 OMPs adhered to purified human nasal mucin in all the strains studied. Lane 9 demonstrates a lower molecular weight protein that binds, which is not P6. (b) Binding of human middle ear mucin and human nasal mucin to outer membrane proteins of *M. catarrhalis*. The overlay binding technique demonstrates that only one purified protein, the CD protein, which is ∼57 kDa, binds to purified mucins.

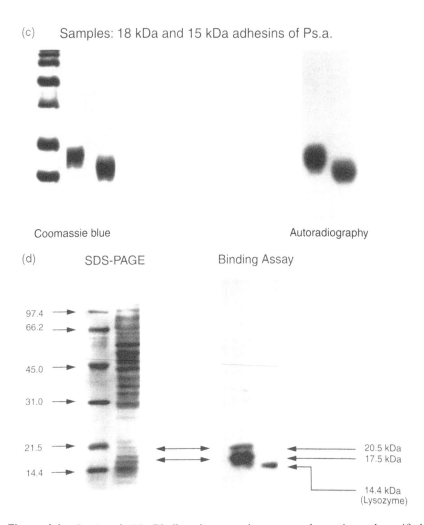

(c)   Samples: 18 kDa and 15 kDa adhesins of Ps.a.

Coomassie blue   Autoradiography

(d)   SDS-PAGE   Binding Assay

97.4
66.2

45.0

31.0

21.5   20.5 kDa
                                                             17.5 kDa
14.4

                                                             14.4 kDa
                                                             (Lysozyme)

Figure 4.1 *Continued* (c) Binding between human nasal mucin and purified *P. aeruginosa* adhesins. The overlay technique demonstrates that purified 15 and 18 kDa proteins of the OMP of *P. aeruginosa* bind specifically to human nasal mucin. These two proteins are nonpilus proteins. (d) Binding of human nasal mucin to components of *S. pneumoniae*. Specific binding of purified nasal mucin to two specific low molecular weight proteins. These proteins have molecular weights of 17.5 and 20.5 kDa.

only trace amounts of binding to human tracheobronchial mucin and no binding to salivary mucin, either the high molecular weight MG1 or the low molecular weight MG2 from saliva (Table 4.1).

    To further examine the selectivity and specificity of mucin-bacterial inter-action, binding studies employing OMPs of *M. catarrhalis, P. aeruginosa,* and

Table 4.1 Summary of Binding Studies—Bacterial Adhesins

Purified mucins	Pilus protein	Nonpilus protein		NTHI	
		15 kDa	18 kDa	P_2	P_5
MG1	No	No	Yes	No	No
MG2	Yes	No	No	No	No
HNM	No	Yes	Yes	Yes	Yes
HMEM	ND	No	Yes	Yes	Yes
HTBM	No	No	Yes	Trace	Trace

	M. catarrhalis	*S. pneumoniae*	
	CD protein, 57 kDa	17.5 kDa	20.5 kDa
MG1	No	No	No
MG2	No	ND	ND
HNM	Yes	Yes	Yes
HMEM	Yes	Yes	Yes
HTBM	Trace	No	No

S. pneumoniae were performed on the five different mucins. Of the several OMPs of *M. catarrhalis*, HNM, and HMEM bound to a single OMP of the size of ~57 kDa [Fig. 4.1(b)].

The 57 kDa component was identified as the CD protein of *M. catarrhalis*. Similarly, binding of ^{125}I-HNM to two nonpilus proteins of *P. aeruginosa* was examined. ^{125}I-HNM bound to the adhesins of *P. aeruginosa* with molecular weights of ~15 and 18 kDa [Fig. 4.1(c)].

Similar to the binding NTHI, the binding of *M. catarrhalis* to human tracheobronchial mucin was present in only trace amounts and there was no binding to saliva (Table 4.1).

The binding of *S. pneumoniae* to HNM and HMEM is limited to two lower molecular weight proteins of 17.5 and 20 kDa [Fig. 4.1(d)]. It is interesting to note that *S. pneumoniae* does not bind to human tracheobronchial mucin or to saliva (Fig. 4.2).

A summary of the specific bacterial-mucin interactions is given in Table 4.1.

Use of asialo-HNM or -HMEM in the binding studies resulted in loss of the binding to the OMPs of *M. catarrhalis*, NTHI, and *P. aeruginosa* (Table 4.2).

These studies have not yet been performed with *S. pneumoniae*. The binding of HNM or HMEM to *M. catarrhalis*, NTHI, and *P. aeruginosa* also could be inhibited by the use of O-glycosidically linked oligosaccharides prepared from fetuin. The binding, however, could not be inhibited by either individual monosaccharides such as fucose, galactose, *N*-acetylglucosamine,

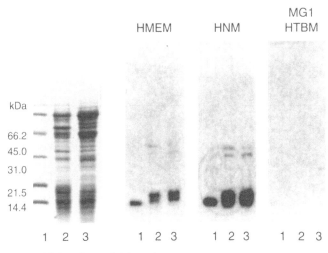

1. Molecular weight markers
2. PBS wash of *S. pneumoniae*
3. PBS extract of *S. pneumoniae*

Figure 4.2   Binding of mucins to *S. pneumoniae*. This figure demonstrates the specific binding of two lower molecular weight proteins to both human middle ear mucin and human nasal mucin, but it also demonstrates the absence of binding to the high molecular weight purified mucin of saliva and human tracheobronchial mucin.

N-acetylgalactosamine, and *N*-acetylneuraminic acid or a mixture of neutral monosaccharides. These results suggest that sialic acid containing oligosaccharides might be receptors for *M. catarrhalis, H. influenzae,* and *P. aeruginosa.*

IV. Discussion

Studies of the characterization of bacterial-mucin interaction may help to identify the true epithelial surface receptors responsible for colonization of bacteria in the upper and lower respiratory tract epithelia. The generation of an immune response to a mucin-binding bacterial protein has the potential to block bacterial adherence and prevent infection and thus, the findings reported here could be important in identifying potential vaccines to prevent colonization of potential pathogens that infect the upper respiratory tract. The results presented here suggest that bacterial-mucin interaction varies between the bacteria being studied and the specific mucin being analyzed. Despite the great number of OMPs of all the bacteria studied, only a few, and in the case of *M. catarrhalis,* only one specific protein binds to purified mucin. It is also interesting to note that the three major pathogens of the upper respiratory tract bind to HNM and

Table 4.2 Binding of Human Midle Ear and Human Nasal Mucins to OMPs of NTHI, *M. catarrhalis*, and *P. aeruginosa*

Inhibitor	Probe	Binding to OMPs
None	^{125}I-mucins	Yes
10 mM galactose	^{125}I-mucins	Yes
10 mM fucose	^{125}I-mucins	Yes
10 mM *N*-acetylglucosamine	^{125}I-mucins	Yes
10 mM *N*-acetylgalactosamine	^{125}I-mucins	Yes
5 mM *N*-acetylneuraminic acid (pH adjusted to 7.2)	^{125}I-mucins	Yes
3.2 mM O-linked type oligosaccharides	Mucins	No
None	Asialo-^{125}I-mucins	No

HMEM, but only in trace amounts to HTBM. Whether or not this lack of binding to HTBM plays a role in the clinical manifestations of pneumonia remains to be evaluated.

P. aeruginosa, a serious pathogen of the lower respiratory tract, particularly in patients with cystic fibrosis, appears to bind by several mechanisms, both with pilus and nonpilus proteins (10,11). It appears that only MG2 binds to the pilus protein of *P. aeruginosa*. One nonpilus protein (18.5 kDa) binds to the high molecular weight salivary mucin (MG1) protein and to all other mucins studied (Table 4.1). The 15 kDa nonpilus protein binds only to HNM.

The attachment of the bacterial organisms to purified mucins is an important biological event. Under normal conditions, these organisms bind to salivary, nasopharyngeal, human middle ear, or tracheobronchial mucins and the latter structures may serve as clearing mechanisms for these organisms. For example, the *P. aeruginosa*–MG1 interaction can be cleared by physical actions such as swallowing, sneezing, and coughing, thus protecting the underlying epithelial cells from bacterial colonization. However, modification of mucin oligosaccharides or changes in the physical properties of the mucous secretions due to disease conditions may result in inefficient binding and clearance of the pathogen. The pathogen can then proliferate in the secretions, penetrate the mucous barrier, and lodge on the epithelial surface, which may lead to colonization and ultimately infection. In this regard, the pathogenesis of otitis media is of particular interest in view of the recent findings of the kinetics of the ascension of NTHI from the nasopharynx of the middle ear coincident with adenovirus-induced compromise in the chinchilla (12). Via fluorescent and transmission electron microscopy, NTHI has been found to preferentially adhere not to the epithelial cells but to the mucous in the eustachian tube and gradually ascend this tubal organ reaching the middle ear ~10 days after intranasal inoculation of adenovirus infected animals. These data confirm our earlier *in vitro* investigation, which suggested that adherence to and growth within stagnant mucous is a possible mechanism by which NTHI, resident in the nasopharynx, gains access to the middle ear to induce otitis media (4).

Although there have been as yet no studies on the exact mechanism of penetration of bacteria into the paranasal sinuses, it has already been suggested that there is a significant improvement in some children with chronic sinusitis following adenoidectomy (13). This finding might suggest that the adenoid is the source of bacteria that is responsible for acute bacterial sinusitis. Recent unpublished data from our laboratory suggest that the organism that is found in the lateral wall of the nose in children with upper respiratory tract infections is identical to that which is found in the adenoid. However, it cannot be proved whether or not the organism in the lateral wall of the nose came from the nasopharynx or originally arose from transmission through the anterior part of the nose after exposure to an infected carrier.

Nevertheless, it would appear that organisms in the nasopharynx are present in the mucin and as with otitis media, it is most likely that the migration of the bacteria from the nasopharynx or nasal cavity into the paranasal sinuses would occur via the mucous rather than from epithelial cell to epithelial cell. These investigations have yet to be done. Finally, of great interest is the finding in this study that *S. pneumoniae* adheres very poorly to human tracheo-bronchial mucous but adheres well to human nasal mucin (Fig. 4.2). It is conceivable that *S. pneumoniae* adheres to nasopharyngeal mucous, but once it is aspirated into the tracheobronchial tree, it may have a better opportunity for adherence and colonization and ultimate infection of the tracheobronchial mucosa resulting in bronchitis or pneumonia.

In summary, the binding of microorganisms to mucins is a prerequisite for the physiological clearance of inhaled bacteria. But this interaction might also be the first step in microbial colonization if mucociliary activity is not functioning properly. This report suggests that the bacterial–mucin interaction displays a wide array of structures. Nevertheless, the mosaics of carbohydrate chains contained in airway mucins can be viewed as having an important role in trapping the inhaled microorganisms before they reach the surface of airway epithelial cells and therefore, have an important role in the defense of the respiratory mucosa (14). However, it is stressed that this protective role only exists if the mucociliary activity is completely efficient. Ciliary disorders, an abnormality in the hydration of periciliary fluid, or abnormalities in mucous production may alter the mucociliary clearance, and a stagnant mucous will allow airway colonization by bacteria.

This is, for instance, the case in ciliary dyskinesia or in the immotile cilia syndrome. This is also the case in chronic bronchial disorders, primary or secondary.

Future work in our laboratory will be directed at characterization of the receptors in nasal and middle ear mucins for adhesins of *S. pneumoniae, M. catarrhalis*, NTHI, and *P. aeruginosa* and the mechanism of this adhesin receptor interaction.

References

1. Davies J, Carlstedt I, Nilsson AK et al. Binding of *Haemophilus influenzae* to purified mucins from the human respiratory tract. Infect Immunol 1995; 63:2485–2492.
2. Reddy MS, Bernstein JM, Murphy TF et al. Binding between outer membrane proteins of non-typable *Haemophilus influenzae* and human nasopharyngeal mucin. Infect Immunol 1996; 64:1477–1479.
3. Forsgren J, Samuelson A, Borrelli S et al. Persistence of non-typable *Haemophilus influenzae* in adenoid macrophages: a putative colonization mechanism. Acta Otolaryngol 1996; 116:766–773.
4. Bernstein JM, Hard R, Cui ZD et al. Human adenoidal organ culture: a model to study non-typable *Haemophilus influenzae* (NTHI) and other bacterial interactions with nasopharyngeal mucosa: implications in otitis media. Otolaryngol Head Neck Surg 1990; 103:784–791.
5. Sirakova T, Kolattukudy PE, Murwin D et al. Role of fimbriae expressed by non-typable *Haemophilus influenzae* in the pathogenesis of and protection against otitis medius and relatedness of the fimbrin subunit to outer membrane protein A. Infect Immunol 1994; 62:2002–2020.
6. Reddy MS, Murphy TF, Faden HS et al. Middle ear mucin glycoprotein: purification and interaction with non-typable *Haemophilus influenzae* and *Moraxella catarrhalis*. Otolaryngol Head Neck Surg 1997; 116:175–180.
7. Murphy TF. *Branhamella catarrhalis*. Epidemiology, surface antigenic structure, and immune response. Microbiol Mol Biol Rev 1996; 60:267–279.
8. Loomis RE, Prakobphol A, Levine MJ et al. Biochemical and biophysical comparison of two mucins from human submandibular-sublingual saliva. Arch Biochem Biophys 1987; 258:452–464.
9. Ramasubbu N, Reddy MS, Bergey J et al. Large scale purification and characterization of the major phosphoproteins and mucins of human submandibular-sublingual saliva. Biochem J 1991; 280:341–352.
10. Reddy MS. Binding between *Pseudomonas* aeruginosa adhesins and human salivary, tracheobronchial and nasopharyngeal mucins. Biochem Mol Biol Int 1996; 40:403–408.
11. Reddy MS, Levine MJ, Paranchych W. Low-molecular mass human salivary mucin, MG2: structure and binding of *Pseudomonas aeruginosa*. Crit Rev Oral Biol Med 1993; 4:315–323.
12. Miyamoto N, Bakaletz LO. Kinetics of the ascension of NTHi from the nasopharynx to the middle ear coincident with adenovirus-induced compromise in the chinchilla. Microb Pathog 1997; 23:119–126.
13. Takahashi H, Honjo I, Fujita A et al. Effects of adenoidectomy on sinusitis. Acta Otorhinolaryngol Belg 1997; 51:85–87.
14. Lamblin G, Roussel P. Airway mucins and their role in defense against microorganisms. Respir Med 1993; 87:421–426.

5

The Eosinophil Cationic Protein: Why We Should and How We Can Control It

Maastricht University,
Maastricht, The Netherlands

I. Introduction

Allergic rhinitis is a type I allergic reaction causing an inflammation of the nasal mucosa. In type I allergies an immediate phase and a late phase of the allergic reaction may occur. The immediate phase is caused by a mast cell degranulation with the release of histamine and other mediators, whereas the late phase is caused by an immigration of inflammatory cells into the mucosa. A cell type with major importance among these inflammatory cells is the eosinophil cell (1–4). During the late phase of the allergic reaction the eosinophil cells are not only attracted but also activated, leading to a release of granular proteins, which cause the mucosal inflammation. These granular proteins are major basic protein, eosinophil peroxidase, eosinophil-derived neurotoxin, and eosinophil cationic protein (ECP) (5). Since the content of ECP in cells other than eosinophil cells is negligible and since it is only released by activated eosinophil cells (6), ECP is a good and specific indicator of eosinophil cell activity and turnover, and possibly of mucosal inflammation (7).

ECP was first purified from human myeloid cells in 1971 (8) and identified as an eosinophil granular protein in 1975 (9). It is a heterogenous protein with molecular weights of the variants from 16 to 24 kDa. It is extremely basic with a pH of 10.8. The gene for ECP is found on chromosome 14 adjacent to other proteins of the ribonuclease family, with which ECP shares some sequence homologies (10). ECP has a variety of biological activities interacting with other immune cells and plasma proteins such as coagulation factors and proteins of the complement system. The cytotoxic activity, however, is the most conspicuous. The different isoforms of ECP seem to have different biological properties with respect to cytotoxicity and the effects on fibroblasts (7). In 1977 a radioimmunosorbent assay was described which allows the detection of ECP in blood serum (11), and in 1991 an improved radioimmunoassay of human ECP (12) followed. The total incubation time of the latter radioimmunoassay is 3.5 h. It is a double-antibody assay with radiolabeled ECP, covering the concentration range of 2–200 µg/L. The detection limit is <2 µg/L and the cross-reactivity with eosinophil protein X is <0.06%. The coefficient of variation within the measuring range is, within assay 4.8–10.4% and total 6.6–12.0%. It can be used for measurement of various body fluids including blood serum, nasal secretions, and bronchoalveolar lavage fluid. Recently, this radioimmuno-assay introduced by Petersen was changed into an enzyme immunoassay.

It was postulated that the release of ECP from activated eosinophil cells causes mucosal inflammation not only in allergic rhinitis but also in allergic asthma and even in nonallergic asthma and chronic obstructive pulmonary disease (COPD) (13–16). Thus, possibly the quantitative analysis of the migration and activation of eosinophil cells by the measurement of ECP levels could simplify the diagnosis of inflammatory allergic and nonallergic diseases of the bronchial or nasal mucosa. To clarify that, different studies on ECP in asthma and COPD were done. There are fewer studies on ECP in allergic rhinitis, and until now there are no studies on ECP in nonallergic rhinitis. However, due to the similarities of ECP mechanisms in the mucosa of the lung and of the nose and due to greater knowledge of ECP in the mucosa of the lung, all different groups of studies will be discussed here.

First, investigations on ECP blood serum levels in three groups of patients (adult patients with asthma and COPD, children with asthma and COPD, children and adult patients with allergic rhinitis) will be discussed; second, investigations on ECP levels in local body fluids (sputum, nasal secretion); third, investigations comparing ECP levels in blood serum and in local body fluids; and finally, investigations on the variation of ECP both in blood serum and in local body fluids.

II. Do ECP Blood Serum Levels Correlate with Disease Activity and Mucosal Hyperreactivity?

A. In Adult Patients with Allergic and Nonallergic Asthma and COPD

Introduction

Numerous investigations deal with ECP blood serum levels in patients with allergic and nonallergic asthma and COPD. However, there is no uniformity with respect to methods and patient populations. Thus, the degree to which ECP blood serum levels correlate with disease activity and mucosal hyperreactivity in these groups of patients has remained controversial until now. However, in distinguishing patients with allergic and nonallergic asthma from patients with COPD, a much more uniform statement can be made.

Patients with Allergic Asthma

In patients with allergic asthma the results of the different studies are quite uniform. Investigations measuring ECP blood serum levels after bronchial allergen challenge in patients with allergic asthma showed a statistically significant correlation between ECP blood serum levels and the late-phase allergic response. One study was performed on 12 allergic asthmatics during a stable phase of their disease (17). After bronchial allergen challenge and resolution of the immediate-phase allergic response, serial measurements of lung function and ECP blood serum levels were made. A statistically significant correlation between the late-phase allergic response of the bronchial mucosa and ECP blood serum levels was found, suggesting either a delayed or a continuous activation of circulating eosinophil cells after bronchial allergen challenge. Another study of 12 patients with allergic asthma also showed an increase of ECP blood serum levels after allergen challenge (18).

In *therapy studies* of allergic asthmatic patients, a statistically significant correlation between ECP blood serum levels and bronchial hyperreactivity was found. In a double-blind investigation of 12 allergic asthmatic patients with known immediate- and late-phase allergic response to allergen challenge, the patients were treated with salmeterol, or placebo as a single dose 10 min before challenge (19). A similar course of ECP blood serum levels and bronchial hyperreactivity was found. After pretreatment with placebo, bronchial hyperreactivity as well as ECP blood serum levels increased statistically significantly 24 and 48 h after allergen challenge, whereas after treatment with salmeterol a decrease in bronchial hyperreactivity and no changes in ECP blood serum levels were found.

Another double-blind study of ECP blood serum levels in allergic asthmatic patients was done on 20 patients allergic to seasonal allergens (15). ECP blood serum levels were monitored outside and during the season, and patients treated with beclomethasone (inhaled) were compared to patients treated with placebo. A statistically significant correlation was observed between ECP blood serum levels, symptom scores, and bronchial hyperreactivity, whereas no correlation with the peak expiratory flow was found.

Patients with Both Allergic and Nonallergic Asthma

In groups of patients with both allergic and nonallergic asthma, the results are nearly as uniform as in studies of patients with allergic asthma alone. In one study ECP blood serum levels in different stages of asthma were evaluated (20). All in all, 123 patients suffering from allergic or nonallergic asthma, which was classified as mild ($n = 49$), moderate ($n = 49$), or severe ($n = 25$), and 31 healthy controls were evaluated. The ECP blood serum levels were statistically significantly higher in the symptomatic than in the asymptomatic patients, and moderate negative correlations, although statistically highly significant, were found between ECP blood serum levels and lung function parameters.

In another investigation an analysis of ECP blood serum levels of 69 patients with allergic and nonallergic asthma and 53 controls showed statistically significantly lower levels in the control group than in the patient group (21).

Therapy studies have shown that ECP blood serum levels can be used in therapy monitoring. One investigation was conducted over a 12-month period in a group of 20 adult patients with both allergic and nonallergic asthma on maintenance inhaled steroid therapy (22). Every 2 months, ECP blood serum levels, spirometry, and bronchial histamine provocation test were obtained from each patient. On the basis of ECP blood serum levels, adjustments in the daily maintenance dose of inhaled steroids were considered. Data were compared with those of a previous 6-month evaluation study of ECP blood serum levels in the same patients. In 10 patients the mean dose of inhaled steroids was decreased. ECP blood serum levels increased slightly, and lung function decreased minimally. In seven patients the mean dose of inhaled or oral ($n = 2$) steroids was increased. In this group, ECP blood serum levels decreased but remained elevated in comparison to normal values and lung function improved. In both groups patients' scores of asthmatic well-being increased significantly. Exacerbation rate remained the same in the decreased and the unchanged group, but was reduced by about 50% in the increased group. It was concluded that adjusting steroid therapy, guided by ECP blood serum levels, may be helpful in tailoring asthma treatment.

A control of ECP blood serum levels in 21 allergic or nonallergic asthmatic patients with acute deterioration of their asthma, 44 stable allergic or nonallergic asthmatic patients on maintenance inhaled steroids, and a control group of 20 stable allergic or nonallergic asthmatics was done recently (23). The first group of patients was treated with oral steroids, which were reduced to zero within 1 week (acute group). In the second group, on the basis of the peak expiratory flow values, adjustments in the doses of steroids were made (reduction group). The control group received a constant dose of inhaled steroids. The ECP blood serum levels in the acute group were statistically significantly higher than in the control group, and a statistically significant decrease of ECP blood serum levels was observed in the acute group after 1 week of oral steroid administration. No statistically significant changes in ECP blood serum levels were observed in the reduction group or in the control group. The conclusion of this study was that the resolution of acute allergic or nonallergic asthma exacerbations during treatment could be followed using ECP blood serum level monitoring.

Patients with COPD

In patients with COPD the correlation between ECP blood serum levels and disease activity or mucosal hyperreactivity remains uncertain. In a cross-sectional study of 18 patients with irreversible bronchial obstruction due to chronic bronchitis, no correlation was found between ECP blood serum levels and the degree of mucosal hyperreactivity as measured by bronchial histamine provocation test and the parameters of airway obstruction (forced expiratory volume in 1 s) (24).

Moreover, no statistically significant difference could be found in the ECP blood serum levels in 10 nonallergic asthmatics with a mild attack and nine COPD patients with acute exacerbation (25). Thus, the measurement of ECP blood serum levels did not appear to be useful in the differential diagnosis of a nonallergic asthma attack and an acute exacerbation of COPD.

In conclusion, there is evidence that ECP blood serum levels correlate with disease activity and mucosal hyperreactivity in allergic and nonallergic asthma patients and that ECP blood serum levels are markers for therapy monitoring in patients with allergic and nonallergic asthma. In COPD, however, a correlation between ECP blood serum levels and disease activity or mucosal hyperreactivity has not yet been proven. Whether such a correlation exists or not should be investigated in further studies. It is possible that in persistent bronchial obstruction, which exists in COPD but not in asthma, changes in the ECP blood serum levels are smaller than in nonpersistent bronchial obstruction. The question as to the necessity of a differentiation between allergic and nonallergic patients is still to be answered.

B. In Children with Allergic and Nonallergic Asthma

Introduction

In children COPD is extremely rare and not the subject of studies on ECP blood serum levels. In children with allergic and nonallergic asthma the results of the different studies are more controversial than in adults. Even in children, however, the methods and populations of the different studies are heterogenous. A distinction between studies of patients with allergic asthma and patients with nonallergic asthma does not offer greater uniformity of the results. However, differences were found in the ECP blood serum levels of children with allergic and nonallergic asthma, and possible explanations can be given for the lack of correlation between ECP blood serum levels, disease activity, and bronchial mucosal hyperreactivity.

Investigations Showing No Correlations

Some investigations showed no correlation between ECP blood serum levels and disease activity measured as clinical parameters in children with allergic and nonallergic asthma. In an allergen challenge study with 32 allergic asthmatic children sensitive to house dust mites and six nonallergic young adult controls, the time course of ECP blood serum levels after bronchial allergen challenge was tested (26). The individual time courses of ECP revealed different characteristic groups of patterns: first, an isolated early blood serum peak during or within the first 60 min after challenge; second, an early plus a late blood serum peak; third, an isolated late blood serum peak 12 h after challenge; fourth, an isolated late blood serum peak 24 h after challenge; and fifth, no statistically significant variation during the 24 h observation period. The hypothesis was formulated that the early peak could be due to short-term changes in eosinophil cell activation, while late peaks may reflect eosinophil cell proliferation, recruitment, subsequent priming, and enhancing of the propensity to release their proteins. No correlation between ECP blood serum levels and clinical parameters such as lung function data was found. It was concluded that the striking groups of time courses of ECP blood serum levels indicate different uniform patterns of eosinophil cell activation during allergen challenge but do not predict the clinical outcome of challenge.

In another publication the same group of authors described the time course of ECP after bronchial allergen challenge in greater detail (27). A rapid increase in ECP blood serum levels up to 30 min after allergen challenge, followed by a rapid decrease nearly to baseline values in the next 30 min, and a steady increase up to 10 h, and even higher levels at 24 h after challenge were found. The authors again concluded that although eosinophil cells are activated in allergic asthmatic children after bronchial allergen challenge, ECP levels are not suitable monitoring variables.

Investigations Suggesting Correlations

Other investigations showed statistically significant correlations in one group of patients, whereas in the other no statistically significant correlation was found. One study was conducted to evaluate the role of ECP blood serum levels as a monitoring parameter in acute exacerbated asthma in children (28). Eleven children (10 allergic, 1 nonallergic) were studied during an acute exacerbation of their disease. Under inhaled corticosteroid therapy, lung function increased statistically significantly on days 1, 14, 28, and 56 as compared to baseline values. ECP blood serum levels decreased statistically significantly on days 28 and 56. Considering the individual ECP blood serum time courses, however, most of the patients did not show a uniform pattern of continuously decreasing values. It was concluded that the measurement of ECP blood serum levels during acute asthma episodes in children may play a role in therapy monitoring in some patients, whereas in others—probably those without acute eosinophil inflammation—monitoring the ECP blood serum levels is of limited value.

Investigations Showing Statistically Significant Correlations

Most investigations showed statistically significant correlations between ECP blood serum levels and disease activity. In a study of children with seasonal allergic asthma which investigated the course of ECP blood serum levels, a seasonal increase of ECP blood serum levels was found (29).

In a therapy study of 27 children with allergic asthma, the relation between ECP blood serum levels and symptom–medication scores and pulmonary function was measured before and at the end of a 3-month inhaled corticosteroid treatment period. Nonasthmatic children with allergic rhinitis served as controls (30). All asthma patients had statistically significantly higher ECP blood serum levels than the rhinitis patients. At the end of the treatment period, symptom–medication scores and pulmonary function improved and ECP blood serum levels were reduced statistically significantly. A statistically significant correlation was found between the improvement of symptom–medication scores, pulmonary function values, and ECP blood serum levels. ECP blood serum levels were considered to be reliable markers of disease activity, particularly in allergic asthma, and to be useful in the follow-up of allergic asthmatic children undergoing inhaled corticosteroid treatment.

In 1998 the results of those investigations suggesting a statistically significant correlation between ECP blood serum levels and disease activity of asthma were confirmed by an investigation of 28 children with allergic asthma (31). It was found that ECP blood serum levels were statistically significantly lower in patients who had been asymptomatic for 3 or 4 weeks before sampling than in patients who had been symptomatic or asymptomatic for only 1 or 2 weeks. In the former group, ECP blood serum levels were statistically significantly higher when patients became symptomatic after sampling than when they remained stable, a finding that suggests that ECP blood serum levels may have a predictive value in certain situations. Although the ECP blood serum level was not proved to be predictive in the latter symptomatic group, the ECP blood serum level was statistically significantly lower when measured again 4 weeks later when the patients' symptoms had resolved. In contrast, ECP blood serum levels were unchanged when patients remained symptomatic, a finding that suggests that ECP blood serum levels reflect the clinical response to therapy.

An article summarizing the clinical experience with the measurement of ECP blood serum levels in children stated the same conclusion, considering ECP blood serum levels to be useful in the management of children with allergic and nonallergic asthma (32).

Explanations for a Lack of Correlation

A possible explanation for the lack of correlation between ECP blood serum levels, disease activity, and mucosal hyperreactivity was offered by an investigation of these parameters (33). Twenty-eight allergic children with pollinosis to birch or grass pollen, but no obvious history of asthma, were studied. Assuming that children with pollinosis often show asthmatic symptoms in addition to symptoms of the upper airways, the ECP blood serum levels, peak expiratory flow rate, and bronchial hyperreactivity (metacholine bronchial provocation test) were measured on three occasions: before, during, and after (autumn) the birch and grass pollen season. Despite the fact that the children had no history of asthma, the majority of the children showed an increased bronchial hyperreactivity. This increase was more pronounced after the season than during it, whereas the ECP blood serum levels and the peak expiratory flow rate increased during the season and decreased after the season. No correlations between ECP blood serum levels and clinical parameters of disease activity and bronchial hyperreactivity were found. The hypothesis was that ECP and other markers of allergic inflammation disappear postseasonally, whereas bronchial hyperreactivity persists, explaining the lack of correlation between the levels of eosinophil cell mediators in blood serum, disease activity, and bronchial hyperreactivity.

Another explanation for the lack of correlation between ECP blood serum levels and disease activity or bronchial hyperreactivity was given by a further study. ECP blood serum levels were determined in 235 allergic and nonallergic children (34). Of these, 36 children had asthma (a history of asthma and at least one objective clinical, lung function or challenge test finding), 33 children had other symptoms of lower airway disease (history of asthma not fulfilling the objective criteria of asthma), and 166 were nonasthmatic. One hundred two children were allergic. The study results were analyzed twice: first, to evaluate the influence of asthma and other symptoms of lower airway disease on the ECP blood serum levels and second, to evaluate the influence of the concomitant existence of allergic sensitization and allergic diseases other than asthma. Sixteen children with asthma received no therapy. They had statistically significantly higher ECP blood serum levels than the control children. Twenty children with asthma who underwent anti-inflammatory therapy (inhaled corticosteroids, inhaled mast cell membrane stabilizers, sympathomimetics) had ECP blood serum levels similar to those of the controls. The children with other symptoms of lower airway disease had statistically significantly lower ECP blood serum levels than the untreated children with asthma, but even higher ECP blood serum levels than the controls. Furthermore, a statistically significant correlation between ECP blood serum levels, allergic sensitization, and allergic disorders other than asthma was found independent of the presence of asthma. The authors concluded that the presence of symptomatic asthma raises ECP blood serum levels, but the concomitant existence of allergic diseases other than asthma or an allergic sensitization seems to raise ECP blood serum levels as well, so that ECP blood serum levels must always be judged in relation to the whole clinical situation, including asthmatic manifestations, the presence of allergic sensitization, other allergic disorders, and the exposure to allergens.

A further investigation confirms the influence of allergic sensitization on ECP blood serum levels. In this investigation a comparison between 27 allergic and nonallergic asthmatic children younger than 5 years was done (35). Fourteen of the children were allergic and 13 nonallergic. The 14 allergic children proved to have statistically significantly higher mean ECP blood serum levels than the 13 nonallergic patients. Seven of the allergic patients required treatment and had a repeat assessment. The mean ECP blood serum levels of these seven allergic patients had fallen statistically significantly after treatment, confirming the correlation between ECP blood serum levels and disease activity.

Our own experience in children with allergic rhinitis and ongoing allergen exposure shows that ECP blood serum levels can increase more slowly than the clinical symptoms of the allergic disease. Although ECP is released after the first allergen exposure, a statistically significant increase in blood serum can be found several days later, so that early seasonal measurements or measurements after allergen challenge may possibly not show a statistically significant correlation to clinical parameters.

In conclusion, there is greater disagreement about the correlation of ECP blood serum levels, disease activity, and mucosal hyperreactivity in children with allergic and nonallergic asthma than in adults. Whether a differentiation of patient groups with different patterns of eosinophil cell activation has to be done must be established in further studies. In seasonal allergic asthma perhaps a persistent increase of mucosal hyperreactivity postseasonally is able to cause a lack of correlation in late measurements. Our own experience in children with seasonal allergic rhinitis shows that at the beginning of the season a delayed increase of ECP can be found, possibly explaining the lack of correlation in early measurements. Most investigations, however, showed ECP blood serum levels to be a reliable marker for monitoring disease activity, mucosal hyper-reactivity, and therapy in children with allergic and nonallergic asthma. The reliability of ECP blood serum measurements in children with asthma can be increased by interpreting the results in relation to the presence of allergic sensitization, other allergic disorders, and exposure to allergens in sensitized children.

C. In Adult Patients with Allergic Rhinitis

Introduction

In allergic rhinitis, measurements of mucosal hyperreactivity are not as established as in allergic and nonallergic asthma. Therefore, investigations of ECP blood serum levels are less directed on mucosal hyperreactivity than on clinical symptoms of allergic rhinitis, which can be considered disease activity. In adults the results of the different studies are not uniform. Two groups of investigations can be distinguished, the first showing ECP blood serum levels not to be a reliable parameter of disease activity in allergic rhinitis, and the second showing the contrary.

Investigations Showing No Correlations

In the group of investigations showing no correlation between ECP blood serum levels and disease activity, an early investigation in 12 patients with nasal allergy demonstrated only a statistically insignificant tendency toward the correlation between ECP blood serum levels and the severity of clinical symptoms (36). However, a statistically significant correlation to the number of blood eosinophil cells was found.

A lack of correlation between ECP blood serum levels and clinical parameters was confirmed by other studies. One investigation was conducted to quantify eosinophil cell activation in perennial allergic rhinitis by measuring ECP blood serum levels (37). Therefore, symptom scores and ECP blood serum levels were measured in patients with perennial allergic rhinitis and in healthy controls. No statistically significant correlation between ECP blood serum levels and clinical parameters was found.

In another investigation 20 patients with allergic rhinitis to grass pollen and 10 healthy controls were examined (38). ECP blood serum levels and symptom scores were studied during and out of the pollen season. In both groups no statistically significant increase of ECP blood serum levels and no correlation between ECP blood serum levels and symptom scores were found.

A further study was performed to examine whether the different forms of rhinitis can be differentiated by measuring ECP blood serum levels (39). The study involved 119 patients with nonrhinitic allergies and different types of allergic and nonallergic rhinitis. The different forms of rhinitis were hyperreactive rhinitis, vasomotor rhinitis, chronic nonallergic sinusitis, nonsymptomatic pollinosis, acute symptomatic pollinosis, perennial allergic rhinitis, combination of perennial and seasonal rhinitis, and nasal polyps in the absence and in the presence of allergy. No statistically significant differences in ECP blood serum levels of the different patient groups were found, so that a differential diagnosis of the different forms of rhinitis does not seem possible using ECP blood serum levels.

Investigations Showing Statistically Significant Correlations

Other studies have shown a statistically significant correlation between ECP blood serum levels and disease activity. An investigation with 28 patients with perennial allergic rhinitis and healthy controls (40) showed statistically significantly higher ECP blood serum levels in the patient group than in the control group, whereas no statistically significant correlation between the number of blood eosinophil cells and ECP blood serum levels was found.

A study of 69 patients with bronchial asthma, 17 patients with allergic rhinitis but no asthma, and 53 controls showed statistically significantly higher ECP serum levels in both the asthma and the rhinitis groups than in the control group (21).

Another investigation had similar results (14). Serum ECP levels of 21 patients with seasonal allergic rhinitis (16 rhinitis alone, 5 rhinitis and asthma) and 17 controls were studied. ECP blood serum levels were statistically significantly higher in the patient group than in the control group. No statistically significant difference was found between ECP levels in patients from the rhinitis and rhinitis plus asthma groups, although the mean ECP blood serum level was higher in the latter group. A statistically significant correlation between total IgE and ECP blood serum levels was found in the patients.

In a further study ECP blood serum levels in three groups of patients were compared (41). The investigation involved 28 patients with seasonal allergic rhinitis (16 symptomatic, 12 extraseasonally), 11 patients with chronic sinusitis, and 20 healthy controls. ECP blood serum levels were statistically significantly increased in patients with symptomatic seasonal rhinitis, whereas no increase of ECP blood serum levels could be found in the other patients and healthy controls.

Recently, an investigation was conducted on the relationship of ECP blood serum levels to disease activity in seasonal allergic rhinitis (40). Forty-nine rhinitis patients allergic to both birch and grass pollen were investigated during the birch pollen season, during the grass pollen season, and after the seasons. Symptom–medication diaries were filled out and ECP blood serum levels were measured. An increase of ECP blood serum levels was observed from the birch pollen season to the grass pollen season, followed by a decrease from the grass pollen season to after the pollen seasons. A partial least square analysis was performed showing a statistically significant correlation between symptom–medication scores and ECP blood serum levels. However, the variation in ECP blood serum levels could explain only a part of the total variation in symptoms. In summary, a statistically significant relationship between the disease activity measured as severity of allergic symptoms and ECP blood serum levels was found, but could account for only a part of the variation in the patients' evaluation of their disease.

In a therapy study of 63 patients with seasonal allergic rhinitis to grass pollen, one group was treated with topical corticosteroids, while the other group was treated with placebo (42). During the season a statistically significantly lower symptom score and lower ECP blood serum levels were found in the corticosteroid group than in the placebo group.

In a study of the effect of immunotherapy on ECP blood serum levels in patients with perennial allergic rhinitis, statistically significantly higher levels were found in patients than in healthy controls (43). The mean ECP blood serum levels in patients who had undergone more than 2 years of immunotherapy were statistically significantly lower than that of the untreated group and not different from that of the control group. ECP blood serum levels were statistically significantly correlated with the duration of immunotherapy.

In conclusion, there is disagreement about the correlation of ECP blood serum levels and disease activity in adult patients with allergic rhinitis. Variations in ECP blood serum levels seem to explain only part of the variation of the disease activity. Other factors influencing the disease activity need to be defined by additional studies. The smaller increase of ECP blood serum levels in patients with allergic rhinitis than in patients with asthma possibly results in a greater influence of these other factors in allergic rhinitis. However, therapy studies showed ECP blood serum levels to be reliable markers for monitoring therapy efficacy. Whether there are differences between patients with allergic and nonallergic rhinitis is not yet certain.

D. In Children with Allergic Rhinitis

Introduction

Unfortunately, few investigations have been performed involving the correlation between ECP blood serum levels and disease activity in children with allergic rhinitis. Although there is some contradiction concerning the measurement of ECP blood serum levels in children with allergic rhinitis, a clearer concept than in adult patients can be developed.

Investigations Showing No Correlations

One therapy study involved 38 children with perennial allergic rhinitis to house dust mites. All children were treated over a period of 3 weeks. One group ($n = 13$) was treated with nasal corticosteroids, one group with nasal mast cell membrane stabilizers ($n = 15$), and one group with placebo ($n = 10$) (44). Before and after treatment ECP blood serum levels showed no statistically significant difference between patients and healthy controls, while ECP levels in nasal secretions and clinical symptoms showed statistically significant differences between patients and controls and were statistically significantly reduced in treated children. In this study ECP blood serum levels were not considered to be useful markers for monitoring therapy efficacy in children with perennial allergic rhinitis.

Investigations Showing Statistically Significant Correlations

One investigation was conducted to study ECP blood serum levels in allergic diseases of the respiratory system during exacerbation and during the remission of symptoms for the purpose of monitoring the course of the disease (45). ECP blood serum levels were determined in 111 children with allergic bronchial asthma and/or allergic rhinitis and 19 controls. In all patients—even in the group of patients with allergic rhinitis alone—ECP blood serum levels were statistically significantly increased during clinical exacerbation of symptoms and parallel with the clinical score of symptoms, so that ECP blood serum levels were recommended for monitoring allergic inflammation in childhood allergic rhinitis and asthma.

In another study of 73 children (13 seasonal allergic rhinitis, 44 seasonal allergic rhinitis and asthma, 16 healthy controls) ECP blood serum levels were measured during and after the pollen season (46). Even after the pollen season, ECP blood serum levels of children with seasonal allergic rhinitis and asthma were statistically significantly higher than in the other two groups. After the season there was no statistically significant difference between the children with allergic rhinitis alone and the controls. During the season the highest values of ECP blood serum levels were again observed in the group of children with seasonal allergic rhinitis and asthma, but even in children with seasonal allergic rhinitis alone, statistically significantly higher levels than in the controls were found. A statistically significant increase of ECP blood serum levels was found in all groups. ECP blood serum levels were recommended as disease activity parameters in children with hay fever.

These results were confirmed by a study of the influence of allergic sensitization and of other allergic disorders in children with asthma (34), in which it was shown that children with allergic rhinoconjunctivitis have statistically significantly higher ECP blood serum levels than healthy controls.

In conclusion, although there are some contradictory results, there is evidence that in children with allergic rhinitis ECP blood serum levels could be a marker for monitoring disease activity. Whether ECP blood serum levels are reliable markers for monitoring therapy efficacy remains uncertain and must be established in further studies.

III. Do ECP Levels in Local Body Fluids (Sputum, Nasal Secretion) Correlate with Disease Activity and Mucosal Hyperreactivity?

A. In Children and Adult Patients with Allergic and Nonallergic Asthma and COPD

Introduction

The correlation between ECP levels in sputum or bronchoalveolar lavage fluid and disease activity or mucosal hyperreactivity in asthma is less controversial than that between ECP blood serum levels and disease activity or mucosal hyperreactivity. In most investigations a statistically significant correlation was found, and only few investigations showed no or statistically insignificant correlations. Just as in measuring ECP blood serum levels, the investigations showing no or statistically insignificant correlations were done in patients with COPD or measured ECP levels in bronchoalveolar lavage fluid shortly after allergen challenge. Few investigations studied ECP levels in sputum or bronchoalveolar lavage fluid in children, but some investigations could demonstrate that childhood asthma has an immunopathology similar to that of asthma in adults (47,48).

Patients with Both Allergic and Nonallergic Asthma

In patients with both allergic and nonallergic asthma, the ECP levels in sputum or bronchoalveolar lavage correlated statistically significantly with disease activity and mucosal hyperreactivity. One study was done to clarify the extent to which ECP levels in sputum relate to indices of asthma severity in chronic stable allergic and nonallergic asthma (49). Forty-six clinically stable patients with mild to severe chronic asthma (34 allergic, 12 nonallergic) and 12 normal nonallergic controls were investigated. ECP levels in sputum were statistically significantly greater in asthmatics than in normal subjects. Moreover, they were statistically significantly greater in patients with severe asthma than in patients with mild asthma. The relationship between the ECP level in sputum and lung function parameters was statistically insignificant.

Another investigation was conducted to evaluate the role of eosinophil cells and eosinophil cell activation in allergic and nonallergic asthma (13). Forty-three patients with chronic asthma (24 allergic, 2 intolerant to aspirin, 17 nonallergic) were compared to 10 healthy controls. A statistically significant increase of the number of eosinophil cells and of the ECP level in bronchoalveolar lavage fluid was found in the patients but not in the controls. Numbers of eosinophil cells and ECP levels were statistically significantly correlated with the clinical severity of asthma.

The aim of another study was to evaluate the correlation between the ECP level and the number of eosinophil cells in sputum and to evaluate the correlation between the ECP level and the degree of activation of eosinophil cells in sputum (50). It was not mentioned whether or not the patients were allergic. In this study a differentiation was made between ECP levels in sputum supernatant and ECP levels in sputum lysed cell pellet and a ratio of both was calculated: 24 patients with stable asthma ($n = 9$), exacerbation of asthma ($n = 5$), COPD ($n = 7$), bronchiectasis ($n = 3$) and seven healthy controls were investigated. ECP levels in sputum lysed cell pellet, but not ECP levels in sputum supernatant, correlated statistically significantly with the number of eosinophil cells in sputum. Both were statistically significantly increased in all patients. The ratio of ECP levels in sputum supernatant to ECP levels in sputum lysed cell pellet was statistically significantly increased in asthma exacerbations, COPD, and bronchiectasis, but not in stable asthma. The ECP ratio was judged to correlate statistically significantly with the eosinophil cell activation. The increased ECP levels in COPD were interpreted to reflect a nonselective accumulation of eosinophil cells in this condition.

In therapy studies, ECP levels in sputum and in bronchoalveolar lavage fluid were found to be reliable parameters of disease activity and mucosal hyperreactivity. In one study the effect of immunotherapy was investigated. Two groups of birch pollen allergic patients with seasonal rhinoconjunctivitis and asthma were followed during two consecutive birch pollen seasons. One group (10 patients) was followed during a season with high pollen load, and one group (15 patients) during a season with low pollen load (51). Half the patients of each group were treated with immunotherapy for 3 and 4 years, respectively. The other half of the patients served as the control group. Bronchoalveolar lavage was performed before and during each pollen season. In both seasons the control group had statistically significantly higher numbers of eosinophil cells and ECP levels than the immunotherapy group. Furthermore, in the control group numbers of eosinophil cells and ECP levels in bronchoalveolar lavage fluid increased statistically significantly within the season with a high pollen load, but not within the season with a low pollen load. The treated group showed no increase in either season. ECP blood serum levels were measured, too, and a statistically significant correlation between ECP blood serum levels and ECP levels in bronchoalveolar lavage was found.

In another therapy study the number of eosinophil cells and the ECP levels in bronchoalveolar lavage fluid were measured. Twenty-two asthmatic patients (21 allergic, 1 nonallergic) and 12 nonallergic healthy controls were investigated (52). Eleven patients (all allergic) were treated occasionally with inhaled bronchodilatators (beta-2-receptor-agonist) and 11 patients (10 allergic, 1 nonallergic) were treated regularly with inhaled corticosteroids. In both asthmatic groups, statistically significantly increased numbers of eosinophil cells were found, whereas the ECP level was only statistically significantly increased in the group of patients treated occasionally with inhaled bronchodilatators. The fact that in the corticosteroid group no increased ECP levels but statistically significantly increased numbers of eosinophil cells were found was explained by the ability of inhaled corticosteroids to prevent activation of eosinophils. It was assumed that ECP levels in bronchoalveolar lavage fluid better reflect eosinophil cell activity and thus are more specific markers for disease activitiy than the number of eosinophil cells.

Patients with COPD

In patients with COPD no correlation was found between ECP levels in sputum and airway obstruction or mucosal hyperreactivity. In a study of 18 COPD patients who had no blood eosinophilia but high mucosal hyperreactivity ECP levels in sputum, the degrees of airway obstruction (forced expiratory volume in 1 s) and of mucosal hyperreactivity (bronchial histamine challenge) were measured (24). No correlation between the three parameters was found.

Bronchoalveolar Challenge Tests

Bronchoalveolar challenge tests in allergic asthmatic patients showed contradictory results. In an investigation of 12 allergic asthmatic patients, bronchoalveolar allergen challenge was performed during a stable phase of the patients' disease (17). After resolution of the immediate-phase allergic response, bronchoalveolar lavage was performed 2 and 24 h postchallenge. The numbers of eosinophil cells and levels of ECP were assessed in the two lavages. Serial measurements of lung function were also done. It was found that although the recoveries in bronchoalveolar lavages of eosinophil cells and ECP tended to increase during the trial, none of the variables predicted the emergence of the late-phase allergic response.

In conclusion, it can be said that ECP levels in sputum and bronchoalveolar lavage fluid correlate statistically significantly with disease activity and mucosal hyperreactivity in allergic and nonallergic asthma. It may be assumed that this correlation can be found in children as well. To date, no investigation shows ECP levels in sputum to be more or less reliable than those in bronchoalveolar lavage fluid, but one study could demonstrate that ECP levels in sputum cell pellet lysate correlate better with the absolute number of eosinophil cells than ECP levels in sputum supernatant. Furthermore, the ratio of supernatant to pellet ECP levels in sputum can possibly be used as an index of eosinophil cell activation. In COPD, ECP levels in sputum or bronchoalveolar lavage fluid cannot be judged as a reliable monitoring variable of disease activity or mucosal hyperreactivity.

B. In Adult Patients with Allergic Rhinitis

Introduction

The results of studies on the correlation between the ECP levels in nasal secretions and disease activity or mucosal hyperreactivity in adults with allergic rhinitis are uniform. Many investigations have been conducted in adults, all showing a statistically significant correlation in both seasonal and perennial allergic rhinitis. No difference can be found between studies measuring ECP levels in nasal secretions after intranasal challenge and studies measuring ECP levels in nasal secretions under natural pollen exposure. Due to the uniformity of the results, only the most representative studies are presented here. Four groups of investigations can be differentiated in the literature. The studies measured ECP levels: after allergen challenge; under natural allergen exposure; in different inflammatory nasal and paranasal sinus diseases; and under therapy.

ECP Levels in Nasal Secretions After Allergen Challenge

In one study 10 patients with previously proven seasonal allergic rhinitis were challenged intranasally (53). A rechallenge was done 24 h later and ECP levels were determined in two nasal lavages performed immediately prior to the challenges. As expected, a statistically significant increase in nasal reactivity upon rechallenge was found. In addition, a statistically insignificant tendency for an increase of ECP levels in nasal lavage fluid was observed. The amount of ECP in the nasal lavage on the second day correlated statistically significantly with the N-alpha-tosyl-L-argimime methyl ester (TAME) esterase activity in the same lavage. Because TAME esterase activity is a marker of ongoing inflammatory activity, the participation of the eosinophil cell in the inflammatory response to allergens was suggested, which can be measured by ECP levels in nasal lavage fluid.

In a further investigation a quantitative determination of ECP in nasal secretions was performed and correlated with complaints and counts of eosinophil cells in the same secretions (54). Eighteen asymptomatic patients with seasonal allergic rhinitis outside the pollen season, 40 symptomatic patients with seasonal allergic rhinitis during the pollen season, and 10 healthy nonallergic subjects were investigated. Allergen challenge was performed in the 18 asymptomatic allergic patients. Seventeen patients had an immediate response of nasal symptoms. One hour later, a simultaneous, statistically significant increase was seen both in the percentage of the eosinophil cells and in the ECP level in nasal secretion. The number of eosinophil cells reached a peak 2 h after nasal allergen challenge with a duration of 8 h, while the highest ECP level was reached only after 24 h with no clear-cut plateau. In the 40 symptomatic allergic patients, the measurement of ECP in nasal secretion was done intraseasonally. Statistically significantly higher ECP levels in nasal secretions than the baseline values of the patients outside the pollen season were observed.

In another study ECP levels in nasal secretions and threshold doses in nasal histamine challenges from 20 patients with seasonal allergic rhinitis were measured (55). An inverse, statistically significant correlation was found between the threshold dose and the ECP levels. Furthermore, the ECP levels after a positive allergen challenge indicated a statistically significant correlation with the strength of the challenge reaction.

ECP Levels in Nasal Secretions Under Natural Allergen Exposure Within the Season

One study examined ECP levels in the nasal lavage fluids obtained from patients with seasonal allergic rhinitis (56). Nine patients with seasonal allergic rhinitis and five normal, nonallergic controls were studied before and during the pollen season. During the pollen season, ECP levels in nasal lavage fluid were increased to a statistically significant degree in the patients but not in the controls.

Another investigation examined 20 patients with seasonal allergic rhinitis to grass pollen and 10 healthy controls (38). ECP levels in nasal secretions and symptom scores were studied during and out of the pollen season. A statistically significant increase of ECP levels in nasal secretions was found in the patients but not in the controls, and the correlation between ECP levels in nasal secretions and symptom scores was determined to be statistically significant. The measurement of ECP levels in nasal secretions was recommended for monitoring disease activity and for monitoring the effects of therapy in allergic rhinitis.

To clarify the clinical–pathological role of ECP in nasal allergy, the ECP levels in nasal secretions and the symptom scores of 22 patients with seasonal or perennial allergic rhinitis were measured (36). A statistically significant correlation was found between ECP levels in the nasal secretions and the severity of clinical symptoms, especially the degree of nasal obstruction. ECP levels were also shown to have a statistically significant correlation to the score of eosinophil cells in the nasal secretions.

A further study was conducted to quantify eosinophil cell activation in perennial allergic rhinitis (37). Therefore, symptom scores and ECP levels in nasal secretions were measured in patients with perennial allergic rhinitis and in healthy controls. A statistically significant correlation between ECP levels in nasal secretions and clinical severity of symptoms was found, and ECP levels in nasal secretions were judged to be a clinical parameter of disease activity in perennial allergic rhinitis.

In an investigation conducted by our group, the natural course of allergic rhinitis was evaluated in 146 grass pollen allergic patients and 33 birch pollen allergic patients. Twelve healthy volunteers served as the control group. ECP was measured in nasal secretion samples using standardized absorbent rubber foam samplers (57). ECP in nasal secretion was determined in each patient before the start of the season, then 1, 2, 3, and 4 weeks intraseasonally, and 4 weeks postseasonally. In the control group we found no statistically significant changes in ECP levels within the study period. Preseasonally, there was no statistically significant difference between the control group and the two patient groups. One week after the start of the season a statistically significant increase of ECP in nasal secretions was found in both patient groups. Even within the following 3 weeks, a statistically significant increase of ECP levels was found. Four weeks postseasonally a statistically significant decrease of ECP levels was found; however, the decrease did not reach preseasonal levels. The increase of ECP levels showed no close time relation to the increase of allergic symptoms like rhinorrhea, sneezing, and nasal obstruction. After 3 weeks of pollen exposure ECP levels were reached which, in an *in vitro* model, were shown to reduce beat frequency of ciliated nasal epithelial cells (58), possibly even causing structural damage and destruction of these cells (6). These data support the results of the other studies which recommend ECP for monitoring disease activity in allergic rhinitis.

ECP Levels in Nasal Secretions in Different Forms of Rhinitis

Whether the different forms of rhinitis can be differentiated by measuring ECP levels in nasal secretions was investigated by several studies. In one study ECP levels in nasal secretions were measured in 119 patients with nonrhinitic allergies and different types of allergic and nonallergic rhinitis (39). The different forms of rhinitis were hyperreactive rhinitis, vasomotor rhinitis, chronic nonallergic sinusitis, asymptomatic pollinosis, acute symptomatic pollinosis, perennial allergic rhinitis, combination of perennial and seasonal rhinitis, and nasal polyps in the absence and in the presence of allergy. In all patient groups except for the vasomotor rhinitis group, ECP levels in nasal secretions differed statistically significantly from the normal controls. No statistically significant differences between the different forms of rhinitis but a statistically significant correlation between nasal eosinophil cells and ECP in nasal secretion was found.

In a further study the ECP levels in nasal secretions in three groups of patients were compared (41). In 28 patients with seasonal rhinitis (16 symptomatic, 12 asymptomatic), 11 patients with chronic sinusitis, and 20 healthy controls ECP levels in nasal secretions were controlled. ECP levels in nasal secretions were statistically significantly higher in the patients than in the controls, and the highest ECP levels in nasal secretions were found in the patients with symptomatic seasonal rhinitis.

A prospective study was carried out in 183 healthy volunteers and 515 patients with different inflammatory nasal and paranasal sinus diseases (94 perennial allergic rhinitis, 131 seasonal allergic rhinitis extraseasonally, 177 seasonal allergic rhinitis intraseasonally, 49 chronic sinusitis without allergic rhinitis, 36 chronic sinusitis with perennial allergic rhinitis, 28 nasal polyps). ECP levels in nasal secretions were measured (5). The analysis of ECP in nasal secretions showed in all patients statistically significantly higher ECP levels than in the controls. Moreover, ECP levels differed among the diseases investigated and were statistically significantly higher in patients with seasonal allergic rhinitis intraseasonally and patients with perennial allergic rhinitis than in patients with seasonal allergic rhinitis extraseasonally and patients with chronic sinusitis without allergic rhinitis. ECP levels in nasal secretions were judged to be a reliable marker for the assessment of disease activity in inflammatory nasal and paranasal diseases and possibly an adjunct to current diagnostic measures.

ECP Levels in Nasal Secretions Under Therapy

In a therapy study 14 patients with seasonal allergic rhinitis were challenged outside the pollen season after a 3-week pretreatment with placebo or slow-release theophylline (59). ECP levels in nasal lavage fluids and symptom scores were measured. The ECP levels in nasal lavage fluid did not increase during the immediate-phase allergic reaction. Five hours after challenge, ECP levels in nasal lavage fluid and symptom scores in the placebo group increased to a statistically significant degree, whereas no statistically significant increase was observed during the theophylline treatment. Theophylline treatment also reduced the nasal symptoms statistically significantly. ECP levels in nasal secretions were judged to be a parameter for controlling therapy efficacy in seasonal allergic rhinitis.

Another therapy study was carried out to study the effect of nasal allergen provocation on the level of ECP in nasal lavage fluid, with and without glucocorticoid pretreatment (60). Twenty grass pollen sensitive volunteers were provoked outside the pollen season on two consecutive days after a 2-week pretreatment with nasal glucocorticoids or placebo. There was no statistically significant increase of ECP levels in nasal lavage fluid during the immediate-phase allergic response, and a late occurring, statistically significant increase of the ECP levels in nasal lavage fluids after 6–24 h was found in the placebo group. A complete inhibition of this increase was observed as well as a statistically significant reduction of the prechallenge ECP levels in nasal lavage fluids by glucocorticoid pretreatment. It was concluded that allergen provocation in the nose results in a late occurring, statistically significant increase of ECP in nasal lavage fluid. One of the therapeutic effects of topical glucocorticoid treatment may be an inhibition of the allergen-induced increase of this cytotoxic molecule.

In conclusion, ECP levels in nasal secretions have been shown to be reliable markers of disease activity and for monitoring therapy efficacy in patients with allergic rhinitis. Both the late allergic response after allergen challenge and the ongoing allergic reaction within the season are correlated to the ECP levels in nasal secretions in a statistically significant manner. Whether a differentiation of the various forms of inflammatory nasal and sinus diseases is possible is not yet clear and has to be clarified in further studies.

C. In Children with Allergic Rhinitis

Introduction

Fewer investigations have been performed in children, but the results of the different studies are as uniform as in adults showing a statistically significant correlation in both seasonal and perennial allergic rhinitis.

ECP Levels in Nasal Secretions Under Natural Allergen Exposure Within the Season

One study evaluated the intraseasonal and postseasonal course of ECP blood serum levels and ECP levels in nasal secretions in seasonal allergic rhinitis (46). In 73 children (13 seasonal allergic rhinitis, 44 seasonal allergic rhinitis and asthma, 16 healthy controls) ECP blood serum levels and ECP levels in nasal secretions were measured during and after the pollen season. The results were equal for both. During the season the highest values of ECP levels were observed in the group of children with seasonal allergic rhinitis and asthma, but even in children with seasonal allergic rhinitis alone statistically significantly higher levels than in the controls were found. A statistically significant increase of ECP levels intraseasonally was found in all groups. Even after the pollen season, the ECP levels in children with seasonal allergic rhinitis and asthma were statistically significantly higher than in the other two groups. After the season there was no statistically significant difference between the children with allergic rhinitis alone and the controls. Both ECP blood serum levels and ECP levels in nasal secretions were recommended as disease activity parameters in children with seasonal allergic rhinitis.

ECP Levels in Nasal Secretions Under Therapy

A therapy study involving 38 children with perennial allergic rhinitis to house dust mites showed similar results (44). All children were treated over a period of 3 weeks. One group ($n = 13$) was treated with nasal corticosteroids, one group ($n = 15$) with nasal mast cell membrane stabilizers, and one group ($n = 10$) with placebo. Before treatment ECP levels in nasal secretions were statistically significantly higher in all patients as compared to the controls. ECP levels in nasal secretion decreased, and clinical symptoms improved statistically significantly in the group of patients treated with nasal corticosteroids, but not in the group treated with mast cell membrane stabilizers. No statistically significant variation was found in the placebo group. It was concluded that ECP levels in nasal secretions may be used to evaluate the activity of eosinophil cells and monitor the anti-inflammatory efficacy of therapy in perennial allergic rhinitis in children. In the same study ECP blood serum levels were not found to be useful for the same purpose.

In conclusion, even in children ECP levels in nasal secretions have been shown to be reliable markers of disease activity and for monitoring therapy efficacy in patients with allergic rhinitis.

IV. Do ECP Blood Serum Levels Correlate with ECP Levels in Local Body Fluids (Sputum, Nasal Secretion)?

A. Introduction

Investigations on the correlation between ECP blood serum levels and ECP levels in local body fluids are extremely rare. More investigations have been conducted concerning the correlation between disease activity or mucosal hyperreactivity and both ECP blood serum levels and ECP levels in local body fluids, but not involving the correlation between these two ECP levels. In these studies, only the results concerning the measurement of ECP blood serum levels and the measurement of ECP levels in local body fluids can be compared.

B. Correlation Between ECP Blood Serum Levels and ECP Levels in Sputum or Bronchoalveolar Lavage Fluid

Introduction

The results of studies investigating both ECP blood serum levels and ECP levels in sputum are uniform, all showing similar results for blood serum and sputum. Some of these studies have been previously mentioned in the appropriate chapters.

Clinical Studies

In clinical studies on the use of ECP measurements in allergic and nonallergic asthma and COPD, the results of ECP blood serum measurements and of ECP measurements in sputum or bronchoalveolar lavage fluid were similar. One investigation (24) found no correlation between both ECP blood serum levels and ECP levels in sputum and the degree of hyperreactivity in patients with COPD.

Another study (25) was performed to clarify whether ECP levels are useful markers in the differential diagnosis of asthma attack and acute exacerbation of COPD. The same results for ECP blood serum levels and ECP levels in bronchoalveolar lavage were shown again; both were judged not to be useful markers in the differential diagnosis of asthma attack and acute exacerbation of COPD.

These results were supported by a study whose objective was to clarify the extent to which ECP levels in sputum relate to indices of asthma severity in chronic stable allergic and nonallergic asthma (49). The results for both ECP blood serum levels and ECP levels in sputum were the same, being statistically significantly higher in asthmatic than in normal subjects. Both were judged to be useful indicators of disease activity in allergic and nonallergic asthma.

Therapy Studies

In therapy studies similar correlations were found between ECP blood serum levels and ECP levels in sputum or bronchoalveolar lavage fluid. One therapy study monitored the effect of theophylline in patients with allergic and nonallergic asthma (61). A statistically significant decrease of both ECP blood serum levels and ECP levels in sputum under therapy was found.

In another therapy study on the effect of treatment with bronchial corticosteroids in patients with allergic and nonallergic asthma, the ECP blood serum levels and the ECP levels in bronchial washes were measured (62). Twenty asthmatic patients and 16 healthy controls were investigated weekly over a period of 10 weeks. Before treatment, statistically significant elevated ECP levels were detected in bronchoalveolar lavage, bronchial wash, and blood serum of the patients as compared to the controls. Under therapy a statistically significant decrease of ECP levels in bronchial wash and blood serum was observed, whereas the decrease of ECP in bronchoalveolar lavage was not considered statistically significant. There were no changes in the nontreated group of patients.

Finally, in a study on the effect of immunotherapy two groups of birch pollen allergic patients with seasonal allergic rhinoconjunctivitis and asthma were followed (51). One group had been treated with immunotherapy for 3 or 4 years, the other group served as control. Intraseasonally, the control group had statistically significantly higher ECP blood serum levels and ECP levels in bronchoalveolar lavage fluid than the immunotherapy group. Furthermore, in seasons with high pollen load ECP blood serum levels and ECP levels in bronchoalveolar lavage fluid increased statistically significantly intraseasonally in the control group, but not in the immunotherapy group. A statistically significant correlation between ECP blood serum levels and ECP levels in bronchoalveolar lavage was found.

Direct Control of the Correlation

A direct control of the correlation between ECP blood serum levels and ECP levels in bronchoalveolar lavage fluid showed a statistically significant correlation (52). The constituents of bronchoalveolar lavage fluids in terms of cell profiles and released ECP were measured in allergic and nonallergic asthmatic patients and healthy controls. Both the increased ECP blood serum levels and the ECP levels in bronchoalveolar lavage fluid were found to be statistically significant in patients treated occasionally with inhaled bronchodilators, but not in the patient group regularly treated with inhaled corticosteroids. A statistically significant correlation between ECP blood serum levels and ECP levels in bronchoalveolar lavage fluid was found and both parameters were judged to be more specific markers for disease activity than the number of eosinophil cells in allergic and nonallergic asthma.

In conclusion, a statistically significant correlation between ECP blood serum levels and ECP levels in sputum or bronchoalveolar lavage fluid was found in patients with allergic and nonallergic asthma. In COPD both ECP blood serum levels and ECP levels in sputum or bronchoalveolar lavage fluid are not statistically significantly correlated to disease activity or mucosal hyperreactivity.

C. Correlation Between ECP Blood Serum Levels and ECP Levels in Nasal Secretions

Introduction

Little is known about the correlation between ECP blood serum levels and ECP levels in nasal secretions. The results of the investigations in which both ECP blood serum levels and ECP levels in nasal secretions are measured are not uniform.

Investigations Showing No Correlation

Some studies show different results for ECP blood serum levels and ECP levels in nasal secretions in the same study population. In one investigation, symptom scores and ECP levels of patients with perennial allergic rhinitis and healthy controls were measured (37). A statistically significant correlation was observed between ECP levels in nasal secretion and the clinical severity of symptoms, but not between ECP blood serum levels and the clinical severity of symptoms. Only the ECP levels in nasal secretions were judged to be a clinical parameter of disease activity in perennial allergic rhinitis.

In an investigation which was done with 20 patients with seasonal allergic rhinitis to grass pollen and 10 healthy controls, ECP blood serum levels and symptom scores were studied during and out of the pollen season (38). In both groups no statistically significant increase of ECP blood serum levels and no correlation between ECP blood serum levels and symptom scores was found, but the raised ECP levels in nasal secretions and the correlation between ECP levels in nasal secretions and symptom scores were determined to be statistically significant.

Another investigation in patients with seasonal allergic rhinitis showed statistically significant higher ECP levels in nasal secretions than in blood serum. ECP levels in nasal secretions but not ECP blood serum levels seemed to have a statistically significant correlation to the cumulative pollen concentration of the 3 days preceding the sampling procedure (5).

A therapy study compared the effect of nasal corticosteroids, nasal mast cell membrane stabilizers, and placebo (44). Before and after treatment no statistically significant difference in ECP blood serum levels between patients and healthy controls was found, while ECP levels in nasal secretions and clinical symptoms showed statistically significant differences between patients and controls. The reduced levels in treated children were also found to be statistically significant. Only the ECP levels in nasal secretions were considered to be useful markers for monitoring disease activity in children with perennial allergic rhinitis.

Investigations Suggesting Correlations

Other studies show partially uniform results for ECP blood serum levels and ECP levels in nasal secretions in the same study population. In a study which was done to clarify the clinical–pathological role of ECP in nasal allergy, a slight tendency toward a correlation between ECP blood serum levels and the severity of clinical symptoms could be observed, but a statistically significant correlation was seen between ECP levels in nasal secretions and the severity of clinical symptoms (36).

An investigation of ECP blood serum levels and ECP levels in the nasal secretion of patients with symptomatic seasonal allergy, patients with asymptomatic seasonal allergy, and patients with chronic sinusitis showed for both ECP blood serum and ECP in nasal secretions statistically significant higher levels in the patients with symptomatic seasonal allergy (41). In the entire patient group, only the ECP levels in nasal secretions but not ECP blood serum levels were statistically significant higher than in controls.

A study of 28 patients with perennial allergic rhinitis and healthy controls showed both raised ECP blood serum levels and ECP levels in nasal secretion in the patient group to be statistically significant, whereas a statistically significant correlation between the number of eosinophil cells and ECP levels was found only in nasal secretions (63).

In a therapy study 63 patients with seasonal allergic rhinitis to grass pollen were investigated (42). One group was treated with topical corticosteroids, while the other group was treated with placebo. During the season ECP blood serum levels, but not ECP levels in nasal secretions, were statistically significantly increased in the placebo group. Under therapy both ECP blood serum levels and ECP levels in nasal secretions decreased to a statistically significant level.

In conclusion, a correlation between ECP blood serum levels and ECP levels in nasal secretions has not yet been proven. Whether such a correlation exists or not should be investigated in further studies.

V. Variation of ECP Levels

A. Variation of ECP Blood Serum Levels

Introduction

ECP blood serum levels can be influenced by several factors both *in vivo* and *in vitro*. *In vivo* these factors are mainly environmental influences such as the time of day, the time of the allergy seasons or smoking, whereas *in vitro* these factors are mainly caused by methodological influences.

In Vivo

An *in vivo* study of the diurnal variation of ECP blood serum levels in normal subjects and in patients with allergic and nonallergic asthma showed a similar diurnal variation in ECP blood serum levels in both groups (64). The ECP blood serum levels in both groups showed the highest level in the early evening, and it was thus concluded that this may be a result of hormonal or other influences.

An investigation of ECP blood serum levels in a general population of 379 individuals was done in 1997 (65). Skin prick tests and methacholine challenges determined 137 of the patients to be allergic. A statistically significant seasonal variation in ECP blood serum levels was found in the group of birch pollen positive subjects, but not in the nonallergic or birch pollen negative allergic group. The mean ECP blood serum level in birch pollen positive subjects was about twice as high in June as in birch pollen allergic subjects examined during the other months. It was concluded that seasonal variation in birch pollen positive subjects must be taken into account when using ECP blood serum levels clinically or in epidemiological research.

Another investigation of the relationship of ECP blood serum levels to smoking history and lung function alteration showed a linear association of

ECP blood serum levels with daily cigarette consumption and forced expiratory volume in 1 s (66).

In Vitro

An *in vitro* study showed an interaction between ECP, which is highly cationic, and heparin, which is highly anionic (67). This interaction can lead to a formation of a complex between the two molecules, which may result in decrease of ECP in heparin plasma samples.

Another study showed that the level of ECP in blood samples is influenced by the method with which the samples were treated (68). Three different blood samples were stored (blood serum, heparin plasma, and EDTA plasma) and ECP levels were measured hourly. A time-dependent and statistically significant increase of ECP levels in blood serum samples or heparin plasma samples was found within the first 2 h. This increase was considered to be due to active *in vitro* release of ECP from eosinophil cells. In addition, ECP levels in blood serum were temperature dependent, being higher at 37°C than at 25°C. On the other hand, ECP levels in EDTA plasma did not change statistically significantly, and these levels of ECP were considered to have been released into the blood *in vivo*. ECP levels were always in the order of serum greater than heparin plasma greater than EDTA plasma. The time-dependent change of ECP levels in blood serum after storage at room temperature was confirmed by another study (69).

A further investigation could show that not storage time alone, but also temperature and anticoagulants have a statistically significant influence on the levels of ECP in blood samples (70). In this investigation the ECP levels were measured in EDTA plasma, heparin plasma, and serum without anticoagulant of five patients with allergic and nonallergic asthma and five healthy controls. In serum and in heparin plasma a temperature-dependent, statistically significant increase of ECP levels was found within 1 h, whereas in EDTA plasma no temperature-dependent variation of ECP levels was found. There were no differences between ECP determination in serum and in heparin plasma under the same conditions of time and temperature.

In children as well, ECP was not released in EDTA plasma during storage, whereas in both heparin plasma and serum a statistically significant temperature-dependent increase of ECP levels was found (71).

In conclusion, different factors influence ECP blood serum levels both *in vivo* and *in vitro*. *In vivo* some factors are known such as diurnal variation or smoking history, but many other factors probably remain unknown, thus requiring more investigations. *In vitro* there is evidence that ECP levels can change depending on the time and temperature. ECP levels in EDTA plasma tend to be more stable than in heparin plasma or in blood serum. However, more studies are needed to clarify the mechanism of ECP release *in vitro* and a stricter protocol for obtaining blood ECP samples has to be defined.

B. Variation of ECP Levels in Sputum and Bronchoalveolar Lavage Fluid

In Vivo

Investigations on the variation of ECP levels in sputum are rare. Whether a variation of ECP levels in sputum *in vivo* is caused by similar factors such as the variation of ECP blood serum levels is not yet known. However, such an influence is quite probable.

In Vitro

In vitro some studies show ECP levels in sputum to be dependent on time and temperature influences. In one investigation, the sputa of 12 patients with stable allergic and nonallergic asthma were homogenized using ultrasonification and then centrifuged (72). Supernatants were evenly divided and stored for 1, 6, 24, or 72 h at either 4°C or 25°C and then frozen at −80°C. The ECP levels were compared with immediately frozen samples. A statistically significant influence of time on ECP levels in sputa was found, and a statistically significant influence of temperature was found when comparing the specimens stored at 4°C with those stored at 25°C. Looking at individual time points, a statistically significant decrease in ECP levels was only seen at 25°C after 24 and 72 h. It was concluded that ECP levels in sputum decrease in a time- and temperature-dependent process, so that specimens should be stored in a refrigerator at 4°C until ECP is measured if sputa cannot be processed immediately after obtaining the specimens.

The aim of another study was to investigate the diagnostic value of the analysis of selected sputum (plugs) and of entire sputum (73). The sputum of 18 allergic and nonallergic asthmatics and eight healthy controls was analyzed, and the ECP levels in supernatant were measured. Statistically significantly higher ECP levels were found in selected sputum as compared with entire sputum. ECP levels were statistically significant and increased similarly in both selected and entire sputum of asthmatic subjects, independent of the method of sputum analysis. The authors concluded that the selected sputum method may provide a higher level of ECP. However, both the selected sputum and the entire sputum methods have the same diagnostic value in distinguishing asthmatics from healthy subjects.

In conclusion, evidence exists showing that ECP levels in sputum can change in both a time- and a temperature-dependent manner. To what degree environmental factors have an influence on ECP levels in sputum is not clear, which should be the subject of future studies.

C. Variation of ECP Levels in Nasal Secretion and Nasal Lavage Fluid

In Vivo and In Vitro

Until now, we know of no study investigating factors disturbing the measurement of ECP levels in nasal secretions *in vivo* or *in vitro*. So, whether these factors are the same in nasal secretions as in sputum is not yet known. However, this is quite probable.

Influence of Sampling Methods

One investigation centers on the impact of different sampling methods. This investigation was done to define norm values of ECP in nasal secretion and to evaluate the clinical use of the different sampling methods of nasal secretions in patients with allergic rhinitis (74). A total of 839 healthy individuals were evaluated using seven different sampling methods: blowing the nose ($n = 82$), suction ($n = 69$), the Okuda microsuction technique ($n = 93$), absorbent cotton wool samplers ($n = 156$), rubber foam samplers ($n = 193$), nasal lavage ($n = 112$), and nasal spray washing ($n = 134$). Missing values occurred in more than 60% for the methods of blowing the nose, suction, and Okuda microsuction technique, so that no norm range was defined for these methods. Normal range for ECP in nasal secretion was 5–46 ng/mL for absorbent cotton wool samplers, 7–41 ng/mL for rubber foam samplers, 4–51 ng/mL for nasal spray washing, and 3–31 ng/mL for nasal lavage.

In conclusion, the methods based on absorption or nasal washing are more reliable than other methods for collecting nasal secretions and determining ECP levels. Other influences on ECP levels in nasal secretions *in vivo* or *in vitro* have to be clarified.

VI. Summary

Allergic rhinitis is the most common allergic disease of the upper respiratory tract. Its incidence is rising, and its prevalence in children is rated as high as 42% (75). The main objective of treatment is to halt the progression of allergic rhinitis to serious medical complications. Therapy is complicated, time-consuming, and not always successful, especially in children. Complications of therapy are possible. An optimally effective therapy with as few side effects as possible can be achieved only if the severity of the disease is precisely assessed. Up to now, this has been accomplished above all by recording disease symptoms on the basis of case history and clinical examination. The degree of activity of the allergic inflammation, however, is only partly recorded. For theoretical considerations, the measurement of ECP levels in nasal secretion offers a solution to this problem. Measurements of ECP blood serum levels, which are easier to perform, may also be suitable for this purpose. However, they register the entire range of manifestations of an allergic disease, for example, the degree of allergic inflammation activity of the bronchial mucous membrane in patients with allergic rhinitis and asthma.

Optimum control of the applied therapy in its lowest dosage can only be achieved if the efficacy of treatment is recorded precisely. Case history and clinical examination, however, also have their limits, while ECP levels in nasal secretion could represent a reliable parameter for monitoring therapy efficacy. ECP blood serum levels likewise would be suitable to a certain degree, since interference with allergic manifestations in other organs could occur.

Even though more examinations of ECP blood serum levels have been performed in asthma and COPD than in allergic rhinitis, a similar behavior can be observed in both diseases. Comparative investigations between both patient groups in fact show higher ECP blood serum levels in asthma, yet both groups have significantly higher levels in comparison to healthy subjects. In spite of several contradictory results, a significant correlation between disease activity and ECP blood serum levels was proven for both diseases. In both cases the possibility of therapy monitoring on the basis of ECP blood serum levels appears to exist. Evidence is available showing that a chronification of the disease limits the validity of ECP measurements in blood serum and that in allergic patients raised ECP levels and possibly a better correlation between disease activity and ECP blood serum levels exist compared to nonallergic patients. In principle, ECP measurements in blood serum taken under allergen provocation appear to be less reliable than those taken during the natural course of the disease. The relationships between ECP blood serum levels and disease activity have been found to be similar in children and adults. Here, too, the ECP measurements taken under allergen provocation have proven to be less reliable, while they have been shown to be sensitive during the natural course of the disease or under therapy.

In asthma and COPD, the measurement of ECP in sputum and broncho-alveolar lavage is judged to be a reliable parameter in determining disease activity and for therapy monitoring. Publications to the contrary concern patients with irreversible bronchial obstruction without blood eosinophilia. In allergic rhinitis, it appears that the measurement of ECP in nasal secretion both under allergen provocation as well as during the natural course of the disease can serve as a reliable parameter for assessing disease activity. Investigations on ECP levels in nonallergic rhinitis are not available as yet. The comparison between ECP blood serum levels and ECP levels in sputum of patients with asthma and COPD has not shown one method superior to the other, whereas in allergic rhinitis a statistically significant superiority of the ECP measurement in nasal secretion was found.

ECP can be determined with the help of reliable immunoassays. Evidence is available indicating that the measurement in EDTA plasma causes the least falsifications due to the influences of temperature or time. In nasal secretion it has been shown that methods based on absorption (absorbent cotton wool samplers, rubber foam samplers) or lavage (nasal lavage, nasal spray washing) ensure the most reliable results. Deviations dependent on the time of day or year as well as external influences such as smoking must be taken into consideration.

Acknowledgments

I am grateful to G. Kittel, BA, Cologne, Germany, for her help in setting up the manuscript and for proofreading and Prof. J. J. Manni, Maastricht, the Netherlands, for reviewing and criticizing the text.

References

1. Bascom R, Pipkorn U, Gleich G, Lichtenstein IM, Naclerio RM. The influx of inflammatory cells into nasal washings during the late response to antigen challenge. Effect of systemic corticosteroids. Am Rev Respir Dis 1988; 138:406–412.
2. Dahl R. Eosinophil and eosinophil products. In: Mygind N, Pipkorn U, eds. Allergic and Vasomotoric Rhinitis: Pathophysiological Aspects. Copenhagen, Denmark: Munksgaard, 1987:136–139.
3. Klementsson H. Time relation between allergen-induced changes in nasal responsiveness and eosinophil granulocytes. Rhinology 1994; 32:90–91.
4. Linder A, Venge P, Deuschl H. Eosinophil cationic protein and myeloperoxidase in nasal secretion as markers of inflammation in allergic rhinitis. Allergy 1987; 42:583–590.
5. Klimek L, Rasp G. Cell activation markers in rhinitis and rhinosinusitis. Eosinophilic cationic protein (ECP). Laryngorhinootologie 1996; 48:377–382.
6. Venge P. Soluble markers of allergic inflammation. Allergy 1994; 49:1–8.
7. Venge P, Bystrom J. Eosinophil cationic protein (ECP). Int J Biochem Cell Biol 1998; 30:433–437.
8. Olsson I, Venge P. Cationic proteins of human granulocytes. II. Separation of the cationic proteins of the granules of leukemic myeloid cells. Blood 1974; 44:235–246.
9. Olsson I, Venge P, Spitznagel JK, Lehrer RI. Arginine-rich cationic proteins of human eosinophil granules. Comparison of the constituents of eosinophilic and neutrophilic leukocytes. Lab Invest 1977; 36:493–500.
10. Hamann KJ, Ten RM, Loegering DA, Jankins RB, Heise MT, Schad CR, Pease LR, Gleich GJ, Barker RL. Structure and chromosome localisation of the human eosinophil-derivated neurotoxin and eosinophil cationic protein genes: evidence for intronless coding sequences in the ribonuclease gene superfamily. Genomics 1990; 7:535–546.
11. Venge P, Roxin LE, Olsson I. Radioimmunoassay of human eosinophil cationic protein. Br J Haematol 1977; 37:331–335.
12. Peterson CG, Enander I, Nystrand J, Anderson AS, Nilson L, Venge P. Radioimmunoassay of human eosinophil cationic protein (ECP) by an improved method. Clin Exp Allergy 1991; 21:561–567.
13. Bousquet J, Chanez P, Lacoste JY, Barncon G, Ghavanian N, Enander I, Venge P, Ahlstedt S, Simony-Lafontaine J, Godard P et al. Eosinophilic inflammation in asthma. N Engl J Med 1990; 323:1033–1039.
14. Sin A, Terzioglu E, Kokuludag A, Sebik R, Kabakci T. Serum eosinophil cationic protein (ECP) levels in patients with seasonal allergic rhinitis and allergic asthma. Allergy Asthma Proc 1998; 19:69–73.

15. Vatrella A, Ponticiello A, Parrella R, Romano L, Zofra S, DiLeva A, Barrifi F. Serum eosinophil cationic protein (ECP) as a marker of disease activity and treatment efficacy in seasonal asthma. Allergy 1996; 51:547–555.
16. Venge P. Monitoring of asthma inflammation by serum measurements of eosinophil cationic protein (ECP). A new clinical approach to asthma management. Respir Med 1995; 89:1–2.
17. Schmekel B, Venge P. Markers for eosinophils and T-lymphocytes as predictors of late asthmatic response. Allergy 1993; 48:94–97.
18. Dahl R, Venge P, Olsson I. Variations of blood eosinophils and eosinophil cationic protein in serum in patients with bronchal asthma. Studies during inhalation challenge test. Allergy 1978; 33:211–215.
19. Pedersen B, Dahl R, Larsen BB, Venge P. The effect of salmeterol on the early- and late phase reaction to bronchial allergen and postchallenge variation in bronchial reactivity, blood eosinophils cationic protein, and serum eosinophil protein X. Allergy 1993; 48:377–382.
20. Parra A, Prieto I, Sanz ML, Dieguez I, Resano A, Oehling AK. Serum ECP levels in asthmatic patients: comparison with other follow-up parameters. Allergy Asthma Proc 1996; 17:191–197.
21. Alvarez-Gutierrez FJ, Rodriguez-Portal JA, Valenzuela-Mateos F, Capote-Gil F, Sanchez-Gil R, Castillo-Gomez J. Inflammation mediators (eosinophilic cationic protein, ECP) in a normal population and in patients with bronchial asthma or allergic rhinitis. Arch Bronconeumol 1995; 31:280–286.
22. Wever AM, Wever-Hess J, Hermans J. The use of serum eosinophil cationic protein (ECP) in the management of steroid therapy in chronic asthma. Clin Exp Allergy 1997; 27:519–529.
23. Kunkel G, Ryden AC. Serum eosinophil cationic protein (ECP) as a mediator of inflammation in acute asthma, during resolution and during the monitoring of the stable asthmatic patients treated with inhaled steroids according to a dose reduction schedule. Inflamm Res 1999; 48:94–100.
24. Chazan R, Jaworski A, Grubek-Jaworska H, Droszcz W. Correlation of ECP levels in sputum and blood with parameters of airflow obstruction and hyperreactivity in patients with irreversible bronchial obstruction due to chronic bronchitis. Pol Arch Med Wewn 1995; 94:300–306.
25. Gursel G, Turktas H, Gokcora N, Tekin IO. Comparison of sputum and serum eosinophil cationic protein (ECP) levels in nonatopic asthma and chronic obstructive pulmonary disease. J Asthma 1997; 34:313–319.
26. Kleinau I, Niggemann B, Wahn U. Individual time-courses of ECP and EPX during allergen provocation tests in asthmatic children. Pediatric Allergy Immunol 1995; 6:109–118.
27. Niggeman B, Kleinau I, Schmitt M, Wahn U. Twenty-four-hour time course of eosinophil granule proteins ECP and EPX during bronchial allergen challenges in serum of asthmatic children. Allergy 1994; 49:74–80.
28. Niggeman B, Ertel M, Lanner A, Wahn U. Relevance of serum measurements for monitoring acute asthma in children. J Asthma 1996; 33:327–330.
29. Zapalka M, Kopriva F, Szotkowska J. Monitoring of serum eosinophil cationic protein (ECP) level and its clinical value in pediatric practice. Acta Univ Palacki Olomuc Fac Med 1998; 141:21–33.

30. Turktas I, Demisirsoy S, Koc E, Gokora N, Elbeg S. Effects of inhaled steroid treatment on serum eosinophilic cationic protein (ECP) and low affinity receptor for IgE (Fc epsilon RII/sCD23) in childhood bronchial asthma. Arch Dis Child 1996; 75:314–318.

31. Fujisawa T, Terada A, Atsuta J, Iguchi K, Kamiya H, Sakurai M. Clinical utility of serum levels of eosinophil cationic protein (ECP) for monitoring and predicting clinical course in childhood asthma. Clin Exp Allergy 1998; 28:19–25.

32. Zimmermann B. Clinical experience with the measurement of ECP: usefulness in the management of children with asthma. Clin Exp Allergy 1993; 23(suppl 2): 8–12.

33. Ferdousi HA, Dreborg S. Asthma, bronchial hyperreactivity and mediator release in children with birch pollinosis. ECP and EPX levels are not related to broncheal hyperreactivity. Clin Exp Allergy 1997; 27:530–539.

34. Remes S, Korppi M, Remes K, Savolainen K, Mononen I, Pakkanen J. Serum eosinophil cationic protein (ECP) and eosinophil protein X (ECP) in childhood asthma: the influence of atopy. Pediatr Pulmonol 1998; 25:167–174.

35. Zimmermann B, Enander I, Zimmermann R, Ahlstedt S. Asthma in children less than 5 years of age: eosinophils and serum levels of eosinophil proteins ECP and EPX in relation to atopy and symptoms. Clin Exp Allergy 1994; 24:149–155.

36. Satoh K, Takagi I, Itoh H, Baba S. Study on eosinophil cationic protein (ECP) and arysulfatase B in nasal secretions and sera from patients with nasal allergy. Nippon Jibiinkoka Gakkai Kaiho 1991; 94:786–793.

37. Hisamatsu K, Ganbo T, Goto R, Nakazawa T, Murakami Y. Eosinophil cationic protein in perennial allergic rhinitis. Auris Nasus Larynx 1995; 22:165–171.

38. Di Lorenzo G, Mansueto P, Melluso M, Candore G, Colombo A, Pelliteri ME, Drago A, Potestio M, Caruso C. Allergic rhinitis to grass pollen: measurement of inflammatory mediators of mast cell and eosinophils in native fluid lavage and in serum out of and during pollen season. J Allergy Clin Immunol 1997; 100:832–837.

39. Rasp G, Thomas PA, Bujia J. Eosinophil inflammation of the nasal mucosa in allergic and non-allergic rhinitis measured by eosinophil cationic protein levels in native nasal fluid and serum. Clin Exp Allergy 1994; 24:1151–1156.

40. Winter L, Moseholm L, Reimert CM, Skov PS, Poulsen LK. Basophil histamine release, IgE, eosinophil counts, ECP, and EPX are related to the severity of symptoms in seasonal allergic rhinitis. Allergy 1999; 54:436–445.

41. Rasp G, Bujia J. Diagnosis of allergic rhinitis by determining of tryptase and eosinophil cationic protein in nasal secretions. Acta Otolaryngol Esp 1994; 45:437–440.

42. Nielsen LP, Bjerke T, Christensen MB, Skamling M, Peterson CG, Mygind N, Dahl R. Eosinophil markers in seasonal allergic rhinitis. Intranasal fluticasone propionate inhibits local and systemic increases during the pollen season. Allergy 1998; 53:778–785.

43. Ohashi Y, Nakai Y, Kakinoki Y, Ohno Y, Sakamoto H, Kato A, Tanaka A. Effect of immunotherapy on serum levels of eosinophil cationic protein in perennial allergic rhinitis. Ann Otol Rhinol Laryngol 1997; 106:848–853.

44. Sensi LG, Seri A, Siracusa A, Petrici L, Marcucci F. Allergic rhinitis in children: effects of flunisolide and disodium cromoglycate on nasal eosinophil cationic protein. Clin Exp Allergy 1997; 27:270–276.

45. Marcianiak D, Tomaszewicz-Fryca J, Plussa T, Chcilowski A. Eosinophil cationic protein in children with allergic diseases of the respiratory tract in exacerbation and remission of symptoms. Pol Merkuriusz Lek 1998; 4:75–77.

46. Cichoka-Jarosz E, Lis G, Pietrzyk JJ. Diagnostic value of selected activity parameters in children with hay fever. Przegl Lek 1997; 54:607–613.

47. Rao R, Frederick JM, Enander I, Gregson RK, Warner JA, Warner JO. Airway function correlates with circulating eosinophil, but not mast cell, markers of inflammation in childhood asthma. Clin Exp Allergy 1996; 26:789–793.

48. Venge P. Role of eosinophils in childhood asthma inflammation I. Pediatr Pulmonol 1995; (suppl 11):34–35.

49. Ronchi MC, Piragino C, Rosi E, Stendardi L, Tanini A, Galli G, Duranti R, Scano G. Do sputum eosinophils and ECP relate to the severity of asthma? Eur Respir J 1997; 10:1809–1813.

50. Gibson PG, Wooley KL, Carty K, Murree-Allen K, Saltos-N. Induce sputum eosinophil cationic protein (ECP) measurement in asthma and chronic obstructive airway disease (COAD). Clin Exp Allergy 1998; 28:1081–1088.

51. Rak S, Björnson A, Hakanson L, Sörenson S, Venge P. The effect of immunotherapy on eosinophil accumulation and production of eosinophil chemotactic activity in the lung of subjects with asthma during natural pollen exposures. J Allergy Clin Immunol 1991; 88:878–888.

52. Ädelroth E, Rosenhall L, Johansson SA, Linden M, Venge P. Inflammatory cells and eosinophil activity in asthmatics investigated by bronchoalveolar lavage. Am Rev Respir Dis 1990; 142:91–99.

53. Andersson M, Andersson P, Venge P, Pipkorn U. Eosinophils and eosinophil cationic protein in nasal lavages in allergen-induced hyperresponsiviness: effects of topical glucocorticosteroid treatment. Allergy 1989; 44:342–348.

54. Wang D, Clement P, Smitz J, de-Waele M, Derde MP. Correlations between complaints, inflammatory cells and mediator concentrations in nasal secretions after nasal allergen challenge and during natural allergen exposure. Int Arch Allergy Immunol 1995; 106:278–285.

55. Linder A, Venge P, Deuschl H. Eosinophil cationic protein and myeloperoxidase in nasal secretion as markers of inflammation in allergic rhinitis. Allergy 1987; 42:583–590.

56. Svensson C, Andersson M, Persson CGA, Venge P, Alkner U, Pipkorn U. Albumin, bradykinins, and eosinophil cationic protein on the nasal mucosal surface in patients with hay fever during natural allergen exposure. J Allergy Clin Immunol 1990; 5:828–833.

57. Klimek L, Eggers G. Olfactory dysfunction in allergic rhinitis is related to nasal eosinophilic inflammation. J Allergy Clin Immunol 1997; 100:158–164.

58. Scherer PW, Hahn II, Mozell MM. The biophysics of nasal airflow. Otolaryngol Clin North Am 1989; 22:265–278.

59. Aubier M, Neukirch C, Maachi M, Boucara D, Engelstatter R, Steinijans V, Samoyeau R, Dehoux M. Effect of slow-release theophylline on nasal antigen challenge in subjects with allergic rhinitis. Eur Respir J 1998; 11:1105–1110.

60. Bisgaard H, Gronborg H, Mygind N, Dahl R, Lindquist N, Venge P. Allergen-induced increase of eosinophil cationic protein in nasal lavage fluid: effect of the glucocorticoid budesonide. J Allergy Clin Immunol 1990; 85:891–895.

61. Tohda Y, Muraki M, Iwanaga T, Kubo H, Fukuoka M, Nakajima S. The effect of theophylline on blood and sputum eosinophils and ECP in patients with bronchial asthma. Int J Immunopharmacol 1998; 20:173–181.

62. Robinson DS, Assoufi B, Durhm SR, Kay AB. Eosinophil cationic protein (ECP) and eosinophil protein x (EPX) concentrations in serum and bronchial lavage fluid in asthma. Effect of prednisolone treatment. Clin Exp Allergy 1995; 25:1118–1127.

63. Beppu T, Ohta N, Gon S, Sakata K, Inamura K, Fukase S, Kimura Y, Koike Y. Eosinophil and eosinophil cationic protein in allergic rhinitis. Acta Otolaryngol (Stockh) 1994; (suppl 511):221–223.

64. Dahl R, Venge P, Olsson I. Blood eosinophil leucocyts and eosinophil cationic protein. Diurnal variation in normal subjects and patients with bronchial asthma. Scand J Respir Dis 1978; 59:323–325.

65. Janson C, Bjornsson E, Enander I, Hakanson L. Seasonal variation in serum eosinophilic cationic protein (S-ECP) in a general population sample. Respir Med 1997; 91:347–349.

66. Jensen EJ, Pedersen B, Schmidt E, Venge P, Dahl R. Serum eosinophilic cationic protein and lactoferrin related to smoking history and lung funciton. Eur Respir J 1994; 7:92–93.

67. Fredens K, Dahl R, Venge P. *In vitro* studies of the interaction between heparin and eosinophil cationic protein. Allergy 1991; 46:27–29.

68. Kurihara K, Yamada T, Saito H, Iikura Y. Basic research into the measurement of eosinophil cationic protein (ECP) in blood samples. Arerugi 1992; 41:512–518.

69. Wantke F, Demmer CM, Gotz M, Jarisch R. Changes in serum ECP levels after storage at room temperature. Allergy 1994; 49:483.

70. Rubira N, Rodrigo MJ, Pena M, Nogueiras C, Cruz MJ, Cadahia A. Blood sample processing effect on eosinophil cationic protein concentration. Ann Allergy Asthma Immunol 1997; 78:394–398.

71. Pena M, Rubira N, Botey J, Rodrigo MJ, Alonso R, Eseverri JL, Marin A, Ras RM. Effect of conditions in obtaining blood samples for ECP testing in children. Allerg Immunol Paris 1996; 28:39–43.

72. Grebski E, Graf C, Hinz G, Wuthrich B, Medici TC. Eosinophil cationic protein in sputum is dependent on temperature and time. Eur Respir J 1998; 11:734–737.

73. Spanevello A, Beghe B, Bianchi A, Migliori GB, Ambrosetti M, Neri M, Ind PW. Comparison of two methods of processing induced sputum: selected versus entire sputum. Am J Respir Crit Care Med 1998; 157:665–668.

74. Klimek L, Rasp G. Norm values for eosinophil cationic protein in nasal secretions: influence of specimen collection. Clin Exp Allergy 1999; 29:374–376.

75. Wright AL, Holberg CJ, Martinez VD. Epidemiology of physician-diagnosed allergic rhinitis in childhood. Pediatrics 1994; 94:895–901.

6

Allergic Rhinitis and Nasal Provocation: Correlation among Objective Symptoms, Mediators, and Eosinophils during the Early- and Late-Phase Reaction after Nasal Provocation in Allergic Patients

PETER A. R. CLEMENT

Free University of Brussels
  (Vrije Universiteit Brussel),
Brussels, Belgium

DE-YUN WANG

The National University of Singapore,
Singapore, Republic of Singapore

Today, the most commonly used sample technique to collect nasal secretions is the nasal lavage technique. With this technique it has been only possible to give qualitative data because of an unknown dilution factor. Biewenga et al. (1) designed a new aspiration system to evaluate protein and immunoglobuline concentrations in human nasal secretions. This direct aspiration system combines the advantages of minimal irritation of the nasal mucosa with the convenience of determine mediator concentrations per gram of secretion. With this technique in mind the authors tried to determine the exact concentrations of selected mediators in the nasal secretions by using the nasal microsuction technique before and after nasal allergen challenge (NAC). It was also attempted to correlate this quantitative data with objective nasal symptoms. In 10 normal test subjects they found the following concentrations for five different mediators: histamine 19 ng/g (range 7.5–32), tryptase 0.0 µU/g (range 0–11), leukotriene C4 (LTC4) 5.7 ng/g (range 3.6–13), prostaglandin D2 (PGD2) 477 pg/g (range 220–788), and eosinophil cationic protein (ECP) 105 ng/g (range 2–281).

First, the authors (2) studied quantitatively the changes within 1 h after nasal allergen challenge of several important mediators such as histamine, tryptase, and LTC4 and they correlated these measures with the objective nasal symptoms such as: the number of sneezes, the weight of the secretions (rhinorrhea), and nasal resistance measured by passive anterior rhinomanometry.

Twenty-six patients with seasonal allergic rhinitis were enrolled outside the pollen season. All measurements were performed before (as a baseline control) and at 1, 10, 30, and 60 min after NAC (Fig. 6.1). The results show that, after NAC, the maximal mediator concentration was already reached after 1 min for histamine (124 ng/mg), 5 min for tryptase (56 μU/g), and 5–10 min for LTC4 (40 ng/g) (Table 6.1). Itching and sneezing started as early as 20–30 s after nasal challenge and they were predominant symptoms within 5 min. Rhinorrhea and nasal obstruction started a few minutes after NAC and lasted until >1 h (Table 6.2). There was no significant correlation between any single mediator and nasal symptoms during the sampling period. This study demonstrates that during early phase reaction the presence of nasal symptoms involves a complex mechanism, reflecting the interaction between the mediators released by inflammatory cells and the receptors on different target organs. When evaluating symptoms during the EPR, one must consider not only the severity of these symptoms but also the time period within which these symptoms occur. For the symptoms of nasal obstruction and rhinorrhea, the early phase reaction lasted >1 h.

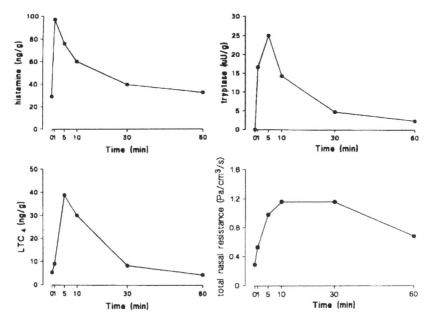

Figure 6.1   Median total nasal resistance and concentrations of histamine, tryptase, and LTC4 in nasal secretions before (time zero) and at different times (min) after nasal allergen challenge in 26 atopic patients outside pollen season. For mediators, baseline recording (time zero) was performed 15 min before challenge.

Table 6.1 Median Maximum Values of Total Nasal Resistance and Concentrations of Histamine, Tryptase, and LTC4 in Nasal Secretions and Time When These Maximum Values Were Reached Within 1 h After Allergen Challenge in 26 Atopic Patients Outside the Pollen Season

Nasal symptoms mediators	Maximum value	Time when maximum reached (min)
Total nasal resistance (Pa/cm^3 per second)	1.4	10–30
Histamine (ng/g)	124	1
Tryptase (μU/g)	56	5
LTC4 (ng/g)	40	5–10

Note: Values of number of sneezes and weight of secretions are not applicable, because they were collected only over sampling period (i.e., 0–1 and 1–5 min).

In another study, the authors, using the same microsuction technique, again determined quantitatively the concentrations of chemical mediators in the nasal secretions after NAC in 18 students with hay-fever and in a control group of 10 healthy volunteers (3). The authors again compared the quantitative data of the mediators with objective nasal findings counting the number of sneezes and recording nasal resistance with passive anterior rhinomanometry (Fig. 6.2). At the same time a sampling of nasal secretion protocol was designed with a follow-up of 3 days after NAC in order to investigate both early and late allergic mediators (Fig. 6.3). Again these data were compared with the objective nasal symptoms. The median base line concentration of five major mediators in the patient group were: histamine 36 ng/g, LTC4 6.4 ng/g, tryptase 0.1 μU/g, PGD2 410 pg/g, ECP 160 ng/g. Significant increases in histamine (214 ng/g), LTC4 (20 ng/g), and tryptase (28 μU/g) were found.

Table 6.2 Median Number of Sneezes and Weight of Secretions Recorded Before (Time Zero) and During Successive Sampling Periods After Nasal Allergen Challenge in 26 Atopic Patients Outside the Pollen Season

Period (min)	Median no. of sneezes (range)	Median weight (g) of secretions (range)	Median weight (g) of secretions/min
0–1	5 (0–22)	0.045 (0–2.1)	0.045
1–5	5 (0–17)	0.280 (0–1.6)	0.070
5–10	0 (0–7)	0.230 (0–2.2)	0.046
10–30	0 (0)	0.705 (0.1–3.7)	0.035
30–60	0 (0)	0.255 (0–2.4)	0.008

Note: Median weight of secretions per minute was also estimated as follows: total median weight of secretions divided by time (min) of each sampling period.

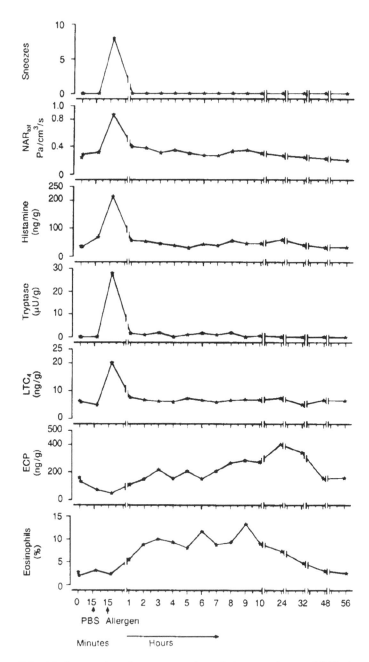

Figure 6.2 Median number of sneezes, total nasal airway resistance (NAR$_{tot}$), concentrations of mediators, and percentage of eosinophils in nasal secretions before (time zero) and after PBS and allergen challenge in 17 atopic patients.

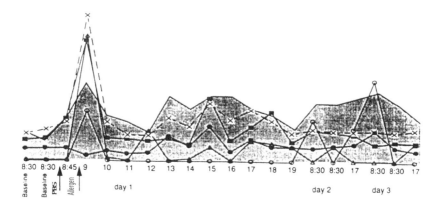

Figure 6.3 Correspondence of mediator peaks with nasal airway resistance (gray background) in a 26-year-old male with atopic rhinitis after nasal allergen challenge (O = number of sneezes, ● = ECP, Δ = tryptase, □ = histamine, and × = LTC4).

At the same time, a significant decrease occurred in ECP (47 ng/g) and PGD2 (226 pg/g) immediately after NAC in the patients studied, probably due to rhinorrhea. Most ECP concentration (94%) increased slowly 1 h after NAC and reached a significantly higher level 24 h later (410 ng/g) (Table 6.3).

Table 6.3 Median Concentrations of Five Mediators During Early and Late Phases (8 and 24 h After Nasal Allergen Challenge) in Nasal Secretions of Patients ($n = 17$) (Wilcoxon Rank Sum Test)

			Late phase	
Mediator	Baseline	Early phase (5 min)	8 h	24 h
Histamine (ng/g)	36 ($p < 0.01$)	214	56 (NS)	60 ($p < 0.01$)
(range)	(22–69)	(77–592)	(21–103)	(23–1502)
Tryptase (μU/g)	0.1 ($p < 0.01$)	28	1.9 (NS)	0.1 (NS)
(range)	(0–6.9)	(0–253)	(0–22)	(0–15)
LTC4 (ng/g)	6.4 ($p < 0.01$)	20	6.6 (NS)	7.5 (NS)
(range)	(2.5–27)	(3.7–128)	(3.2–16)	(3.4–25)
PGD2 (pg/g)	410 ($p < 0.01$)	226	374 (NS)	366 (NS)
(range)	(39–941)	(3–469)	(78–619)	(10–1329)
ECP (ng/g)	160 ($p < 0.01$)	47	267 (NS)	401 ($p < 0.01$)
(range)	(6–1475)	(2–237)	(21–1978)	(32–2298)

In evaluating nasal symptoms, sneezes were present in a high percentage of cases (76%) during the early phase but were uncommon during the late phase (29%). Total nasal obstruction occurred in 94% during the early phase. In contrast, unilateral nasal obstruction presented in 82% during the late phase, whereas total nasal obstruction was present only in 41% during the same late phase. The most common type of late phase nasal obstruction shown by passive anterior rhinomanometry (PAR) was the alternating nasal obstruction (Fig. 6.3).

In a third study (4), a quantitative determination of the inflammatory mediators was performed and correlated with complaints and the measurement of the inflammatory cells in nasal secretions of 18 seasonal allergic rhinitis patients (group 1) outside the pollen season and 40 symptomatic patients (group 2) with seasonal allergic rhinitis during the pollen season. Ten nonallergic subjects (group 3) were also studied as a normal control group. In group 1, 17 (94%) out of 18 patients had an immediate response of nasal symptoms accompanied by a significant increase of histamine, LTC4, and tryptase 5 min after NAC. One hour later, a simultaneous increase was seen both in the percentage of the eosinophils and in the ECP concentration. The eosinophil count reached a peak 2 h after NAC with a duration of 8 h, while the highest ECP level was reached only after 24 h with no clear-cut plateau. In group 2, a high percentage of eosinophils was observed. Mostly one observed significantly ($p > 0.01$) higher concentrations than the baseline values of group 1 of ECP, LTC4, and histamine but not of tryptase (Tables 6.3–6.5). The authors concluded that during the pollen season allergic rhinitis reflects mainly a chronic state of allergic inflammation of the nasal mucosa involving various inflammatory components induced by one or more episodes of early-phase type allergic reaction. Infiltration of eosinophils and consequently release of the various late-phase inflammatory mediators into the nasal secretions are certainly believed to be the predominant pathophysiologic condition in these patients.

The authors also investigated (5,6) the activity of recent antiallergic drugs in the treatment of seasonal allergic rhinitis (Table 6.6). Two experiments were

Table 6.4 Median Baseline Concentrations and Range Between Brackets of Four Mediators in Nasal Secretions of Atopic Patients (Group 1) Outside of the Pollen Season, in Atopic Patients (Group 2) During the Pollen Season, and in Nonallergic Subjects (Group 3)

	Histamine (ng/g)	Tryptase (μU/g)	LTC4 (ng/g)	ECP (ng/g)
Group 1	36	0.1	6.4	160
	(22–69)	(0–6.9)	(2.5–27)	(6–1475)
Group 2	51.5	0	23	410
	(4–146)	(0–84)	(11–77)	(6–2380)
Group 3	19	0	5.7	105
	(7.5–32)	(0–11)	(3.6–13)	(2–281)

Table 6.5 Baseline Percentages of the Leukocytes in Nasal Secretions of Atopic Patients (Group 1) Outside of the Pollen Season, of Atopic Patients (Group 2) During the Pollen Season, and of Nonallergic Subjects (Group 3)

	Neutrophils	Eosinophils	Lymphocyte	Mast cells/basophils
Group 1	96.3	2.7	1	0
	(51–99.7)	(0–45)	(0–5.6)	
Group 2	86	13.5	0	0
	(13–99)	(1–85)	(0–9)	(0–1)
Group 3	99.7	0	0.3	0
	(99–99.7)	(0.06)	(0–0.6)	

performed during the pollen season to study the activity of different antiallergic drugs in the treatment of seasonal allergic rhinitis. NAC was performed to mimic an acute attack of allergic rhinitis and to objectively evaluate the effect of the drugs on the early-phase reaction during season. The first study assessed the effect of an anti-H1 (cetirizine 10 mg a day) and of a combination of an anti-H1 (cetirizine 10 mg) plus an anti-H2 (cimetidine 800 mg a day) antagonists on nasal symptoms, mediator release, and eosinophil count in a group of 16 patients with seasonal allergic rhinitis. During the same season, a second study compared in a randomized way (two parallel groups), the effect of budesonide (Rhinocort Aqua) and azelastine (Allergodil nasal spray) in a group of 14 patients. Results showed that both antihistamines, applied topically or dosed orally, reduced sneezing even when significant increases of histamine concentration in nasal secretions were evidenced immediately after NAC. When a combination of cetirizine and cimetidine was administered, a significant ($p < 0.01$) reduction of nasal airway resistance after NAC was demonstrated as well. In addition, topical application of budesonide showed a strong ($p < 0.01$)

Table 6.6 Effect of Different Drugs on the Subjective Symptoms Before the Allergen Challenge and Objective Nasal Symptoms After the Allergen Challenge

	Subjects symptoms score before NAC					Objective symptoms after NAC
	Sneezing	Itching	Rhinorrhea	Congestion	NAR_{tot}	Sneezing
Cetirizine	++	+	+	+	−	++
Ceterizine and cimetidine	++	++	++	+	++	++
Budesonide	−	−	−	−	+	−
Azelastine	+	+	+	+	+	+

Note: −, not significant; +, $p < 0.05$; ++, $p < 0.01$; NAR_{tot}, total nasal airway resistance.

downregulation of the infiltration and activation of eosinophils during the season, and on tryptase release after NAC. These effects lasted at least for 1 week after therapy.

Finally, the authors studied the onset of action of fluticasone propionate aqueous nasal spray (FPANS) on 28 patients with seasonal allergic rhinitis at the end of the pollen season (7). At that time, the patients were still primed and very sensitive to nasal provocation. They did not receive any medication for the last 2 weeks and they did not have any corticosteroids 30 days prior to nasal provocation. This study was conducted utilizing two periods (7 days) of FPANS 200 µg once daily and placebo in a randomised, double blind, placebo-controlled and cross-over design. The patients were followed for each period of 7 days and multiple NAC were performed. During that week the patients used fluticasone propionate according to the recommendations of the company. This study demonstrated that FPANS has a significant effect on the inflammatory condition of the nasal mucosa characterised by reduction of eosinophils and ECP release induced by allergen challenge. This effect can start after about 48 h and becomes more pronounced after 7 days of treatment. There was also a significant, or almost significant, improvement in the change of symptoms score after allergen challenge, which sets in after 48 h after the start of the treatment and shows a clear cut effect on all the symptoms after seven days. From this study it also appears that the effect of fluticasone propionate aqueous nasal spray on mediator release during the early phase reaction induced by allergen challenge and the relief of acute nasal symptoms had not reached its full effect after 1 week of treatment.

In conclusion, one can state that the allergic nasal reaction is a very complex reaction consisting of an early- and a late-phase reaction. During season the complexity increases because consecutive nasal challenges occur even before a steady state late phase reaction can be reached. It is also obvious that the nasal reaction especially during the late phase is not mediated by only one mediator or one cell population. From our studies it was also clear that after an allergen exposure the only drug that can give fast relief for the patient is an anti-H1 drug. On the other hand, an antihistamine only blocks the antihistamine receptor and does not induce a clear cut change in any mediator concentration or in the eosinophilic inflammation. Only topical corticosteroids have a much broader action, as well on symptoms as on mediator release and eosinophilic infiltration. Unfortunately, they start to act after 2–3 weeks reaching a maximum effect only after a week.

References

1. Biewenga J, Stoop AE, Baker HE, Swart SJ, Nauta JJP, van Kamp FJ, Vander Baan S. Nasal secretions from patients with polyps and healthy individuals, collected with a new aspiration system: evaluation of total protein and immunoglobulin concentrations. Ann Clin Biochem 1991; 28:260–266.

2. Wang D, Smitz J, Waterschoot S, Clement P. An approach to the understanding of the nasal early-phase reaction induced by nasal allergen challenge. Allergy 1997; 52:162–167.
3. Wang D, Clement P, Smitz J, Derde MP. Concentrations of chemical mediators in nasal secretions after nasal allergen challenges in atopic patients. Eur Arch Otolaryngol 1995; 252(suppl 1):S40–S43.
4. Wang D, Clement P, Smitz J, De Waele M, Derde MP. Correlations between complaints, inflammatory cells and mediator concentrations in nasal secretions after nasal allergen challenge and during natural allergen exposure. Int Arch Allergy Immunol 1995; 106:278–285.
5. Wang D, Clement P, Smitz J, De Waele M, Derde MP. The activity of recent antiallergic drugs in the treatment of seasonal allergic rhinitis. Acta Otolaryngol Belg 1996; 50:25–32.
6. Wang D, Clement P, Smitz J. Effect of H1 and H2 antagonists on nasal symptoms and mediator release in atopic patients after nasal allergen challenge during the pollen season. Acta Otolaryngol (Stockh) 1996; 116:91–96.
7. Wang D, Duyck F, Smitz J, Clement P. Efficacy and onset of action of fluticasone propionate aqueous nasal spray on nasal symptoms, eosinophil count, and mediator release after nasal allergen challenge in patients with seasonal allergic rhinitis. Allergy 1998; 53:375–382.

7

Anatomy and Development of the Nasal Septum in Relation to Septal Surgery in Children

CAREL D. A. VERWOERD and **HENRIETTE L. VERWOERD-VERHOEF**

Erasmus University Medical Center,
Rotterdam, The Netherlands

I. Introduction

In most textbooks of otorhinolaryngology little attention is paid to development of the nasal septum in children with respect to nasal surgery. The child-specific features of the nasal septum were disregarded as it was generally accepted to postpone septo(rhino)plasty in children until the young patient had reached the age of 16 years and nasal growth had dropped to a minimum. This "tradition" was based on numerous reports of defective growth of the nose after partial submucous septal resection at a young age.

Following the introduction of more conservative surgical techniques in rhinosurgery, the tendency to introduce these techniques in children has increased considerably. It was even suggested that contrary to the previously performed partial submucous *resection* of the septum, submucous *correction* would not interfere with nasal growth and thus, may be considered as a "safe" procedure in children (1–6).

Certainly, the discussion between opponents and advocates of nasal surgery in children is still not closed (7,8). It seems, therefore, appropriate to review the present knowledge of anatomy and developmental mechanics of the child's nose in relation to the surgical management of pathology of the growing nasal skeleton and the nasal septum in particular.

II. Specific Anatomy of the Infant Nose

It is important to recognize that the face of an infant is not a miniature, small-scale edition of the adult face. Characteristic for the head of neonates is the relatively large size of the neurocranium and orbits. This is related to the rapid growth rate during fetal life of the brain and eyes, in particular, in comparison to the nose, maxilla, and mandible. This combination of a proportionally large brain skull and a smaller facial part outlines the specific "baby face" of the young child [Fig. 7.1(a) and (b)]. Compared to the adult nose, the infant nose

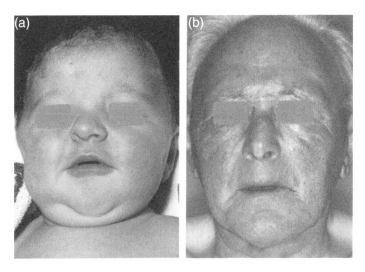

Figure 7.1   (a) Face of newborn. (b) Adult face.

shows less frontal projection, a shorter dorsum, a larger nasolabial angle [Fig. 7.2(a) and (b)], a shorter columella, a flat tip, and round nares [Fig. 7.3(a) and (b)].

During postnatal growth, the nose, maxilla, and mandible grow faster than the brain skull, transforming the "baby face" into the adult physiognomy (Fig. 7.2).

In the newborn the anatomy of the nasal skeleton differs significantly from the adult nose (9,10). The cartilaginous septum reaches from columella to crista Galli and sphenoid (Fig. 7.4) whereas the perpendicular plate has not yet been formed (11). The ventrocaudal end of the cartilaginous septum is connected to the anterior nasal spine through the septospinal ligament. The triangular non-cartilaginous part of the septum, which is bordered by the basal rim of the septal cartilage, the palatal bone and the posterior (choanal) edge of the nasal septum, consists of connective tissue with irregular lamellae of bone, representing the anlage of the *inferior* part of the vomer (12). On both sides of the basal rim of the cartilaginous septum a process of intramembranous ossification produces bony wings as *superior* part of the vomeral bone. These wings make a longitudinal medial gutter enfolding the basal rim of the septal cartilage, and merge with the inferior midline anlage to form the total vomer (Fig. 7.5). In this stage the

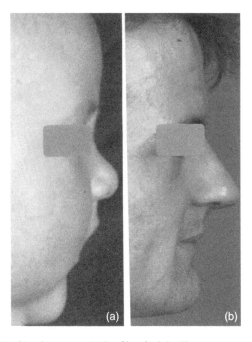

Figure 7.2   (a) Profile of neonate. (b) Profile of adult. The upper one-third of the face of the infant (brain skull) is enlarged to the dimensions of the adult face. Middle (midface) and lower (jaws) one-third are proportionally larger in the adult.

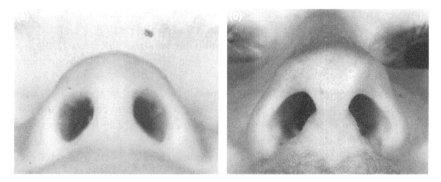

Figure 7.3 Basal view of the nose. A young child (a) usually has rounder nares with shorter columella and more flat tip, than the adult (b).

vomer anlage, however, plays no supporting role for the cartilaginous septum. The latter is still primarily based on the sphenoid.

The mechanical function of the septal part of the dorsoseptal cartilage is reflected in the regional differences in thickness of the tissue (Fig. 7.4). A zone of thicker cartilage (2.5–3.5 mm) spreads from the sphenoid to the nasal dorsum (13). A second zone of equally thick cartilage is found in the basal rim of the septum, reaching from sphenoid to anterior nasal spine. The centroventral

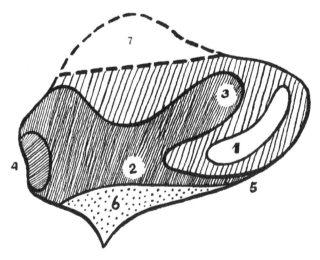

Figure 7.4 Schematic representation of nasal septum in the newborn. Regional differences in thickness of the neonatal septal cartilage. (1) Centroventral zone; (2) sphenospinal zone; (3) sphenodorsal zone; (4) sphenoid bone; (5) anterior nasal spine; (6) vomer; (7) crista Galli.

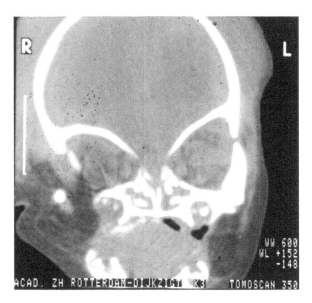

Figure 7.5 CT scan of nose and orbita in frontal section (late fetal stage). There are no osseous structures in the medial part of anterior cranial base; inferior part of vomer with wings on both sides of the basal rim of septal cartilage (median gutter); bilateral osseous skeleton of concha superior, media, and inferior.

area is by far the thinnest part of the septum (0.4–0.5 mm). Actually, the configuration of thicker and thinner zones strongly suggests that in the neonate the nasal dorsum is primarily supported by the sphenodorsal column of thick cartilage within the septum (14). The columellar rim is only slightly thickened compared to the centroventral area; its contribution to supporting the nasal dorsum will, therefore, be minimal at this stage.

Unlike in the adult, the upper lateral cartilages of the newborn [Fig. 7.6(a) and (b)] fully extend under the nasal bones and are united with the cartilaginous anlage of the paramedial parts of the anterior cranial base (15). The septum and upper lateral cartilages are not separated anatomical entities. Together they are one T-bar-shaped structure (Fig. 7.7). This is the dorsoseptal cartilage, which acts as a supporting framework for the external nose (14). In theory, such a T-bar is much stronger than a simple plate-like structure, and therefore, more suitable to buttress the developing nasal dorsum.

In the human newborn the alar cartilages, which have developed separately from the dorsoseptal cartilage, are very thin and relatively broad. They show the same topographic relationship to the upper lateral cartilages and septum as in the adult. Mostly in newborns the soft tissues covering the nasal skeleton include a thick layer of subcutaneous fat [Fig. 7.6(a)].

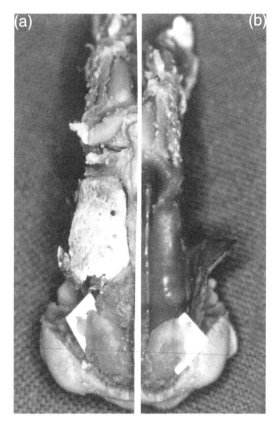

Figure 7.6 Anatomical dissection of the nose of a neonate in two stages: (a) after removal of skin and (b) removal of nasal bone, with alar cartilage (on paper), upper lateral cartilage reaching the cartilaginous anterior cranial base and supraseptal groove.

III. Postnatal Development of the Nose

During childhood the proportions in the face change considerably. The nose, maxilla, and mandible grow more rapidly and over a longer period than the brain skull. The baby face is converted into the adult face through a more prominent profile of nose, upper and lower jaw. In frontal view an elongation of the middle and lower part of the face can be observed [Figs. 7.1(a), (b) and 7.2(a), (b)]. In a longitudinal study the (adolescent) growth spurt of the nose has been reported to take place around puberty (16). In general, the process of nasal development ends later in the male adolescent (18–20 years) than in the female (16–18 years), but growth may well continue into the third decade of life.

Apart from the increase in the dimensions of the nose, postnatal development is characterized by marked changes in the anatomy of the nasal skeleton. The cephalic part of both upper lateral cartilages shows a gradual regression in

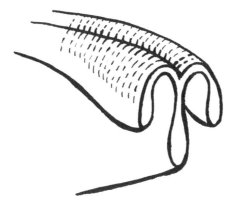

Figure 7.7 T-bar-shaped dorsoseptal cartilage.

caudal direction (Fig. 7.7). As a result, the part of the upper lateral cartilage remaining under the nasal bone is in the adult reduced to a small and variable strip (3–15 mm) of cartilage (17). In the meantime, the crista Galli is transformed into bone by endochondral ossification and the osseous anlage of both ethmoid complexes are formed.

Endochondral ossification of the cartilaginous septum starts in the area adjacent to the crista Galli and will proceed in ventrocaudal direction [Figs. 7.8(a–c) and 7.9(a–c)], forming the perpendicular plate of the ethmoid (12,18).

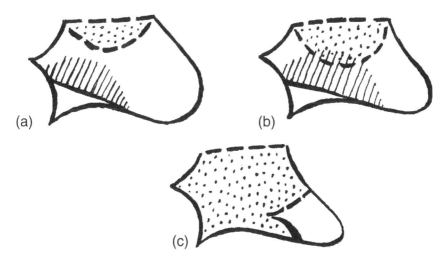

Figure 7.8 Progressive ossification (dotted) of the cartilaginous septum with fusion of perpendicular plate and vomer. Change in support of the cartilaginous nasal dorsum from sphenoid in infant (a) to caudal rim of perpendicular plate (c); intermediate stage with vomeral wings (striped) overlapping the ossifying perpendicular plate (b).

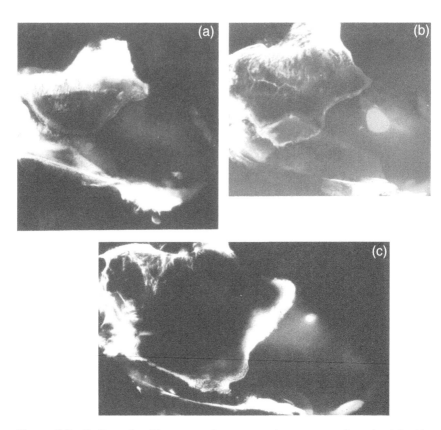

Figure 7.9 Radiographs of human nasal septum specimens, as seen from the right side. Only the thickened rim of the bone of the perpendicular plate is demonstrated; the central parts are too thin to produce contrast. (a) Five years of age: zone of not yet ossified cartilage between perpendicular plate and vomer wing. (b) Aged 17 years: overlap of perpendicular plate and vomer wing. (c) Aged 30 years: rim of thick cartilage on the caudal side of the perpendicular plate (a firm base for the septal cartilage) and bony canal for sphenoid tail. See also Figs. 7.8 and 7.10.

The enlarging perpendicular plate will ultimately reach to and extend between the vomer wings (alae) establishing the ethmoido-vomeral junction [Fig. 7.9(b)]. This junction shows many developmental variations (19). The alae of the vomer often develop asymmetrically, or can even be absent on one side (Fig. 7.10). Occasionally, the basal rim of the cartilaginous septum is deviated from the midline, and the vomer follows this deviation (20). At rhinoscopia anterior the resulting deformity is presented as a spina vomeri or crista.

In young children, there is no direct relation between septal crista or vomeral spine and deviation of the nasal dorsum as the growing dorsoseptal cartilage is still mainly based on the sphenoid and not on the vomer (Fig. 7.8).

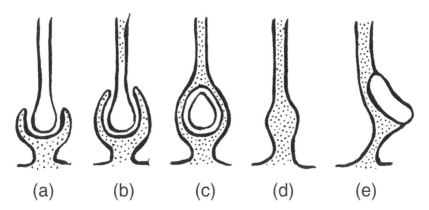

Figure 7.10 Variations of ethmoido-vomeral junction; (a) septal cartilage with thin basal rim in vomeral gutter; (b) ossifying front of perpendicular plate has not reached the vomer wings; (c) fusion of perpendicular plate and partial overlap with vomeral alae, resulting in a canal containing the basal rim of cartilage (sphenoid tail); (d) complete ossification of basal rim leading to complete fusion of vomer wings and perpendicular plate; (e) ethmoido-vomeral (dis)junction; persistent cartilage (sphenoid tail) is only covered by the vomer ala on one side.

The median position of the nasal dorsum is further ensured by the upper lateral parts of the dorsoseptal T-bar construct.

When the perpendicular plate is increasing in size through endochondral ossification, the cartilaginous septum gradually looses contact with the sphenoid. Instead, the cartilage becomes firmly anchored to the broad ventral rim of the perpendicular plate (Fig. 7.9). The cartilage which remains present between vomer alae and perpendicular plate shows a varying degree of ossification. It is sometimes even found in the adult as a cartilaginous elongation extending to the sphenoid (sphenoid tail), in other cases it is completely ossified (Figs. 7.9 and 7.10).

In case of a unilateral cleft of lip, alveolus, and palate the basal rim of the septal cartilage becomes gradually deviated to the cleft side with increasing age (Fig. 7.11). Consequently, the vomer (the inferior part), extending between the palatal process on the non-cleft side and the deviated septal rim, will adopt a semi-horizontal position, giving the impression of a broadened nasal floor on this side (12,21,22).

IV. Mechanisms of Facial Development

Surgical procedures in face and nose of a child hold the risk of interfering with the processes of facial growth. The various parts of the facial skeleton and bony skull do influence each other during growth. Some parts appear to be dominant, whereas others tend to adapt to neighboring structures. Knowledge of these

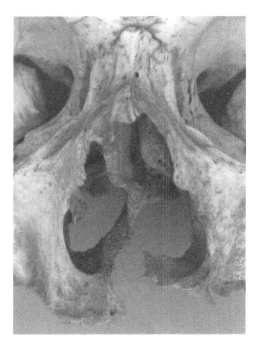

Figure 7.11   Frontal view of human skull with unilateral cleft of upper jaw and palate. Semi-horizontal position of the inferior part of the vomer, broadening the nasal floor on the right non-cleft side.

complex developmental interrelations, as far as the face and nose are concerned, was still fragmentary. Animal studies, however, demonstrated clearly that the dorsoseptal cartilage plays a dominant role in postnatal development of the nose and neighboring parts of the midface. Some conclusions regarding the mechanisms of facial growth derived from animal experiments are the following:

1. An intact dorsoseptal cartilage is mandatory for the normal development of nose and maxilla. Local defects of dorsoseptal cartilage, either in septum or upper lateral, change the pattern of growth of the total cartilaginous structure, and indirectly of the nasal bones, the vomer, and to some extent the maxilla. The dorsoseptal cartilage is considered to be a growth center during childhood (12,23). In particular, growth of the cartilage in the sphenodorsal zone is held responsible for the increasing prominence of the nasal dorsum (Fig. 7.4). Growth in the sphenospinal zone contributes to the forward expansion of the maxilla.

2. The bony structures, on the other hand, also exert an influence on the growing dorsoseptal cartilage. When growth of the frontonasal (23) or premaxillo-maxillary suture (24) is impeded on one side, it will result in an apparent asymmetry of the nose and maxilla.

In healthy young animals, unilateral excision of the premaxillo-maxillary suture leads to a specific syndrome of abnormal nasal and midfacial growth. A similar abnormal facial development is observed in patients with an untreated cleft of lip, alveolus, and palate. Subtotal resection of the nasal bone(s), without injuring the suture, does not alter the growth pattern of the dorsoseptal cartilage (23).

V. Nasal and Facial Development After Loss of Septal Cartilage

The above-mentioned morphogenetic mechanisms which have been elaborated in more detail by animal studies, can explain some, at first sight contradictory, observations in adolescent or adult patients who had a septal injury in early childhood.

In general, in patients with a septal perforation in the thin centroventral area, dating back to a nasal trauma at a young age, a normal nasal dorsum is found [Fig. 7.12(a)]. The explanation is that the thin centroventral

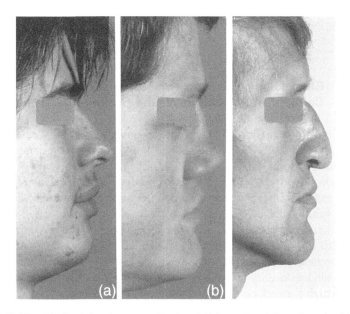

Figure 7.12 (a) Nasal development after (partial) loss of septal cartilage in childhood. Nasal dorsum is normally developed despite traumatic perforation in the centroventral area of the septum. (b) Irregular flattening and broadening of the bony and cartilaginous nasal dorsum, retroposition of the anterior nasal spine and underdevelopment of the maxilla, ascribed to loss of sphenodorsal and sphenospinal zones in the cartilaginous septum at a young age. (c) Normal bony part of the nasal dorsum, underdevelopment of the cartilaginous dorsum and maxilla with retroposition of the anterior nasal spine after loss of the ventrobasal part of the septum, at a young age.

area bears no morphogenetic significance; nose and maxilla will grow normally as long as the thick sphenodorsal and sphenospinal zones are intact, see also Fig. 7.4.

The most typical form of posttraumatic nasal maldevelopment in patients is seen as an irregular flattening and broadening of the bony and cartilaginous nasal dorsum, combined with an underdevelopment of the upper jaw and a retroposition of the anterior nasal spine [Fig. 7.12(b)]. These patients often have a history of a septal abscess or haematoma following trauma, during one of the first years of life. It is assumed that damage to the growing sphenodorsal zone of thick cartilage accounts for the maldevelopment of the nasal dorsum whereas injury to the sphenospinal zone explains a later retroposition of the nasal spine and the maxilla. The relative prominence of the nasal tip is due to the support by the alar cartilages, which are independent of the septum.

Another type of post-traumatic facial maldevelopment includes the combination of a normal bony nasal dorsum, a low cartilaginous dorsum, and a retroposition of the anterior nasal spine and maxilla [Fig. 7.12(c)]. This malformation can be ascribed to the loss of the ventrobasal part of the septal cartilage, and must not be confused with the hump nose, which is due to an increased sagittal dimension of the bony and/or cartilaginous dorsum.

VI. Biomechanical Properties of the Growing Septal Cartilage in Relation to Wound Healing After Trauma

During surgical exploration of a malformed septum, next to local defects in the cartilage, overlap and/or angulation of the fractured parts is a current finding in children. The local defect points to the very restricted capacity of cartilage regeneration. The reason for overlapping edges and angulations is more complex, and refers to biomechanical properties of cartilage and specific features of wound healing (25).

Resilience and strength are typical features of the septal cartilage. Gibson (26) and later, Fry (27) have ascribed these mechanical properties to a balanced system of interlocked stresses. In other words, it is hypothesized that the water-binding quality of proteins in the cartilage cells and matrix build up a stress, which is interlocked in a three-dimensional network of collagen fibers, stretching out between the dense (sub)perichondrial fibrous zone on each side of the septum.

It is suggested that one-side injury to this network of collagen fibers results in disruption of the balanced system of interlocked stresses and thus, in an immediate bending of the septum, as observed in isolated septa of rabbits and human septa (27). The immediate overlap of cut edges after transection of the septum *in vivo* and *in situ*, as observed in animal experiments [Fig. 7.13(a)], is thought to be another effect of the release of interlocked stresses within

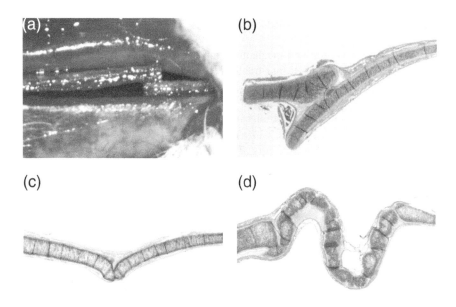

Figure 7.13 (a) Illustrations from animal experiments (young rabbits). Immediate overlap of the cut edges after transection of the nasal septal cartilage (dorsal view). (b) Side-to-side reconnection of septal fragments. (c) Angulation (deviation) after transecting the septum. (d) Septal deviation after implantation of crushed cartilage.

hyaline cartilage (25). This phenomenon prevents an end-to-end reconnection of separated parts.

In a short time, cut or fractured edges of septal cartilage are covered by regenerating perichondrium (28). Reconnection of the straight approximated or overlapping ends takes place by end-to-end or side-to-side union of the perichondrial layers [Fig. 7.13(b)]. The site of fusion and/or overlap remains a mechanically weak point. During later development, progressive angulation at these sites will regularly occur [Fig. 7.13(c) and (d)].

VII. Septal Deviations

Deformities (deviation, crista, spina vomeri) of the nasal septum can be the result of "spontaneous," variations of the development such as those previously discussed in relation to the septo-vomeral or ethmoido-vomeral junction.

On the other hand, external trauma to the nose can cause complete fractures, or incomplete when the perichondrium on one side is preserved. These injuries, often not recognized by parents or physicians, can lead to apparent deformities during further growth.

VIII. Preferred Fracture Lines

In view of the structural and mechanical inhomogeneity of the nasal septum in children it may be expected that fractures occur preferably at sites which have the least mechanical strength (Fig. 7.4) (29). In case of dislocation of the caudal end of the septum—a common septal deformity in children—the fracture line is located in the area of thin cartilage, cephalic and semi-parallel to the thickened columellar rim [Fig. 7.14(a) and (b)].

A C-formed fracture line (Fig. 7.15) has also been observed in the septum of a child (29). The fracture runs through the thin part of the septum, superior to the thick basal rim, to reach the fragile central part of the perpendicular plate. From there, the fracture line takes a cephalic and, later, anterior directed course. A rupture between the perpendicular plate and septal cartilage is apparently prevented by their firm connection.

IX. Neonatal Septal Deviations

In newborns, the incidence of septal deformities has been reported by most authors to be less than 4% (Fig. 7.16). Spontaneous straightening of the septum seemed to occur in half of the cases. The deviations were described as "bends" in the cartilaginous nasal septum (30). Such a deviation, appearing as a smooth concavity/convexity, is most probably due to bending in the weak zone superior to the basal rim (Fig. 7.4).

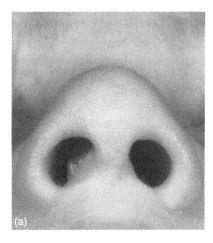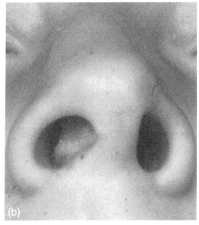

Figure 7.14   (a) Luxation of caudal end of the septum in the right nostril, columella void of septal cartilage, midline tip supported by alar cartilages. (b) Anterior septal deviation, caudal rim in columella, deviated tip. In (a) and (b) septum fracture semi-parallel to columellar rim.

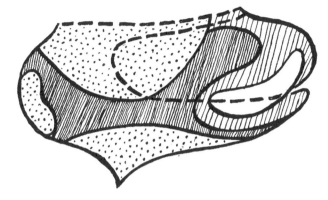

Figure 7.15 Schematic presentation of a C-formed septal fracture through centroventral zone of thin cartilage and perpendicular plate, as observed in a 4-year-old boy. (Courtesy Dr. J. van Loosen.)

X. Developmental Aspects of Septal Correction: Conclusions from Morphological and Experimental Studies

How the nose grows after septal surgery is determined by: (a) the genetic condition determining facial development, (b) the previously existing pathology, and (c) surgery. The effects on nasal growth of various surgical interventions have been assessed in a series of animal experiments (24,25,28,31–34). Conclusions, as far as they are relevant to septoplasty, are summarized as follows:

1. Elevation of the mucoperichondrium on one or two sides may be considered a safe procedure; no disadvantages in terms of disturbed

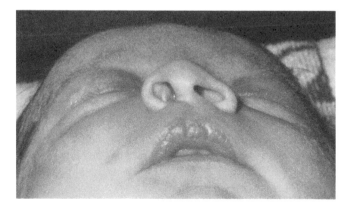

Figure 7.16 Septal deviation in the newborn.

growth were demonstrated, on condition that the cartilage itself is not injured.

2. The elevated perichondrium can be stimulated by blood to produce extra fibrocartilage, which is different in morphology from the hyaline cartilage of the septum. This fibrocartilage, like scar tissue, shows hardly any growth, which can lead to maldevelopment of the dorsoseptal cartilage and ultimately, of the nose. Therefore, intraseptal collection of blood should be avoided.

3. Substantial defects in the thick sphenodorsal and/or sphenospinal zone will result in underdevelopment (too low, too short) of the nose.

4. Transecting the septal cartilage bears the risk of overlapping cut edges and the promotion of angulations during further growth. Therefore, it is strongly advised to carefully adapt (and suture) the edges.

5. Closing a cartilage defect by reimplantation of crushed [Fig. 7.13(d)] or noncrushed autologous cartilage grafts helps to prevent septal perforation and excessive scar formation. Then, some improvement of nasal growth can be achieved. It certainly does not result in a normalization of growth, mainly due to bending and dislocation of the implanted material in relation to the nonmobilized parts of the septum.

6. Alloplastic or biomaterials, in general, are not capable of growth. Therefore, allogenic non-growing implants in a growing septum induce a severe "stunting" of the growing septum and consequently, a maldevelopment of the nose.

7. A deviated basal rim of the septal cartilage can be partly resected without a risk for disturbing the outgrowth of the nasal dorsum. The septospinal ligament should be kept intact.

8. The vomer is not essential for nasal development, and therefore can be (partially) resected as long as the perpendicular plate and the septal cartilage are preserved.

9. Be aware of the progressing endochondral ossification of the cartilaginous septum. In younger children the greater part of the septum is cartilaginous; the caudal border of the perpendicular plate has a highly variable position and cannot function as a landmark during the dissection of the septum. Beware of injuries to the cartilaginous cranial base!

10. Try to avoid posterior chondrotomy or resection of the ventral rim of the perpendicular plate since this area is of permanent importance for the support of the cartilaginous nasal dorsum and the increasing prominence of the nasal dorsum during childhood.

11. Unilateral loss of an upper lateral cartilage causes progressive deviation of the nasal dorsum and the nasal septum to the non-injured side. This underlines the importance of:

    (a) preventing the loss of an upper lateral cartilage in case of a dorsum haematoma,

    (b)   repositioning the upper lateral cartilage which was dislocated as a result of the ruptured connection with the bony nasal aperture,

    (c)   suturing the upper lateral(s) to the septum in case of surgical or traumatic separation.

12.   The development of the nose (and dorsoseptal cartilage) is not disturbed by osteotomies and mobilization of the nasal bones.

13.   To date, there are no experimental observations warning against the open-approach for septorhinoplasty, as far as scars in the soft tissue are concerned. Uncertain is the developmental potential of the (radically) reconstructed septum which will determine the ultimate nasal form (35).

XI. Concluding Remarks

In recent years the biological basis of surgical treatment for nasal septal pathology in children has been broadened by new data concerning developmental anatomy, developmental mechanisms and wound healing. Still, the effects of surgery on nasal (midfacial) development are not completely predictable. A well-organized follow-up of all surgical cases is then of very great importance. Clinical and experimental data should be studied comparatively and over a long period.

A future challenge is to develop the concept of growth-correcting surgery, next to functional and aesthetic rhinosurgery. Growth-correcting surgery must be based on thorough knowledge of the developmental mechanisms of the midface. Currently, the restricted regenerative capacity of cartilage seems to be the limiting factor. Further research aiming at improvement of wound healing, probably with the local application of growth factors and the use of tissue-engineered cartilage (36–38), might open new avenues for surgery dealing with the injured or deformed cartilaginous nasal framework in growing children.

Acknowledgments

We acknowledge the cooperation in research of Dr. J. van Loosen, Dr. C. A. Meeuwis, Dr. G. J. Nolst Trenité, and Dr. R. M. L. Poublon.

References

1.   Bailey BJ. Nasal fractures. In: Bailey BJ, ed. Head and Neck Surgery. Otolaryngology. Vol. 78. Lippincott Comp., 1993:1004–1005.

2.   Farrior RT, Conolly ME. Septorhinoplasty in children. Otolaryngol Clin North Am 1990; 109:454–460.

3. Gross ChW, Boyle TR. Nasal surgery for congenital and acquired disease. In: Smith JD, Bumsted R, eds. Pediatric Facial Plastic Surgery and Reconstructive Surgery. Vol. 3. New York: Raven Press, 1993:31–41.

4. Ortiz-Monasterio F, Olmedo A. Corrective rhinoplasty before puberty: a long-term follow-up. Plast Reconstr Surg 1981; 381–391.

5. Stucker FJ, Bryarly RC, Shockley WW. Management of nasal trauma in children. Arch Otolaryngol 1984; 110:190–192.

6. Tardy ME, Broadway D. Septorhinoplasty in the preadolescent. In: Healy G, ed. Common Problems in Pediatric Otolaryngology. Chicago: Yearbook Medical Public, 1990.

7. Pirsig W. Open questions in nasal surgery in children. Rhinology 1986; 24:37–40.

8. Potsic WP, Cotton RT, Handler SD. Nasal deformity. In: Surgical Pediatric Otolaryngology. Vol. 13. New York: Thieme Medical Publishers Inc, 1997:168–180.

9. Fairbanks DNF. Embryology and anatomy. In: Bluestone CD, Stool SE, eds. Pediatric Otolaryngology. Vol. 28. WB Saunders Comp., 1990:611–617.

10. Stool SE, Marasovich WA. Postnatal craniofacial growth and development. In: Bluestone CD, Stool SE, eds. Pediatric Otolaryngology. Vol. 2. WB Saunders Comp, 1990:17–31.

11. Loosen van J, Verwoerd-Verhoef HL, Verwoerd CDA. The nasal septal cartilage in the newborn. Rhinology 1988; 26:161–165.

12. Verwoerd CDA, Loosen van J, Schütte HE, Verwoerd-Verhoef HL, Velzen van D. Surgical aspects of the anatomy of the vomer in children and adults. Rhinology 1989; (suppl 9):87–91.

13. Loosen van J, van Velzen D, Verwoerd-Verhoef HL, Verwoerd CDA. Growth characteristics of the human nasal septum. Rhinology 1996; 34:78–82.

14. Verwoerd CDA, Verwoerd-Verhoef HL. Rhinosurgery in children: surgical and developmental aspects. In: Nolst Trenité GJ, ed. Rhinoplasty. Vol. 20. 2nd ed. The Hague, The Netherlands: Kugler, 1998:210–211.

15. Poublon RML, Verwoerd CDA, Verwoerd-Verhoef HL. Anatomy of the upper lateral cartilages in the human newborn. Rhinology 1990; 28:41–46.

16. Graber TM. Postnatal development of cranial, facial and oral structures: the dynamics of facial growth. In: Orthodontics; Principles and Practice. Vol. 2. Philadelphia: WB Saunders, 1966:69–78.

17. Lang J. Clinical Anatomy of the Nose, Nasal Cavity and Paranasal Sinuses. New York: Thieme Verlag, 1989.

18. Schultz-Coulon HJ, Eckermaier L. Zum postnatalen Wachstum der Nasenscheidewand. Acta Otolaryngol 1976; 82:131–142.

19. Takahashi R. The formation of the nasal septum and its evolutionary paradox. Acta Otolaryngol 1988; (suppl 443):1–160.

20. Takahashi R. The evolution of the nasal septum and the formation of septal deformity. Rhinology 1988; 6:1–23.

21. Verwoerd CDA, Mladina R, Nolst Trenité GJ, Pigott RW. The nose in children with unilateral cleft lip and palate. Int J Ped Otorhinolaryngol 1995; 32:S45–S52.

22. Verwoerd-Verhoef HL, Verwoerd CDA. Nasal malformations. In: van Cauwenberge P, Wang DY, Ingels K, Bachert C, eds. The Nose. The Hague, The Netherlands: Kugler, 1998:335–342.

23. Verwoerd-Verhoef HL, Verwoerd CDA. Sinonasal surgery and growth: an experimental study review. In: Tos M, Thomsen J, eds. Rhinology: a State of the Art. Amsterdam, New York: Kugler, 1995:195–201.
24. Verwoerd CDA, Urbanus NAM, Verwoerd-Verhoef HL. Growth mechanisms in skulls with facial clefts. Acta Otolaryngol (Stockh) 1979; 87:335–339.
25. Verwoerd CDA, Verwoerd-Verhoef HL, Meeuwis CA. Stress and wound healing of the cartilaginous nasal septum. Acta Otolaryngol (Stockh) 1989; 107:441–445.
26. Gibson T, Davis WB. The distortion of autogenous cartilage grafts: its cause and prevention. Br J Plast Surg 1958; 10:257–274.
27. Fry HJH. Nasal skeletal trauma and the interlocked stresses of the nasal septal cartilage. Br J Plast Surg 1967; 20:46–158.
28. Verwoerd-Verhoef HL, Ten Koppel PGJ, van Osch GJVM, Meeuwis CA, Verwoerd CDA. Wound healing of cartilage structures in the head and neck region. Int J Ped Otorhinolaryngol 1998; 43:241–251.
29. van Velzen D, van Loosen J, Verwoerd CDA, Verwoerd-Verhoef HL. Persistent pattern of variations in thickness of the nasal septum: implications for stress and trauma as illustrated by a complex fracture in a 4-year-old boy. Adv Oto-Rhino-Laryngology 1997; 51:46–70.
30. Kent SE, Reid AP, Brain DJ, Nairn ER. Neonatal septal deviations. J Royal Soc Med 1988; 81:132–135.
31. Meeuwis JA, Verwoerd HL, Verwoerd CDA. Normal and abnormal nasal growth after partial submucous resection of the cartilaginous septum. Acta Otolaryngol (Stockh) 1993; 113:379–382.
32. Nolst Trenité GJ, Verwoerd CDA, Verwoerd-Verhoef HL. Reimplantation of autologous septal cartilage in the growing nasal septum I and II. Rhinology 1997; 25:225–237(I), 1988; 26:25–32(II).
33. Verwoerd-Verhoef HL, Meeuwis CA, van der Heul RO. Wound healing of the nasal septal perichondrium in young rabbits. ORL 1990; 52:180–186.
34. Verwoerd-Verhoef HL, Meeuwis CA, van der Heul RO, Verwoerd CDA. Histologic evaluation of crushed cartilage grafts in the growing nasal septum of young rabbits. ORL 1991; 53:305–309.
35. Crysdale WS, Tatham B. External septorhinoplasty in children. Laryngoscope 1985; 95:12.
36. Pirsig W, Bean JK, Lenders H, Verwoerd CDA, Verwoerd-Verhoef HL. Cartilage transformation in a composite graft of demineralized bovine bone matrix and ear perichondrium used in a child, for the reconstruction of the nasal septum. Int J Ped Otorhinolaryngol 1995; 32(2):171–183.
37. Ten Koppel PGJ, van Osch GJVM, Verwoerd CDA, Verwoerd-Verhoef HL. Efficacy of perichondrium and a trabecular demineralized bone matrix for generating cartilage. Plast & Rec Surg 1998; 102:212–220.
38. Verwoerd-Verhoef HL, Bean JK, van Osch GJVM, Ten Koppel PGJ, Meeuwis JA, Verwoerd CDA. Induction in vivo of cartilage grafts for craniofacial reconstruction. Am J Rhinol 1998; 12:27–31.

8

Air Pollution and the Child

DE-YUN WANG and YOKE TEEN PANG

The National University of Singapore,
Singapore, Republic of Singapore

I. Introduction

Air is one of the basic elements essential for the survival and quality of life of human being. There is no doubt that fresh, clean, and clear air is much more preferable to polluted air with dusts, burning smoke, harmful gases, and chemical particles. However, the air that we breathe every day is not a single substance, but a mixture of nitrogen, oxygen, carbon dioxide, and other gases with varying amounts of water vapor. The proportion in which they are present differs from place to place (Fig. 8.1).

During the last decades, there is an increasing awareness of air pollution as a major contributing factor to the increase of human diseases. The increased number of motor vehicles in urban areas has particulary contributed to the rise

- *78% Nitrogen gas*
- *21% Oxygen gas*
- *1% Nitrogen gas*
- *0.03% Carbon dioxide gas*
- *Water vapour*
- *Gases from industrial and natural pollution*

Figure 8.1 Some properties of the main gases in air.

in air pollution. The exhaust fumes from the engines of automobiles contain a number of pollutants, including carbon monoxide, a variety of complex hydrocarbons, nitrogen oxides, and other compounds. It is one of the major causes of respiratory distress in children, elder people, and those suffering from pre-existing respiratory disease.

In addition, environmental factors such as indoor and outdoor pollution play an important role in the clinical expression of allergic disease, which is estimated in approximately 30–40% of world population. These pollutants may exert their influence directly on allergic disease either by acting as a co-factor for an IgE response to common allergens so increasing the prevalence of atopy, or by exacerbating already existing disease, so increasing its severity (1).

II. What is Air Pollution?

Air pollution, by definition, is the presence of harmful gases or solid particles in the air. Air pollution occurs when the rates of release of finely divided solids, or finely dispersed liquid aerosols into the atmosphere exceed the capacity of the atmosphere to dissipate them or to dispose of them through incorporation into solid or liquid layers of the biosphere. Air pollution results from a variety of causes, not all of which are within human control. Dust storms in desert areas and smoke from forest, volcanic eruption and grass fires contribute to chemical and particulate pollution of the air.

Air pollution is a side effect of modern life, contributed by increasing industries, motor vehicles, and power stations, among others. The types and sources of the pollutants can be classified in a variety of ways. Two general categories are commonly used, namely outdoor and indoor pollutants (Table 8.1). They encompass a wide range of chemicals, gases, and particulates (Table 8.2).

The common outdoor pollutants in the air include carbon monoxide, sulfur dioxide, oxides of nitrogen, lead compounds, and chlorofluorocarbons (CFCs) (Fig. 8.2). The increase of these pollutants has led to the increase of health problems, the greenhouse effect, thinning of the ozone layer, and acid rain.

Indoor air pollutants can also be important in the genesis of respiratory disease, considering that town dwellers spend less than 1 h a day outdoors (an

Table 8.1 The Sources of Air Pollutants

Outdoor	Indoor
Power stations	Wood and coal burning
Industrial works	Tobacco smoke
Transport	Gas and kerosene heaters
Diesel vehicles	Photocopiers, laser printers
Waste incinerators	Insulation and furnishing
Secondary pollutants (i.e., ozone, ...)	Detergents

average of 0.7 h), the rest of the time being at home, at work or in some means of transport (2). Exposure to oxides of nitrogen from space heaters or gas ovens may promote respiratory tract infections in children. Tobacco smoke inhalation by smokers and nonsmokers impairs respiration and had led to increases in lung cancer and chronic obstructive pulmonary disease. On the other hand, in developing countries, disease may be caused by inhalation of fungi from roof thatch materials or by the inhalation of smoke when the home contains no chimney.

III. Influence of Pollutants on Human Health Problem

To date there are sufficient evidences pointing to a causal relationship of air pollution and human health problem. Many studies have demonstrated that increased air pollution were associated with a higher mortality of cardiovascular diseases, emergency visits of asthmatic children, lung cancer, chronic obstructive pulmonary disease, damage in nasal respiratory epithelium, viral infection and/or emotional stress (3–13).

The mechanisms of action, exposure–response relationship, and pollutant interactions remain to be completely elucidated. The literature suggests that the increased incidence of the upper and lower respiratory tract symptoms is significantly associated with high levels of pollutants such as ambient ozone levels. One explanation is that some pollutants can either impair defense mechanisms in the airways rendering them more susceptible to viral and/or bacterial infection, or

Table 8.2 The Distinction of Air Pollutants

Sulphur dioxide (SO_2)	Nitrogen oxides (NO_x, NO_2, O_3)	Particulates
Power stations	Power stations	Wood and coal burning
Industrial works	Industrial works	Tobacco smoke
Diesel vehicles	Transport	Gas and kerosene heaters

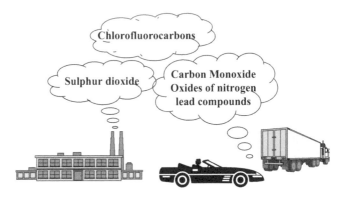

Figure 8.2 Pollutants in air.

cause an immunological toxicity in the airways (Fig. 8.3) (14). However, there is still a lack of evidence to support this hypothesis.

Epidemiological data from London in 1952 demonstrated a good case in point. The occurrence of thick fog together with the attendant high levels of sulfur dioxide and particulate pollution (and probably also sulfuric acid) led to the deaths of more than 4000 people during that week and the subsequent 3 weeks. Many, but not all, of the victims already had chronic heart or lung disease.

Also, in 1952 a different kind of air pollution was seen for the first time in Los Angeles. The large number of automobiles in that city, together with the bright sunlight and frequently stagnant air, led to the formation of a photochemical smog. This began with the emission of nitrogen oxide during the morning commuting hour, followed by the formation of nitrogen dioxide by oxygenation,

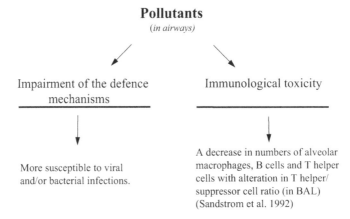

Figure 8.3 Possible relationship between air pollution and immune defense function.

and finally, through a complex series of reactions in the presence of hydrocarbons and sunlight, to the formation of ozone and peroxyacetyl nitrite and other irritant compounds. Eye irritation, chest irritation with cough, and possibly the exacerbation of asthma occurred as a result.

It is now recognized that ozone is an important air pollutant. It is the most irritant gas known. In controlled exposure studies, it reduces the ventilatory capability of healthy people in concentrations as low as 0.12 ppm. Ozone is found in significant quantities in many large cities of the world. In Mexico City, Bangkok, Sao Paulo and in many large cities in the world, ozone regularly exceeds this level. The main reasons are high automobile population and favorable meteorological conditions for photochemical oxidation.

Although acute episodes of communal air exposure leading to demonstrable mortality are unlikely, there is much concern over the possible long-term consequences of brief but repetitive exposures to oxidants and acidic aerosols; exposures which are now common in millions of people. Their impact has not yet been precisely defined.

Tobacco smoking is a widespread source of indoor pollution in both the developed and developing countries. The negative health consequences of active smoking have been clearly documented in epidemiological, clinical, and basic research studies (15). In recent years, many studies showed that exposure to environmental tobacco smoke is associated with higher prevalence of respiratory infections and respiratory symptoms in children (16). Both active and passive smoking may facilitate the development of airway disease, especially in children.

IV. Effect of Air Pollution on Children's Health

Children are highly susceptible to deleterious effects of environmental toxins. Those who live in underprivileged communities may be particularly at risk because environmental pollution has been found to be disproportionately distributed among these communities. Mounting evidence suggests that asthma rates are rising and that this disease can be caused or aggravated by air pollution (17).

Children are not just little adults; they are uniquely vulnerable. Pediatric medicine shows that children are uniquely vulnerable to environmental toxicants because of their greater relative exposure, less developed metabolism, and higher rates of cell production, growth, and change (18). The environmental insults of childhood may manifest themselves over a lifetime of growth to adulthood and senescence. In addition to physiologic vulnerabilities, children may have great social vulnerabilities as well. Poverty, malnutrition, and environmental injustice are our collective responsibility. It is therefore very important to investigate the effect of indoor and outdoor pollution on children's health. This will provide not only a better understanding of the relationship between environmental exposures and health outcomes in children, but also to delivering a clear and workable program for its prevention.

It has recently been reported that 3–4 million children and adolescents in USA live within 1 mile of a federally designated hazardous waste disposal site and are at risk of exposure to chemical toxicants released from these sites into air, groundwater, surface water, and surrounding communities (19).

There was a prospective study performed in southwest metropolitan Mexico City (20). In this study, nasal biopsies at the posterior portion of the inferior turbinate were obtained from 87 children who are repeatedly exposed to high levels of a complex mixture of air pollutants (including ozone, particulate matter, aldehydes, metals, and nitrogen oxides), and 12 controls from a low-polluted coastal town. Detection of a major mutagenic lesion producing GT transversion mutations using an immunohistochemical method and DNA single strand breaks (ssb) using the single cell gel electrophoresis assay as biomarkers of oxidant exposure was performed. The results suggest that DNA damage is present in nasal epithelial cells in Mexico City children. Persistent oxidative DNA damage may ultimately result in a selective growth of pre-neoplastic nasal initiated cells in this population and the potential for nasal neoplasms may increase with age. The combination of 8-OHdG and DNA ssb should be useful for monitoring oxidative damage in people exposed to polluted atmospheres.

There is need, however, for more research that will assess patterns of children's exposures to hazardous chemicals from pollutants; quantify children's vulnerability to environmental toxicants; assess causal associations between environmental exposures and pediatric disease; and elucidate the mechanisms of environmental disease in children at the cellular and molecular level.

V. Air Pollution and Allergic Diseases

Most epidemiological data have demonstrated in recent years that the prevalence and severity of allergic diseases such as asthma and rhinitis have increased greatly especially in children and young adults. The increase mirrored the rise in the air pollution around the world. The complete etiologic mechanism for the development and expression of atopic disease is not yet understood. Zeiger and Heller (21) have summarized the intricate interactions between the genetic and environmental factors responsible for the phenotypic expression of atopic disease. Both genetic and environmental factors (including air pollutants) influence the expression of allergic disease.

Allergic rhinitis is frequently caused by exposure to perennial or seasonal allergens which exist in our living environment of the home, offices, workplaces, and polluted air. The common allergens responsible for allergic rhinitis are pollens, house-dust mites, molds, pets, cockroaches, insect-related allergens, and animal proteins. The prevalence of allergic rhinitis in an atopic individual will depend on exposure to a specific allergen with a high sensitizing capacity. Particulate allergens such as pollen vary in size from 10 to 100 μg, such particles escape the anterior filter of nasal hairs. They are however, ideally sized for entrapment on the ciliated nasal mucosa. Therefore, water-soluble proteins from the atmosphere readily leached out into the nasal mucus where they become available to trigger cells sensitized by IgE antibodies (22).

The clinical expression of allergic disease has been reported to be influenced by geographic variations, climate, socioeconomic conditions, family structure or history, infant diet, excessive allergen exposure especially during the early life, cigarette smoking, specific and early infections with viruses, and exposure to products of pollution. Amongst these factors, air pollution plays a significant role either by acting as direct or as a cofactor for the development of allergic diseases. Air pollution is a frequently quoted adjuvant factor for allergic sensitization and cause of increased prevalence rates of allergic disease in industrialized countries. In addition to already identified allergens, exposure to high levels of pollutants including oxides of nitrogen, ozone, sulfur dioxide, black smoke—large particulate matter, small particulates, carbon monoxide, and volatile organic compounds have been considered as important contributing factors in both the exacerbation and etiology of allergic airway disease (14,23,24).

From the epidemiological data, it is still not clear that the increase of the prevalence of allergic disease is distinctly different between the areas with higher or lower degree of the air pollution. On the other hand, the epidemiology of allergic disease such as asthma and allergic rhinitis is still incomplete, probably due to the problems of definition and diagnostic criteria of these diseases by both patients and doctors over time.

The quantity and type of pollutants also influence development of allergic disease. This has already been explained by an epidemiological study performed in two cities of Germany. Von Mutius et al. (25) have studied a total of 7653 children in Munich ($n = 5030$) and in Leipzig ($n = 2623$). In the latter city, there was a considerably higher degree of air pollution with sulfur dioxide produced by coal, while, an "automobile-type" pollution was found in Munich. The prevalence rate of allergic rhinitis, asthma, and of positive skin tests to aero-allergens were significantly lower in Leipzig (2.7%, 3.9%, and 18.2%) than in Munich (8.6%, 5.9%, and 36.7%). Therefore, it has been suggested that effective pollution control policy will require an understanding of how measures to alter emissions from different sources influence personal exposure, and hence health outcomes (26). A more powerful epidemiological study is needed and must be performed on the basis of prospective settings in several regions, and with unique investigational criteria to assess the prevalence and severity of allergic disease.

VI. The Impact of Air Pollution on Allergic Disease

To date, however, the exact mechanism by which pollutants may exert their influence on the development of allergic disease is still not entirely understood (26). A number of studies had demonstrated that diesel exhaust particles and their associated polyaromatic hydrocarbons are a major component of ambient air pollution and have adjuvant activity for IgE production both in mice and human airways (27,28).

Several clinical and experimental studies have demonstrated that pollutants may affect disease processes (14,23,27,29–32) (Fig. 8.4): (1) among several mixtures of pollutants, especially organic compounds, substances may be found with a great impact on IgE formation; (2) different pollutants may enhance several important mediator (such as histamine, leukotriene C_4, prostaglandins) production or release from different inflammatory cells; (3) decreased ciliary beat leads to decreased allergen clearance; (4) increased production of cytokines resulting in an increased production of IgE and in an increased activity of inflammatory cells; and (5) air pollution can enhance allergic sensitization to aero-allergens by exerting their irritant effects upon skin and respiratory mucosa. Therefore, air pollutants may play a direct or indirect role in the pathophysiology and the development of allergic diseases.

VII.   Indoor Environment and Allergic Rhinitis in Children

Exposure of indoor allergens in our house environment, such as house-dust mites, molds, pets, cockroaches, insect-related allergens, and animal proteins are common causes of perennial allergic rhinitis. Young children especially spend most of their time inside the house. It is true that when a high concentration of one or more allergens is present in the house, the risk of allergenic sensitization in the early life will increase consequently. Therefore, a better understanding of the role of the house environment in the expression of allergic disease will ultimately lead to a better prevention of allergic rhinitis.

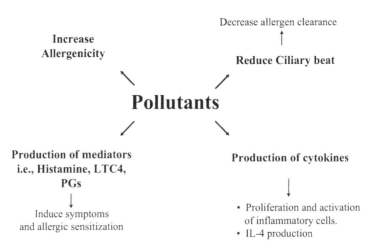

Figure 8.4   Possible relationship between air pollution and allergic disease.

House dust is a heterogeneous mixture, which varies according to region and household. It consists of various allergenic substances, consisting primarily of the somatic and metabolic allergens of mites, and secondarily of allergens derived from domestic animals, human skin scales, and domestic insects such as cockroaches. In addition, fungal spores or mycelia and other products of animal or vegetable origin such as feathers, wool, and natural fibers, may be sources of dust allergens. Animals are also an important source for inducing indoor symptoms; not only domesticated cats and dogs but also rodents (e.g., mice, guinea pigs, hamsters, etc.) introduced into the house as pets. The allergens come from four different sources: the saliva, feces, urine, and dander of the animal.

The knowledge of the geographical distribution of the Pyroglyphidae has recently progressed considerably, but the map of their distribution remains incomplete. Nevertheless, numerous investigations to date have confirmed that *Dermatophagoides pteronyssinus* predominates over all other species in most countries, and that *Dermatophagoides farinae* and *Euroglyphus maynei* may also be present in numbers which vary according to climate (33). Several factors in our dwelling houses, such as increased temperature, the use of fitted carpets, tighter insulation, and detergents effective in cool water, have improved the conditions for dust mites propagation (34). The identification and definition of mite allergens are mainly described in two main groups. The group I allergens are found in the fecal pellets, and the group II allergens are derived from both the mite bodies and feces (35). The threshold exposure concentration of group I mite allergens has been recognized as 2 $\mu g/g$ dust (36,37).

Some prospective studies have clearly demonstrated that high mite-allergen exposure (≥ 2 $\mu g/g$) increased the risk of specific sensitization and the development of asthma in atopic children and young adults (34,36). Studies from England, Australia, France, Denmark, USA, and Germany have all demonstrated that children growing up in houses with a concentration higher than 2 μg of group I mite allergen per gram of dust are at risk for developing positive skin test responses and serum IgE antibodies (38).

There is a need for effective measures to remove or reduce the allergen exposure, as well as the exposure to other adjuvant factors in the home. In addition to a simple removal of the allergen source, it is now possible to reduce the concentration of house-dust mites either by chemicals (tannic acid or solidified benzyl benzoate) or bedding encasings. In this way, Lau et al. (36) obtained an allergen reduction of at least 80% in most houses to achieve allergen concentrations lower than 2 $\mu g/g$ and a reduction of the sensitization risk in mite-sensitive patients.

VIII. Conclusion

In the light of recent explosion in knowledge on air pollution and its interactions with the individual, air pollution certainly plays an important part if not pivotal role in the pathogenesis of allergic and respiratory diseases. We will need to put more work into identifying which pollutants have an health impact on humans and in which subgroups, and the mechanism for disease production. This will need to include pathways of chemical, molecular, and cellular interactions.

Having understood these, we will then be able to deliver a comprehensive and effective program for the masses. Global cooperation and the willingness to set aside political and economic differences are vital to the success of large-scale changes in manufacturing and lifestyle. We have seen some success in the reduction of CFC release into the atmosphere and in the use of nonleaded motor fuel in many countries. Much work is still to be performed and the collaboration between the scientist who discover the pathway of diseases and the politicians and administrators who can implement and legislate practices is vital to the success of any preventive program.

References

1. Wardlaw AJ. Introduction. Clin Exp Allergy 1995; 25(suppl 3):7–8.
2. Molina CL. Respiratory manifestations induced by indoor air. In: Godard Ph, Bousquet J, Michel FB, eds. Advances in Allergology and Clinical Immunology. Lancs: The Parthenon Publishing Group, 1992:377–386.
3. Anderson HR, Spix C, Medina S, Schouten JP, Catellsague J, Rossi G, Zmirou D, Touloumi G, Wojtyniak B, Ponka A, Bacharova L, Schwartz J, Katsouyanni K. Air pollution and daily admissions for chronic obstructive pulmonary disease in 6 European cities: results from the APHEA project. Eur Respir J 1998; 11:992–993.
4. Calderon-Garciduenas L, Osnaya N, Rodriguez-Alcaraz A, Villarreal-Calderon A. DNA damage in nasal respiratory epithelium from children exposed to urban pollution. Environ Mol Mutagenesis 1997; 3:11–20.
5. Garty BZ, Kosman E, Ganor E, Berger V, Garty L, Wietzen T, Waisman Y, Minouni M, Waisel Y. Emergency room visits of asmathic children, relation to air pollution, weather and airborne allergens. Ann Allergy Asthma Immunol 1998; 81:563–570.
6. Katsouyanni K, Pershagen G. Ambient air pollution exposure and cancer. Cancer Causes Control 1997; 8:284–291.
7. Kunzli N, Braun-Fahrlander C, Rapp R, Ackerman-Liebrich U. Air pollution and health causal criteria in environmental epidemiology. German. Schweizerische Medizinische Wochensschrift. J Suisse Med 1997; 127:1334–1344.
8. Lipfert FW. Air pollution and human health: perspectives for the '90s and beyond. Risk Anal 1997; 17:137–146.
9. Romieu I, Borja-Aburto VH. Particulate air pollution and daily mortality: can results be generalized to Latin American countries? Salud Publica Mexico 1998; 39:403–411.
10. Smrcka V, Leznarova D. Environmental pollution and the occurrence of congenital defects in a 15-year period in a south Moravian district. Acta Chirurgiae Plasticae 1998; 40:112–114.
11. Timonen KL, Pekkanen J. Air pollution and respiratory health among children with asthmatic or cough symptoms. Am J Respir Crit Care Med 1997; 156:546–552.

12. Yang CY, Cheng MF, Tsai SS, Hung CF, Lai TC, Hwang KC. Effects of indoor environmental factors on risk for acute otitis media in a subtropical area. J Toxicol Environ Health 1999; 56:111–119.

13. Zmirou D, Schwartz J, Saez M, Zanobetti A, Wojtyniak B, Touloumi G, Spix C, Ponce de Leon A, Le Moullec Y, Bacharova L, Schouten J, Ponka A, Katsouyanni K. Time-series analysis of air pollution and cause-specific mortality. Epidemiology 1998; 9:495–503.

14. Krishna MT, Mudway I, Kelly FJ, Frew AJ, Holgate ST. Ozone, airways and allergic airways disease. Clin Exp Allergy 1995; 25:1150–1158.

15. US Public Health Service. The Health Consequences of Smoking: Chronic Obstructive Disease. A Report of the Surgeon. General Washington, DC: US Government Printing Office, 1984.

16. US Department of Health and Human Services. The Health Consequences of Smoking: Chronic Obstructive Disease. A Report of The Surgeon. General Washington, DC: US Government printing Office, 1986.

17. Claudio L, Torres T, Sanjurjo E, Sherman LR, Landrigan PJ. Environmental health sciences education. A tool for achieving environmental equity and protecting children. Environ Health Perspect 1998; 106(suppl 3):849–855.

18. Carlson JE. Children's environmental health research: an introduction. Environ Health Perspect 1998; 106(suppl 30).

19. Landrigan PJ, Suk WA, Amler RW. Chemical wastes, children's health, and the superfund basic research program. Environ Health Perspect 1999; 107:423–427.

20. Calderón-Garcidueñas L, Lian WW, Zhang YJ, Rodriguez-Alcaraz A, Osnaya N, Villarreal-Calderón A, Santella RM. 8-Hydroxy-2′-deoxyguanosine, a major mutagenic oxidative DNA lesion, and DNA strand breaks in nasal respiratory epithelium of children exposed to urban pollution. Environ Health Perspect 1999; 107:469–474.

21. Zeiger RS, Heller S. The development and prediction of atopy in high-risk children. Follow-up at age seven years in a prospective randomized study of combined maternal and infant food allergen avoidance. J Allergy Clin Immunol 1995; 95:1179–1190.

22. Norman PS. Allergic rhinitis. J Allergy Clin Immunol 1985; 75:531–545.

23. Devalia JL, Wang JH, Rusznak C, Calderón M, Davies RJ. Does air pollution enhance the human airway response to allergen? In vivo and in vitro evidence. ACI News 1994; 6:80–84.

24. Utell MJ, Samet JM. Particulate air pollution and health; new evidence on an old problem. Am Rev Respir Dis 1993; 147:1334–1335.

25. Von Mutius E, Martinez FD, Nicolai T, Roell G, Thieman H-H. Prevalence of asthma and atopy in two areas of West and East Germany. Am J Respir Crit Care Med 1994; 149:358–364.

26. Ashmore M. Human exposure to air pollutants. Clin Exp Allergy 1995; 25(suppl 3):12–22.

27. Diaz-Sanchez D, Saxon A. The effect of diesel exhaust particles on allergic disease. ACI Int 1996; 8:57–59.

28. Muranaka M, Suzuki S, Koizumi K, Takafuji S, Miyamoto T, Ikemori R, Tokiwa H. Adjuvant activity of diesel-exhaust particulates for the production of IgE antibody in mice. J Allergy Clin Immunol 1986; 77:616–623.

29. Bascom R. Air pollution. In: Mygind N, Naclerio R, eds. Allergic and Non-Allergic Rhinitis. Copenhagen: Munksgaard, 1993:32–45.

30. Behrendt H, Friedrichs K-H, Krämer U, Hitzfeld B, Becker W-M, Ring J. The role of indoor and outdoor air pollution in allergic diseases. In: Johansson SGO, ed. Progress in Allergy and Clinical Immunology. Germany: Hogrefe & Huber Publishers, 1995:83–89.
31. Burkholter D, Schiffer P. The epidemiology of atopic diseases in Europe—A review. ACI News 1995; 7:113–125.
32. Ring J, Behrendt H, Schäfer T, Vieluf D, Krämer U. Impact of air pollution on allergic disease: clinical and epidemiologic studies. In: Johansson SGO, ed.. Progress in Allergy and Clinical Immunology. Germany: Hogrefe & Huber Publishers, 1995:74–182.
33. Fain A. Morphology, systematics and geographical distribution of mites responsible for allergic disease in man. In: Fain A, Guerin B, Hart BJ, eds. Mites and Allergic Disease. France: Allerbio, 1990:7–10.
34. Sporik R, Holgate ST, Platts-Mills TAE, Cogswell J. Exposure to house dust mite allergen (Der p I) and the development of asthma in children: a prospective study. N Engl J Med 1990; 323:502–507.
35. Naspitz CK, Rizzo MC, Arruda LK, Fernandez-Caldas E, Solé D, Chapman MD, Platts-Mills TAE. Enviromental control of mite allergy. In: Johansson SGO, ed. Progress in Allergy and Clinical Immunology. Germany: Hogrefe & Huber Publishers, 1995:334–339.
36. Lau S, Falkenhorst G, Weber A, Werthmann I, Lind P, Buettner-Goetz P, Wahn U. High mite-allergen exposure increases the risk of sensitization in atopic children and young adults. J Allergy Clin Immunol 1989; 84:718–725.
37. Platts-Mills TAE, Sporik RB, Ward GW, Heymann PW, Chapman MD. Dose–response relationships between asthma and exposure to indoor allergens. In: Johansson SGO, ed. Progress in Allergy and Clinical Immunology. Germany: Hogrefe & Huber Publishers, 1995:90–96.
38. Platts-Mills TAE, Sporik RB, Wheatley LM, Heymann PW. Is there a dose–response relationship between exposure to indoor allergens and symptoms of asthma? J Allergy Clin Immunol 1995; 96:435–440.

9

Correlation between Respiratory Diseases and Histologic Alterations Due to Urban Pollution

TANIA MARIA SIH

University of Sao Paulo,
Sao Paulo, Brazil

I. Introduction

Contamination of the atmosphere is the most important factor affecting the environment. Environmental pollution is recognized as a respiratory health hazard and some epidemiological studies have focused on the prevalence of respiratory illnesses in adults and in children exposed to outdoor air pollution (1–3). The initial studies by Lunn (4) and Melia (5) provided evidence that the number of diseases was increasing in proportion to the poor quality of the atmosphere.

It appears that the elderly and infants are the most sensitive population groups (6). Moreover, children may be more susceptible than adults because their organs are still growing (7–9).

Over the past decades, human activities have been dangerously modified with striking alterations in atmospheric conditions due to the introduction of gaseous and particulate substances potentially dangerous to human health. Traffic in big cities and waste products from industrial plants pollute the air with sulfur dioxide, nitrogen dioxide, carbon monoxide, lead, hydrocarbons, particulate matter, etc.

The influence of air pollution on health of the inhabitants of urban areas has been extensively investigated in the last 30 years (5). However, it has not been possible to precisely determine the levels of specific air pollutants that can be accepted by the population, since it is difficult for both experimental and epidemiological studies to define a direct cause–effect relation, especially in situations of chronic exposure to low levels of pollutants.

Some studies demonstrated histopathological alterations produced by air pollutants, particularly on mucociliary activity (10,11). Studying sulfuring aerosol effects on respiratory tracts of mice, Fairchild (12) found a reduction in mucociliary clearance rate. Inhalation of organic peroxides may induce functional changes in the nasal mucosa. It is possible that chronic stimulation with lower doses can affect the nasal mucosa in a similar way. In animal experiments, exposure to ozone, automobile fumes, or city air, increase the susceptibility to diseases and particularly to respiratory infections (13,14).

The aim of this study was to determine the possible relationship between children's respiratory health and urban air pollution and its consequences, and also correlate those findings with structural alterations of the respiratory tract in animals exposed to the atmospheric pollution of São Paulo city.

II. Material and Methods

A. Studying the Children

In order to understand the role of environment in relation to infections and allergy, a survey was conducted with 2000 children (age range 7–14 years). The study period was between November 1996 and February 1997. In order to have similar socio-economic conditions for all subjects, all children attended São Paulo state public schools. The school children were divided into two groups with 1000 children each:

1. Red group from São Paulo (capital city of the state)—17,000,000 inhabitants (schools close to a local airport, highly polluted area)
2. Green group from rural area around Tupã (pollution-free environment).

A standardized anamnesis questionnaire was used to ascertain clinical symptoms, infectious and allergic respiratory diseases as well as related aspects and predisposing factors.

Clinical Symptoms

The frequency of the following clinical symptoms, respiratory infections, and allergic diseases and their related aspects was investigated: blocked nose, running nose, nocturnal cough, sinusitis, rhinitis (having been mentioned by a physician, with positive symptoms of nose itching, sneezing episodes, and perennial clear nose secretion), currently under treatment with antiallergic management or antibiotic for respiratory allergy or infection, recurrent throat infections (every episode treated with antibiotic), upper respiratory infections (URI) related to sudden weather change, absenteeism (missing school) at least one day (previous month) because of respiratory disease, and previous ear, nose, and throat (ENT) surgeries.

Predisposing Factors

The frequency of the following predisposing factors was investigated: passive smoking, house humidity (mould), room/cohabitant ratio (more than three people sleeping in the same room), pets inside the house, and insecticide used indoors and outdoors.

The data were analyzed with the statistical software program EPI-INFO 6.0 (Centers for Disease Control and Prevention, Atlanta, GA). Logistic regression was carried out, using the software program EGRET ANALYSIS MODULE-PECAN-0,26.6 (SERC and CYTEL, 1991), to control for potential confounding variables.

B. Studying the Animals

Saldiva et al. from the Laboratório de Poluição Atmosférica Ambiental da Faculdade de Medicina da Universidade de São Paulo, SP, Brazil, conducted the animal experiments. The measured levels of environmental pollutants during the exposure of the animals in São Paulo, provided by CETESB (environmental state agency) were: CO, 1.25 ppm; ozone, 11.08 ppb; particulates, 35.18 $\mu g/m^3$; SO_2, 29.05 $\mu g/m^3$.

A total of 69 male Wistar rats (2 months old at the beginning of the study) were maintained for 6 months in São Paulo, while 56 control animals were housed in the rural area during the same period. Thirty animals of the rural area and 24 rats of São Paulo were studied. In both places, the animals were fed the same balanced food, and were matched in terms of space and ventilation as well as possible.

Ultrastructural Studies

Samples of tracheal and right main bronchus epithelium were collected from four animals in each group. The samples were fixed in 2.5% glutaraldehyde and osmium tetroxide, and were processed according to the routine procedures for electron microscopy. Araldyte-embedded sections, stained with lead citrate and uranyl-acetate, were examined in a Philips 400 transmission electron microscope, with special emphasis on ciliary apparatus.

Optical Microscopy

Samples of nasal epithelium were collected from the rats in both groups. For this purpose, the nasal septum was fixed in buffered 10% formalin solution and pH of 2.5, processed according to routine histological procedures. With this technique, neutral and acid glycoproteins were stained in red and blue, respectively.

Scanning Electron Micrography

Samples of nasal epithelium were collected from the rats in each group. The tissue was fixed in 2% OsO_4 and post-fixed in 4% glutaraldehyde.

III. Results

A total of 2800 questionnaires were distributed and 2000 were used in the study. Frequency of symptoms from URIs and allergic and infectious diseases, plus related aspects according to groups of children (Red, Green) are shown in Table 9.1. Statistical significance of the associations is expressed in terms of p-values.

Nasal obstruction, running nose, rhinitis, sinusitis, recurrent throat infection, URI related to sudden weather changes, currently under antibiotic or

Table 9.1 Association Between Frequencies of Symptoms from Upper Respiratory Infections (URI) and Allergic Diseases with Its Related Aspects by Groups of Children

Symptoms of URI and allergic diseases and related aspects	Group of children (%)		p-Value
	Red ($n = 1000$)	Green ($n = 1000$)	
Blocked nose	19	9	<0.005
Running nose	8	5	<0.005
Nocturnal cough	14	8	<0.005
Rhinitis	7	4	<0.005
Sinusitis	12	8	<0.005
Throat infections	15	13	<0.045
URI related to sudden weather changes	28	20	<0.005
Currently under treatment with antiallergic drug(s) or antibiotic(s)	9	5	<0.084
Absenteeism from school	17	9	<0.006
Previous ENT surgeries	4	2	<0.005

antiallergic treatment, absenteeism from school, and previous ENT surgeries were prevalent in the Red group (*p* statistically significant).

Frequency of possible predisposing factors for respiratory allergic and infectious diseases in each group is shown in Table 9.2.

Among predisposing factors, passive smoking, insecticide use, pet kept inside the house, mould (house humidity), episodes of URI related to sudden weather changes, and crowding (more than three people sleeping in the same room) were more frequently found in the urban area of São Paulo.

Logistic regression was carried out for sinusitis (Table 9.3) and rhinitis (Table 9.4), in order to control for potential confounding effects of smoking, mould, insecticide, and pets inside the home.

In the univariate analysis, the Red group of children had a higher probability (40%) of having had sinusitis than children from the Green group. The OR became even slightly larger (50%) after controlling for potential confounding variables using logistic regression.

In the univariate analysis, the Red group of children had a higher probability (30%) of having had rhinitis than children from the Green group. The OR became even slightly larger (40%) after controlling for potential confounding variables using logistic regression.

Ultrastructural studies in the rat population detected abnormal cilia of tracheal epithelium more frequently found in animals of São Paulo. In these animals, the presence of composite cilia microtubular defects and vesicle cilia were frequently seen, as well as a marked decrease in the microvilli of the luminal membrane (Fig. 9.1).

Optical microscopy showed normal nasal epithelium (Fig. 9.2) in control rats (rural area). In rats exposed to urban pollution, the epithelium showed areas with squamous epithelium (Fig. 9.3) and chronic inflammatory process with secretory hyperplasia (Fig. 9.4).

Scanning electron nasal micrography in the rat population detected lack of cilia from nasal epithelium more frequently found in animals from São Paulo (Fig. 9.5).

Table 9.2 Frequency of Possible Predisposing Factors for Respiratory Diseases by Groups of Children

	Group of children (%)		
Predisposing factors	Red (*n* = 1000)	Green (*n* = 1000)	*p*-Value
Passive smoking	58	52	<0.005
Mould	18	8	<0.005
Insecticide	32	34	<0.005
Pet inside the house	31	36	<0.005
Room/cohabitant ratio	28	17	<0.005

Table 9.3 Crude and Adjusted Odds Ratios[a] for Sinusitis, by Group of Children

	Crude OR	(95% CI)	p	Adjusted OR	(95% CI)	p
Red	1.40	(1.10–1.77)	0.005	1.50	(1.18–1.91)	0.001
Green	1.05	(0.83–1.34)	0.067	1.06	(0.83–1.36)	0.65

[a]Adjusted for smoking, mould, insecticide, and pets inside the home.

IV. Discussion

The present epidemiological investigation assessed the frequency of some respiratory diseases (allergy and infections) in children exposed to urban polluted environment. The use of "self-administered" questionnaires in the screenings and the definition of the illnesses under study were validated in previous studies (10,12).

Our data confirm the relevance of nasal and laryngo-tracheo-bronchial symptoms depicted in Table 9.1: nasal obstruction, running nose, and nocturnal cough appear to be relevant in air polluted urban environment. Studying 1177 children in a polluted district of Poland, Gryczynska (15) found chronic cough in 45%, frequently accompanied by nasal obstruction and running nose. In this group, the cough characteristics were nocturnal, paroxysmal, often similar to whooping cough and rather dry, lasting for several months. In fact, respiratory mucosae tend to react as a whole to the various infective, allergic, and environment aggressions.

In an epidemiological survey conducted on 2304 Italian children from urban schools, rhinitis was present in 8.2% (3). Our survey showed 7% for the polluted environment of São Paulo and 4% for rural areas without any pollution.

Chronicity of the stimulation and immaturity of the defense system make children prone to respiratory allergy (3). In atopic children, sensitization to one or more prevalent allergens can take place and will be followed by the appearance of allergy symptoms. Air pollution could act as a factor which favors the sensitization of atopic children, causing allergic symptoms (16).

Our findings showed high prevalence of respiratory infectious diseases, like sinusitis, recurrent throat infections and URI in air polluted urban environment. Surveys carried out in Japan compared nasal conditions of rural and urban children in two different periods (17). In the first period, 1952–1955, the incidence of

Table 9.4 Crude and Adjusted Odds Ratios[a] for Rhinitis, by Group of Children

	Crude OR	(95% CI)	p	Adjusted OR	(95% CI)	p
Red	1.00	(0.53–0.91)	0.008	1.00	(0.45–0.83)	0.002
Green	0.67	(0.51–0.88)	0.004	0.62	(0.45–0.85)	0.003

[a]Adjusted for smoking, mould, insecticide, and pets inside the home.

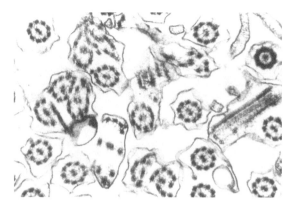

Figure 9.1   Ultrastructural aspect of tracheal epithelium of rat exposed to São Paulo urban pollution. Note the marked ciliary abnormalities, with incomplete microtubular structures and loss of orientation of microtubular pairs ($\times 82,500$).

chronic sinusitis in rural communities was over six times higher that in urban communities. Rapid changes in social and environmental conditions resulting from the high growth of the nation's economy anticipated a new problem: air pollution. Another rhinologic investigation was conducted between 1972 and 1975. This second study revealed that the rate of sinusitis among urban children was 19.2% and 8.9% among rural children. Our findings were similar: sinusitis was present in 12% of the children in the polluted urban area as compared to 8% in the pollution-free rural area.

When compared with the rural areas, the higher incidence of URI in city children is strongly correlated with the environment (14). Children living in polluted air environments presented more absenteeism from school, had more

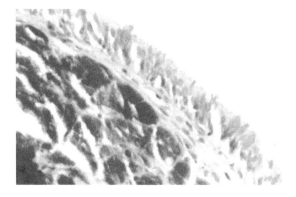

Figure 9.2   Normal nasal epithelium in control rats (rural area).

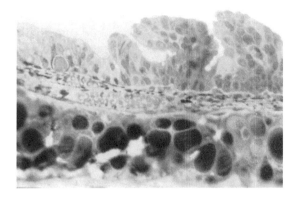

Figure 9.3 Nasal mucosa of rats exposed to urban pollution showed squamous epithelium.

antibiotic or antiallergic treatments, had more hospitalizations due to respiratory complications and a higher number of previous ENT surgeries.

Our survey confirms the relevance of some predisposing factors for respiratory allergic and infectious diseases like passive smoking, house humidity with mould, sudden weather changes and URI, insecticide use, room/cohabitant ratio. All these predisposing factors were prevalent in the urban group where respiratory allergy and infections were higher (urban air). Passive smoking is often cited as a contributory factor in respiratory troubles and appears to play a major influence on respiratory diseases (2).

Air pollutants affect the respiratory mucosa, particularly impairing the mucociliary system, causing alterations in the ciliary structure (11).

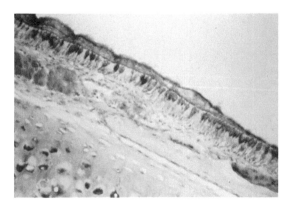

Figure 9.4 Nasal mucosa of rats exposed to urban pollution showed areas with secretory hyperplasia, chronic inflammatory infiltrate in the lamina propria, and thickening of the epithelium basement membrane.

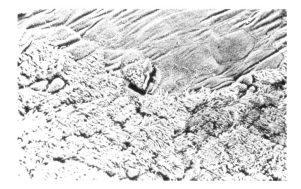

Figure 9.5   Nasal epithelium of rats from urban area showed lack of cilia.

The most significant functional alteration of air pollution-exposed rats was the dysfunction of mucociliary apparatus. Animals maintained in São Paulo (18) presented a significantly lower mucus output from the trachea, in the presence of widespread secretory cell hyperplasia. This association points to contraction of pulmonary infections. The reasons for the disturbance of the mucus clearance are multiple. Ultrastructural studies of the airways of these rats revealed high frequency of ciliary abnormalities, comprising composite cilia and microtubular disarrangements, alterations that are compatible with ciliary regeneration (19).

Our data showed that a high prevalence of allergic and infectious respiratory symptoms and diseases in children exposed to urban pollution is correlated with important histological abnormalities in animals exposed to the same environment, causing respiratory disorders. Children's quality of life and health suffer from the impact of air pollution. As physicians and scientific researchers, it is our task to correlate the noxious effects of environmental alteration on society's health.

Acknowledgment

I am grateful to Dr. Paulo Saldiva and colleagues from the Laboratório de Poluição Ambiental da Faculdade de Medicina de São Paulo, who contributed with the histological results.

References

1. Committee on Environmental Health. Ambient air pollution: respiratory hazards to children. Pediatrics 1993; 91:1210–1213.
2. Fergusson D, Horwood L, Shannon F. Parental smoking and respiratory illness in infancy. Arch Dis Child 1980; 55:358–361.

3. Porro E, Calamita I, Rana L, Criscione S. Atopy and environmental factors in upper respiratory infections: an epidemiological survey on 2304 school children. Int J Pediatr Otorhinolaryngol 1992; 24:111–120.
4. Lunn J. Patterns of respiratory illness in Sheffield infant school children. Br J Prev Soc Med 1987; 21:7–16.
5. Melia E. Respiratory illness in British school children and atmospheric smoke and sulfur dioxide, 1973–1977 cross sectional findings. J Epidemiol Commun Health 1981; 35:161–167.
6. Barker D, Osmond C. Childhood respiratory infection and adult chronic bronchitis in England and Wales. Br Med J 1986; 293:1271–1275.
7. Burchfield C, Higgins M, Keller J, Howatt F, Butler W, Higgins I. Passive smoking in childhood: respiratory conditions and respiratory function in Tecumseh, Michigan. Am Rev Respir Dis 1986; 133:966–973.
8. Ronchetti R, Martinez F, Criscione S, Macri F, Tramutoli G. Respiratory function and environmental factors in children. Bull Eur Physiopathol Respir 1980; 16:3–4.
9. Scotti P. Indoor air pollution as a risk factor of respiratory illness in childhood. In: Fior R, Pestalozza G, eds. The Child and the Environment. Amsterdam, London: Excerpta Medica, 1993:230–232.
10. Guney E, Tanyeri Y, Kandemir B, Yalcin S. The effect of wood dust on the nasal cavity and paranasal sinuses. Rhinology 1987; 25:273–277.
11. Passali D, Lauriello M. Air pollution and nasal allergy. In: Fior R, Pestalozza G, eds. The Child and the Environment. Amsterdam, London: Excerpta Medica, 1993:224–229.
12. Fairchild G, Kane P, Adams B, Coffin D. Sulfuric acid and streptococci clearance from respiratory tracts of mice. Arch Environ Health 1975; 30:538.
13. Dart R, Stretton R. Microbiological Aspects of Pollution Control. Amsterdam, London: Elsevier, 1977.
14. Pukander J, Luotonen J, Sipila M, Karma P. Incidence of acute otitis media. Acta Otolaryngol (Stockh) 1982; 93:447–453.
15. Gryczynska D, Krawczynski A, Zakrzewska J. Clinical evaluation of children's nasal obstruction in a highly polluted district of Poland. In: Fior R, Pestalozza G, eds. The Child and the Environment. Amsterdam, London: Excerpta Medica, 1993:233–237.
16. Ronchetti R, Martinez F, Criscione S, Macri F, Tramutoli G. Influence of familial and environmental factors on the prevalence of asthmatic and bronchitic syndromes of children (epidemiological survey of 2500 roman pupils). Riv Ital Pediatr 1982; 8:755–756.
17. Takahashi R. Environmental factors in the development of infection and allergy of the nose and paranasal sinuses. Proceedings of International Symposium on Infection and Allergy of the Nose and Paranasal Sinuses (ISIAN), Tokyo, 1976:21–26.
18. Saldiva PHN, King M, Delmonte VLC, Macchione M, Parada MAC, Daliberto ML, Sakae RS, Criado PMP, Silveira PLP, Zin WA, Böhm GM. Respiratory alterations due to urban air pollution: an experimental study in rats. Environ Res 1992; 57:19–33.
19. Breeze RG, Wheeldom EB. The cells of the pulmonary airways. Am Rev Respir Dis 1977; 116:705–777.

10

Nasal Polyposis: Cytokines, Recruitment of Eosinophils, and Epithelial Remodeling

JOEL M. BERNSTEIN

State University of New York,
Buffalo, New York, USA

I. Introduction

Nasal polyposis represents a chronic inflammatory disease of the lateral wall of the nose and the anterior ethmoidal air cells. In the last decade, a truly significant effort has been made to understand the pathogenesis, growth, persistence, and recurrence of nasal polyps. Two textbooks have appeared within the last year exclusively devoted to nasal polyps and their epidemiology, pathogenesis, and treatment (1,2).

The condition of nasal polyposis has been an enigma in the recorded history of mankind. It is found in a wide number of diseases and has varied histological components determined by the basic disease state. Thus, it may represent a common pathological endpoint in a number of disease processes and offers a spectrum of severity ranging from discrete localized lesions to massive diffuse mucosal change producing significant facial deformity.

The history of nasal polyps goes back to a period of over 4000 years to ancient Egypt and this condition may perhaps be the earliest recorded disease for which we know the names of both the patient and the physician (3). A complete review of nasal polyps is beyond the scope of this chapter because it would include epidemiology, histopathology, chemical mediators, the relationship to asthma, immunohistopathology, pathophysiology, and treatment.

The purpose of this chapter is to highlight recent developments in the molecular biology and electrophysiology of nasal polyposis. Based on this new information and recent advances in our understanding of the alteration of the cystic fibrosis transmembrane regulator protein (CFTR), the cyclic AMP-controlled chloride channel at the apical surface of the respiratory epithelial cell and its relation to the amiloride-sensitive sodium channel, a new model for the pathogenesis of nasal polyps will be developed.

II. Histopathology

The major differences between nasal polyps and normal nasal mucosa consist of four consistent attributes: (1) eosinophilia, (2) edema, (3) alteration in epithelial regrowth, and (4) development of new gland formation [Figs. 10.1, 10.2, and 10.3(a), (b)]. It is emphasized that the histopathology of nasal polyps is different from that of nasal mucosa. Therefore, any theory describing the development of nasal polyps must consider the alterations in the above-mentioned characteristics. The critical point to be made is that nasal polyposis is not edema of normal nasal mucosa, but a *de novo* new inflammatory development which is the result of an upregulation of inflammatory mediators, cytokines, adhesion molecules, and endothelial counter-receptors.

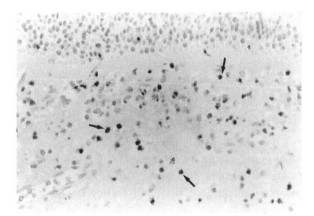

Figure 10.1 Typical morphology of a nasal polyp with respiratory epithelium covering a very edematous stroma with multiple inflammatory cells which are mainly eosinophils (arrows) (H and E, ×200).

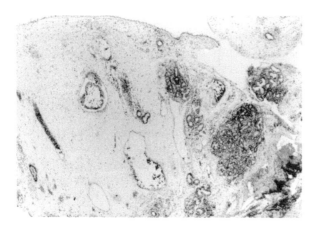

Figure 10.2 Photomicrograph of a polyp arising from middle turbinate mucosa. On the right are typical sero mucinous glands found in the middle turbinate. Adjacent to these glands, on the left, are large cystically dilated abnormal glands of a nasal polyp with tremendously edematous stroma (H and E, ×100).

III. Eosinophilia

Although fibroblasts, epithelial cells, and endothelial cells make up the most common constitutive cells of the nasal polyp, eosinophils are the most common inflammatory cells in the nasal polyps (4). The presence of eosinophilia

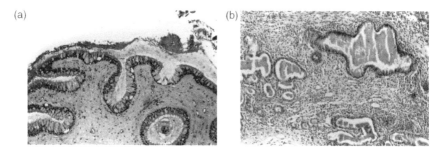

Figure 10.3 (a) Photomicrograph of a nasal polyp demonstrating significant remodeling of surface epithelium. Goblet cells have almost totally replaced the epithelium. There is significant mucous production as a result of the increased goblet cells on the surface of the epithelium. Edema is a principle pathological feature in the lamina propria (H and E, ×200). (b) High power photomicrograph of cystically dilated glands with inspissated mucus. There are multiple inflammatory cells within the lamina propria. These large distorted glands are totally different than the morphology of the normal sero mucinous glands in the lamina propria of the inferior middle turbinates. This finding strongly suggests that the glands represent a part of the *de novo* inflammation of nasal polyps.

in the tissue of nasal polyps does not appear to depend on the presence of allergy or IgE-mediated hypersensitivity (5) but is related to the upregulation of appropriate cytokines and growth factors which specifically attract eosinophilic precursors from the microvasculature (6).

Our laboratory has been studying a number of cytokines that are present in nasal polyps including IL-1β, tumor necrosis factor alpha (TNF α), macrophage-granulocyte colony stimulating factor (MG-CSF), vascular cell adhesion molecule-1 (VCAM-1), α4 β1 integrins (VLA-4), lymphocyte function antigen-1 (LFA-1) (αL β2) and intercellular adhesion molecule-1 (ICAM-1). All of these cytokines have a direct or indirect effect on the rolling, adherence, and transmigration of eosinophils from the microvasculature into the lamina propria of nasal polyps (Fig. 10.4). Once the eosinophils are present in the interstitium of the nasal polyp, they become activated, degranulate, and, in addition to releasing inflammatory mediators which will be mentioned below, also release cytokines IL-3 and IL-5 (7). These two cytokines are responsible for increased recruitment of eosinophils in an autocrine upregulated fashion. Furthermore, these cytokines are responsible for decreasing apoptosis, leading to increased survival of eosinophils (8).

VCAM-1 is increased on the lining endothelium of medium-sized blood vessels of nasal polyps as compared to patients' inferior turbinates (Fig. 10.5). There is also an increase in the avidity of VLA-4 to VCAM-1 in nasal polyps and this appears to be controlled by granulocyte macrophage colony stimulating factor (GM-CSF) (9).

The mechanisms of inflammatory eosinophil recruitment have been well studied and appear to involve a multistep model for leukocyte extravasation, as summarized in Fig. 10.4. In the first step, free-flowing leukocytes within the lumin of venules attach to the endothelial cells. This initial adhesion is

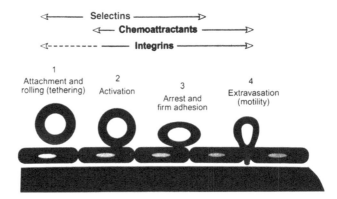

Figure 10.4 Diagram of the overlapping role of selectins, chemoattractants, and integrins in leukocyte attachment, rolling, firm adhesion and extravasation (see text for details).

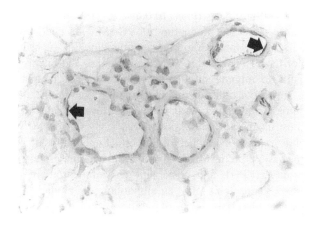

Figure 10.5 Vascular cell adhesion molecule-1 (VCAM-1) is shown on the lining endothelium of a medium-size blood vessel in the nasal polyp (closed arrows). When compared to the patient's inferior turbinates, VCAM-1 was significantly increased.

mediated by the selectin family of adhesion molecules that recognize specific cell-surface carbohydrates. The three members of the selectin family are L-selectin expressed on circulating leukocytes and E- and P-selectin expressed on activated endothelium. This initial adhesion is independent of leukocyte activation and is relatively loose under shear stress; it enables slow rolling of interacting leukocytes along the vessel wall. In the second step, activation of integrins on rolling leukocytes is initiated by G-protein-coupled chemo attractant receptors (10). In this process, chemokines are believed to complex with and to be presented by endothelial glycosaminoglycans, thereby triggering, within seconds, firm adhesion of rolling phase of leukocytes through integrin activation. $\alpha 4$, $\beta 1$ integrins (VLA-4) are expressed on lymphocytes, monocytes, and eosinophils but not on neutrophils. Recent reports have shown that $\alpha 4$ integrins not only mediate firm adhesion but are also involved in the initial rolling phase of leukocytes, which suggests that even greater diversity exists in the process of extravasation (11).

When the leukocyte finally adheres firmly, subsequent paracellular migration through the endothelial junction occurs. This event probably is directed by a chemotactic gradient formed by chemoattractants in combination with leukocyte binding to PCAM-1 (platelet/endothelial cell adhesion molecule) (12).

Prior to the activation of eosinophils on the blood vessels, it is necessary for the counter-receptors on the endothelial cells to be upregulated. This upregulation appears to be the function of IL-1β and TNF α. We, along with others, have demonstrated that the message for IL-1β and TNF α is upregulated in the constitutive cells of the nasal polyp including the epithelial cells and endothelial cells and fibroblasts (Figs. 10.6 and 10.7). IL-1β and TNF α, when upregulated, cause increased production of VCAM-1 on endothelial surfaces. This latter molecule, a member of the immunoglobulin superfamily, is the counter receptor for VLA-4. In this way, the cytokines and integrins interact to allow eosinophils to migrate through the blood vessels. It appears that the cytokines that are responsible for this upregulation are significantly increased in allergic rhinitis, asthma, and nasal polyposis. However, quantitatively, they appear to be most increased in nasal polyposis.

Eosinophils release a number of important mediators of inflammation including major basic protein (MBP), eosinophilic cationic protein (ECP), eosinophilic peroxidase (EPO), and eosinophil-derived neurotoxin (EDN) (13). Although these basic proteins play an important role in the elimination of helminthic disease, they also cause significant inflammatory response in mucosa. Most important for our discussion in the pathogenesis of nasal polyps, however, is the fact that major basic protein is responsible for the increased chloride secretion at the apical surface of the respiratory mucosal cell (14), as well as an increased sodium flux into the cell. Therefore, eosinophils play a role in inflammation as well as electrolyte and water transport.

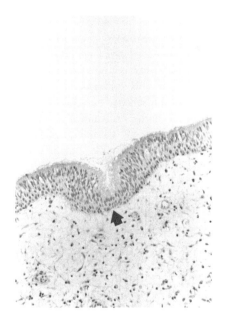

Figure 10.6 Photomicrograph of nasal polyp demonstrating TNF α in the epithelium of the nasal polyp (arrow). The message for this cytokine was also demonstrated to be present in the epithelium and the endothelial cells as well as in fibroblasts (data not shown).

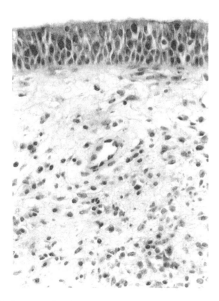

Figure 10.7 IL-1β is seen in the epithelium of nasal polyp. This cytokine was significantly increased in the nasal polyp as compared to the inferior turbinate epithelium. mRNA for this cytokine was upregulated in the nasal polyp in comparison to the inferior turbinate (data not shown).

IV. Abnormal Airway Epithelial Ion and Liquid Transport in Nasal Polyps

Cystic fibrosis (CF) is the model that best explains some of the events that occur with net ion flow across airway epithelia under basal conditions and after stimulation with certain mediators of inflammation. In normal airway epithelia, there is usually a net active sodium absorption and very little chloride secretion (15).

At least three major defects occur in the respiratory epithelial cell in CF; an increased active sodium absorption across the epithelial surface, increased sodium/potassium/ATPase sites on the baso-lateral membrane (16), and an absence of the c-AMP-mediated luminal membrane chloride conductance associated with a dysfunctional CFTR. An alternate chloride conductance that is calcium dependent is, however, present in normal and CF respiratory epithelia. Because nasal polyps occur in 30–50% of children with CF, we sought to compare the bioelectrical events associated with polyps from CF patients and polyps from non-CF patients. In addition, we compared the electrophysiological parameters of the homologous inferior turbinate mucosa as internal controls. In collaboration with Dr. James Yankaskas, our laboratory has studied the voltage (V_t), resistance (R_t) and the short circuit currents (I_{eq}) of cultured polyp and inferior turbinate epithelial cells (17,18). Most polyp specimens cultured in collagen matrix support dishes produce measurable and significant bioelectrical properties. The maximal voltage, resistance, and short circuit currents of these cultures are summarized in Table 10.1.

The most striking observation is the increased voltage and short circuit current in polyp cells as compared to turbinate cells. We have found these alterations in both patients with CF and non-CF polyps. To evaluate the regulatory pathways of ion transport, specimens have been evaluated in Using chambers under basal conditions and during exposure to selected chemicals such as amiloride, isoproterenol, and ATP. The overall results are summarized in Table 10.2. The basal current was significantly decreased by amiloride and was increased by both isoproterenol and ATP. Turbinate cultures had similar but smaller responses. Similar studies on CF cultures (data not shown) demonstrated the ion transport regulatory properties that characterize CF. In particular, amiloride caused a dramatic decrease in I_{eq} and there was no response to isoproterenol, but the ATP response was retained.

These findings suggest that there was a significant increase in sodium absorption across the cell in nasal polyps in both CF and non-CF patients. Furthermore, the chloride channel in patients who do not have CF is normal because it responds to isoproterenol. It is possible that the increased sodium absorption could be one of the fundamental defects in nasal polyps. The increased sodium absorption would allow water to be absorbed through the epithelium into the interstitial space and might account for the edema which is a classic hallmark of the nasal polyp.

V. Remodeling of Human Nasal Polyp Epithelium

Recently, it has been shown that in non-CF polyp epithelia there is restructuring of the airway epithelia (19,20). Basal cell hyperplasia, squamous metaplasia, and goblet cell hyperplasia often are present in non-CF polyp epithelia (Figs. 10.8–10.11). These three alterations following the regeneration of injured

Table 10.1 Maximal Bioelectric Properties of Cultured Human Nasal Polyp and Turbinate Epithelial Cells

	n	V_t (mV)	R_t (Ω cm^2)	I_{eq} (μA/cm^2)
CF				
Polyp (8 patients)	13	-20.4 ± 6.8	242 ± 33	106.3 ± 30.4
Turbinate (8 patients)	13	-17.9 ± 4.1	213 ± 20	86.1 ± 20.2
Non-CF				
Polyp (12 patients)	37	-11.2 ± 1.5	243 ± 315	43.6 ± 4.2
Turbinate (7 patients)	9	$-5.3 - 1.4$	187 ± 24	28.5 ± 5.7

Table 10.2 Bioelectric Properties of Cultured Human Nasal Polyp and Turbinate Epithelial Cells

	Polyps (n = 21)			Turbinates (n = 3)		
	V_t (mV)	R_t (Ω cm^2)	I_{eq} (μA/cm^2)	V_t (mV)	R_t (Ω cm^2)	I_{eq} (μA/cm^2)
Basal	7.8 ± 1.2	173 ± 16	44.1 ± 6.2	−2.4 ± 1.0	103 ± 17	20.8 ± 6.0
Amiloride hydrochloride, 10^{-4} mol/L	−4.0[a] ± 0.5	208[a] ± 20	20.6[a] ± 2.0	−1.1 ± 0.4	104 ± 15	10.4 ± 1.5
Isoproterenol, 10^{-5} mol/L	−4.3[a] ± 0.5	194[a] ± 15	22.8[a] ± 2.2	−1.3 ± 0.4	100 ± 16	12.7 ± 2.9
ATP, 10^{-4} mol/L	−6.7 ± 1.1	142[a] ± 13	64.0[a] ± 11.4	−1.7 ± 1.8	77 ± 15	30.0 ± 11.1

[a]Significant change from preceeding value, p, 0.01, paired t-test.

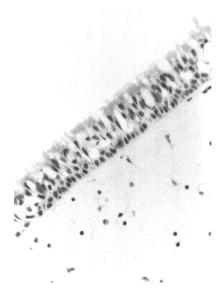

Figure 10.8 Classification of different morphological subtypes of the surface epithelium of human nasal polyps. Normal pseudostratified surface epithelium mainly composed of ciliated cells, mucous cells and one layer of basal cells (H and E, ×200).

nasal polyp epithelia result in defective CFTR location and is phenotypically similar to the genetic defect in CF. Thus, in nasal polyposis, there is defective sodium absorption through the amiloride-sensitive apical sodium channel, even in the absence of CF. We have not been able to demonstrate any defect in chloride secretion. If the CFTR protein is not functioning because the protein is diffusely present in the cytoplasm and not localized to the apex as it normally should be, this dysfunctional CFTR protein will then have an effect on the regulation of the sodium channels by increasing the number of open channels. It also will have an effect on decreasing the function of the outwardly rectifying chloride channel (ORCC) (21).

There is evidence that the eosinophilic mediator major basic protein has an effect on altering the amount of mucus secreted by the respiratory epithelium (22), and furthermore, major basic protein has an effect on increasing chloride secretion and increasing sodium absorption (14). All of these events could alter the surface epithelium of the non-CF polyp. In as much as the CFTR protein may not be functioning, chloride secretion may be decreased and sodium chloride would then be pumped into the interstitium. Water would then follow this increased movement of sodium into the lamina propria. This movement of sodium could account for the movement of water with resultant edema, and it is edema which is a major pathologic feature of nasal polyposis.

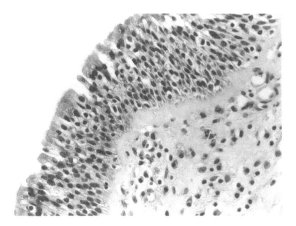

Figure 10.9   Basal cell hyperplasia representing at least three layers of basal cells in the epithelium of a nasal polyp (H and E, ×200).

VI.   Summary

A model for the development of nasal polyps and, perhaps, the growth of nasal polyps can be now considered. The microenvironmental theory of inflammation has been championed by the McMaster group for the last decade (23). Our laboratory has confirmed these findings, suggesting that the constitutive cells of the nasal polyp produce a greater amount of inflammatory cytokines, as compared to homologous inferior turbinate mucosa. The inflammatory cytokines then lead to an upregulation of receptors on the surface of vascular endothelia and

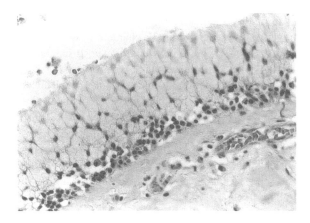

Figure 10.10   Mucous cell hyperplasia in which the entire mucous membrane has been replaced by goblet cells. There is also slight hyperplasia of the basal cell layer as well (H and E, ×400).

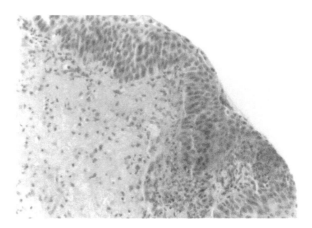

Figure 10.11 Squamous metaplasia characterized by the presence of multi-layered flattened cells (H and E, ×400).

integrins on the surface of inflammatory cells. The paradigm for rolling, adhesion, and transmigration of eosinophils has been discussed and accounts for the increase in the number of eosinophils seen in the lamina propria of nasal polyps. The release of mediators from eosinophils can recruit more eosinophils. The increased recruitment, activation, and survival of eosinophils lead to increased production of basic granule proteins which in turn have an effect on mucus production as well as ion flux. The movement of sodium and water from the lumen into the cell and then into the lamina propria may account for edema that is seen in nasal polyps. The second potential model for the development of nasal polyps is summarized in Fig. 10.12. Damage to the surface epithelium by inflammatory mediators from eosinophils and other inflammatory cells, leads to regeneration of new epithelia characterized by goblet cell hyperplasia, squamous metaplasia, or basal cell hyperplasia. It has been shown that in these altered epithelia, CFTR protein, which is necessary for chloride secretion, is not located in the correct position at the apex of the cell. This defect causes an imbalance of sodium channels so that there may be more open channels allowing for increased sodium absorption and water retention (14). Thus, there are two arms of the model for the development of nasal polyposis (Fig. 10.12). One caused by cytokine upregulation leading to increased eosinophil degranulation and the other mechanism is one of injury to the airway epithelial cells induced by allergen, virus, or trauma, leading to defective CFTR. Both eosinophilic degranulation and defective CFTR migration lead to alteration of sodium and chloride flux in the epithelial cell lining the nasal mucosa in the lateral wall of the nose resulting in the major pathological finding in nasal polyps, edema.

In conclusion, the new information in molecular biology and inflammation in nasal polyps coupled with the data on sodium and chloride ion fluxes may lead

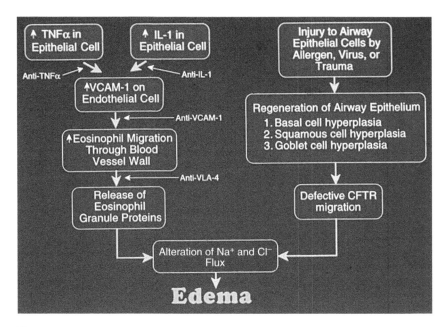

Figure 10.12 Alternative hypotheses for the development of edema in nasal polyposis. On the left-hand side of the figure, TNF α and IL-1β are upregulated in the epithelium. The cause of this upregulation is not known but presumably could be due to virus, bacteria, allergen or an alternative irritative mechanism. These two inflammatory cytokines may be responsible for the upregulation of VCAM-1 on endothelial cells and for the increased expression of VLA-4 on the surface of eosinophils. This receptor-counter receptor interaction allows for the increased migration of eosinophils into the lamina propria of nasal polyps. The release of eosinophil granule proteins, particularly major basic protein, may lead to an alteration in the sodium and chloride flux in the surface epithelium leading to absorption of sodium and water and the ultimate development of edema. On the right side of the figure is an alternative method by which edema can be produced. Injury to the airway epithelial cells by the same triggers that upregulate cytokines, can lead to regeneration of airway epithelium, particularly basal cell hyperplasia, stratified squamous cell hyperplasia and goblet cell hyperplasia. This may lead to defective migration of the cystic fibrosis transmembrane regulator protein which then can produce an increased number of open sodium channels with resultant water absorption and finally, edema. On the left-hand side of the diagram, various antibodies are shown which could theoretically inhibit the effect of various cytokines on the migration of eosinophils into the nasal polyp lamina propria.

to new therapies in the treatment of nasal polyposis. For example, in addition to the use of the classical anti-inflammatory drugs such as corticosteroids, there may now be a role for the use of amiloride or furosemide as sodium channel inhibitors to prevent the influx of sodium, and the use of uridine triphosphate (UTP) to increase chloride secretion. There may also be a role for antibodies directed against VCAM-1 and VLA-4 which can downregulate the recruitment and migration of eosinophils. It is exciting to consider the role of molecular biology and specific antibodies against cell surface receptors in the treatment of nasal polyposis in the 21st century.

References

1. Mygind N, Lildholdt T. Nasal Polyposis; an Inflammatory Disease and Its Treatment. Copenhagen: Munksgaard, 1997:13–183.
2. Settipane G, Lund V, Bernstein J, Tos M. Nasal Polyps: Epidemiology, Pathogenesis and Treatment. Providence, RI: Oceanside Publications Inc, 1997:1–190.
3. Brain TJ. Historical background of nasal polyps. In: Settipane G, Lund V, Bernstein J, Tos M, eds. Nasal Polyps, Epidemiology, Pathology, Treatment. Providence, RI: Oceanside Publications Inc, 1997:1913.
4. Hamilos DL, Leung DYM, Wood R et al. Chronic hyperplastic sinusitis; association of tissue eosinophilia and a RNA expression of granulocyte-macrophage colony-stimulating factor and interleukin-3. J Allergy Clin Immunol 1993; 92:39–48.
5. Ruhno J, Howie K, Anderson M, Andersson B et al. The increased number of epithelial mast cells in nasal polyps at adjacent terbinates is not allergy-dependent. Allergy 1997; 45:370–374.
6. Sriramarao P, Butcher EC, Boeurdon MA, Broide DH. L-selectin and very late antigen-4 integrin promote eosinophil rolling at physiological shear rates in vivo. J Immunol 1994; 153:4238–4246.
7. Allen JS, Eismar, Leonard G, Kreutzer D. Interleukin-3, interleukin-5, and granulocyte-macrophage colony-stimulating factor expression in nasal polyps. Am J Otolarygol 1997; 18:239–246.
8. Morita M, Lamkhioued B, Soussi, Gounni A, Aldeberdt et al. Induction by interferons of human eosinophil apoptosis and regulation by interleukin-3, granulocytes-macrophage colony-stimulating factor and interleukin-5. Eur Cytokine Network 1996; 7:725–732.
9. Sung KL, Li Y, Elices M, Gang J, Sriramarao P, Broide DH. Granulocyte-macrophage colony-stimulating factor regulates the functional adhesive state of very late antigen-4 expressed by eosinophils. J Immunol 1997; 158:919–927.
10. Murphy PM. The molecular biology of leukocyte chemoattractant receptors. Ann Rev Immunol 1994; 12:593–633.
11. Alon R, Kassner PD, Carr MW, Finger EB, Hemler ME, Springer TA. The integrin VLA-4 supports tethering and rolling in flow on VCAM-1. J Cell Biol 1995; 128:1243–1253.
12. Liao F, Huinh HK, Eiroa A, Greene T, Polizzi E, Muller WA. Migration of monocytes across endothelium and passage through extracellular matrix involves separate molecular domains of VCAM-1. J Exp Med 1995; 182:1337–1343.
13. Venge P. Human eosinophil granule proteins; structure, function and release. In: Smith H, Cook MR, eds. Immunophamacology of Eosinophils. London: Academic Press, 1993:43–56.
14. Jacoby DB, Ueki IF, Widdicombe JH, Loegering DA, Gleich G, Nadol J. Effect of human eosinophil major basic protein on ion transport in dog tracheal epithelium. Am Rev Respir Dis 1988; 137:13–16.

15. Smith JJ, Welsh MJ. Fluid and electrolyte transport by cultured human airway epithelia. J Clin Invest 1993; 91:1590–1597.
16. Stutts MJ, Canessa CM, Olsenj C, Hamrick M, Cohn JA et al. CFTR as a c-AMP dependent regulator of sodium channels. Science 1995; 269:847–850.
17. Bernstein JM, Cropp GA, Nathanson I, Yankaskas JR. Bioelectric properties of cultured nasal polyp in turbinate epithelial cells. Am J Rhinol 1990; 4:45–49.
18. Bernstein JM, Yankaskas JR. Increased ion transport in cultured nasal polyp epithelial cells. Arch Otolaryngol Head Neck Surg 1994; 120:993–996.
19. Brezillon S, Dupuit F, Hinnrasky J, Marchand F, Kalin N, Tummler B, Puchelle E. Decreased expression of the CFTR protein in remodeled human nasal epithelium from non-cystic fibrosis patients. Lab Invest 1995; 72:191–200.
20. Dupuit F, Kalin N, Brezillon S, Hinnrasky J, Tummler B, Puchelle E. CFTR and differentiation markers expression in non-CF and Δ F508 homozygous CF nasal epithelium. J Clin Invest 1995; 96:1601–1611.
21. Jovov B, Ismailov I, Berdiev BK, Fuller CM, Sorscher J et al. Interaction between cystic fibrosis transmembrane conductance regulator and outwardly rectified chloride channels. J Biol Chem 1995; 270:2194–2200.
22. Lundgren JD, Davey RT, Lundgren B, Mullol J, Marom Z et al. Eosinophil cationic proteins stimulates and major basic protein inhibits airway mucous secretion. J Allergy Clin Immunol 1991; 87:689–698.
23. Denburg J, Dolovich J, Ohtoshi T, Cox G, Gaulidi J, Jordana M. The micro environmental differentiation hypothesis of airway inflammation. Am J Rhinol 1990; 4:29–32.

B. Diagnosis

11

Anatomic Terminology and Nomenclature of the Paranasal Sinuses and Quantification for Staging Sinusitis

ERIN D. WRIGHT

University of Western Ontario,
London, Ontario, Canada

WILLIAM E. BOLGER

University of Pennsylvania Health System,
Philadelphia, Pennsylvania, USA

DAVID W. KENNEDY

University of Pennsylvania,
Philadelphia, Pennsylvania, USA

I. Introduction

The last 15 years has seen a tremendous advance in the technology available for the diagnosis and treatment of paranasal sinus disease. The resolution of current imaging techniques and the level of surgical precision provided by endoscopic techniques are unparalleled in history. The opportunity for precise surgical intervention makes accurate communication between radiologists and surgeons imperative. Therefore the need for standardized anatomic nomenclature is essential. Additionally, international communication between otolaryngologists would be greatly facilitated by a uniform system for anatomic terminology. Further, detailed knowledge of paranasal sinus anatomy forms the basis for the current understanding of the pathophysiology of sinus inflammatory disease.

Recent years have seen the development of a standardized anatomical nomenclature for the paranasal sinuses. An International Conference was convened in Princeton, New Jersey, USA in 1993 to attempt to standardize the anatomical terms used in the paranasal sinuses. This conference was followed in 1995 by a formal report that documented this effort to develop a unified system of nomenclature (1). This chapter constitutes a synopsis of these endeavors, which has been supplemented by the more recent literature and evolving understanding of paranasal sinus anatomy. Prior to discussing the anatomic nomenclature of the paranasal sinuses, a review of the functionally relevant embryology will be presented.

II. Embryology of the Lateral Nasal Wall

The ethmoid turbinates appear in the 9th and 10th weeks of fetal development. Initially, the appearance of the lateral nasal wall consists of six ridges or ethmo-turbinals. Corresponding furrows separate the ethmoturbinals. As the appearance of the ethmoturbinals matures, they can be observed to acquire separate anterior (ascending) and posterior (descending) portions.

The first ethmoturbinal has a rather complicated development that deserves special mention. Its ultimate fate is dual. The ascending portion remains as the agger nasi (nasoturbinal), while the descending portion becomes the uncinate process. The furrow between the first and second ethmoturbinals also has a dual fate. The descending portion gives rise to the ethmoidal infundibulum while the ascending portion gives rise to the frontal recess. Pneumatization from the frontal recess into the frontal bone gives rise to the frontal sinus.

The second ethmoturbinal gives rise to the middle turbinate while the third ethmoturbinal gives rise to the superior turbinate. The fourth and fifth ethmoturb-inals fuse together and give rise to the supreme turbinate. The inferior turbinate arises from the maxilloturbinal. This maxilloturbinal represents a separate bone which is attached to the lateral nasal wall but that is unrelated to the ethmoturbinals.

The embryological origin of the bulla ethmoidalis is rather complicated. It is felt to arise as a secondary lateral nasal wall evagination related to but separate from the maxilloturbinal ethmoturbinal (2). These evaginations have also been termed secondary or accessory conchae.

The basal lamella of the middle turbinate (second basal lamella) is a critical reference point when considering the development of ethmoid pneumatization. Cells that begin pneumatizing from a point anterior to the second basal lamella are termed anterior ethmoid cells while cells that begin to pneumatize posterior to the basal lamella are termed posterior ethmoid cells. In other words, the relation-ship to the basal lamella of the second ethmoturbinal determines the site of drai-nage of the ethmoid air cells. Thus, despite considerable variation with respect to the pneumatization of ethmoid air cells, they have a fixed point of reference, which is their ostium. It is from this fixed reference point that pneumatization occurs. This then explains the adult anatomy where the anterior ethmoid cells drain into the middle meatus while the posterior ethmoid air cells drain into the superior meatus, behind the basal lamella of the middle turbinate.

A surgically useful summary and extension of these embryological relation-ships is to consider the basal lamellae of the ethmoturbinals. The uncinate process is actually the basal lamella of the first ethmoturbinal. The ethmoidal bulla arises from a secondary concha related to the first ethmoturbinal while the middle turbinate arises from the second ethmoturbinal. The surgical usefulness is that they generally correspond to the order in which structures are taken down during endoscopic sinus surgery using the Messerklinger technique (3).

III. Anatomical Philosophy

The recent evolution in the nomenclature of paranasal sinus anatomy has been based on several philosophical principles. The first of these principles was to drop the individual names or eponyms associated with anatomical structures and to use the more accurate, descriptive anatomical term. Generally, the English nomenclature, based on the traditional Latin Nomina Anatomica, has been adopted for international use except for rare instances where the Latin term has been universally accepted. The International Conference on Sinus Disease also took the position that anatomical variants generally did not require specific nomenclature (e.g., paradoxically curved middle turbinate). Finally, topographic and directional instructions (e.g., superior, inferior) refer to the standard anatomical position with the person standing.

IV. Ethmoid Sinuses

As outlined previously, the ethmoid air cells are classified as belonging to either anterior or posterior systems. This relates to their previously described embryology as well as the patterns of drainage and mucociliary flow. The anatomical definition states that the basal lamella of the middle turbinate is the dividing line between anterior and posterior ethmoid complexes. Cells that drain anterior and inferior to the basal lamella are said to belong to the anterior complex while cells that drain posterior and superior to the basal lamella belong to the posterior ethmoid complex. The obvious and notable exception to this rule is the sphenoid sinus that has a separate ostium that drains into the sphenoethmoidal recess. "Middle ethmoid cells" and related terms such as "middle ethmoid" are historical terms that can be used currently to refer to the retrobullar and suprabullar recesses.

V. Basal Lamella of the Middle Turbinate

This anatomically complex structure is the embryological derivative of the basal lamella of the third ethmoturbinal and is outlined in the sagittal plane in Fig. 11.1. The tortuous course of the basal lamella begins most anteriorly and superiorly at the crista ethmoidalis of the maxilla. The most posterior and inferior end attaches to the crista ethmoidalis of the perpendicular process of the palatine bone (lamina perpendicularis).

Between the aforementioned origins, the course of the basal lamella can be conceptualized into three portions. The first third is that portion that inserts

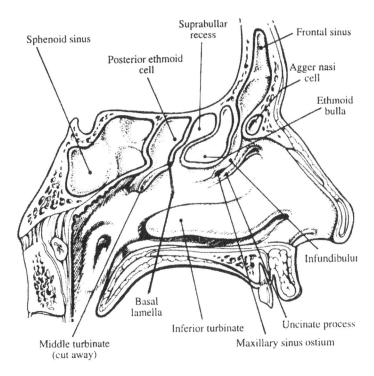

Figure 11.1   Sagittal section through the nose and ethmoid sinuses. The basal lamella divides ethmoid air cells into anterior and posterior and forms an integral part of the middle turbinate. From International Conference on Sinus Disease: Terminology, Staging, Therapy. In: Kennedy DW, ed. Ann Otol Rhinol Laryngol 1995; (suppl 167) 104(10):1–31. (Reproduced with permission.)

vertically into the skull base at lateral edge of the cribriform plate. The middle portion of the basal lamella twists laterally to insert into the lamina orbitalis (also termed the lamina papyracea) where it courses in a posteroinferior direction. The final portion runs in a horizontal plane and attaches to the crista ethmoidalis ossis palatini, as mentioned previously. Thus the basal lamella can be seen to run in three different planes, initially in the sagittal plane, and subsequently in the oblique frontal plane. The final third is more or less horizontal and attaches to the either the medial wall of the orbit or the medial wall of the maxillary sinus, or both. The middle turbinate is thus a relatively stable structure owing to its fixation in three planes.

The middle portion of the basal lamella of the middle turbinate deserves additional description since it will be traversed and opened during the dissection of a total ethmoidectomy. Although conceptualized as running smoothly and obliquely in a posteroinferior direction, it may often be indented by well-pneumatized anterior ethmoid cells. This middle portion may thus be seen to run in the posterosuperior direction dorsally. Conversely, posterior ethmoid cells can create an anterior bulge in the midsection of the basal lamella.

A final comment regarding the nomenclature of the basal lamella of the middle turbinate is that terms like ground lamella are misnomers and should not be used lest they create confusion. This statement was emphasized and supported by the report of the International Conference (1).

VI. Anterior Ethmoidal Region

The anterior ethmoid air cells and their surrounding structures are complex and play a fundamental role in our current understanding of the pathophysiology of chronic sinusitis. It is this single area of the paranasal sinuses, along with the frontal recess, that has generated the most confusion with respect to nomenclature over the years. The related structures including the uncinate process, agger nasi, sinus lateralis, hiatus semilunaris, and infundibulum will be discussed along with the ethmoid bulla.

A. Uncinate Process

Translated from Latin, this structure is the "hooked outgrowth" that represents the remnant of the descending portion of the first ethmoturbinal. This thin bony leaflet is oriented sagittally and runs from anterosuperior to posteroinferior (Fig. 11.2).

The posteroinferior free margin is concave and parallel to the anterior surface of the ethmoid bulla. The posterior and inferior attachments of the uncinate process include the perpendicular process of the palatine bone and the ethmoid process of the inferior turbinate. It also attaches anteriorly where its convex anterior margin ascends to the lacrimal bone. When curved medially to a significant degree, the uncinate process may protrude into or out of the middle meatus, giving rise the so-called "double middle turbinate." This outdated term, with its potential for confusion, is clearly a misnomer and should not be used in the future.

B. Agger Nasi

Taken from Latin and meaning "nasal mound," this structure is a superior remnant of the first ethmoturbinal. This mound or crest is located immediately anterior and superior to the middle turbinate. If pneumatized, it is referred to as an agger nasi cell and should not be confused with the more posterior ethmoid bulla or more superior frontal cells. Agger nasi cells drain into the ethmoidal infundibulum. When well pneumatized, the agger nasi cell may be seen to extend laterally and result in narrowing of the frontal recess.

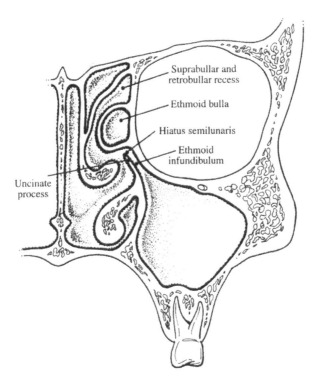

Figure 11.2 Coronal section at the level of the uncinate process. Ethmoid bulla, hiatus semilunaris and ethmoid infundibulum are demonstrated. From International Conference on Sinus Disease: Terminology, Staging, Therapy. In: Kennedy DW, ed. Ann Otol Rhinol Laryngol 1995; (suppl 167) 104(10):1–31. (Reproduced with permission.)

C. Ethmoid Bulla

The Latin term bulla refers to a thin-walled (bony) prominence or blister. In the case of the ethmoid bulla, this refers to the most constant and largest group of ethmoid air cells. Formed by pneumatization of the bulla lamella (a secondary evagination between the first and second ethmoturbinals) the ethmoid bulla sits like a bleb or blister on the lamina orbitalis. It has been demonstrated to be variably pneumatized and to lack a discrete posterior bony wall (4).

D. Retrobullar and Suprabullar Recess

These structures have been previously known as the sinus lateralis of Grunwald (5) and the susbullar cell of Mouret (6) and may be called the middle ethmoid pneumatization. The suprabullar recess refers to the space created when the bulla lamella fails to attach to the skull base. The space created superior to the bulla below the skull base is the suprabullar recess (Fig. 11.1). The suprabullar recess may open into the frontal recess if the bulla lamella fails to reach the skull base. The retrobullar recess is that space located posterior to the bulla lamella and anterior to the basal lamella of the middle turbinate posteriorly. The suprabullar recess, on rare occasion, may be continuous with the retrobullar recess posteriorly (Fig. 11.1).

E.   Hiatus Semilunaris

The hiatus semilunaris is the term describing the two-dimensional cleft in the sagittal plane between the posterior free edge of the uncinate process and the anterior face of the ethmoid bulla (Fig. 11.2). It therefore does not represent a true space but is, in fact, a crescent-shaped gap that provides an entranceway into the three-dimensional space that is the ethmoidal infundibulum.

F.   Ethmoid Infundibulum

This term refers to a funnel-shaped space bordered medially by the uncinate process and laterally by the lamina orbitalis (Figs. 11.1 and 11.2). The report of the International Conference refers to this space as being analogous to an inverted segment of a grapefruit with the wider edge facing posteriorly. The anterior end of the infundibulum ends blindly in an acute angle while posteriorly the infundibulum extends to the anterior face of the ethmoid bulla. At this point it opens into the middle meatus through the hiatus semilunaris.

G.   Maxillary Sinus Ostium

The ostium of the maxillary sinus is found at the floor and lateral aspect of the infundibulum towards its posterior end. Thus, the natural ostium of the maxillary sinus is hidden from the middle meatus by the uncinate process, located infero-laterally in the ethmoid infundibulum.

H.   Nasal Fontanelles

This term is derived from French and refers to membrane-covered spaces remaining in the incompletely ossified skull. In the paranasal sinuses it refers to areas of the lateral nasal wall where no bone exists but rather that a mucosal and periosteal barrier separates the maxillary sinus from the middle meatus. They are typically located immediately above the insertion of the inferior turbinate. If the mucoperiosteal barrier breaks down or does not form, these fontanelles can form accessory ostia into the maxillary sinus. The posterior fontanelle is more commonly seen clinically and is located superior and posterior to the part of the uncinate process that fuses with the medial wall of the maxillary sinus. The anterior fontanelle is located anterior and inferior to the uncinate process.

The posterior fontanelle is important surgically since this accessory ostium is often confused with the natural ostium resulting in two openings into the maxillary sinus. Failure to recognize this situation will result in mucous recirculation from the natural ostium into the accessory or iatrogenic ostium with persistence of inflammation and infection.

I. Frontal and Maxillary Infundibula

Both of these structures refer to a funnel-shaped narrowing of the respective sinuses that are located within the sinuses as they approach their natural ostia. In the case of the frontal sinus this is a significant narrowing toward the floor of the sinus while in the maxillary sinus the lumen does not typically narrow significantly towards its ostium.

J. Ethmoid Roof

Technically speaking, the ethmoid roof is formed by the frontal bone. The entire complex, however, has a step-like configuration (Fig. 11.3). Beginning medially, the ethmoid roof complex is formed by the cribriform plate. At the lateral aspect of the cribriform plate, where the middle turbinate also inserts, the skull base turns upward in the sagittal plane. This *lateral lamella* of the cribriform meets the medial extension of the true ethmoid roof. The step-like structure created forms a groove in which the olfactory bulb sits.

The configuration of the ethmoid roof has been classified by Keros (7) into three types. The basis for the classification is the length of the lateral lamella of the cribriform plate and by extension the depth of the olfactory groove. The clinical significance of this classification is that the lateral lamella is the thinnest bone in the entire skull base and is the most common site for iatrogenic cereberospinal fluid (CSF) leaks in endoscopic sinus surgery. As outlined in Fig. 11.3, a Keros type I skull base has an olfactory fossa that measures 1–3 mm in depth and therefore has a short or almost nonexistent lateral lamella which puts the ethmoid roof in almost the same plane as the cribriform plate. A Keros type II skull base refers to a longer lateral lamella and an olfactory fossa that is 4–7 mm deep. The Keros type III skull base has an olfactory fossa that measures 8–16 mm deep and thus the ethmoid roof lies significantly above the cribriform plate.

It can therefore be seen that a Keros type III skull base will pose the greatest risk for iatrogenic injury, a fact that has pre-operative significance when reviewing the computed tomography (CT) scan prior to surgical intervention.

K. Anatomical Variants of the Anterior Ethmoid

A concha bullosa is the term used to refer to a pneumatized middle turbinate. For the middle turbinate, the pneumatization has been described as originating from the frontal recess or from the agger nasi. An interlamellar cell is the term used to refer to pneumatization of the vertical lamella of the middle turbinate, which originates from the superior meatus. The infraorbital ethmoid cell is historically referred to as a Haller's cell. These cells originate from the ethmoid system and grow into the bony orbital floor/maxillary sinus roof (Fig. 11.4). From a

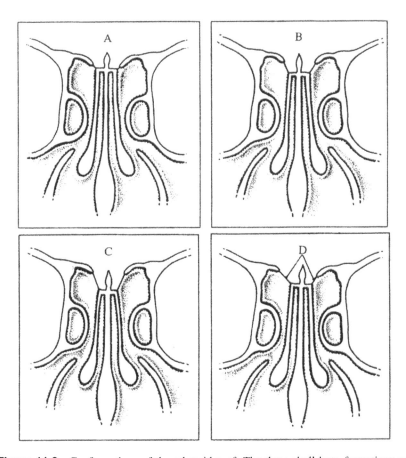

Figure 11.3 Configurations of the ethmoid roof. The three skull base formations are (A) type 1, in which the olfactory fossa is 1–3 mm deep, (B) type 2, in which it is 4–7 mm deep, and (C) type 3, in which it is 8–16 mm deep. (D) Asymmetric skull base is an anatomic variant that should be identified with preoperative computed tomography to avoid skull base injury. Note the thin lateral lamella of the cribriform plate. From International Conference on Sinus Disease: Terminology, Staging, Therapy. In: Kennedy DW, ed. Ann Otol Rhinol Laryngol 1995; (suppl 167) 104(10):1–31. (Reproduced with permission.)

pathophysiologic perspective these cell can be significant due to their creation of a narrowed ethmoid infundibulum or maxillary sinus ostium.

L. Ostiomeatal Complex

The current conceptualization of the ostiomeatal complex (OMC) is that of a functional entity of the ethmoid complex that represents the final common pathway for the drainage and ventilation of the frontal, maxillary, and anterior

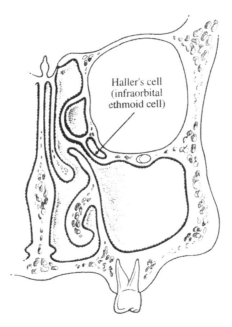

Figure 11.4   Infraorbital ethmoid cell. Also known as Haller's cell, this ethmoid cell is positioned inferiorly and lateral to the ethmoid bulla and is intimately related to the ethmoidal infundibulum. From International Conference on Sinus Disease: Terminology, Staging, Therapy. In: Kennedy DW, ed. Ann Otol Rhinol Laryngol 1995; (suppl 167) 104(10):1–31. (Reproduced with permission.)

ethmoid air cells (Fig. 11.5). Disease of anyof the cells or related structures and their dependent sinuses contributes to the pathophysiology of sinusitis.

VII.   Frontal Recess and Frontal Sinus

Deserving of separate discussion, the frontal recess is the most complex and variable structure in the anterior ethmoid complex. The term refers to the most anterior and superior portion of the complex that leads to and communicates with the frontal sinus. As pointed out in the report of the International Conference, this structure is *not* synonymous with the nasofrontal duct.

The boundaries of the frontal recess are as follows. The medial border is the most anterior and superior part of the middle turbinate (vertical portion that attaches to the skull base). The lateral border is formed by the orbital plate of the frontal bone and the lamina orbitalis. Posteriorly, the border is formed by skull base as it slopes anteriorly and superiorly with potential contribution from the ethmoid bulla. A well-pneumatized bulla may form the posterior limit of the frontal recess resulting in narrowing of the recess thus leading to a

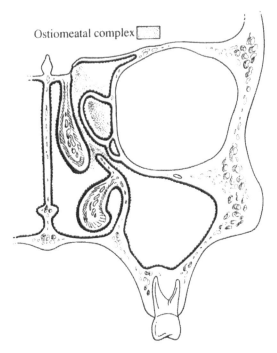

Figure 11.5 The ostiomeatal complex is the functional unit that comprises the maxillary sinus ostium, the anterior ethmoid cells and their ostia, ethmoid infundibulum, hiatus semilunaris and middle meatus. From International Conference on Sinus Disease: Terminology, Staging, Therapy. In: Kennedy DW, ed. Ann Otol Rhinol Laryngol 1995; (suppl 167) 104(10):1–31. (Reproduced with permission.)

tubular appearance, which is the reason for the historical and erroneous label of nasofrontal duct. Anteriorly, the frontal recess is bordered by the agger nasi, which, when pneumatized, may narrow or obscure the recess (Fig. 11.1).

The frontal recess, when seen in sagittal section, has the shape of an inverted funnel. Therefore, when combined with the frontal infundibulum, the combined shape is that of an hourglass with the constriction at the level of the natural ostium of the frontal sinus.

The frontal recess receives drainage of several cells aside from the frontal sinus proper. Supraorbital ethmoid cells, as well as frontal cells, may drain into the recess. The agger nasi has been previously discussed but the supraorbital ethmoid cell and frontal cells warrant additional comment.

A. Supraorbital Ethmoid Cell

This represents an ethmoid cell that pneumatizes the orbital plate of the frontal bone posterior to the frontal recess and posterolateral to the frontal sinus (8).

This cell can thus result in displacement of the posterior wall of the frontal sinus with resultant encroachment of the frontal sinus drainage pathway.

B. Frontal Cells

These represent cells that are derived from the anterior ethmoid system behind the agger nasi. They are seen to pneumatize the frontal recess above the agger nasi and may result in obstruction of the frontal sinus drainage or the frontal sinus itself (9).

VIII.   Posterior Ethmoidal Region

Discussed in this section will be the posterior ethmoid cells, the sphenoid sinus and anatomical variants related to these two sinus areas. Intimately related in to these sinuses is the optic nerve, which will be given special attention.

A. Posterior Ethmoid Cells

These cells have been defined by the International Conference to comprise the cells of the superior meatus and, if present, the cells and clefts underneath the supreme (4th) turbinate. As outlined previously, the formal posterior ethmoid cells are less numerous than the anterior ethmoid cells and drain under the superior turbinate.

B. Sphenoethmoidal Recess

This space is the site of drainage for the sphenoid sinus. It is bordered laterally by the superior turbinate and medially by the nasal septum. The superior border of the sphenoethmoidal recess is the roof of the nose while the anterior face of the sphenoid forms the posterior border. Typically, during sphenoethmoidectomy, the natural ostium of the sphenoid sinus is found immediately posterior and medial to the mid-portion of the superior turbinate.

C. Sphenoethmoid Cell

Previously known as an Onodi cell, this cell refers to the most posterior ethmoid cell that pneumatizes posteriorly into the region of the sphenoid. The pneumatization can occur laterally or superiorly to the sphenoid. The corollary to this is that the sphenoid is therefore located inferior and medial to the sphenoethmoid cell. This variable pneumatization can assume great clinical significance. The optic nerve can be present within a sphenoethmoidal cell (Fig. 11.6) as can the carotid artery. Failure to recognize this anatomical fact can result in serious vascular compromise or blindness.

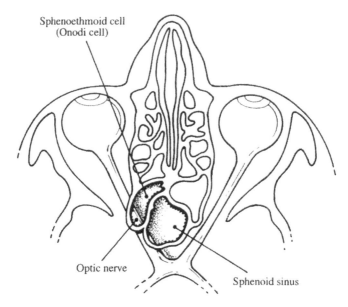

Figure 11.6 Sphenoethmoid cell. Also known as an Onodi cell, this posterior ethmoid cell is lateral and superior to the sphenoid sinus and frequently has an intimate relationship with the optic nerve. From International Conference on Sinus Disease: Terminology, Staging, Therapy. In: Kennedy DW, ed. Ann Otol Rhinol Laryngol 1995; (suppl 167) 104(10):1–31. (Reproduced with permission.)

D. Optic Nerve Tubercle

This structure is the anatomical bulge of the medial aspect of the bone surrounding the optic foramen. Due to the potentially variable anatomy of the sphenoethmoidal region, this structure may be located in the posterior ethmoid, in the sphenoid sinus or at the transition point between the two.

IX. Quantification for Staging

A. Overview—The Need for Staging Systems

In the last 10–15 years, there has been a significant changes in our ability to diagnose and treat sinusitis. The widespread use of nasal endoscopy and newer generation CT scanning has greatly enhanced our ability to evaluate the sinonasal cavity. With the advent of endoscopic sinus surgery, we are now able to provide improved management to our patients with even recalcitrant chronic sinusitis.

In an effort to facilitate accurate communication between otolaryngologists in the scientific literature, attempts have been made in recent years to develop evaluation scales and staging systems for sinusitis. These staging systems were originally based on CT scan data and appeared to have prognostic value. More recent developments in the objective staging of chronic sinusitis have begun to incorporate data concerning coexistent and related illnesses as well as surgical data.

In addition to facilitating communication between otolaryngologists, the development of objective staging systems is necessary for the study and improved understanding of chronic sinusitis. Without a standardized system for recording data and reporting results, the study of this chronic illness would be fragmented and open to personal bias and might fail to generate adequate numbers for more widespread use. Further, to properly understand the disease processes at work, patients must be classified with respect to the severity of their disease, including possible etiologic factors. This requires a universally accepted staging system.

Finally, in our current health care environment, with its economic and resource-related constraints, therapeutic results must be demonstrated to be cost-effective. We believe that such evaluations should include an objective evaluation of outcome results, as well as subjective measures. Because of the long time lag between objective evidence of persistent disease and the development of symptoms and complications of sinus disease, such objective reporting is particularly important in this disorder.

B. Objective Measures/Staging Systems for Sinusitis

The evaluation of patients with chronic sinusitis incorporates both symptomatology and objective analyses. As otolaryngologists, we base a large part of our diagnosis on hard findings such as those seen on physical examination/endoscopy and the radiological investigations such as the CT scan. Such findings lend themselves well to quantification and numerical staging. Numerous attempts have been made in recent years to develop objective systems for the evaluation of chronic sinusitis. The first significant step forward was the staging system suggested by Kennedy in 1992 (10). More recently the Lund–MacKay staging system (11) was modified based on recommendations of the Rhinosinusitis Task Force and has since been endorsed by this body for use in future outcomes research (12).

Prognostic Factors, Outcomes, and Staging—The Kennedy System (10)

The staging system of Kennedy was based on his initial close observation of an early cohort of subjects undergoing endoscopic sinus surgery. Based on his findings over a follow-up period of 18 months, several recommendations were made and an initial staging system was proposed.

With respect to prognostic factors several findings were noted. The presence of allergy had no impact on the objective outcome. When initially examined, the presence of previous ethmoid surgery, acetyl salicylic acid (ASA) sensitivity, and the presence of asthma seemed to impart a poorer prognosis.

However, when the extent of disease based on CT and endoscopy was considered, these previously listed factors were not demonstrated to be predictive of outcome, at least with the numbers of patients in each category available in the study. The only factor demonstrated to be predictive of objective outcome was the radiological and surgical extent of disease.

In devising the initial staging system, the parameters examined included the extent of radiographic disease as well as the degree of surgical mucosal disease. As outlined in Table 11.1, stage I disease included patients in whom anatomical abnormalities were identified, those with unilateral disease and those with bilateral disease limited to the ethmoid cavities. Stage II disease included patients having bilateral ethmoid disease with involvement of one dependent sinus. Stage III were those patients having two or more dependent sinuses involved on each side while stage IV incorporated those patients with diffuse nasal polyposis.

The Need for a More Comprehensive System

While demonstrated to be statistically valid and having certain rationality and logic, the initial staging system proposed by Kennedy was recognized by the author to have some limitations. There was no accounting for the presence of systemic illnesses that contribute to chronic sinus disease such as cystic fibrosis and ciliary dyskinesias as well as immunologic disorders. The grading system proposed by Lund and MacKay in 1993 (11) and subsequently modified by the International Conference on Sinus Disease (12) and by the AAO-HNS Rhinosinusitis Task Force (13) served to improve upon pre-existing staging systems and address some of the limitations of the original staging system suggested by Kennedy.

The Modified Lund–MacKay System (AAO-HNS Rhinosinusitis Task Force) (13)

The original Lund–MacKay staging system was based primarily on a numerical score derived from analysis of CT scan information (Table 11.2).

Table 11.1   Staging for Chronic Rhinosinusitis (Kennedy)

Stage I	Anatomic abnormalities
	All unilateral sinus disease
	Bilateral disease limited to ethmoid sinuses
Stage II	Bilateral ethmoid disease with involvement of one dependent sinus
Stage III	Bilateral ethmoid disease with involvement of two or more dependent sinuses on each side
Stage IV	Diffuse sinonasal polyposis

Source: Adapted from Kennedy (10).

Table 11.2 Radiological Staging of Chronic Rhino-sinusitis (Lund–Mackay)

Sinus	Left	Right
Maxillary		
Anterior ethmoid		
Posterior ethmoid		
Sphenoid		
Frontal		
Ostiomeatal complex		
Total for each side		

Scoring: Sinuses—0 = no abnormalities, 1 = partial opacification, 2 = total opacification.
OMC—0 = not occluded, 2 = occluded.
Source: Adapted from Lund and Mackay (11).

Through its various modifications, the last of which was made by the Rhinosinusitis Task Force, additional information has been included. In its current incarnation, the Lund–MacKay system recommends recording demographic data (Table 11.3) which includes a nasal diagnosis as well as any systemic diagnosis which may have an impact on the upper airways and infection or inflammation thereof.

The radiographic data was expanded to include the presence of anatomical variants that may contribute to the development of chronic sinusitis (Table 11.4).

A surgery score is also included which tabulates the procedures that were performed, thus providing in a tabular format the extent of surgery required for the individual patient (Table 11.5).

For patient follow-up, a symptom score was incorporated into the system which records key sinus related symptoms on a visual analog scale (0–10).

Table 11.3 Demographic Information (Rhinosinusitis Task Force)

Last name: _____	Operation: _____
First name: _____	Date of surgery: _____
Sex: _____	Surgeon: _____
Date of birth: _____	Nasal diagnosis (0–4): _____
Age: _____	Systemic diagnosis: _____
Hospital number: _____	Anesthetic duration (min): _____
Postoperative medications: _____	Complications: _____

Nasal Diagnosis: 1 = chronic rhinosinusitis, 2 = recurrent acute, 3 = nasal polyposis, 4 = miscellaneous.
Source: Adapted from Lund and Kennedy (13).

Table 11.4 Radiological Grading: Anatomic Variants (Rhinosinusitis Task Force)

Anatomic variant	Left	Right
Absent frontal sinus		
Concha bullosa		
Paradoxical middle turbinate		
Everted uncinate process		
Haller cells		
Agger nasi cells		

Scoring: 0 = no variant, 1 = variant present.
Source: Adapted from Lund and Kennedy (13).

These key symptoms include nasal congestion, facial pain, headache, and altered sense of smell, as well as nasal discharge, sneezing and an overall symptom experience. These values are recorded at various time intervals beginning pre-operatively and continuing at 3 months, 6 months, 1 year, and 2 years postoperatively (Table 11.6).

Although not formally included at this time the Task Force did suggest the recording of endoscopic appearances at similar time intervals to the symptom data (Table 11.7).

Endoscopic findings thought to be important include the presence of polyps, edema and discharge as well as the presence of scarring and crusting. Current thinking is placing a significant emphasis on these endoscopic findings, which can often predate and herald a recurrence before the patient begins to experience recurrent symptoms. The prognostic value of the endoscopic appearance thus appears significant and future outcome studies are likely to validate this contention.

Table 11.5 Surgery Score (Lund–Mackay/Rhinosinusitis Task Force)

Surgical procedure	Left	Right
Uncinectomy		
Middle meatal antrostomy		
Anterior ethmoidectomy		
Posterior ethmoidectomy		
Sphenoidotomy		
Frontal recess surgery		
Reduction of middle turbinate		
Total for each side		

Scoring: 0 = no procedure, 1 = procedure done (range 1–14).
Source: Adapted from Lund and Kennedy (13).

Table 11.6 Symptom Score (Lund–Mackay/Rhinosinusitis Task Force)

	Before surgery	After surgery			
Symptom		3 Months	6 Months	1 Year	2 Years
Nasal blockage/congestion					
Headache					
Facial pain					
Altered sense of smell					
Nasal discharge					
Sneezing					
Overall symptom					
Total points					

Scoring: Visual analog scale for each symptom (0–10), 0 = not present, 10 = most severe.
Source: Adapted from Lund and Kennedy (13).

It was the opinion of the Rhinosinusitis Task Force that the modified Lund–MacKay staging system is a simple method that is easy to apply and reproduce. It thus can theoretically be used internationally by many investigators and in the opinion of the Task Force "... seems highly suited to the validation of outcomes research in large clinical studies."

Table 11.7 Endoscopic Appearance (Lund–Mackay/Rhinosinusitis Task Force)

Characteristic	Baseline	3 Months	6 Months	1 Year	2 Years
Polyp, left					
Polyp, right					
Edema, left					
Edema, right					
Discharge, left					
Discharge, right					
Scarring, left*					
Scarring, right*					
Crusting, left*					
Crusting, right*					
Total points					

Scoring: Polyps: 0 = absence of polyps, 1 = middle meatal polyps, 2 = beyond middle meatus.
Edema/Scarring/Crusting: 0 = absent, 1 = mild, 2 = severe.
Discharge: 0 = no discharge, 1 = clear, thin discharge, 2 = thick, purulent discharge.
*Postoperative scores to be used for outcomes assessment only.
Source: Adapted from Lund and Kennedy (13).

C. Subjective vs. Objective Evaluation—Significance for Prognosis

As stated previously, objective endoscopic evaluation during the postoperative period has been suggested for inclusion in the modified Lund–Mackay staging system. Although not formally included in the staging system, current thinking is placing significant emphasis on these endoscopic findings since they often predate symptomatic recurrence in patients with chronic hyperplastic sinusitis (10,14).

Short- and medium-term (18 months) follow-up data for endoscopic sinus surgery consistently demonstrates excellent subjective results (10). The symptomatic improvement does not however, necessarily correlate with objective endoscopic findings (10,15). Furthermore, it has been recently demonstrated that patients who have endoscopic evidence of a normalized sinus cavity at 18–24 months following ESS are much less likely to recur and thus require revision surgery (16). The corollary to this conclusion is that endoscopic evaluation may permit the early detection of significant yet potentially reversible or treatable recurrent disease while it is still asymptomatic (14).

It can thus be concluded that the prognostic value of the postoperative endoscopic appearance is significant and that future outcomes studies are likely to validate this contention. It is also likely that these future studies will demonstrate that staging systems, particularly those incorporating objective endoscopic evaluations, are not as important in predicting subjective outcomes but are critically important in terms of objective outcomes and, more importantly, for long-term results.

D. Subjective Evaluation Scales—Outcomes Research

Subjective evaluation scales play a significant and useful role in outcomes research and are important for health management organizations in evaluating short-term cost-efficacy. These evaluation scales are classified as general health status instruments and disease-specific instruments.

A commonly used general health evaluation tool is the Medical Outcomes Study Short Form-36 (SF-36) (17). While not specifically designed for sinusitis, this evaluation tool provides information concerning the functional well being of the individual and the evaluation of the overall response to treatment.

For the evaluation of the subjective effects of chronic sinusitis and response to therapy, several tools have been developed. Examples of these disease-specific tools include the Chronic Sinusitis Survey (CSS) (18), developed at the Massachusetts Eye and Ear Infirmary as well as the Chronic Sinusitis TyPE Specific Questionnaire developed by the Health Outcomes Institute (19). Both of these systems are duration-based and serve to monitor both patient symptoms and requirement for medical therapy over the previous 8-week period. Both of these forms have been accepted as being reliable and sensitive to clinical change over time. They are both simple and easy to use and provide information over time regarding the efficacy of a therapeutic intervention. The TyPE Specific questionnaire has been recommended by the AAO-HNS Rhinosinusitis Task Force for thorough evaluation (20).

References

1. Stammberger HR, Kennedy DW. Paranasal sinuses: anatomic terminology and nomenclature. The anatomic terminology group. Ann Otol Rhinol Laryngol 1995; (suppl 167):7–16.
2. Libersa C, Laude M, Libersa J. The pneumatization of the accessory cavities of the nasal fossae during growth. Anat Clin 1981; 2:265–273.
3. Stammberger H. Functional Endoscopic Sinus Surgery. Philadelphia, PA: BC Decker, 1991.
4. Wright ED, Bolger WE. The bulla ethmoidalis—lamella or a true cell? J Otolaryngol 2001.
5. Grunwald L. Deskriptive und topographische Anatomie der Nase und ihrer Neben-hohlen. In: Denker A, Kahler O, eds. Handbuch der Hals-Nasen-Ohrenheilkunde. Berlin: Springer-Bergmann, 1925:1–95.
6. Mouret J. Anatomie des cellules ethmoidales. Rev Hebdomad Laryngol Otol Rhinol 1898; 31:913–924.
7. Keros P. Uber die praktische Bedeutung der Niveauunterschiede der lamina cribrosa des eethmoids. Laryngol Rhinol Otol (Stuttg) 1965; 41:808–813.
8. Owen RG Jr, Kuhn FA. Supraorbital ethmoid cell. Otolaryngol Head Neck Surg 1997; 116(2):254–261.
9. Bent JP, Cuilty-Siller C, Kuhn FA. The frontal cell as a cause of frontal sinus obstruction. Am J Rhinol 1994; 8(4):185–191.
10. Kennedy DW. Prognostic factors, outcomes and staging in ethmoid sinus surgery. Laryngoscope 1992; 102(12 Pt 2 suppl 57):1–18.
11. Lund VJ, Mackay IS. Staging in rhinosinusitus. Rhinology 1993; 31(4):183–184.
12. Lund VJ, Kennedy DW. Quantification for staging sinusitis. The Staging and Therapy Group. Ann Otol Rhinol Laryngol 1995; (suppl 167):17–21.
13. Lund VJ, Kennedy DW. Staging for rhinosinusitis. Otolaryngol Head Neck Surg 1997; 117(3 Pt 2):S35–S40.
14. Kennedy DW, Wright ED, Goldberg AN. Objective and subjective outcomes in surgery for chronic sinusitis. Laryngoscope 2000; 110(3 Pt 3):29–31.
15. Vleming M, de Vries N. Endoscopic paranasal sinus surgery: results. Am J Rhinol 1990; 4(1):13–17.
16. Senior BA, Kennedy DW, Tanabodee J, Kroger H, Hassab M, Lanza D. Long-term results of functional endoscopic sinus surgery. Laryngoscope 1998; 108(2):151–157.
17. Ware JE Jr, Sherbourne CD. The MOS 36-item short-form health survey (SF-36). I. Conceptual framework and item selection. Med Care 1992; 30(6):473–483.
18. Gliklich RE, Metson R. Techniques for outcomes research in chronic sinusitis [see comments]. Laryngoscope 1995; 105(4 Pt 1):387–390.
19. Hoffman SR, Mahoney MC, Chmiel JF, Stinziano GD, Hoffman KN. Symptom relief after endoscopic sinus surgery: an outcomes-based study [see comments]. Ear Nose Throat J 1993; 72(6):413–414, see also pp. 419–420.
20. Leopold D, Ferguson BJ, Piccirillo JF. Outcomes assessment. Otolaryngol Head Neck Surg 1997; 117(3 Pt 2):S58–S68.

12

The Diagnosis of Nasal Allergy in Children

GLENIS K. SCADDING

Royal National Throat, Nose and Ear Hospital,
London, UK

I. Introduction

Rhinitis is common in childhood and is increasing in prevalence. Symptoms of nasal running, blocking, sneezing, and itching have effects upon the quality of life and the comorbid associations of rhinitis such as sinusitis, otitis media, and asthma can affect school attendance and examination performance. Unfortunately rhinitis in childhood is often misdiagnosed and mistreated (1).

Allergic rhinitis is clinically defined as a symptomatic alteration of the nose, induced by an IgE-mediated inflammation after exposure of the nasal mucosa. Allergic rhinitis with its symptoms of itching, rhinorrhea, sneezing, and nasal obstruction have been previously classified according to time and circumstance of exposure in perennial, seasonal or occupational (2). The new

209

classification (3) of allergic rhinitis (Fig. 12.1):

- considers quality of life symptoms and parameters;
- is based on duration of clinical manifestations and is classified into "intermittent" or "persistent" rhinitis;
- severity may be "mild" or "moderate-severe," depending on the intensity of symptoms and the impact on the quality of life of patients.

The immunological reactions underlying rhinitis are illustrated in Fig. 12.2 where it will be seen that there is an early phase due to mediator release from mast cells. This reaction follows quickly (within minutes), upon allergen exposure and is usually easy to recognize. The late-phase reaction with its cellular infiltration and inflammation is mainly characterized by nasal obstruction and is less clinically obvious. Seasonal rhinitis or intermittent allergen contact involves more early phase reactions; perennial allergen contact causes a practically continuous late-phase response and can easily be confused with other causes of nasal blockage such as hypertrophic adenoids. Another confounding factor is the frequent occurrence of viral rhinitis in children, with a normal child having six to eight colds per year.

The major differential diagnosis of nasal allergy in childhood are shown in Table 12.1.

Many conditions present with rhinorrhea and nasal obstruction in children. Most children have from six to eight viral upper respiratory tract infections per year. This can be difficult to differentiate from perennial allergic rhinitis. Hypertrophic adenoids cause upper airway obstruction with or without rhinorrhea, but itching and sneezing are not found. Chronic rhinosinusitis often presents

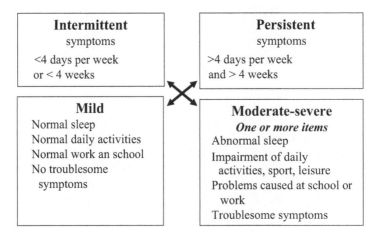

Figure 12.1   Classification of allergic rhinitis [according to ARIA (3), 2001].

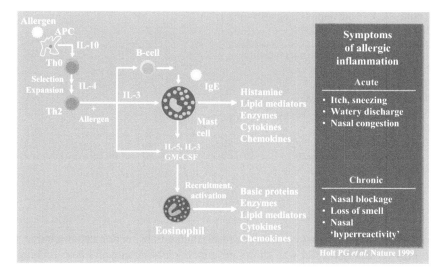

Figure 12.2 The basic mechanisms underlying allergic rhinitis. Allergic sensitization takes place at a mucosal surface causing T-cell IL4 driven IgE production by B-cells and subsequent "arming" of mast cells. The immediate reaction is caused by mast cell degranulation and mediator release after allergen combined with IgE on the mast cell surface. This results in nasal itch, sneezing, and rhinorrhea. In some cases, especially with the large allergen dose, an inflammatory late-phase response ensues with ingress of eosinophils, neutrophils, mast cells, and T-lymphocytes. In chronic allergen stimulation, this phase predominates and the major clinical complaint is of nasal obstruction.

persistent nasal discharge. Minor immune defects such as low IgA or IgG subclass deficiencies are relatively common in childhood and frequently present with a chronic or recurrent purulent nasal discharge. Other causes of this are mucociliary impairment such as occurs in primary ciliary dyskinesia or cystic fibrosis. In small children, nasal obstruction can be caused by congenital abnormalities such as choanal atresia or an encephalocoele. Foreign bodies, especially foam are a common cause of unilateral nasal obstruction, often accompanied by secondary infection and mucopurulent discharge.

II. Diagnosis

The diagnosis of allergy is made on history plus clinical examination together with confirmation from tests such as skin prick test or RAST (4,5).

History taking is the most important modality and should include all the symptoms and signs together with the timing of their occurrence and whether there is any seasonal or diurnal pattern or any particular exacerbating factor

Table 12.1 Differential Diagnosis of
Nasal Allergy in Childhood

1. Viral upper respiratory tract infections
2. Hypertrophic adenoids
3. Chronic rhinosinusitis
4. Minor immune deficiency
5. Foreign body (usually unilateral)
6. Choanal atresia
7. Encephalocoele
8. Primary ciliary dyskinesia
9. Cystic fibrosis

or factors. Although many conditions result in nasal obstruction and discharge it is only the allergic child who shows prominent nasal itching and nose rubbing. Associated symptoms such as itchy eyes, wheezing, or skin irritation also suggest underlying atopy. Use of a questionnaire (see Appendix), helps to speed the consultation. If this can be sent to the parents beforehand then they have a chance to observe their child for a while and may be alerted to underlying allergens by the questions on the form.

The most offending symptom should be noted and whether or not this is permanent or intermittent. Nasal allergy rarely causes symptoms that are totally unvarying, or unilateral. Thus, a unilateral nasal blockage is more likely to be caused by choanal atresia if present since birth or a foreign body if occurring later on, especially if the discharge is malodorous. Complete bilateral nasal blockage may be due to rhinitis but could also be caused by nasal polyps (which in childhood should stimulate the search for cystic fibrosis), or by grossly hypertrophied adenoids. In small babies nasal blockage and clear rhinorrhea can be due to an encephalocoele.

The past medical history is also important and this should include a birth history with details of pregnancy, birth weight, birth month, early feeding, and whether there was any colic or other feeding problems especially early eczema. A history of bronchiolitis, croup, or asthma should be sought. A past or family history of atopy makes allergic rhinitis more likely.

The family history should also be taken looking for atopic diseases in any first degree relative. Environmental allergen exposure should also be assessed and important questions include the age of the home, the presence of damp or mould, recent building works, whether there are carpets and central heating present, the type of bedding used, presence of pets in the house, and whether the parents smoke.

The child's eating habits should also be noted plus whether there are any foods which cause rashes around the mouth, stomach aches, mouth ulcers, abnormal behavior, eczema, asthma, or nasal symptoms.

Finally, an inquiry should be made about treatments used thus far for the child's nasal symptoms, compliance with these and whether or not they have proved effective.

III. Examination

Much can be gained by simply observing the child and parent whilst talking to them. An allergic crease may be visible across the lower third of the nose or an allergic salute (Fig. 12.3), by either the child or even the parent. The skin may show signs of atopic dermatitis and the eyes may be reddened with conjunctivitis or have an extra allergic crease beneath them or allergic shiners.

The child may be breathing chronically through his or her mouth. The nasal airway can be tested simply (though not very accurately), by misting of a metal nasal spatula held beneath the nostrils whilst the mouth is closed. Airway assessment is possible with peak flow measurement in children $\geq 3-4$ years old (Fig. 12.4). Acoustic rhinometry is possible in older children and gives more accurate results.

Internal examination of the lower part of the nose is easily done by asking the child to look up and simply elevating the nasal tip with a finger and shining a light inside. The nature of the mucosa can be seen; usually in allergy it is pale and bluish, and wet. However, if children have been on nasal sprays then the mucosa tends to be reddened. Uncomplicated allergic rhinitis usually gives nasal secretions that are clear, watery, and excessive, however, plentiful eosinophils

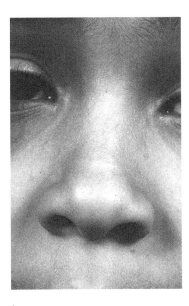

Figure 12.3 The allergic crease.

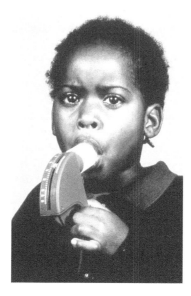

Figure 12.4   Airway assessment in the clinic: peak flow measurement should be undertaken in children with rhinitis as soon as they are old enough to manage to blow into the machine (3–4 years old).

may result in yellowish, thickened secretions. Greenish discoloration usually suggests bacterial infection. It is relatively simple to take a nasal smear with the rhinoprobe to examine the cell content of nasal discharge. Staining with Wright's Giemsa allows identification of eosinophils. (Fig. 12.5).

Optic fiber endoscopy is possible in the cooperative older child without anesthetic provided it is done very gently. Initial examination without using local anesthetic/decongestant is frequently possible. This means that mucosal appearance and function are not altered and smears, scrapings for ciliary beat

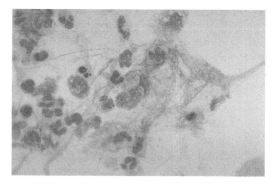

Figure 12.5   Nasal smear showing eosinophils.

frequency and mucosal function for saccharin time (Fig. 12.6), are all preserved. When these tests have been undertaken then local anesthetic/decongestant can be used and after 5 min the middle meatus can be examined for the presence of polyps or purulent secretions suggestive of an infective sinusitis, the posterior choana can be examined for patency and for obstructing adenoid tissue.

One-quarter of a grain of saccharin is placed one centimeter back on the anterior end of the inferior turbinate after the child has blown their nose. The time taken to taste the saccharin is recorded and is usually under 20 min. Sniffing or snorting the saccharin back must be avoided otherwise a false reading is given. This test is obviously only suitable for older children. Delayed nasal mucociliary clearance time can be due to a primary defect in cilia or mucus or can be secondary to chronic infection. In the latter case the clearance time should improve following treatment with antibiotics.

It is important to examine not only the nose but also to check the throat and ears looking for evidence of tonsillitis and of otitis media. The state of the eardrum if retracted may give a clue that Eustachian tube function is compromised. Examination of the chest should also be made looking for abnormal shape such as Harrison's sulcus, checking that there is good lateral chest expansion which is bilateral and equal and listening for normal breath sounds together with any added sounds such as wheezing. In children over 3 years of age, the peak flow reading should be taken and the best of three attempts recorded.

It is important to record the child's height and weight since therapy with corticosteroids may be necessary.

IV. Confirmatory Tests

By this time the clinician will usually have a reasonable idea of the likely diagnosis and, if this is allergic rhinitis, of the likely allergen involved. The simplest

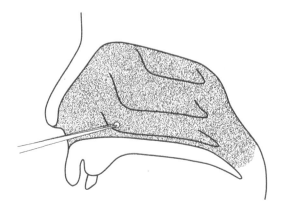

Figure 12.6   Measurement of saccharin time.

method of confirmation is by skin prick testing which can be done in children of any age provided a few simple rules are observed. In those with a previous history of anaphylaxis testing is best avoided and blood tests substituted. False negative responses are likely to occur in children taking antihistamines, this can be covert since many will receive cough medicines containing antihistamines bought over the counter and given them by their parents at night (6). Careful enquiry should be made about this prior to testing. In children with moderate to severe atopic dermatitis, skin prick tests can cause itching and exacerbation of their condition and are best avoided with blood tests substituted.

It is usual to employ a small number of skin prick tests initially; in the UK, grass pollen, cat, dog, and house dust mite are the most frequent inhalant allergens. In smaller children, foods such as cow's milk, egg, soya may be responsible for rhinitis, though other conditions such as asthma and eczema, or gastrointestinal problems are usually associated. A negative control (saline), and a positive control (histamine), should always be employed. Anxious children may do better if testing is carried out on their back rather than on the forearm.

Positive results are those 3 mm greater than the negative control. Skin prick tests (Fig. 12.7), must always be interpreted in the light of the history.

Wheals over 3 mm diameter, larger than the negative control (saline) are regarded as positive, but must be interpreted together with the history. The positive control (histamine) is included to ensure that a response can occur. Many children receive antihistamines, often in the form of cough mixtures, which will reduce the skin prick test results.

Blood testing for specific IgE can be substituted if skin prick testing is not possible due to fear, atopic dermatitis, previous anaphylaxis, or antihistamine use, but is more expensive and no more reliable.

Cap RAST is a simple blood test which can identify specific IgE. It is useful when skin prick testing is not possible, but is no more sensitive. It is also expensive and has the disadvantage of lack of immediacy. The power of positive skin prick testing to influence compliance with allergen avoidance has never been tested but clinical suspicion suggests that it is potent.

Allergic diseases such as rhinitis start by mucosal sensitization and local switching of B-cells to IgE production has now been demonstrated (6). This

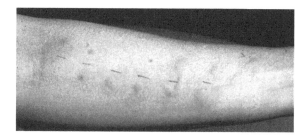

Figure 12.7   Skin prick test on forearm.

means that it is possible for a child to have allergic rhinitis with local IgE production but negative skin prick tests. This situation will probably obtain until sufficient IgE is produced to spill over into the general circulation and sensitize skin mast cells. Thus, negative skin prick tests or cap RAST in the light of a very suggestive history should not prevent a trial of antiallergy therapy.

V. Other Tests

Nasal smears can be stained with Wright Giemsa and examined for eosinophils (Fig. 12.5). If infection is present, a neutrophilia is usually noted; however, after antibiotic therapy the underlying allergic eosinophilia might be revealed.

Nasal allergen challenge in skin prick test negative patients with a suggestive history is practised in adults but is rarely done in childhood. However, removal of dietary allergens for a week or two followed by their reintroduction is a possible procedure and is relatively simple with respect to cow's milk. This should be removed for 2–3 weeks whilst a careful symptom score chart is kept, then reintroduced to see whether symptoms recur. This must be done under medical supervision where the child has had previous anaphylaxis. If the test proves positive, then a prolonged period of cow's milk protein restriction will be necessary and this should be undertaken with the help of a dietician who will ensure that the diet contains sufficient calcium. Food allergy is usually found in smaller children (<3 years), with rhinitis in addition to other disorders such as asthma, eczema, failure to thrive, and gut problems.

VI. Blood Tests

If the major problem is one of chronic purulent nasal discharge and blood is being taken for IgE testing then it is sensible to obtain a full blood count, differential white cell count including eosinophils at the same time together with immunoglobulins and IgG subclasses. These tests may reveal an underlying immune deficiency which is usually transient (eg) low levels of IgA may persist until approximately 12 years of age.

VII. Subsequent Visits

Having been alerted to the possibility of allergy at the first visit, the parent may well prove a good source of information about likely allergens at the subsequent interview. The effect of removing certain items from the diet or from the child's bedroom (such as a furry toy collection) can also be assessed. Cooperation is vital in the diagnosis and the treatment of allergy therefore patient and parent education is a vital part of the consultation. This time-consuming effort is frequently best undertaken by a specialized nurse.

VIII. Conclusion

The diagnosis of nasal allergy in children requires time spent talking to the patient and his or her family plus a few relatively simple and inexpensive investigations. It is time well spent because allergic rhinitis is frequently associated with comorbid disorders such as sinusitis, otitis media with effusion and asthma and also reduces quality of life, and educational ability.

References

1. Albert D. Nasal obstruction and rhinorrhea in infants and children. In: Adams DA, Cinnamond MJ, eds. Paediatric Otolaryngology. Scott-Brown's Otolaryngolgy. 6th ed. Oxford: Butterworth Heinemann, 1996.
2. Vuurman E, Van Veggel L, Utterwijk M, Leutner D, O'Hanlon J et al. Seasonal allergic rhinitis and antihistamines effects on children's learning. Ann Allergy 1993; 71:121–124.
3. Allergic Rhinitis and Its Impact on Asthma Initiative (ARIA) in cooperation with WHO (World Health Organization). Panel of Experts: Jean Busquet (President), Paul van Cauwenberge (Co-President), Nikolai Khaltaev (Secretary). Other members: Aït-Khaled N, Annesi-Maesano I, Bachert C, Baena Cagnani CE, Bateman E, Bonini S, Canonica GW, Carlsen KH, Demoly P, Durham SR, Enarson D, Fokkens WJ, Gerth van Wijk R, Howarth P, Ivanova NA, Kemp JP, Klossek JM, Lockey RF, Lund V, MacKay Ian, Malling HJ, Meltzer EO, Mygind N, Okuda M, Pawankar R, Price D, Scadding GK, Simons FER, Szczeklik A, Valovirta E, Vignola AM, Wang DY, Warner JO, Weiss KB. J Allergy Clin Immunol 2001; 108:148–336.
4. Scadding GK. BSACI Rhinitis Management Guidelines 1998. 2nd ed.
5. Van Cauwenberge P, Bachert C, eds. Managing Allergic Rhinitis EAACI Position Paper. Allergy 2002.
6. Durham SR, Scadding GK. Nasal immunology. In: Jacob, Philips, Hilges, eds. Disorders of the Head, Neck and Throat. London: Arnold, 1998.

Appendix

Questionnaire

Allergy Questionnaire used at the Royal National Throat, Nose and Ear Hospital—Pediatric Rhinitis Clinic.

PLEASE FILL IN AS FULLY AND ACCURATELY AS POSSIBLE AND BRING WITH YOU TO THE CLINIC

Child's

Surname ....

First Names ....

Date of Birth ....

Address ....

....

Telephone Number ....

N.H.S. Number ....

What is the main reason for referral to the clinic?

....

....

....

Are there any other problems or difficulties which may be relevant?

....

....

....

Please circle any of the following which apply to your child.

Running nose

Clear nasal discharge

Thick nasal discharge, often green/yellow

Sneezing

Blocked nose   left size   right size   both sides

Snoring

Mouth breathing at night

Itchy nose

Rubs nose with fingers/hand

Lack sense of smell

Lack sense of taste

When did these symptoms start?

....

....

....

Are they worse at any particular time of year?   Yes/No

If so, when?

....

....

Are they worse at any particular time of day?   Yes/No

If so, when?

....

....

Is there anything that you know of which will make the

symptoms worse?   Yes/No

If so, what?

....

....

Are they worse at any particular time place?   Yes/No

If so, where?

....

....

Does your child

Wheeze?	Yes/No
Get out of breath easily?	Yes/No
Have a frequent dry cough?	Yes/No
Cough at night?	Yes/No
Suffer from frequent chest infections?	Yes/No
Suffer from frequent ear infections?	Yes/No
Have a lot of sore throats?	Yes/No
Have difficulty in hearing?	Yes/No
Do you think your child was/is late in talking?	Yes/No
Do you think your child is difficult to understand?	Yes/No/Sometimes

Birth History

Was the pregnancy normal?   Yes/No

If not, please specify what problems occurred

....

....

....

Labour	Normal	Rapid	Prolonged	
Delivery	Normal	Forceps	Breech	Cesarean

Full term   Yes/No

If not, at how many weeks? ....

Birth weight .... 1b/oz .... Kg

Condition at birth   Normal   Difficulty with breathing   Jaundice

Feeding

Breast-fed?   Yes/No

                                              If no, for how long? ....

Bottle-fed?   Yes/No

When was bottled milk first given? ....

Type of milk used ....

Did the baby feed well   Yes/No

If not, what problems occurred ....

....

....

....

Any colic   Yes/No

When was weaning first started? ....

Which foods were introduced? ....

Has your child suffered from any severe illness?   Yes/No

Which? ....

....

Has your child had any operations?   Yes/No

Nature of operation (s) and date(s) ....

....

....

....

Family History

Are there any other children in the family?   Yes/No

Please give the age and sex of each child: ....

....

....

....

Does anyone in the family have allergies?   Yes/No

(Asthma, eczema, hay fever, urticaria, food allergy, drug allergy, infantile eczema, etc)

Please specify: ....

....

....

....

....

Does any in the family suffer from repeated infections?   Yes/No

Please specify: ....

....

....

Potential Allergens:

Please tick any of the following which are in your home:

Carpets	Furry Toys
Central Heating	Feather Pillows
Pets	Feather/down duvet
Damp	Wool Blankets
Mould	Cigarette Smoke
Trees	

Any food fads or fancies?   Yes/No

If so please specify: ....

....

....

Does your child eat much dairy products?   Yes/No

Does your child eat much junk food?   Yes/No

Do any food upset your child?   Yes/No

Does your child attend school or nursery?   Yes/No

Medications:

What treatments has your child tried?

....

....

....

Has your child ever reacted to medicine?   Yes/No

Please specify: ....

....

....

Which, if any, have proved helpful?

....

....

13

The Role of Allergy in Chronic Pediatric Rhinosinusitis

GLENIS K. SCADDING

Royal National Throat, Nose and Ear Hospital,
London, UK

I. Introduction

Chronic rhinosinusitis in children is a hotly debated topic (1). Since the natural history is only partly known, it is difficult to evaluate treatments which range from complete nonintervention through medical therapy to sinus surgery, which these days is likely to be endoscopic. A recent consensus report has encouraged the definition of pediatric rhinosinusitis on clinical grounds, without the necessity of a computed tomography (CT) scan (1).

A definition of rhinosinusitis is:

- nasal running (anterior/posterior)
- nasal sneezing/itching
- nasal blocking.

II. Prevalence

The diagnosis of chronic rhinosinusitis is not easy in childhood since symptoms may consist largely of vague ill health or may (cough, wheeze, sputum), appear to involve the lower respiratory tract. Older children may be able to indicate that they have a headache. The presence of a purulent nasal discharge was always associated with sinusitis on a magnetic resonance imaging (MRI) scan in a recent survey by Gordts et al. (2), who studied 100 children with central nervous system disease. They found that 45% of the children had sinusitis, that it tended to be more severe than in adults, and that the pattern was different with the sphenoid and posterior ethmoids being affected in addition to the anterior ethmoids and maxillary sinuses. The incidence of sinusitis on MRI in children with different nasal findings is shown in Table 13.1; even allowing for the fact that MRI scans tend to over diagnose sinus disease pediatric rhinosinusitis is obviously a common condition. This is not surprising since normal children have between six and eight viral upper respiratory tract infections (URTIs) per year and these involve not only the nasal lining but those of the sinuses as well. According to three separate studies there appears to be a spontaneous decrease in prevalence of pediatric rhinosinusitis after 7 years of age (3–5).

III. Underlying (Predisposing) Factors

The major factors responsible for rhinosinusitis are shown in Fig. 13.1 (6). This applies to both adults and children, but the importance of individual factors probably varies with age.

IV. Immune Deficiency

Small children (<2 years) are not fully immunocompetent. There is a trough in immunoglobulin levels at around 6 months of age when maternal

Table 13.1   MRI Findings in a Non-ENT Population

Pediatric Rhinosinusitis	
Gordts study	Sinusitis on MRI (%)
Nasal obstruction	50
Recent URTI	81
Bilateral mucosal swelling	80
Purulent secretions[a]	100

[a]A total of 35% without purulent secretions showed opacification and/or fluid level.

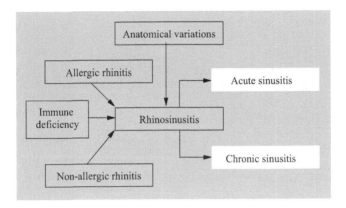

Figure 13.1 Factors underlying or predisposing recurrent/chronic rhinosinusitis.

immunoglobulin has disappeared and the baby's own levels are gradually rising. IgG subclasses appear at different times with IgG-2 being relatively late, reaching normal levels at around 2 years. This is probably relevant to the upper respiratory tract since IgG-2 is the major protective antibody against carbohydrate-coated organisms such as *Staphylococcus aureus*, *Streptococcus pneumoniae*, and *Haemophilus influenzae*. Delayed maturation of IgA "mucosal antiseptic paint" and IgG, is also common (Fig. 13.2) and in a proportion of children adult levels may not be reached until 12 years of age (7).

Mutations in mannose binding lectin (MBL) is relatively common (approximately 5%), in the Caucasian population. This is an opsonin which facilitates phagocytosis and is especially important in children with low IgG-2 levels. Recent studies have shown that children presenting with infection to a casualty department are more likely to be MBL deficient than those presenting for other reasons (8). Deficiencies of one or more IgG subclasses, sometimes together with IgA deficiency, are relatively common in the childhood population attending ENT clinics. This may account for the observation that children with tonsillitis are more likely to have acute otitis media and sinus infections and vice versa (9) (Fig. 13.3).

Children with frequent or severe URTIs should have immunoglobulins, IgG subclasses and mannose binding lectin analysed from a peripheral blood sample.

IV. Muco-Ciliary Clearance

The most important defense mechanisms in the upper respiratory tract are the innate factors of ciliary beating with mucus production and clearance. This is obvious from the fact that children with defects in cilia (primary ciliary dyskinesia, PCD), or mucus (cystic fibrosis), suffer from recurrent upper as well as lower respiratory tract problems. Secondary problems with muco-ciliary clearance can occur due to allergy or chronic infection (*vide infra*).

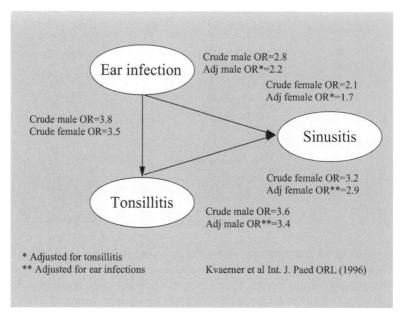

Figure 13.2 Children with tonsillitis are more likely to have acute otitis media and sinus infections and vice versa.

V. Nitric Oxide

This colorless, odourless gas is continually produced in the sinuses at levels which are toxic to bacteria, fungi, and tumor cells. It appears to be intimately linked to ciliary beating and in primary ciliary dyskinesia (PCD) very low

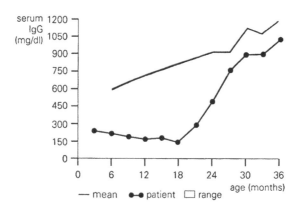

Figure 13.3 Delayed maturation of IgG.

levels (<100 ppb, normal range 450–900 in our laboratory) are found. The fact that all PCD patients lack inducible nitric oxide synthase (iNOS), even those individuals with normal ciliary ultrastructure and disorganized beating, suggests that lack of iNOS may be the primary defect (10).

VI. Atopy

There is some dispute about whether allergic rhinitis predisposes to infantile rhinosinusitis. Sanderson and Warner (11) showed that children presenting for ENT operations were more likely to be atopic than age and sex matched controls who were undergoing orthopedic procedures. They also demonstrated that such children responded better to medical than to surgical treatment.

There are probably many factors underlying the increased infections seen in children with allergy, the most obvious being the boggy, hypertrophied mucosa, which leads to ostial obstruction. This is more likely to be relevant in perennial rhinitis where the late-phase reaction predominates (see chapter on Diagnosis of Nasal Allergy in Children).

Allergic reactions also affect muco-ciliary clearance. Ciliary beat frequency was decreased to 20 min following positive house dust mite challenge compared to controls with the negative response to the allergen (12). Although the decrease was small, it was probably sufficient to allow bacterial adherence to epithelial cells and establishment of infection. Bacteria themselves produce factors which decrease ciliary beat frequency further (13). Improvement in beating can be seen in adults with chronic rhinosinusitis following prolonged antibiotic treatment (14).

Eosinophils are the cardinal cells in the allergic response. The prime purpose of eosinophil recruitment and activation is probably for the killing of metazoan parasites, not because of their size, by phagocytosis, but by extracellular lysis. Eosinophils possess very toxic products including major basic protein, eosinophil-derived neurotoxin, free oxygen radicals and cysteinyl leukotrienes. Exfoliation of epithelial cells and ciliary damage in cell cultures have been reported after the addition of activated eosinophils (15). Thus, the allergic response can probably damage the sinus mucosa in the same way as it does the bronchial mucosa in asthma.

Cellular infiltration to the inflammatory site is regulated by cytokines and adhesion molecules. One of the latter, ICAM-1, has been found to be the receptor for rhinoviruses (16) which are responsible for approximately 30% of viral URTIs. Upregulation of ICAM-1 occurs on the epithelium, and not only on the vascular endothelium. Thus, there is a possible route for increased viral infection in atopics, with subsequent secondary bacterial infection. As yet this is unproven.

It is conceivable that in some patients an allergic reaction can take place to bacteria or to bacterial products. In our clinic we find children with gross nasal eosinophilia, muco-purulent discharge and chronic infection, usually with *S. aureus*, who respond to long-term penicillin by losing all these manifestations.

Evidence for an increase of atopy in chronic upper respiratory infection in children and adults is present in our clinics where approximately 60% of such individuals are skin prick test positive, roughly double the population percentage. Spontaneous manufacture of IgE by tonsil specimens from 12 of 18 children with tonsillitis was reported by Peter Amlot (unpublished data).

If allergy promotes infection then the treatment of nasal allergy should reduce the prevalence of chronic rhinosinusitis. There is little good evidence for this as yet although our recent open study using topical corticosteroids in children with recurrent otitis media with effusion does suggest that long-term treatment with 100 μg of beclamethasone daily to reduce minimal persistent inflammation was associated with fewer colds and less need for antibiotics as well as better hearing and fewer ear infections (17) (Fig. 13.4). Similar results have been obtained by Canonica and his colleagues (18) using oral terfenadine over 1 year. Double-blind, placebo-controlled trials are in progress in our department with intranasal corticosteroids in the treatment of chronic recurrent otitis media with effusion and in children with tonsillitis and adenoid hypertrophy who are on the waiting list for operations.

VII. Conclusion

Pediatric chronic rhinosinusitis is a common disorder, which usually remits spontaneously with age. There are many underlying factors, immune deficiency and allergy are probably two of the major ones. Social factors such as parental

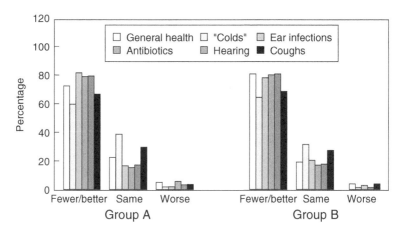

Figure 13.4 Parental perception, as assessed by anonymous questionnaire, of symptomatic changes in their children who had chronic/recurrent OME as a result of therapy with A topical corticosteroids plus allergen avoidance or B topical corticosteroids alone. In both groups, there were fewer colds and ear infections, better hearing, and less need for antibiotics with no significant difference between the two groups.

smoking and early day care attendance are probably also relevant, as they are for acute otitis media. The importance of several predisposing factors changes with increasing age (19,20).

Surgical intervention in this group of children is very rarely necessary since "there is more to pediatric rhinosinusitis than anatomical abnormalities and ostio-meatal complex obstruction" (21). It is primarily a mucosal problem and further research and carefully controlled trials of medical and surgical therapies are needed (1).

References

1. Clement PAR, Bluestone CD, Gordts F et al. Management of rhinosinusitis in children. Arch Otolaryngol Head/Neck Surg 1998; 124:31–34.
2. Gordts F, Clement PAR, Estryker A, Desprechins B, Kaufman L et al. Prevalence of sinusitis signs on MRI in a non-ENT paediatric population. Rhinology 1997; 35:154–157.
3. Clement PAR, Buissenet T, Desprechins B, Kaufman L, Derde M et al. Age related CT scan study of the incidence of sinusitis in children. Am J Rhinol 1992; 6:45–48.
4. Manning SC, Biavati MJ, Philips D et al. Correlation of clinical sinusitis signs and symptoms to imaging findings in pediatric patients. Int J Pediatr Otorhinolaryngol 1996; 37:65–74.
5. Otten FW, Van-Aarem A, Grote JJ et al. Long-term follow up of chronic therapy resistant purulent rhinitis in children. Clin Otolaryngol 1992; 17:32–33.
6. Evans KL. Diagnosis and management of sinusitis. B Med J 1999; 309:1413–1422.
7. Taylor B, Fergusson DM, Mahoney GN, Hartley WA, Abbott J et al. Specific IgA and IgE in childhood asthma, eczema and food allergy. Clin Allergy D 1981; 56(12):939–942.
8. Summerfield JA, Sumiya M, Levin M, Turner MW et al. Association of mutation in mannose binding protein with childhood infection in hospital series. Br Med J 1997; 314:1229–1232.
9. Kvaerner KJ, Tambs K, Harris JR, Mair IW, Magnus P et al. Otitis media: relationship to tonsillitis, sinusitis and atopic disease. Int J Pediatr Otorhinolaryngol 1996; 35(2):127–141.
10. Wodehouse T. PhD. thesis, University College, London, UK, 2000.
11. Sanderson J, Warner JO. Previous ear, nose and throat surgery in children presenting with allergic perennial rhinitis. Clin Allergy 1987; 17(2):113–117.
12. Holmstrom M, Lunds VJ, Scadding GK et al. Nasal ciliary beat frequency after nasal allergen challenge. Am J Rhinol 1992; 6(3):101–105.
13. Wilson R, Cole PJ. The effect of bacteria products on ciliary function. Am Rev Respir Dis 1988; 138:549–553.
14. Scadding GK, Lund VJ, Darby YC et al. The effect of long-term antibiotic therapy upon ciliary beat frequency in chronic rhinosinusitis. J Laryngol Otol 1995; 109:24–26.
15. Abdelaziz MM, Devalia JL, Khair OA, Bayram H, Prior AJ, Davies RJ et al. Effect of fexofenadine on eosiniphil-induced changes in epithelial permeability and cytokine release from nasal epithelial cells of patients with seasonal allergic rhinitis. J Allergy Clin Immunol 1980; 101(3):410–420.

16. Staunton DE, Merluzzi VJ, Rothein R et al. A cell adhesion molecule, ICAM-1, is the major surface receptor for rhinosinusitis. Cell 1989; 56:849–853.

17. Parikh A, Scadding GK, Alles R, Hawk L, Darby YD et al. Topical corticosteroids for children with otitis media with effusion and allergic rhinitis. J Audiol Med 2000; 3:231–235.

18. Canonica W. Paper presented at EAACI, 1998. Birmingham, England.

19. Van Der Veken PJ, Clement PAR, Buisseret TH et al. Age-related CT scan study of the incidence of sinusitis in children. Am J Rhinol 1992; 6:45–48.

20. Yaniv E, Oppenheim D, Fuchs C. Chronic rhinitis in children. Int J Pediatr Otorhinolaryngol 1992; 23:51–57.

21. Younis RT, Lazar RH. Criteria for success in pediatric functional endonasal sinus surgery. Laryngoscope 1996; 106:869–873.

14

How to Monitor Nasal Allergy in Children

DESIDERIO PASSÀLI,
LUISA BELLUSSI, and
VALERIO DAMIANI

Medical School, University of Siena,
Siena, Italy

FRANCESCO MARIA PASSÀLI and
GIULIO CESARE PASSÀLI

Medical School, University of Genova,
Genova, Italy

I. Introduction

The alteration of vasomotility of nasal mucosa can be included in the term "nasal hyperreactivity syndrome." This phrase includes all those diseases based on a vaso-motor disequilibrium, which can be caused by a specific, or a nonspecific stimulus.

We distinguish between specific vasomotor rhinopathy and nonspecific vasomotor rhinopathy. Specific vasomotor rhinophaty can replace the old term allergic rhinitis that to us does not seem to be appropriate enough.

In fact, in our experience, the term rhinopathy presumes the existence of a pathological systemic condition that has its shock organ in the nose. The word "rhinitis" stresses only the local condition, not the general one. The term "specific" represents the possibility of finding a specific agent, a specific allergen that is responsible for the reaction that in general is an expression of hypersensitivity of the first type. We call the rhinopathy "nonspecific" when an IgE mediated reaction does not exist.

In Italy, the prevalence of specific rhinopathy is 20–25% in young adults and 3% in the elderly. The most frequent allergens are Graminaceae (36%), Dermatophagoides (33%), and Parietaria (12%), but also the mixed forms have a high incidence (1).

It is important to stress the fact that, unfortunately, the incidence of nasal allergy is increasing. It is due to a lot of factors, such as: pollution, cigarette smoke and in particular air conditioning systems in houses. Due to the "priming effect," (2) all the aforementioned factors change the permeability and reactivity of nasal mucosa so that allergens can provoke all the typical symptoms of allergy more easily in predisposed subjects.

The clinical phase of allergic rhinitis usually starts in children aged between 8 and 12 years (3), allergic inflammation starts when allergens bind to IgE molecules linked to the mast cells, causing cellular degranulation and releasing a great number of inflammatory mediators which are responsible for early- and late-phase responses.

The early-phase response depends on the release of preformed mediators such as histamine and newly generated mediators such as leukotriene C4 or prostaglandin D2.

The most important one is histamine. Its release stimulates sensory nerves, causing pruritus of the nose, palate, and conjunctiva. The concomitant stimulation of parasympathetic reflexes contributes to vasodilatation and mucous hypersecretion. The typical symptoms are in fact nasal obstruction, rhinorrhea, itching, and sneezing, which are just the epiphenomena of the internal imbalance of the system ruling nasal reactivity. Allergic rhinitis, however, does not stop here, as there is also a late phase that adds up to the early phase. The late-phase response is present in the majority of the patients, and entails a process of cell-infiltration and activation with a duration of 4–24 h.

It begins when autacoid mediators and cytokines released from mast-cells during the early-phase response, upregulate the expression of endothelial adhesion molecules in the postcapillary venules of the nose.

Postcapillary venules are also the site of blood cell extravasation. Once the blood cells are in the submucosal tissue, they release their own mediators. This perpetuates the inflammatory response.

The chronic inflammation caused by repeated allergen exposure lowers the threshold for new provocations. So, allergic people, because of this "priming effect," react more strongly to low levels of primary allergen and to other allergens to which they are only mildly sensitive, or to some nonspecific "triggers" such as cigarette smoke and cold air.

On the other hand, some adhesion molecules such as ICAM-1 are specific receptors for viral infections. So the importance of the late-phase response is to start the process of "minimal persistent inflammation" represented by upregulation of adhesion molecules, present and persistent even outside the allergic attack (4). For all these reasons we must emphasize the importance of a correct monitoring method for nasal hyperreactivity, that has a relevant social and economic impact, in order to treat it in the best way.

II. Clinical Examination

History and clinical examination are important, if not fundamental to make a proper diagnosis of allergic rhinitis, but are not sufficient to find the etiologic agent. Nasal obstruction, pruritus, sneezing are the classic symptoms. Although any symptom can prevail depending on the case, on the whole we are dealing with aspecific protective responses whose purpose is to keep irritating particles and substance away, preventing their penetration into the lower airways.

It is important to find out whether the symptoms are seasonal or not, if they occur under particular conditions, the presence of a familiar history, or if specific environmental conditions cause the attacks.

After history taking and anterior rhinoscopy, it is necessary to complete the examination through methods that test nasal function. These methods are: active anterior rhinomanometry (AAR), acoustic rhinometry (AR), and determination of muco-ciliary transport time (MCTt).

A. Active Anterior Rhinomanometry

AAR gives us important information about nasal ventilation. It should be performed according to recommendations of the Standardization Committee (5,6). Two parameters are recorded in a dynamic way (breathing): pressure gradient and airflow. We carry out this examination using a face mask specific for children: one nostril is sealed off to record the naso-pharyngeal pressure, and the airflow of the other nasal cavity is recorded. There is a minimal or no nasal valve deformation with this technique, little chance of leakage at the level of the nostril and active ventilation through each nasal cavity separately is recorded. Through a computerized elaboration of results, we obtain the value of the resistance of the left and the right nasal cavity and of the total resistance at a fixed pressure that was determined at 150 Pa. In case of allergic rhinitis all these values increase. We consider values of unilateral resistance $<0.50\,\mathrm{Pa/cm^3}$ per second normal for adults (>16 years old), $<1.20\,\mathrm{Pa/cm^3}$ per second normal for children younger than 8 years old, $<1\,\mathrm{Pa/cm^3}$ per second normal for children aged between 8 and 12 years, and $<0.70\,\mathrm{Pa/cm^3}$ per second normal for children between 12 and 16 years of age.

It is also necessary to carry out the nasal decongestion test (NDT) by administering two puffs of a nasal decongestant for each nostril, waiting 5 min, and repeating the same administration of decongestant again, and then, after 5 min, repeating the AAR. In case of functional stenosis of the nose, as in allergy, the resistance values decrease significantly.

B. Acoustic Rhinometry

This method is performed with a particular instrument that can compare the incident acoustic wave with the one reflected by the physiological and/or pathological geometry of each nasal cavity, obtaining data which the computerized system uses for the measurement of the cross-sectional area at different distances from the nostrils (7,8). The wave tube is set in the working plane with a fixed angulation of 60°. This examination, according to our experience, is performed with the use of an ophtalmologic-type craniostat that permits the exact repositioning of the patient's head with respect to the rhinometer, reducing the errors caused by the test procedure itself. The base of the instrument slides along two rails, allowing antero-posterior movements, in the sagittal plane only, of the patient's head, which is positioned with the chin and forehead against the craniostat. For the exact positioning of the patient's head in the sagittal plane, reference is made to the line joining the superior margin of the external auditory meatus and the anterior nasal spine. This line is oriented relatively to the axis of the wave tube, with which it must form a fixed angle of 120° (9).

Through this technique, we can measure the cross-sectional area at varying distances from the nostril (e.g., at the level of the head of the inferior turbinate). After administration of a nasal decongestant or during nasal challenge testing, the profile of the acoustic rhinogram changes.

C. Muco-ciliary Transport Time

Muco-ciliary transport system is, together with filtration, the most important factor of the aspecific defence of the nose. The most voluminous particles (>50 μm) are filtered by the vibrissae, particularly sensitive hair that protudes into the lumen of the nostril orifice. Particles with a diameter <10 μm are eliminated by the muco-ciliary transport system. It consists of a ciliated epithelium covered by a continuous layer of mucus. All the cilia move in the same direction (backwards to the nasopharynx) but in a different phase, permitting the progression of a carpet of mucus lining, in a metachronous movement.

A single cilium makes the movement in two stages: during the first, or propultion phase, it emerges from the fluid layer and reaches the mucus, in the second slower phase it returns to its resting position. For a good ciliary transport, the presence of a particular fluid medium is essential. It is divided into two strata: the surface (gel), which lines the cilia and is like a conveyor belt for the trapped particles and the deeper layer (sol) in which cilia are immersed and make their movements possible. Muco-ciliary transport time is linked to the physical properties of the nasal secretions and to the integrity of the cilia and so of the nasal mucosa. To have complete information on nasal function, it is useful to determine the value of MCTt. Many methods for determining MCTt have been suggested, with radioactive, radiopaque, or inert substances. We use a mixture of inert substances consisting of charcoal powder and saccharin. Charcoal and saccharin are in the proportion of 3%. Saccharin, as a soluble marker, dissolves in the sol layer, providing data on clearance time, understood to be a more complex reaction of the mucosa to the extraneous particles. Charcoal, a nonsoluble marker, does not spread out but merely adheres to the mucous carpet, so it provides a time corresponding more closely to the time of actual mucociliary transport (10). This test gives obtain an objective value (the duration before the examiner sees the charcoal in the oropharynx) and a subjective measurement (sensation of sweetness reported by the patient due to the saccharin). This test is capable of revealing alterations in transportation even when the appearance of the mucosa has not yet undergone obvious modifications. Normal times in physiological conditions are: 13 ± 2 min in adults and 8 ± 3 min in children for charcoal powder and 17 ± 5 min in adults and 11 ± 6 min in children for saccharin. The MCTt is considered to be blocked when after 30 min the charcoal has not appeared in the pharynx and/or there is no sensation of sweetness due to saccharin (11).

In allergic rhinopathies, the efficiency of the system is impaired: in seasonal forms the sol and gel phases of the mucus are altered because of the increased glandular secretion; in perennial forms the ciliar carpet is severely damaged, because of a metaplastic transformation into squamous epithelium.

III. Allergy Tests

When we suspect an allergic rhinitis and after a complete anatomic and functional evaluation of the nose, we follow a particular diagnostic program that allows us to confirm the clinical diagnosis and to create an adequate preventive and therapeutic program. The diagnostic program consists of:

- first level investigations;
- second level investigations;
- third level investigations (12).

The first level investigations consist of skin tests. To confirm specific vasomotor rhinopathy, caused by allergen reactions of the first type, a prick test can be used. This is carried out on the skin of the volar side of the forearm to have a quicker and more uniform cutaneous reactivity the one of the skin of the back. In the majority of people, we manage to find the allergens responsible for the allergy. In some subjects, however, negative results on the skin tests can contrast with the history, which is suggestive of an allergic disease.

In this case it is necessary to resort to second and/or third level investigation.

Second level investigations: total IgE dosage (PRIST or ELISA) in the serum is not very specific and consequently has a limited application.

An interesting contribution could be given, on the other hand, by the total IgE dosage in the nasal secretion (the target organ). However, this method has not been well standardized yet.

Presently, the most significant laboratory test that can be routinely administered is the specific IgE dosage (RAST or ELISA), both in the serum and in the nasal secretion.

Third level investigations: the direct application of the allergen to the nasal mucosa can be considered, at least from a theoretical point of view, as the most correct and direct etiological and quantitative method for the diagnosis of allergic rhinitis.

So the nasal provocation test allows us to show beyond any doubt the relationship between a particular allergen and the outcome of typical symptoms in the shock organ. In fact, the clinical symptoms of allergic rhinitis depend on the prevalent or exclusive localization of the previously primed mastocytes in the shock organ.

In specific vasomotor rhinopathy, the nose is the meeting point of the allergens and specific IgE presented by the mastocytes. It is here that they are concentrated. The surplus circulates in the bloodstream and colonizes distant organs with a high content of mastocytes, such as the skin.

It is therefore possible that the reactivity of the shock organ does not correlate well with the cutaneous reactivity or with serum positivity for a transitory or permanent deficit of IgE in circulation or residing at a distance.

In our experience, we demonstrated a specificity and a predictive positive value (PPV) of nasal provocation test equal to 100% for the most common allergens in Italy.

In order to obtain high levels of reliability and reproduction, we follow specific guidelines. First of all, we try to obtain a uniform distribution of the allergens during the administration. This goal can be reached by using a nebulizer dosimeter, which delivers a known quantity of solution or simple devices that release powder containing lyophilized extract dispersed in lactose. In this way we avoid all the problems induced by the use of aqueous solutions administered by means of squeeze bottles, or poor stability of the content and difficulty in administering the allergen. To evaluate the results of the test, we not only record the symptoms of the patient during increasing dosage with allergen, but we also measure specific parameters of functional aspects of the nose that give this test a high reliability (13). Following are the steps we follow:

1. Determination of a baseline value using AAR to exclude a nasal stenosis incompatible with the test.
2. Administration of lactose into the nose with the appropriate insufflator and, after 10 min, AAR is repeated. The fossa to be studied is the one that presents the best respiratory patency during the rhinomanometric examination.
3. Administration of the powder containing the lyophilised allergen. This test consists of insufflation of progressively increasing dosage of the allergen (2.5, 5, 10, 20, 40, 60, 80 UA/cps) into the selected nasal cavity until, in the case of positive results, an increment of nasal resistance $\geq 100\%$ is obtained together with the appearance of clinical symptoms.

IV. Conclusion

Allergic rhinitis is a widespread disease, and reaches its highest incidence in the first years of life. Even though it is not a life-threatening disease, it has a remarkable social impact. In fact, a substantial number of patients with hay-fever develop asthma at a later age, with an increased risk of death, a diminished quality of life, and an increase in the expenses related to the pharmacological treatment and hospitalization.

For this reason, a correct diagnostic and therapeutical approach starting from the first years of life is of fundamental importance.

The treatment of allergic rhinitis in childhood is based on an adequate environmental prevention, symptomatic treatment, and eventually specific immunotherapy both by systemic and local administration in order to prevent the involvement of the lower respiratory tract.

However, before starting any antiallergic therapy and during it, to monitor the degree of mucosal inflammation, it is necessary to be informed of nasal function with AAR, AR, and MCTt. After that, the allergy tests are performed, following different levels of investigation. The last step, which is the nasal provocation test, confirms the nose to be the shock organ of the allergic reaction; it is the best way to confirm the prevalent allergen at the nasal level and establishes the threshold of sensitization.

References

1. Passàli D. Screening of allergic rhinitis. Rhinology 1983; 21:32–38.
2. Connel JT. Quantitative intranasal pollen challenge II. Effects of daily pollen challenge, environmental pollen exposure and placebo challenge in nasal membrane. J Allergy 1968; 41:153–157.
3. Passàli D. Allergy in childhood. Rhinology 1986; 24:25–28.
4. Canonica GW, Ciprandi G, Buscaglia S, Pesce G, Bagnasco M. Adhesion molecules of allergic inflammation: recent insights into their functional roles. Allergy 1994; 35–141.
5. Clement PAR. Committe report on standardization of rhinomanometry. Rhinology 1984; 22:151–153.
6. Clement PAR. Rhinomanometry. Rhinology 1991; (suppl 14).
7. Grymer LF, Hilberg O, Elbron O, Pederson OF. Acoustic rhinometry: evaluation of the nasal cavity with septal deviations, before and after septoplasty. Laryngoscope 1989; 99:1180–1183.
8. Grymer LF, Hilberg O, Pederson OF, Rasmussen TR. Acoustic rhinometry: values from adults with subjects with free nasal patency. Rhinology 1991; 29:35–40.
9. Passàli D, Biagini C, Di Girolamo S, Bellussi L. Acoustic rhinometry: practical aspects of measurement. Acta Otorhinolaryngol Belg 1996; 50:41–45.
10. Passàli D, Bellussi L, Bianchini Ciampolini M, De Seta E. Our experience in nasal mucociliary transport time determination. Acta Otorhinoloryngol Scand 1984; 97:319–323.

11. Passàli D, Bianchini Ciampolini M. Normal values of mucociliary transport time in young subjects. Int J Pediar Otorhinolaryngol 1985; 9:151–156.

12. Errigo E. Il Memorandum della SIAIC Sulla Diagnostica delle Allergopatie. In: Pallestrini E, Pàssali D, eds. Allergie in Otorinolaringoiatria: Tecniche Diagnostiche e Terapeutiche. Genova: Scuola Sup. di Oncologia e Scienze Biomediche, 1992:19–24.

13. Bellussi L. I Test di Provocazione Nasale. In: Pallestrini E, Passàli D, eds. Allergie in Otorinolaringoiatria: Tecniche Diagnostiche e Terapeutiche. Genova: Scuola Sup. di Oncologia e Scienze Biomediche, 1992:123–133.

15

Imaging of Paranasal Sinus Disease in Children

LALITHA SHANKAR

University of Toronto,
Toronto, Canada

I. Introduction

Messerklinger has demonstrated that ventilation and drainage of the anterior ethmoidal sinus, the maxillary sinus, and the frontal sinus are dependent on the patent "ostiomeatal complex".

Most sinus infections are rhinogenic in origin and spread from the ostiomeatal complex to secondarily involve the frontal and the maxillary sinuses. The ostiomeatal complex in the lateral nasal wall is easily narrowed or occluded by mucosal edema. This results in impaired ventilation and poor mucociliary clearance and the stagnation of mucus and pus in the larger paranasal sinuses (1–6).

II. Plain Radiographs

Radiographs reflect the general condition of the larger paranasal sinuses (especially the frontal, maxillary, and sphenoid sinuses). Very little information can be obtained on the ethmoidal air cells and the ostiomeatal complex. This is in most instances the primary site of disease. Hence, plain radiographs are inadequate prior to functional endoscopic sinus surgery.

Conventional or plain radiographs usually involve four projections (adults):

1. *Caldwell's projection*: It is useful to assess all the sinuses except the sphenoid sinuses.
2. *The lateral projection*: Under the age of 3 it is of little use as the sphenoid sinus is not fully developed.
3. *Waters' projection*: This is the most important view for the paranasal sinuses.
4. *The submentovertical projection*: Large turbinates and nasal secretions prevent adequate visualization of the ethmoid sinuses in this projection.

In children the Waters' and the lateral projections are more commonly used.

The following points may justify the usage of plain radiographs:

1. Primary care physicians use routine X-rays for documenting acute sinusitis prior to initiation of diagnosis or referral to an ENT specialist as it is easily available.
2. When the clinical diagnosis is equivocal, radiographs readily confirm the presence of an air–fluid interface or a totally opacified sinus at a lower cost.
3. Serial radiographs for the follow-up of an uncomplicated acute sinusitis are not necessary.

Plain X-rays may be inconclusive and CT scans may be necessary in chronic or chronic recurrent sinusitis. Office nasal endoscopy is the primary line of investigation prior to CT scans (7,8):

1. The radiograph may merely show a normal sinus or replacement of an air–fluid level by mucosal thickening. This does not shed any light on the ostiomeatal complex or the ethmoid sinuses.
2. Pre-existing developmental anomalies in larger sinuses such as the maxillary sinuses may be misleading.
3. In children plain X-rays may not only be inconclusive, but also misleading.
4. Plain films are not useful if orbital or intracranial complications occur with sinusitis.

5. A normal radiograph does not exclude the presence of sinusitis or ethmoidal disease.
6. Computed tomography (CT) enables the surgeon to opt for computer-assisted surgery to avoid intra-operative complications (9,10).

III. Computed Tomography

Coronal plane CT is the optimum imaging modality used most frequently prior to any sinus surgery (11–15). This is easily achieved in cooperative adults but can be a challenge when coronal plane CT examination is attempted in the pediatric population. With the helical CT scanning a lot of the centers scan the uncooperative patients in the axial plane and reconstruct the images in the coronal plane without too much degradation of the images (16–18). Infants and younger uncooperative children are sedated with intravenous nembutol. These children are closely monitored by nurses familiar with the routine. The sedated child is connected to a pulse oximeter. Contrast enhancement is reserved for cases where intraorbital or intracranial spread of benign or malignant sinus disease is suspected (19–27).

IV. Magnetic Resonance Imaging

Magnetic resonance imaging (MRI) is not found to be useful in the evaluation of the bony structures of the sinus. MR is obtained when differentiation between invasive fungal sinusitis and malignancy is in question or when intracranial extension of tumor or infection needs evaluation. The orbital apex and the pterygopalatine fossa are better delineated by MRI (28–37).

V. Normal Anatomy

The sinus anatomy in children is similar to that in adults. Coronal plane CT scans best delineate the anatomy of the lateral nasal wall. A brief description of pertinent structures as seen on CT follows (38–42).

VI. The Frontal Sinus

The frontal sinuses (Fig. 15.1) are asymmetrical paired cavities located between the two tables of the frontal bone. The frontal sinuses are absent at birth and shortly after the second year the frontal bone shows pneumatization and by the sixth to eighth year it is fairly well developed. The adult size is reached after puberty. Congenital absence is common if there is bilateral persistence of the metopic suture (43).

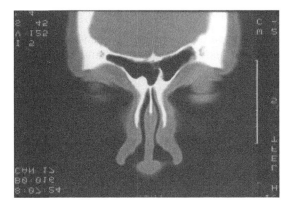

Figure 15.1 This coronal CT examination demonstrates normal frontal sinuses bilaterally, the lateral aspects of the vertical plates of the middle turbinates bilaterally.

The shape and size of the frontal sinus is highly variable and it may be hypoplastic or even absent. Asymmetry of the frontal sinuses is more common in those races with dolichocephalic heads, such as the mongoloid race. Extensive pneumatization of the superciliary portion of the frontal bone is a common variant in both normal individuals and acromegalics. The frontal sinus drains into the nasal cavity via the frontal recess.

A. Normal Frontal Recess

The route of ventilation and drainage of the frontal sinus through the frontal recess (Fig. 15.2) depends on the embryological development (44).

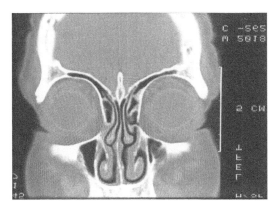

Figure 15.2 This CT scan demonstrates the frontal recesses draining lateral to the middle turbinates.

The frontal recess may open into

1. The premeatal groove anterior to the hiatus semilunaris and therefore drain independently of the ethmoidal infundibulum and the maxillary and ethmoid sinuses.
2. The ethmoid infundibulum, in which case inflammation affecting the maxillary sinus may spread along the infundibulum to affect the frontal sinus.

The frontal recess is rarely visualized at the time of routine, preoperative endoscopy, and CT in the coronal plane is ideal for assessing this region. A short, wide frontal recess may be easily visualized on a single scan. A more tortuous and narrow frontal recess usually cannot be seen on a single scan because the frontal recess runs obliquely with its distal (inferior) end more posterior than its proximal (superior) end. In such a narrow frontal recess, which runs between crowded anterior ethmoidal air cells, minimal swelling can impede the drainage of the frontal sinus and predispose it to recurrent infection.

B. Maxillary Sinus

The maxillary sinus (Fig. 15.3) is the largest of the paranasal sinuses (45). It measures <5 mm at birth. It increases 2 mm/year and measures ~23 mm after 12 years of age. The maxillary sinuses drain into the middle meati through the ethmoid infundibula.

C. Maxillary Sinus Ostium

The natural ostium of the maxillary sinus is located in the supero-medial aspect of the medial sinus wall. The maxillary sinus ventilation and drainage is through the ostium, which opens into the ethmoidal infundibulum (46).

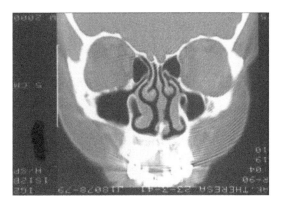

Figure 15.3 Normal maxillary sinus. The maxillary sinus ostia are seen opening into the ethmoid infundibulum, which in its turn opens into a two-dimensional slit-like aperture, the hiatus semilunaris. The hiatus semilunaris drains into the middle meatus.

D. Ethmoid Sinuses

The ethmoid bone lies between the orbits. It consists of a horizontal plate, a vertical plate, and on either side of the latter, the ethmoidal labyrinths. The ethmoid labyrinth is separated from the orbit by the delicate lamina papyracea. Natural dehiscences in the lamina papyracea may allow spread of infection into the orbit. These dehiscences should not be mistaken to be pathological erosions.

The ethmoid labyrinths are divided into an anterior and a posterior group of air cells. The horizontal plate that separates the anterior from the posterior ethmoid sinuses is called the ground or the grand lamellae. The ground lamella curves laterally to project onto the lamina papyracea and forms the roof of the middle meatus. After 1 year of age the ethmoid cells are demonstrated on the plain radiographs. At 12 years the ethmoid sinuses reach adult configuration.

E. The Anterior Ethmoid Sinuses

The anterior ethmoid air cells (Fig. 15.4) are usually smaller and more numerous than the posterior group of air cells. The largest of the anterior ethmoid air cells is called the ethmoid bulla. It is the most prominent structure in the middle meatus. The anterior ethmoid cells drain into the middle meatus whereas the posterior ethmoid cells drain into the superior meatus (47–49).

F. The Cribriform Plate and Fovea Ethmoidalis

The cribriform plate lies at a variable level in relation to the foveolae ethmoidales (Figs. 15.5 and 15.6). The roof of the ethmoid may not be symmetric on the two sides. The cribriform plate and the fovea may lie well below the roof of the nasal

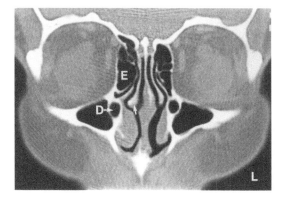

Figure 15.4 Coronal plane CT examination through the anterior ethmoid sinuses (E) demonstrates anterior ethmoid air cells with the air filled nasal lacrimal duct (D) and a normal nasal septum and middle turbinate (arrow).

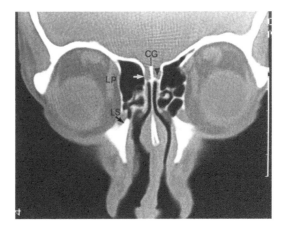

Figure 15.5 Anterior ethmoid sinuses. Normal scan through the anterior part of the sinuses demonstrates the lacrimal sac (LS), lamina papyracea (LP), crista galli (CG), cribriform plate (black arrowhead) and thin lamina lateralis (white arrow).

cavity. In some cases the foveolae ethmoidales may be asymmetric with one side at a lower level than the other. This is well demonstrated by CT in the coronal plane. If sinus surgery is being contemplated, the surgeon will use this information to avoid injury to the cribriform plate. Such injuries can result in permanent anosmia or cerebrospinal fluid rhinorrhea and the risk of intracranial infection.

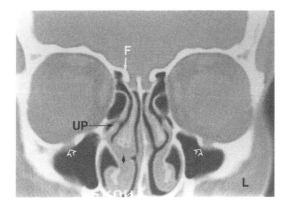

Figure 15.6 Normal cribriform plate fovea ethmoidalis (F) and normal lamina lateralis with vertical insertion of the middle turbinates are noted. The uncinate process (UP) is seen to be normal. There is apposition of hypertrophied middle turbinate against the right inferior turbinate (black arrows). White arrows indicate the site of the infraorbital nerves.

G. Ethmoid Infundibulum

The ethmoid infundibulum (Fig. 15.7) is the slit-like critical drainage channel bounded superolaterally by the ethmoidal bulla, the lamina papyracea, and inferomedially by the uncinate process. It connects the natural ostium of the maxillary sinus to the middle meatus via the hiatus semilunaris. The ethmoidal infundibulum can be compromised by anomalies of the middle turbinate, the uncinate process, or a large ethmoid bulla. Anteriorly and superiorly, the frontal recess may open into the ethmoidal infundibulum.

H. Hiatus Semilunaris

The hiatus semilunaris is a semilunar two-dimensional aperture bounded posteriorly by the anterior surface of the ethmoid bulla and anteriorly by the posterior free margin of the uncinate process. The ethmoidal infundibulum drains into the middle meatus through the hiatus semilunaris.

I. The Middle Meatus

The middle meatus is the space inferolateral to the middle turbinate, into which the anterior ethmoid and the frontal and the maxillary sinuses eventually drain. The most prominent structure within the middle meatus is usually the ethmoidal bulla. The size of the middle meatus can vary, for example, it may be deep when there is maxillary sinus hypoplasia and the posterior fontanelle is retracted laterally. The middle meatus and the nasal cavities are small when the sinuses are well developed.

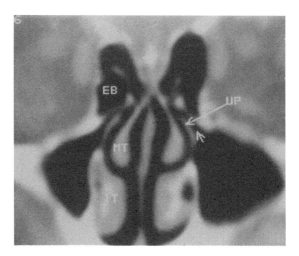

Figure 15.7 Normal ostiomeatal complex. The ostiomeatal complex is the final drainage pathway for the frontal recesses, maxillary sinuses, and anterior ethmoid sinuses. EB = ethmoid bulla, MT = middle turbinate, UP = uncinate process, IT = inferior turbinate, small arrow = ethmoid infundibulum.

The middle meatus may be compromised by a large ethmoid bulla, a deviated nasal septum, a bony septal spur or one of the many variants of the middle turbinates listed in Table 15.1 (52).

The ostiomeatal complex (Fig. 15.7) is a term used to collectively describe that area of the anterior ethmoid into which the frontal, the maxillary, and the anterior ethmoidal sinuses drain. It is composed of the frontal recess, the ethmoid infundibulum, the hiatus semilunaris, and the adjacent portion of the middle meatus (53–55). The anatomy of the anterior ethmoid sinus is variable. These variations are of clinical interest when they cause obstruction of the ostiomeatal complex. Inflammatory disease in the ostiomeatal complex is the key to the development of most inflammatory diseases of the frontal, maxillary, and ethmoid sinuses.

VII. The Ethmoidal Bulla

The largest and most constantly present anterior ethmoidal air cell is the ethmoidal bulla (Fig. 15.4). The anterior wall of the ethmoidal bulla forms the posterior margin of the ethmoidal infundibulum. The roof of the ethmoid bulla may be continuous with the roof of the ethmoid sinus or it may be separated by a suprabullar extension of the lateral sinus. The lateral sinus is an inconstant space seen sometimes between the ethmoid bulla and the ground lamella. When present it drains into the hiatus semilunaris.

VIII. The Posterior Ethmoid Sinuses

The posterior ethmoid air cells (Fig. 15.8) are larger in size than the anterior ethmoid air cells, but fewer in number. They drain into the superior meatus, which is situated inferolateral to the superior turbinate. An inconstant additional turbinate may be situated above the superior turbinate and is called the supreme turbinate. The largest and most posterior of the posterior ethmoid air cells is called the Onodi cell, after the anatomist who first described it (56). It shares a common wall with the adjacent sphenoid sinus. Its importance lies in the fact that the optic nerve may in some instances lie close to its superolateral wall. The posterior ethmoid sinus may expand superiorly into the orbit forming supraorbital cells, or it may expand laterally to encompass the optic nerve (57). These variants, need to be identified preoperatively, as they may pose extreme hazards to the patient's vision. Bony dehiscences also pose greater risk of trauma to the optic nerve at surgery.

IX. The Sphenoid Sinus

The sphenoid sinus (Figs. 15.9–15.11) lies within the sphenoid bone. At birth these sinuses are absent. By the second year the posterior extension of the

Table 15.1 The Important Anatomical Structures of the Ostiomeatal Complex and Their Variations

A. Agger nasi cells (Fig. 15.12)

When present and enlarged agger nasi cells can obstruct the frontal recess

B. Nasal septum

Deviation of the nasal septum

Septal spurs

C. Uncinate process

Medially or laterally deflected

Inferiorly deflected (Fig. 15.13)

Hypertrophy

Pneumatized (Fig. 15.14)

Aplasia or hypoplasia

D. Middle turbinate

Soft tissue hypertrophy (Fig. 15.15)

Concha bullosa (aeration) (Fig. 15.16)

When a turbinate contains an air cell it is referred to as a "concha bullosa"; the air cell of
  such a middle turbinate can be affected by any of the disorders that affect the paranasal
  sinuses (50)

Conditions that can occur in a concha bullosa

  Concha bullitis (an acute bacterial infection)

  Mucocele/pyocele (Fig. 15.17)

  Polyps arising within the concha bullosa (Fig. 15.18)

  Polyps arising from the conchal sinus (the lateral surface of the concha bullosa)

Paradoxically bent middle turbinate

Lateralization of the middle turbinate

Bony hypertrophy of the middle turbinate

Partial or complete agenesis

E. Ethmoidal bulla

The ethmoidal bulla may be the site of inflammatory disease or it may predispose the
  patient to inflammatory disease by obstructing the ostiomeatal complex. It is unusual to
  find isolated ethmoidal bullitis and the ethmoidal bulla is more commonly involved in
  generalized inflammatory disease of the ethmoid sinus (47,51)

  Large: (Figs. 15.19 and 15.20)

    Protrudes into the middle meatus

    Overhangs the hiatus semilunaris

    Obstructs the ethmoid infundibulum

    Obstructs the frontal recess

  Hypoplasia

  Absent

F. Haller's cell (Fig. 15.21)

These cells are thought to arise from the anterior ethmoidal sinus and are located near the
  inferomedial aspect of the orbital floor opposite the natural ostium of the maxillary sinus.
  When present and enlarged a Haller's cell can obstruct the natural ostium of the maxillary
  sinus and the ethmoid infundibulum, thus predisposing to recurrent or chronic
  inflammatory disease in the maxillary and frontal sinuses.

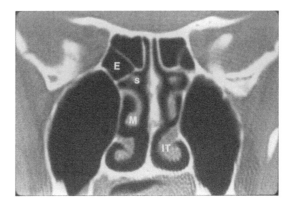

Figure 15.8 Coronal scan of the posterior ethmoid sinuses demonstrates normal posterior ethmoid air cell (E), inferior turbinate (IT), middle turbinate (M), and superior turbinate (S). The space below and inferior to the middle turbinate is the middle meatus. The space above the middle turbinate is the superior meatus.

ethmoid sinus is the first sign of the sphenoid sinus. It grows between the second and the sixth year and reaches adult size around 12 years of age. On either side of the sphenoid sinus lie the cavernous sinuses, which transmit the internal carotid artery and the third, fourth, and sixth cranial nerves. The intracavernous portion of the internal carotid artery passes superiorly alongside the body of the sphenoid sinus. The internal carotid artery may sometimes lie within the lumen of the sphenoid sinus. It is usually separated by a thin plate of bone, but this may be dehiscent.

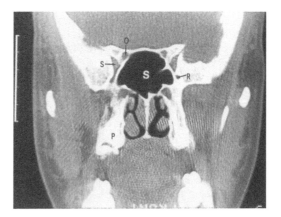

Figure 15.9 Normal sphenoid sinus. The normal structures on the lateral wall of the sphenoid sinuses (S) are optic nerve, superior orbital fissure (s), foramen rotundum (R), and pterygoid plates (P).

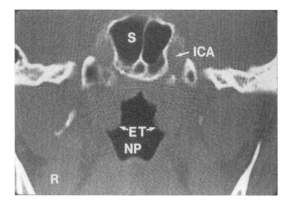

Figure 15.10 Normal sphenoid sinus. The relationship of the internal carotid artery (ICA) along the lateral wall of the sphenoid sinus. Inferior to the sphenoid sinus (S), lie the eustachian tube (ET) and the nasopharynx (NP).

The foramen rotundum and the Vidian canal traverse the body of the sphenoid and are lateral relations of the sphenoid sinus (Figs. 15.9–15.11).

A. Sphenoid Sinus Ostium

The sphenoid sinus drains through a small ostium in the anterior wall, close to the roof of the sinus, into the spheno-ethmoid recess. This is usually not well demonstrated by CT in the coronal plane, but is well demonstrated on scans taken in the axial plane, sagittal reformatted images, or sagittal MR scans. The optic nerve lies above and lateral to the sphenoid sinus and the pituitary gland lies above

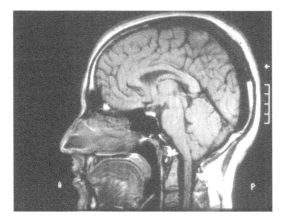

Figure 15.11 Normal sphenoid sinus with the pituitary gland in the roof of the sphenoid sinus.

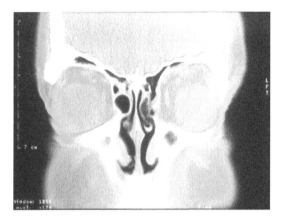

Figure 15.12   A large agger nasi air cell on the right side is seen to compromise the right frontal recess.

the sinus. Inferiorly, the sphenoid sinus is related to the nasopharynx, the eustachian tubes, and eustachian cushions.

X.   The Important Anatomical Structures of the Ostiomeatal Complex and Their Variations

Coronal CT allows the radiologist to determine the site and extent of disease in the paranasal sinuses and to identify those anatomical variants which predispose

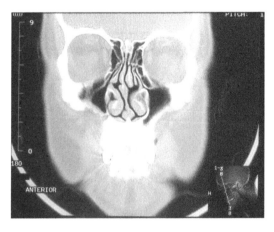

Figure 15.13   This coronal CT scan demonstrates a large uncinate process deflected inferiorly into the left middle meatus. A large Haller cell is also shown. The middle turbinate is hypertrophied on the left side and is seen to focally deflect the nasal septum to the right.

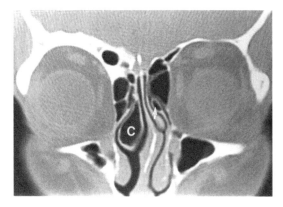

Figure 15.14 The CT examination demonstrates a pneumatized uncinate process (white arrow) on the left side and a large concha bullosa (C) of the middle turbinate on the right side with focal deviation of the nasal septum to the left. There are also changes compatible with fibrous dysplasia in the right frontal bone.

the individual to sinusitis (54,55,58–62). Those structures that are large or deflected from their normal position adjacent to the drainage pathways of the major sinuses can compromise drainage and ventilation (63–69). These important anatomical variants are listed in Tables 15.1 and 15.2.

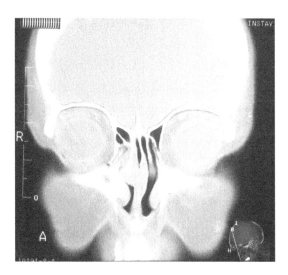

Figure 15.15 A hypertrophied right middle turbinate is seen to narrow the right frontal recess.

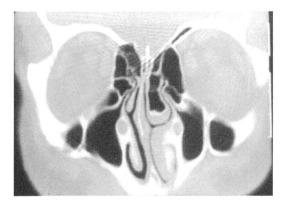

Figure 15.16   A large concha bullosa is seen to fill the entire middle meatus on the left side. There is hypoplasia of the right middle turbinate and the ostiomeatal complex is narrowed bilaterally.

This process is usually reversible and once the ostiomeatal complex is reopened, the secondary disease within the larger maxillary and frontal sinuses usually resolves spontaneously.

The important anatomical structures of the ostiomeatal complex and their variations are as follows:

1. *Agger nasi cells* (Fig. 15.12): When present and enlarged, agger nasi cells can obstruct the frontal recess.
2. *Nasal septum*
    i.   deviation of the nasal septum
    ii. septal spurs
3. *Uncinate process*
    i.   medially or laterally deflected
    ii. inferiorly deflected (Fig. 15.13)
    iii. hypertrophy
    iv. pneumatized (Fig. 15.14)
    v.   aplasia or hypoplasia
4. *Middle turbinate*
    i.   soft tissue hypertrophy (Fig. 15.17)
    ii. concha bullosa (aeration) (Fig. 15.18)
         When a turbinate contains an air cell it is referred to as a "concha bullosa." The air cell of such a middle turbinate can be affected by any of the disorders that affect the paranasal sinuses (50).
         Conditions that can occur in a concha bullosa:
         a.   concha bullitis (an acute bacterial infection)
         b.   mucocele/pyocele (Fig. 15.17)

       c. polyps arising within the concha bullosa (Fig. 15.18)

       d. polyps arising from the conchal sinus (the lateral surface of the concha bullosa)

    iii. paradoxically bent middle turbinate

    iv. lateralization of the middle turbinate

     v. bony hypertrophy of the middle turbinate

    vi. partial or complete agenesis

5. *Ethmoidal bulla*: The ethmoidal bulla may be the site of inflammatory disease or it may predispose the patient to inflammatory disease by obstructing the ostiomeatal complex. It is unusual to find isolated ethmoidal bullitis and the ethmoidal bulla is more commonly involved in generalized inflammatory disease of the ethmoid sinus (47,51).

     i. large (Figs. 15.19 and 15.20)

        protrudes into the middle meatus

        overhangs the hiatus semilunaris

        obstructs the ethmoid infundibulum

        obstructs the frontal recess

    ii. hypoplasia

   iii. absent

6. *Haller's cell* (Fig. 15.21): These cells are thought to arise from the anterior ethmoidal sinus and are located near the inferomedial aspect of the orbital floor opposite the natural ostium of the maxillary sinus. When present and enlarged, a Haller's cell can obstruct the natural ostium of the maxillary sinus and the ethmoid infundibulum, thus predisposing to recurrent or chronic inflammatory disease in the maxillary and frontal sinuses (Figs. 15.19–15.21).

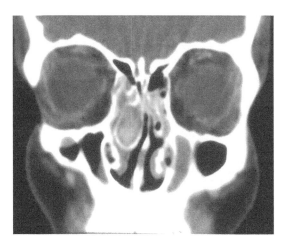

Figure 15.17 A large mucocele is seen to involve the right middle turbinate and a high-density polyp is seen in the lumen of the right middle turbinate.

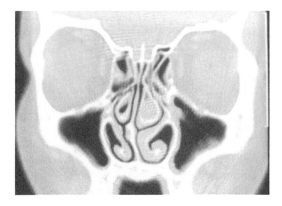

Figure 15.18   Inflammatory polyp is seen in the concha bullosa lumen on the left side. Inflammatory disease is seen is the ostiomeatal complex on the left side.

Failure of resorption of mesodermal plate
   Membranous atresia
Failure of perforation of the buccopharyngeal membrane
   75% associated with other defect

XI.   Maxillary Sinus Hypoplasia

Hypoplasia of the maxillary sinus is a developmental abnormality that can be identified radiologically in patients with and without sinus disease. Bolger and Parsons analyzed a series of 202 consecutively obtained CT scans, and noted a

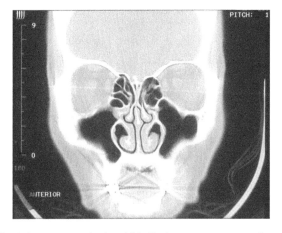

Figure 15.19   A large septated ethmoid bulla is seen to compromise and obstruct the ethmoid infundibulum on the right side.

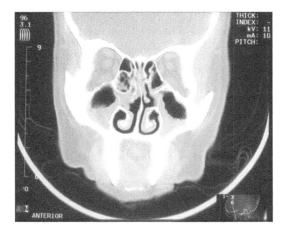

Figure 15.20 Inflammatory disease in a large ethmoid bulla. There is muco-inflammatory disease in the lumen of the ethmoid bulla on the right side. Inflammatory disease is seen in both ostiomeatal complex and in the maxillary sinus.

prevalence of maxillary sinus hypoplasia of 10% (70–72). The superior bone, air, and soft tissue contrast resolution of CT enables the radiologist to accurately diagnose such variants and has led to the finding of the association of hypoplasia of the uncinate process with hypoplasia of the maxillary sinus. They presented a classification system based on the radiographic features of the sinus as seen on CT. The maxillary sinus and the nasal cavity are inversely proportional to one another. The smaller the sinus, the larger the nasal cavity on the same side. Asymmetric sinuses may be demonstrated by plain radiographs.

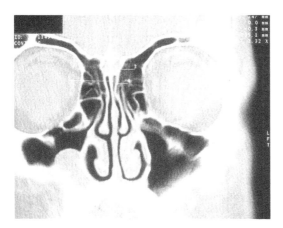

Figure 15.21 A large Haller's cell is seen to compromise the right maxillary sinus ostia. There is pneumatization of the floor of the left orbit.

Table 15.2   The Anatomical Variants That are Best Seen on
CT and Important for the Surgeon to Know Prior to Fess

Dehiscence of the lamina papyracea
Dehiscence of the walls of the orbit (Fig. 15.22)
Low-lying fovea ethmoidalis/cribriform plate (Fig. 15.23)
Dehiscence of the optic nerve canal
Dehiscence of the internal carotid artery bony wall (Fig. 15.24)
Hypoplasia of the maxillary sinus (Figs. 15.25–15.27)
Choanal atresia (Figs. 15.28–15.31)
  Unilateral or bilateral atresia of the nasal cavity
  Bony or membranous atresia

Long-standing atrophic rhinitis can mimic maxillary sinus hypoplasia (73).
The various types of maxillary sinus hypoplasia and their radiological appearance
are discussed in Tables 15.3 and 15.4.

The clinical significance of maxillary sinus hypoplasia include the
following:

1. The smaller sinus may be misinterpreted as a sinus of normal dimen-
    sions with chronic maxillary sinusitis, especially when the patient has a
    history of persistent upper respiratory tract infections. In such circum-
    stances these patients may be erroneously subjected to prolonged
    medical management (75,76).
2. These patients may undergo surgical exploration only to find normal sinus
    mucosa within the smaller sinus cavity. An attempted uncinectomy in
    these patients will lead to inadvertent entry into the orbit through the
    lamina papyracea or orbital floor (Tables 15.3 and 15.4).

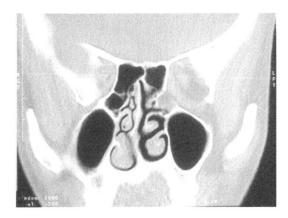

Figure 15.22   Dehiscence of the medial margin of the orbit. This congenital dehiscence
is seen with protrusion of the orbital fat into the superior meatus region on the left side.

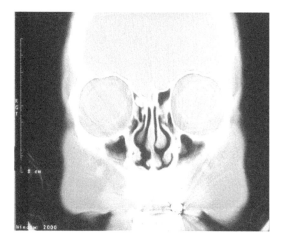

Figure 15.23 Asymmetry of the fovea ethmoidalis. The fovea ethmoidalis is seen to be at a lower plane on the right side when compared to the left side. This is an important anomaly that needs to be mentioned to the surgeon as any trauma to this low-lying fovea ethmoidalis can result in cerebrospinal rhinorrhea or infection spreading intracranially. An osteoma is noted in the right frontal recess.

XII. Sinusitis

A. Radiographic Features of Sinusitis

Acute sinusitis (Figs. 15.32 and 15.33) is characterized clinically by nasal obstruction, purulent nasal discharge, postnasal drip, and facial pain. The pain of frontal sinusitis radiates to the forehead and is usually associated with a

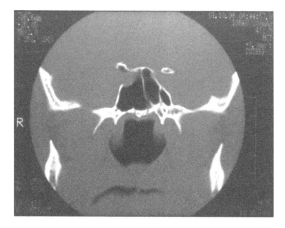

Figure 15.24 Dehiscence of the internal carotid artery bony wall.

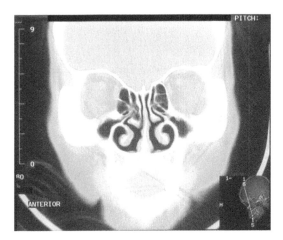

Figure 15.25 Type 1 maxillary sinus hypoplasia. Both maxillary sinuses are small. Uncinate processes and ethmoid bulla are normal.

generalized headache. In acute maxillary sinusitis the pain usually radiates from the inner canthus to the cheek. The pain may also radiate to the alveolar region, mimicking dental disease. Acute ethmoid sinusitis is associated with pain that tends to localize to the bridge of the nose and behind the medial canthus of the eye. It is often cyclical being worse first thing in the morning after rising. In acute sphenoid sinusitis patients experience retro-orbital and posterior occipital headaches.

The following changes are seen on CT, MR, or plain radiographs.

1.   The mucosal lining of the sinus may be thickened and if mucus or pus is collecting in the sinus an air fluid level will be evident.

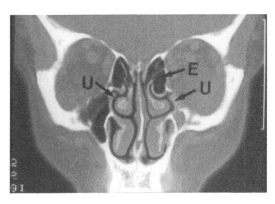

Figure 15.26 Type 2 maxillary sinus hypoplasia. The left hypoplastic uncinate process (U) is plastered against the inferior medial margin of the orbit. The ethmoid bulla (E) is of normal size. The maxillary sinus on the left side is small.

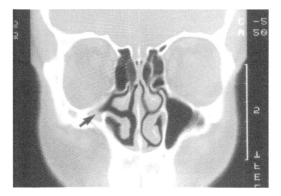

Figure 15.27 Type 3 maxillary sinus hypoplasia. A slit-like maxillary sinus lumen is seen on the right side (arrow). The uncinate process is laterally deviated.

2. In cases of severe sinusitis, the extensive mucosal edema and fluid exudate will make the sinus appear totally opaque. The infection may be confined to one of the larger sinuses, or it may involve all of the sinuses on one side as a "pansinusitis."
3. Spread of infection from the anterior ethmoid complex to the posterior ethmoid sinus is usually through a defect in the ground lamella.
4. The significance of "cloudy sinus" is uncertain. Normal children with no symptoms of sinusitis can present with opacified sinuses. The various factors that cause cloudy sinuses include cystic fibrosis, asthma, and allergic sinusitis.

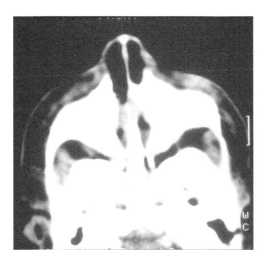

Figure 15.28 Choanal atresia. There is significant narrowing of the nasal cavity bilaterally on this axial plane. Bony atresia is seen posteriorly near the posterior nares.

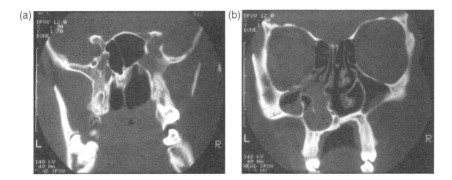

Figure 15.29   (a) Bony and membranous atresia. The posterior choana is narrow on the left side. (b) The right side is normal. The left maxillary sinus and nasal cavity are narrow and there is atretic with soft tissue filling the left nasal cavity.

5. On MRI inflamed sinus mucosa is hyperintense or bright on T2-weighted (T2-W) MR scans. Normal nasal cycle can be seen as hyperintense mucosa and should not be mistaken for inflammatory disease. Hence, careful clinical correlation is essential (3,77,78).

B. Chronic Sinusitis

The symptoms of chronic sinusitis are variable and generally mild. These patients frequently present with recurrent headaches and facial pain. There is usually a combination of nasal obstruction, rhinorrhea, and postnasal drip. Multiple

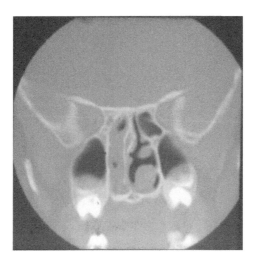

Figure 15.30   Membranous atresia showing dense soft tissue occluding the inferior meatus and nasal cavity region.

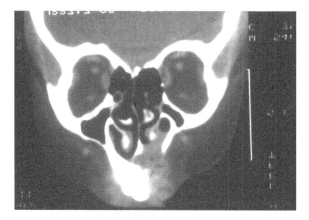

Figure 15.31 Left nasal atresia with cleft palate. This patient has a deformity of the face with cleft palate defect. There is a large defect seen along the floor of the left nasal cavity with a membranous atresia noted within the left nasal cavity. The left maxillary sinus is also noted to be small.

Table 15.3 Hypoplasia of the Maxillary Sinus

Primary maxillary sinus hypoplasia
Type I maxillary sinus hypoplasia (incidence 7%) (Fig. 15.25)
    Mild decrease in the maxillary sinus volume
    Normal uncinate process
    Normal ethmoid infundibulum.
Type II maxillary sinus hypoplasia (incidence 3%) (Fig. 15.26)
    Mild to moderate reduction in the volume of the maxillary sinus
    CT evidence of an absent or hypoplastic uncinate process
    Absent or poorly defined ethmoid infundibulum.
Type III maxillary sinus hypoplasia (incidence 0.5%) (Fig. 15.27)
    The maxillary sinus in primarily absent and consists of only a cleft
    Ethmoid infundibulum is absent
    The uncinate process is absent
    The nasal cavity and orbit on the involved side are usually enlarged.

Secondary maxillary sinus hypoplasia
Trauma
Infection
Radiation
Fibrous dysplasia
Paget's disease
Systemic diseases

Table 15.4 Imaging Findings in Primary Maxillary Sinus
Hypoplasia (74) and Acquired Hypoplasia

Primary maxillary sinus hypoplasia
Enlargement of the ipsilateral orbits
Enlargement of the superior and inferior orbital fissures
Enlargement of the pterygopalatine fossa
Widening of the middle meatus and retraction of the fontanelles
Elevation of the canine fossa
Lateralized infraorbital nerve
Uncinate process hypoplasia and lateralization of the same
Small ethmoid bulla
Asymmetry cribriform plate
Low-lying fovea ethmoidalis

Acquired hypoplasia
The maxilla is of normal size
Inflammatory reaction produces a partial or complete obliteration
    and resorption of the sinus lumen

episodes of acute (recurrent) sinusitis or a prolonged episode of persistent (subacute) infection are classified as "chronic sinusitis." Epistaxis, anosmia or cacosmia, and nasal vestibulitis may be caused by chronic sinusitis.

The key CT features of chronic sinusitis are as follows:

1. The mucoperiosteal thickening, chronic fibrosis with polypoidal
    degeneration of sinus mucosa and retained secretions contribute to
    the opacification of the involved sinuses.

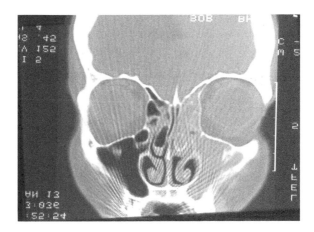

Figure 15.32 Chronic maxillary sinusitis. Left maxillary sinusitis and left anterior
ethmoid sinusitis and ostiomeatal complex disease are noted. There is diffuse
thickening of the left maxillary sinus wall as a result of reactive ostitis. The findings are
compatible with chronic maxillary sinusitis.

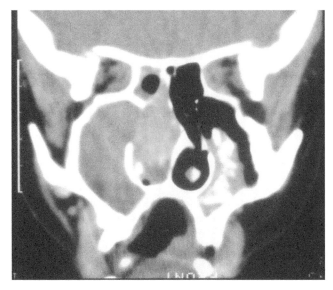

Figure 15.33   Chronic granulomatous sinusitis. This patient presented with chronic nasal obstruction. There is a dense soft tissue mass demonstrated within the left maxillary sinus. There is also erosion of the medial wall of the left maxillary sinus. On the right maxillary sinus there are dense calcifications seen in its lumen. This patient underwent sinus surgery. The final diagnosis was chronic sinusitis with granulomatous reaction in the maxillary sinuses.

2. Recurrent or chronic sinusitis will produce an osteitis with new bone formation along the contours of the sinus cavity. The extent of the osteitis is proportionate to the frequency of infection and the length of the history.
3. The resulting sclerosis can lead to thickening of the sinus wall with decrease in the volume of the sinus cavity. This can result from previous surgery (12).
4. The sinus walls may be eroded by chronic benign inflammation, usually occurring along the medial wall of the maxillary sinus and around the infraorbital canal.
5. If chronic infections occur during childhood, the sinus may remain small and hypoplastic.

The key MR features of chronic sinusitis are as follows. Thickened mucosa which is low to intermediate in signal intensity on the T1-weighted (T1-W) sequences. On proton density weighted (PD-W) and T2-W sequences, the thickened mucosa is hyperintense (brighter) in signal intensity. Following the administration of gadolinium-diethylenetriamine-penta-acetic acid (GD-DTPA) there is intense enhancement of the inflamed mucosa (79–83).

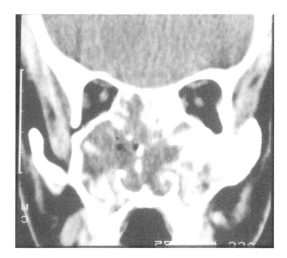

Figure 15.34 Fungal sinusitis. The coronal CT examination demonstrates complete opacification of the sinonasal cavity with dense calcific reaction within the sinonasal cavity. This is fairly classic for fungal sinusitis.

C. Fungal Sinusitis

Fungal sinusitis (Figs. 15.34–15.37) occurs in both the healthy and the immuno compromised population. A high index of suspicion is necessary for the diagnosis and the clinical examination is rarely conclusive. The extramucosal disease

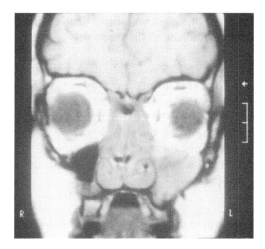

Figure 15.35 MRI of fungal sinusitis. This T1 weighted MR scan demonstrates low signal intensity within the maxillary sinus surrounded by an area of increased signal intensity in the left maxillary sinus.

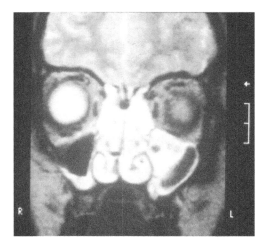

Figure 15.36 MRI of fungal sinusitis. Same patient as in Fig. 15.35. T2 weighted MR; fungal sinusitis demonstrates areas of signal void intensity within the left maxillary sinus lumen. These are changes as a result of ferromagnetic substance that is produced by the fungal metabolism.

presents with symptoms that are similar to chronic sinusitis, with nasal obstruction, purulent rhinorrhea, and facial pain, all of which are resistant to treatment with antibiotics. This may be associated with the growth of a fungus ball within the lumen of the sinus (84,85).

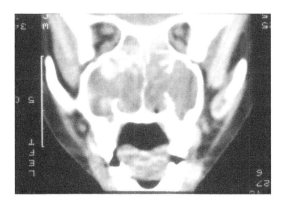

Figure 15.37 Fungal polyposis. This patient has a history of chronic sinusitis and polyposis. This coronal CT examination demonstrates complete opacification of the sinonasal cavity. One or two high-density masses are seen in the left maxillary sinus lumen. These could be either sinonasal polyps or fungal polyposis. Final diagnosis: polyposis with fungal infection.

Table 15.5 Classification of Fungal Sinusitis

Allergic fungal sinusitis
Indolent, slowly progressive invasive disease
Noninvasive local disease: aspergilloma
Fulminant invasive type in the immunocompromised host

These patients are usually investigated by a CT scan to exclude any complications from chronic sinusitis as fungal sinusitis is resistant to conventional medical treatment. Unenhanced CT scans are more sensitive than conventional X-ray in detecting the classical focal areas of hyperdensity and calcification seen in soft tissue masses of fungal sinusitis.

Aspergillosis is the commonest form of fungal infection seen in the population at large. These fungi are commonly found in the soil, decaying fruits, and vegetables. The three classes of aspergillosis that are most commonly responsible for sinus and respiratory infections are *Aspergilus fumigatus* (the most common), *Aspergillus niger*, and *Aspergillus flavus*. The sinonasal and the pulmonary forms of aspergillosis are unrelated, with the pulmonary form occuring primarily among immunocompromised patients (Tables 15.5 and 15.6; Figs. 15.34–15.37).

Plain Radiographs and CT Scan Findings

1. Nodular mucoperiosteal thickening.
2. Absent air fluid levels, clouding of the ethmoid sinuses, and bony erosion.
3. Areas of increased attenuation in a diseased sinus, in the absence of intravenous contrast administration, are readily identified by CT and are highly suggestive of fungal infection. It is the accumulation of heavy metals such as iron and magnesium that are essential components of fungal metabolism that causes the high-density signal on CT.
4. Sclerotic thickening (reactive osteitis) of the bony walls of the sinuses with both remodeling and erosion or destruction can be seen in some cases.
5. When there is extensive bony destruction, fungal sinusitis mimics malignancy.

Table 15.6 Predisposing Factors

Chronic sinusitis and sinonasal polyposis
Immunosuppressed individuals
Diabetes mellitus
Stagnant mucus as a result of poor ventilation,
   decreased mucociliary activity

6. The CT scans demonstrate the ostiomeatal complex compromise as the key factor that predisposes to recurrent infection and fungal sinusitis.

The treatment of fungal sinusitis is surgical debridement, re-establishment of ventilation to sinus, and a combination of systemic antifungal agents in those patients who have invasive fungal disease.

MR Findings of Fungal Sinusitis

1. T1-W sequences usually demonstrate a hypointense mass in the sinus cavity surrounded by fluid.
2. On the PD-W and the T2-W sequences the fungus balls usually show signal void areas, and signal intensities are lower than that which is seen on a T1-W scan.
3. The specimens from fungal infection are rich in iron, magnesium, calcium, and manganese. These heavy metals are also responsible for the increase in the CT number and the hyperdensity seen on the CT scans and the signal void areas on MR scans. The signal void areas are easily mistaken for normal air in the sinus cavity.
4. The sinus mucosa that is inflamed is usually hyperintense.
5. The limitations to MR imaging are teeth, calcifications, and air, which are easily differentiated on CT scans; all produce no signals and can easily go undetected on MR scans. MR will continue to play a major role in sinus imaging, especially where benign lesions such as muco-celes or fungal infections present as aggressive and malignant lesions on CT examinations (Table 15.7).

Mucormycosis

The fulminant form of fungal sinusitis usually occurs in immunosuppressed or uncontrolled diabetic patients with ketoacidosis. This has in the past been primarily attributed to mucormycosis. This form of fungal sinusitis has an aggressive

Table 15.7 Differential Diagnosis of Hyperdense Masses Seen on CT Scans in the Sinonasal Cavity

Thick pus
Desiccated secretions in nasal polyps
Thrombus or intrasinus hemorrhage
Foreign bodies
Fungal sinusitis
Bony tumors surrounded by inflammation
Sarcomas with dystrophic calcification
Dystrophic calcifications in inverting papilloma

evolution with orbital, intracranial, and vascular invasion. Sinus infections in the immunocompromised patient can easily spread intracranially. The clinical features of fever, rhinorrhea, and sinus tenderness may be disproportionately insignificant to the danger they present. Necrosis of the turbinates with black crusting in the nasal cavity is suggestive of this aggressive form of invasive fungal sinusitis. Opaque sinuses may indicate bony involvement with or without destruction by the infection and the outlook is ominous. The symptoms are not severe enough to seek medical attention, which delays diagnosis and treatment. This is followed by gangrenous necrosis with poor response to all kinds of treatment including systemic amphotericin.

The diagnosis can be confirmed by examination of nasal scrapings and mucosal biopsies.

Some of the feared complications include

1. Vasculitis
2. Intracranial mycotic aneurysms
3. Intracranial hemorrhage
4. Internal carotid artery thrombosis
5. Meningitis and cerebral abscess
6. Multiple cranial nerve palsies
7. Orbital apex syndrome

D. Polyps

Polyps (Fig. 15.38) are the most common complication of inflammatory sinusitis. It is often associated with other conditions such as allergies, vasomotor rhinosinusitis, aspirin hypersensitivity, cystic fibrosis, nickel exposure, and diabetes mellitus. Small polyps resolve with medical therapy and treatment of the other associated conditions. Most of the polyps seen in the nasal cavity arise from the ethmoidal area, the most frequent sites of origin being areas of contact between the infundibulum, the middle turbinate, and the uncinate process.

CT is the most appropriate examination for benign sinonasal polyposis. MR is reserved for complex cases of sinonasal polyps, where superimposed fungal sinus infection, intracranial or intraorbital extension of disease are suspected.

Nasal Polyposis

CT and MR Features of Sinonasal Polyposis

1. Most sinonasal polyps are seen as soft tissue masses that occupy one or more of the sinonasal cavities. They may show variable densities depending on the water content: low density where there is more water and higher density where there is higher protein content.

2. Most polyps are of the same signal intensity as that of water: hypointense on T1W-MRI and hyperintense (bright) on T2W-MRI scans. The characteristic

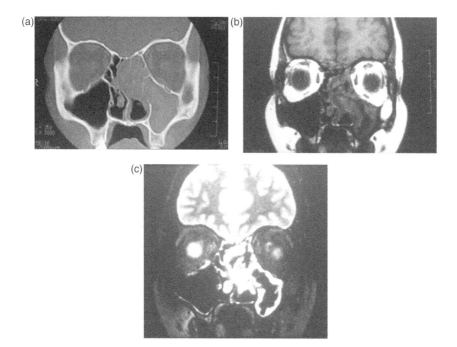

Figure 15.38 (a) Coronal CT examination demonstrates a mass occupying the left ethmoid and maxillary sinus, as well the middle meatus, with varying densities. (b) Coronal MR examination demonstrates several polyps obstructing the sinonasal cavity. These polyps are of mixed signal intensity. (c) On T2W-MRI signal void areas from lack of mobile hydrogen protons are seen. This is seen in polyps with low water content.

MR features of sinonasal polyposis is a reflection of the rich proteinaceous and watery contents of these polyps.

3. As the polyps age the amount of free available hydrogen protons decreases, and as a result the MR characteristics of nasal polyps are variable. Polyps that are bright on T1-W and T2-W MR scans are either due to high protein content or due to hemorrhage within the polyps.

4. Chronic, long-standing polypoidal lesions in the sinonasal cavity undergo biochemical changes. Consequently, their MR appearance changes. There is significant loss of water and with sufficient time there is increase in the protein content in these polyps. This results in shortening of T1 and T2 relaxation times. As a result, there are varying low, intermediate, high signal intensities with areas of signal void. Polyps that are present for a long time can cause pressure erosion of the sinus walls and the roof of the nasal cavity. Despite erosions, the inhomogenous appearance of the lesions in all sequences characterizes the benignity of these lesions. Thus, by the MR features one can confidently predict if the polyps have been present for a long time.

Antrochoanal Polyp

Antrochoanal polyps (Figs. 15.39 and 15.40) are the most common benign sinonasal tumors in children, which have a great tendency to recur if inadequately excised. The etiology of these unilateral polyps is unclear. Of these patients 15–40% present with a history of allergy. Histologically, these polyps are similar to ordinary inflammatory nasal polyps. An antrochoanal polyp has two components: a cystic part in the lumen of the maxillary sinus, which originates most commonly from the posterolateral wall, and a solid part, which extends through the maxillary ostium into the middle meatus. When large, these polyps progressively expand to reach the choana causing severe nasal obstruction.

The CT Scan Appearance of Polyps

Opacification of the maxillary sinus:

1. A soft tissue mass of uniform density in the ipsilateral nasal cavity; large polyps extend to the posterior choanae.
2. A lateral view may demonstrate the smooth posterior margin of the polyp hanging in the nasopharynx.
3. The sinus ostium and the nasal cavity may be widened to accommodate the polyp.
4. Occasionally, the surrounding bone may exhibit a mixture of resorption and reactive osteitis.
5. On MRI scans these polyps are similar to inflammatory polyps.

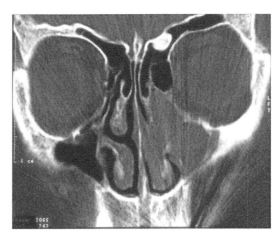

Figure 15.39 A large antrochoanal polyp is seen to arise from the left maxillary sinus lumen extending into the middle meatus. An incidental note is made of a small osteoma in the left frontal recess.

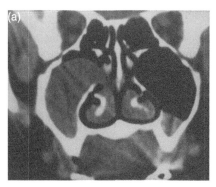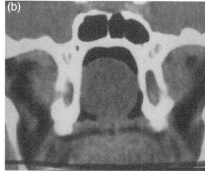

Figure 15.40 Antrochoanal polyp. Coronal CT demonstrates a large polyp arising from the right maxillary sinus. The posterior scan (Fig. 15.40b) demonstrates the large polyp protruding into the nasopharynx.

The differential diagnosis includes hemangioma, juvenile angiofibroma, and inverting papilloma as well as any other relatively slow-growing malignancy.

E. Retention Cysts

These benign, usually asymptomatic, cysts (Fig. 15.41) have multiple causes including trauma, infection, and allergy. Nonsecretory cysts are caused by obstruction of a minor salivary gland. These cysts contain serous fluid and are located in the connective tissue of the mucus membrane. The mucus secreting cyst is lined with respiratory epithelium. Retention cysts may be situated on the infraorbital nerve as it passes through the roof of the maxillary sinus, and cause paresthesia of the infraorbital nerve. Irrespective of their origin their CT and MR features are alike.

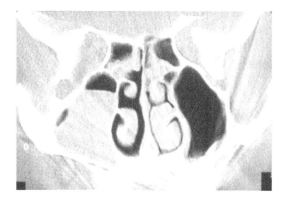

Figure 15.41 A well-defined large retention cyst is noted in the left maxillary sinus. This cannot be differentiated from the sinus polyp.

CT and MR Features of Retention Cysts

1. A dome-shaped density usually arising in the floor of the sinus. However, cysts may arise at any mucosal site.
2. With large cysts bony remodeling may occur and in the sinus cavity a crescentic rim of air above the cyst helps to differentiate it from a mucocele.
3. Retention cysts are hypointense on T1-W and hyperintense on T2-W MR imaging sequences.

XIII. Complications of Sinusitis

The complications of sinusitis result from spreading of infection to the adjacent anatomical structures. The widespread use of antibiotics has significantly impacted the incidence of such complications and these occur more commonly in association with resistant bacteria or immunocompromised patients, such as those with AIDS. Complications of sinusitis can be divided into three groups: local, orbital, and intracranial. The various complications are listed in Table 15.8.

Early diagnosis and treatment prevents permanent ocular and neurological damage.

Predisposing factors that complicate sinusitis include:

1. Congenital deficiencies of the sinus walls (defects in the wall of the sphenoid sinus)
2. Fractures
3. Surgical defects
4. Erosion of the bony walls by infection or tumor
5. Retrograde phlebitis: the retrograde spread of infection through various venous portals including those along the interstitium surrounding the veins, through the emissary foramina and through the diploic veins
6. Extension along pre-existing anatomical pathways: perineural spread may occur around the branches of the olfactory nerve traversing the

Table 15.8 Complications of Sinusitis

Local	Orbital	Intracranial
Empyema	Preseptal cellulitis	Meningitis
Mucocele	Subperiosteal abscess	Epidural empyema or abscess
Pyocele	Intraorbital abscess	Brain abscess
Facial cellulitis	Endophthalmitis	Cavernous sinus thrombosis
Osteitis	Optic neuritis	Superior sagittal sinus thrombosis
Osteomyelitis	Occlusion of central retinal artery	Superior orbital fissure syndrome
		Multiple cranial nerve palsies from meningitis

cribriform plate, via nerves that communicate into the pterygopalatine fossa, the Vidian nerve, or the maxillary division of the trigeminal nerve.

7. Hematogenous spread as part of a generalized septicemia.

Plain radiographs are of no value in the diagnosis of intracranial or intra-orbital complications. CT in both the axial and the coronal planes following the administration of intravenous contrast is the modality of choice.

XIV. Mucoceles of the Paranasal Sinuses

A mucocoele (Figs. 15.42 and 15.43) is the most common expansile lesion seen in the paranasal sinuses. It results from long-standing obstruction of the sinus ostia. The mucosal lining of the sinus cavity continues to secrete a thick, white, clear uninfected mucus, which cannot escape from the sinus. The rising pressure in the sinus causes resorption of the bony walls, erosions, and expansion of the sinus. The sinuses involved in decreasing order of frequency are the frontal, the ethmoid, the maxillary, and the sphenoid sinuses. Occasionally, multiple mucoceles may occur in the same patient.

The causes are multifactorial and include obstruction of the ostium with chronic inflammation or polyps, trauma (surgical or accidental), allergy, and tumor.

A. Radiological Features of a Mucocele

1. Opacified expanded sinus is seen from the contents of the mucocele. On CT or plain radiographs the involved sinuses are isodense or hypodense relative to brain tissue.

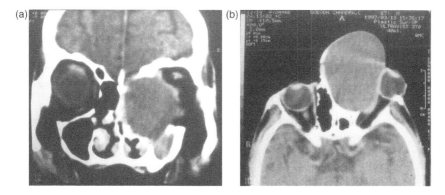

Figure 15.42 (a) A large expansile lesion with thinning and erosion of the sinus wall and the roof of the nasal cavity is noted. This has the classic featurres of a ethmoid sinus mucocele. (b) Axial scan demonstrates the large ethmoid sinus mucocele extending anteriorly with left exophthalmos.

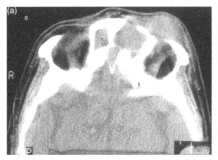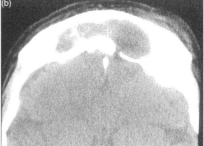

Figure 15.43 Axial scans through the frontal and ethmoid sinuses. Two scans demonstrate an expansile mass with erosion of the posterior wall of the frontal sinus and the anterior wall of the frontal sinuses with extension into the left orbit. This patient had a history of acute onset of fever and is compatible with a mucopyocele.

2. Gradual expansion of the sinus cavity with thinning and loss of the peripheral bony margins is noted.
3. With continuous increase in the intrasinus pressure, bone remodeling is accompanied by bony erosion.
4. There may be reactive sclerosis of the sinus walls.
5. A pyocele is a mucocele which has become secondarily infected. This usually exacerbates the symptoms. The radiological features are similar to those of mucoceles, but following the administration of intravenous contrast there is usually enhancement of the inflamed mucosa while the content remains hypodense.

B. MR Features of Mucoceles

The retained secretion within the sinuses may change its biochemical character- istics over a period of time. The water is slowly absorbed resulting in a thicker fluid. If the obstruction of the sinus continues, then the chronic reaction may stimulate the goblet cells of the lining epithelium to produce a fluid which is rich in protein. The dynamic biochemical and physiological changes in an obstructed sinus form the basic ingredients that will influence the MR appearance of fluid on the various spin–echo sequences of MRI.

1. A mucocele which contains serous secretions (high water content) is hypointense on T1-W, intermediate in signal intensity on PD-W, and hyperintense (bright) on T2-W MR imaging sequences.
2. If the water content of a mucocele is slowly absorbed and is replaced by protein rich secretions from the seromucinous glands then this makes the mucocele intermediate in signal intensity on T1-W and hyperintense on T2-W MR sequences.
3. With further loss of free and mobile hydrogen protons, and an increase in the protein content, the mucocele (content thick and pasty) is hyper- intense on T1-W and T2-W MRI sequences.

4. A long-standing mucocele's content is dry and desiccated. There are no free hydrogen protons, and the mucocele is now seen as a signal void cavity on T1-W and T2-W MR scans. These mucoceles pose a problem as they can be easily misinterpreted as a normal air filled sinus. The differentiation is done by a CT scan, which will demonstrate the desiccated material in the sinus in addition to the expansion of the sinus by the mucocele.

5. Mucosa is enhanced following GD-DTPA administration. Clotted blood, fibrotic scar, mycetomas, calcium, tooth, bone, or a pocket of air can also cause signal void areas in a sinus.

XV. Osteomyelitis

Osteomyelitis affects the frontal bone most commonly, with the maxillary sinus being the second most commonly affected. The sepsis spreads into the bone either by direct extension or via thrombophlebitis of the valveless diploic veins. Osteomyelitis occurs with infection of diploic bone and osteitis is due to infection of compact bone, such as is found in the floor of the frontal sinus. Osteomyelitis of the maxilla may occur in both adults and infants. The commonest cause is dental infection. It leads to subperiosteal abscess spreading across the maxilla. Radiological features are minimal in some cases with slight opacity of the maxillary sinus. In some cases there may be marked sclerosis of the maxilla.

A. Radiographic Appearance of Osteomyelitis

1. Poor definition of the sinus walls with disruption of the mucoperiosteal lining.
2. Rarification of skull bone with multiple lytic lesions appearing in the adjacent bone.
3. Bony sequestra are less common in chronic osteomyelitis of the facial bones or skull.
4. In chronic cases, sclerotic changes are superimposed over areas of rarefaction and the margins of the sinus become indistinct.
5. Following intravenous contrast administration the acutely inflamed mucosa exhibits intense enhancement. This needs to be differentiated from the enhancement of pyoceles. The smooth expansion of the sinus walls associated with pyoceles is usually absent with osteomyelitis.

XVI. Intraorbital Complications

Intraorbital complications (Figs. 15.44 and 15.45) include orbital cellulitis, subperiosteal abscess, orbital abscess, optic neuritis, and central retinal artery occlusion. These complications are usually associated with infection of the frontal or

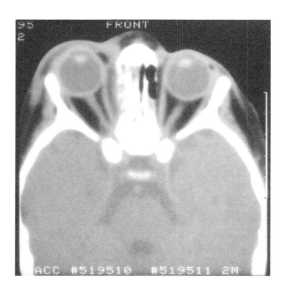

Figure 15.44   A 4-year-old patient with peri-orbital cellulitis. An axial CT examination demonstrates a phlegmon in the right orbit with lateral displacement of the medial rectus muscle.

ethmoid sinuses or with a pansinusitis. Other causes include foreign bodies, trauma, facial infections, and generalized septicemia. The usual route of spread is either through bony dehiscences of the sinus wall or through the venous pathways. Raised intrasinus pressure results in decrease in periosteal blood supply

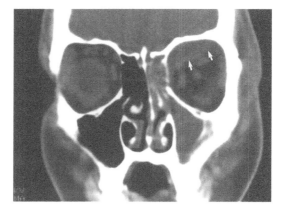

Figure 15.45   Subperiostial abscess. Coronal CT scan of the orbit demonstrates left maxillary and ethmoid sinusitis with extension of the inflammatory process (arrows) into the left orbit.

and necrosis of the lamina papyracea. The patient may become blind if treatment is not given immediately.

An important clinical differentiation must be made in this group regarding the position of the focus of infection in relation to the orbital septum. The orbital septum is the fibrous band that spans from the orbital margins to the tarsal plates. Both preseptal and postseptal orbital inflammation present with swelling of the upper eyelid.

A. Preseptal Orbital Cellulitis

1. CT of preseptal inflammation shows a diffuse increase in density with thickening of the eyelid.
2. Abscess is seen as an area of low density which may or may not exhibit rim enhancement following the administration of intravenous contrast.
3. The globe usually does not exhibit proptosis and occasionally is displaced slightly posteriorly.
4. Preseptal cellulitis may be successfully treated with cellulitis.

B. Postseptal Orbital Cellulitis

Postseptal inflammation requires different management and is divided into three groups:

1. Extraconal
2. Intraconal
3. Combined (both intraconal and extraconal)

C. Features of Extraconal Orbital Cellulitis

1. Proptosis of the globe, restricted eye movements, chemosis of the conjunctiva, and vision may rapidly deteriorate.
2. Aggressive treatment with intravenous antibiotics and surgical drainage of any abscess collection is required.
3. Most medial extraconal inflammation is secondary to ethmoid sinusitis. Anterolateral displacement of the globe with inflammatory exudate in the subperiosteal space is seen.
4. Subperiosteal inflammation or abscess is the accumulation of exudate between the lamina papyracea and the loose periosteum. The infection is limited by the periosteum and it rarely spreads into the intraconal space.
5. CT characteristics are similar for both subperiosteal phlegmon and subperiosteal abscess. The enhancing medial rectus muscle and the elevated enhancing periosteum are displaced laterally by the collection.

D. Features of Intraconal Orbital Cellulitis

1. Clinical features include proptosis, restricted eye movements, chemosis, with or without papilledema of the optic disk, and rapid decrease in visual acuity. There is a grave risk of retrograde infection causing cavernous sinus thrombosis.
2. CT will demonstrate intraconal inflammation as loss of definition of the extraocular muscles and the optic nerve. The fat in the intraconal space is infiltrated with linear strands of inflammatory reaction making it difficult to distinguish the extraocular muscles and the optic nerve. Abscess formation is indicated by the characteristic development of an area of low density with an enhancing rim of air in the orbital fat. Again, treatment consists of aggressive antibiotic therapy and orbital decompression.

E. Features of Diffuse Intraconal and Extraconal Orbital Cellulitis

1. The infection initiates in the intraconal or extraconal compartments.
2. There is severe proptosis, with possibility of spread of infection to the infratemporal fossa and cavernous sinus if left untreated.
3. The CT findings usually demonstrate obliteration of the muscles and of the optic nerve by inflammatory exudate.

XVII. Intracranial Complications

Intracranial complications are rare but life threatening complications of uncontrolled sinus disease, and include meningitis, epidural abscess, subdural abscess, intracerebral abscess, and cavernous sinus thrombosis. These complications usually occur in adolescent males as a consequence of inadequate antibiotic treatment, the presence of resistant bacteria or in patients who are immunocompromised (3,86). The organisms held responsible for intracranial complications are the same as those for ear infections and include *S. pneumoniae,* *H. influenza,* and *M. catarrhalis.*

A. CT Appearance of Intracranial Infection

CT with contrast is invaluable in identifying if and where an intracranial abscess has occurred:

1. *Meningitis*: Sphenoid sinusitis is the most frequent source of meningitis. Meningitis can cause multiple cranial nerve palsies and hydrocephalus. On CT cortical and gyral enhancement may be seen following the administration of intravenous contrast with or without hydrocephalus.

2. *Epidural abscess*: An extradural abscess occurs between the bone of the calvarium and the dura mater. On CT this is seen as a lentiform collection limited

by the dural attachment to the suture lines between the individual skull bones. Both the periosteum and the meninges are enhanced following the administration of intravenous contrast. The adjacent brain may be hypodense because the surrounding tissue is edematous.

3. *Subdural abscess*: An abscess in the subdural space, that is, between the dura and the arachnoid, is semilunar in shape. Subdural abscess is more common than epidural abscess. *Staphylococcus aureus* sinusitis is the most common cause of subdural abscess.

4. *Intracerebral abscess*: An intracerebral abscess may result from the direct spread of infection from the sinus into the cerebral tissue, or septic emboli. With direct spread the abscess is usually in the brain adjacent to the infected sinus. With septic emboli the abscess may be distant from the infected sinus. Frontal sinusitis is frequently responsible for intracerebral abscesses. In the early stage of the abscess formation an ill-defined hypodense area with little enhancement may be seen. If left untreated, this will progress, and a well-demarcated, ring enhancing lesion is seen. The surrounding brain appears hypodense, from the edema. MRI is far more sensitive in detecting early cerebritis, abscess, and meningitis.

5. *Cavernous sinus thrombosis*: Cavernous sinus thrombosis is a rare intracranial complication of sinusitis. The most common organism responsible for cavernous sinus thrombosis is *S. aureus*. On CT a normal cavernous sinus is seen as a brightly enhancing structure surrounding the pituitary fossa, with a sharply defined lateral border. Usually, the intracavernous part of the internal carotid artery is indistinguishable from the surrounding venous structure. In contrast, in cavernous sinus thrombosis the venous structure fails to enhance and the internal carotid arteries will become very prominent as enhanced tubular structure. The other features include outward bulging of the lateral wall of the sinus, and multiple filling defects in the sinus, and dilatation of the superior ophthalmic vein that drains into the cavernous sinus.

References

1. Littlejohn MC, Stiernberg CM, Hokanson JA et al. The relationship between the nasal cycle and mucociliary clearance. Laryngoscope 1992; 102:117–120.
2. Maran AGD, Lund VJ. Clinical Rhinology. New York: Thieme Medical Publishers Inc., 1990.
3. Shankar L, Evan K, Hawke M, Stammberger H. In: An Atlas of Imaging of the Paranasal Sinuses. Martin Dunitz, 1994:41–81.
4. Stammberger H. In: Functional Endoscopic Sinus Surgery. Philadelphia, PA: BC Decker, 1991.
5. Zinreich SJ, Kennedy DW, Rosenbaum AE et al. Paranasal sinuses: CT imaging requirements for endoscopic surgery. Radiology 1987; 163:769–775.
6. Zeifer B. Limited coronal CT: an alternative screening examination for sinonasal update on sinonasal imaging: anatomy and inflammatory disease. Neuroimaging Clin North Am 1998; 8(3):607–630.

7. Mafee MF. Endoscopic sinus surgery. Role of the radiogiist. AJNR Am J Neuroradiol 1991; 12:855–860.
8. Nass RL, Holliday RA, Reede DL. Diagnosis of surgical sinusitis using nasal endoscopy and computed tomography. Laryngoscope 1989; 99:1158–1160.
9. Mosges R et al. Computer-assisted surgery of the paranasal sinuses. J Otolaryngol 1993; 22(2):69–71.
10. Rontal M, Rontal E. Studying whole-mounted sections of the paranasal sinuses to understand the complications of endoscopic sinus surgery. Laryngoscope 1991; 101:361–366.
11. Rao VM et al. Sinonasal imaging. Anatomy and pathology. Radiol Clin North Am 1998; 36(5):921–939.
12. Rowe-Jones J et al. Charing Cross CT protocol for endoscopic sinus surgery. J Laryngol Otol 1995; 109(11):1057–1060.
13. Russell EJ, Czervionke L, Huckman M et al. CT of the inferomedial orbit and the lacrimal drainage apparatus. Normal and pathologic anatomy. AJR Am J Roentgenol 1985; 145:1147–1154.
14. Rubin GD et al. Perspective volume rendering of CT and MR images: applications for endoscopic imaging. Radiology 1996; 199(2):321–330.
15. Schatz CJ, Becker TS. Normal and CT anatomy of the paranasal sinuses. Radiol Clin North Am 1984; 22:107–118.
16. Hudgins PA. Sinonasal imaging. Neuroimaging Clin North Am 1996; 6(2):319–331.
17. Lloyd GAS. CT of the paranasal sinuses: study of a control series in relation to endoscopic sinus surgery. J Laryngol Otol 1990; 104:477–481.
18. Melhem ER et al. Optimal CT evaluation for functional endoscopic sinus surgery. AJNR Am J Neuroradiol 1996; 17(1):181–188.
19. Babbel R, Harnsberger HR, Nelson B et al. Optimization of techniques in screening CT of the sinuses. AJNR Am J Neuroradiol 1991; 12:849–854.
20. Kaluskar SK et al. The role of CT in functional endoscopic sinus surgery. Rhinology 1993; 31(2):49–52.
21. Kopp W et al. Special radiologic imaging of paranasal sinuses. A prerequisite for functional endoscopic sinus surgery. Eur J Radiol 1988; 8(3):153–156.
22. Mafee MF. Modern imaging of paranasal sinuses and the role of limited sinus computerized tomography; considerations of time, cost and radiation. Ear Nose Throat J 1994; 73(8):532–534.
23. Mafee MF et al. Functional endoscopic sinus surgery: anatomy, CT screening, indications, and complications. AJR AJR Am J Roentgenol 1993; 160(4):735–744.
24. Raymond HW, Zwiebel WJ, Harnesberger HR. Essentials of screening sinus computed tomography. Seminars in Ultrasound, CT and MRI 1991; 12(6):526.
25. Rice DH. Endoscopic sinus surgery. Otolaryngol Clin North Am 1993; 26(4):613–618.
26. White PS et al. Limited CT scanning techniques of the paranasal sinuses. J Laryngol Otol 1991; 105(1):20–23.
27. Wigand ME. Endoscopic Surgery of the Paranasal Sinuses and the Anterior Skull Base. New York: Thieme Medical Publishers Inc., 1990.
28. Beahm E, Teresi L, Lufkin R, Hanafee W. MR of the paranasal sinuses. Surg Radiol Anat 1990; 12:203–208.

29. Bingham B, Shankar L, Hawke M. Pitfalls in computed tomography of the paranasal sinuses. J Otolaryngol 1991; 20(6):414–418.
30. Bradley WG Jr. Fundamentals of magnetic resonance image interpretation. In: Bradley WG, Adey WR, Hasso AN, eds. Magnetic Resonance Imaging of the Brain, Head, and Neck: A Text Atlas. Rockville, MD: Aspen, 1984:1–16.
31. Conner BL, Roach ES, Laster W, Georgitis JW. Magnetic resonance imaging of the paranasal sinuses: frequency type of abnormalities. Ann Allergy 1989; 62:457–460.
32. Cook PR et al. Functional endoscopic sinus surgery in patients with normal computed tomography scans. Otolaryngol Head Neck Surg 1994; 110(6):505–509.
33. Curtin HD, Williams R. Computed tomographic anatomy of the pterygopalatine fossa. Radiographics 1985; 5(3):429–435.
34. Daniels DL, Rauschning W, Lovas J et al. Pterygopalatine fossa. Computed tomographic studies. Radiology 1983; 149:511–516.
35. Daniels DL, Pech P, Kay MC et al. Orbital apex. Correlative anatomic and CT study. AJR Am J Roentgenol 1985; 145:1141–1144.
36. Lloyd GAS, Lund VJ, Phelps PD et al. Magnetic resonance imaging in the evaluation of nose and paranasal sinus disease. Br J Radiol 1987; 957.
37. Rak KM, Newell JD, Yakes WJ et al. Paranasal sinuses on MR images of the brain. Significance of mucosal thickening. AJNR Am J Neuroradiol 1990; 11:1211.
38. Bridger MWM, van Nostrand AWP. The nose and paranasal sinuses—applied surgical anatomy. J Otolaryngol 1978; 7(suppl 6).
39. Casiano RR. Correlation of clinical examination with computer tomography in paranasal sinus disease. Am J Rhinol 1997; 11(3):193–196.
40. Lang J. Clinical Anatomy of the Nose, Nasal Cavity and Paranasal Sinuses. New York: Thieme Medical Publishers Inc., 1989.
41. Masala W, Perugini S, Salvolini U, Teatini GP. Multiplanar reconstruction in the study of ethmoid anatomy. Neuroradiology 1989; 31:151–155.
42. Rohen JW, Yokochi C. Color Atlas of Anatomy. Schattauer Verlag, 1983.
43. Gray H. Gray's anatomy. In: Goss CM, ed. Philadelphia, PA: Lea & Febiger, 1973.
44. Wallace R, Salazar JE, Cowles S. The relationship between frontal sinus drainage and ostiomeatal complex disease: a CT study in 217 patients. AJNR Am J Neuroradiol 1990; 11:183–186.
45. Dolan KD, Smoker WRK. Paranasal sinus radiology, part 4A: maxillary sinuses. Otolaryngol Head Neck Surgery 1983; 5:345–362.
46. Dolan K, Smoker WRK. Paranasal sinus radiology, part 4B: maxillary sinus, head and neck surgery. Otolaryngol Head Neck Surgery 1983; 5:428–446.
47. Som PM, Lawson W, Biller HF, Lanzieri CF. Ethmoid sinus disease: CT evaluation in 400 cases. Part one: non-surgical patients. Radiology 1986; 159:591–597.
48. Scuderi AJ et al. Pneumatization of the paranasal sinuses: normal features of importance to the accurate interpretation of CT scans and MR images. AJR Am J Roentgenol 1993; 160(5):1101–1104.
49. Terrier F, Weber W, Ruenfenacht D et al. Anatomy of the ethmoid: CT, endoscopic and macroscopic. AJR Am J Roentgenol 1985; 144:493–500.
50. Zinreich SJ, Mattox DE, Kennedy DW. Concha bullosa: CT evaluation. J Comput Assist Tomogr 1988; 12(5):778–784.
51. Som PM, Lawson W, Biller HF, Lanzieri CF. Ethmoid sinus disease: CT evaluation in 400 cases. Part two: postoperative findings. Radiology 1986; 159:599–604.

52. Khanobthamchai K, Shankar L, Hawke M, Bingham B. The secondary middle turbinate. J Otolaryngol 1991; 20(6):412–413.

53. Shankar L, Hawke M. Principles and objectives of functional endoscopic sinus surgery and CT of the paranasal sinuses. ENT J 1991; 4:1.

54. Zinreich SZ. Paranasal sinus imaging. Radiology 1990; 103(5):863–869.

55. Zinreich SJ. Paranasal sinus imaging. Otolaryngol Head Neck Surg 1990; 103:863.

56. Driben JS et al. The reliability of computerized tomographic detection of the Onodi (sphenoethmoid) cell. Am J Rhinol 1998; 12(2):105–111.

57. Khanobthamchai K, Shankar L, Hawke M, Bingham B. The ethmo-maxillary sinus and hypoplasia of the maxillary sinus. J Otolaryngol 1991; 6(20):425–427.

58. Elahi M et al. Development of a standardized proforma for reporting computerized tomographic images of the paranasal sinuses. J Otolaryngol 1996; 25(2):113–120.

59. Mafee MF. Preoperative imaging anatomy of nasal-ethmoid complex for functional endoscopic sinus surgery. Radiol Clin North Am 1993; 31(1):1–20.

60. Milczuk HA et al. Nasal and paranasal sinus anomalies in children with chronic sinusitis. Laryngoscope 993; 103(3):247–252.

61. Roithmann R, Shankar L, Noyek A et al. CT imaging in the diagnosis and treatment of sinus disease: a partnership between the radiologist and the otolaryngologist. J Otolaryngol 1993; 22(4):253–260.

62. Stoney P, Shankar L, Hawke M et al. CT scanning for functional endoscopic sinus surgery: analysis of 200 cases with reporting scheme. J Otolaryngol 1993; 22(2):72–78.

63. Bolger WE, Butzin CA, Parsons DS. Paranasal sinus bony anatomic variations and mucosal abnormalities. CT analysis for endoscopic sinus surgery. Laryngoscope 1991; 101:56–64.

64. Cooke LD, Hadley DM. MRI of the paranasal sinuses: incidental abnormalities and their relationship to symptoms. J Laryngol Otol 1991; 105:278–281.

65. Flinn J et al. A prospective analysis of incidental paranasal sinus abnormalities on CT head scans. Clin Otolaryngol 1994; 19(4):287–289.

66. Havas TE, Motbey A, Gullane PJ. Prevalence of incidental abnormalities on computed tomographic scans of the paranasal sinuses. Arch Otolaryngol Head Neck Surg 1988; 114:856–859.

67. Kennedy DW, Zinreich SJ, Shaalan H et al. Endoscopic middle meatal antrostomy: theory, technique and patency. Laryngoscope 1987; (suppl)43,94(8,II Part 3):1.

68. Kennedy DW et al. Functional endoscopic sinus surgery. Theory and diagnostic evaluation. Arch Otolaryngol 1985; 111(9):576–582.

69. Laine FJ et al. The ostiomeatal unit and endoscopic surgery: anatomy, variations, and imaging findings in inflammatory diseases. AJR Am J Roentgenol 1992; 159(4):849–857.

70. Bolger WE, Woodruff WW, Morehead J. Maxillary sinus hypoplasia. Classification and description of associated uncinate process hypoplasia. Otolaryngol Head Neck Surg 1990; 103:759–765.

71. Fascenelli Maj FW. Maxillary sinus abnormalities. Arch Otolaryngol 1969; 90:98–101.

72. Furin MJ, Zinreich SJ, Kennedy DW. The atelectatic maxillary sinus. Am J Rhinol 1991; 5(3):79–83.

73. Pace Balzan A, Shankar L, Hawke M. Computed tomographic findings in atrophic rhinitis. J Otolaryngol 1991; 20(6):428–432.

74. Bassoiouny A, Newlands WJ, Ali H et al. Maxillary sinus hypoplasia and superior orbital fissure asymmetry. Laryngoscope 1982; 92:441–448.

75. Modic MT, Weinstein WA, Berlin J, Duschesneau PM. Maxillary sinus hypoplasia visualised with computed tomography. Radiology 1980; 135:383–385.

76. Shankar L, Hawke M et al. Maxillary sinus hypoplasia, embryology and radiology. Arch Head Neck Surg 1993.

77. Moser FG, Panush D, Rubin JS et al. Incidental paranasal sinus abnormalities on MRI of the brain. Clin Radiol 1991; 43:252–254.

78. Zinreich SJ, Kennedy DW, Kumar AJ, Rosenbaum AE et al. MR imaging of the normal nasal cycle: comparison with sinus pathology. J Comput Assist Tomogr 1988; 12(6):1014–1019.

79. Jorgensen RA. Endoscopic and computed tomographic findings in ostiomeatal sinus disease. Arch Otolaryngol Head Neck Surg 1991; 117:279–287.

80. Som PM, Bergeron RT. In: Head and Neck Imaging. 2nd ed. Mosby-Year Book Inc., 1991.

81. Som PM. CT of the paranasal sinuses. Neuroradiology 1985; 27:189–201.

82. Unger JM, Shaffer K, Duncavage JA. Computed tomography in nasal and paranasal sinus disease. Laryngoscope 1984; 94:1319–1324.

83. Yousem DM. Imaging of sinonasal inflammatory disease. Radiology 1993; 188(2):303–314.

84. Shankar L, Roithman, Hawke M, Chapnik J, Kassel E, Noyek AM. Diagnostic imaging of fungal sinusitis: eleven new cases and literature review. Rhinology 1995; 33(2):104–110.

85. Yousem DM, Galetta SL, Gusnard DA, Goldberg HI. MR findings in rhinocerebral mucormycosis. J Comput Assist Tomogr 1989; 13(5):878–882.

86. Valvassori GE, Buckingham RA, Carter BL et al. Head and Neck Imaging. New York: Thieme Medical Publishers Inc., 1988.

16

Pediatric Rhinomanometry and Acoustic Rhinometry

PER DJUPESLAND

Ullevål University Hospital,
Oslo, Norway

RENATO ROITHMANN[*]

Universidade Luterana do Brasil,
Canoas, Brazil

PHILIP COLE

University of Toronto, Toronto,
Ontario, Canada

---

[*]Mount Sinai Hospital, Toronto, Ontario, Canada.

I. Introduction

The nasal airway is the natural and preferred respiratory route for humans at all ages (1). In infants and animals, the elevated position of the larynx secures a functional separation between the airway and the oral alimentary tract. Whereas it enhances suckling and prevents aspiration, this anatomic configuration renders neonates particularly vulnerable to nasal obstruction of the respiratory airway. Both congenital and acquired nasal obstruction may cause severe, life-threatening respiratory distress in neonates (2). The subsequent gradual decent of the larynx, perquisite to accommodate human speech facilitates conversion to oral breathing. Oral breathing complements or replaces nasal breathing, only if the nasal airway becomes obstructed or a need for increased ventilation occurs (1).

The commonest causes of obstruction to nasal breathing in children result from mucosal swelling, adenoid hypertrophy and, more rarely, structural intrusion on the airway (3,4) (Table 16.1).

The high incidence of upper respiratory tract infection (URTI) and allergy in childhood causes immune-activation with consequent mucosal engorgement and hyperplasia of the abundant lymphatic tissues of the upper respiratory tract (1,5). Thus, although nasal and nasopharyngeal obstruction contribute to snoring, mouth breathing, and disturbed sleep at all ages, these pathologies are particularly common in early childhood. Disturbed sleep contributes to

Table 16.1 Diagnostic Categories of 986 Consecutive Children Referred to the ENT Department, Hospital for Sick Children, Toronto for Rhinomanometry.

Diagnosis	Number of cases	% of total
Unobstructed	295	29.9
Mucosal swelling	317	32.1
Adenoid hyperplasia	157	15.9
Septal deviation	93	9.4
Mucosal swelling and adenoid hyperplasia	93	9.4
Nasal valve abnormality	19	1.9
Post pharyngoplasty	6	0.6
Undiagnosed posterior obstruction	6	0.6
Total	986	100

behavioral changes, reduced school performance, growth retardation and even cardiopulmonary changes in severe long-standing cases (1,5).

Despite the obvious deleterious impact of upper airway obstruction on children as well as their parents, the investigative modalities suitable for assessment of the upper airway patency are limited. Although flexible endoscopy is a very useful diagnostic tool in children it does not provide an objective measure of airway patency. Cost and complexity of modern imaging techniques such as computed tomography (CT) and magnetic resonance (MR) limit their application in assessment of infants and children.

Rhinomanometric measurement is unique among methods of nasal assessment in that it provides a sensitive numerical evaluation of how hard it is for a subject to breathe through the nose. The derived value, airflow resistance, is obtained from the ratio between transnasal airflow and associated transnasal differential pressure (6,7). Airflow is measured by means of a pneumotach and pressure by a manometer, modern instrumentation is electronically based and, in many laboratories, computer assisted (Fig. 16.1). Assessment of obstructive nasal disease by rhinomanometry (RM) is a common diagnostic and follow-up procedure in adult and teenage patients. It is less common in young children and requires special attention to their peculiarities.

The requirement for co-operation restricts the use of functional assessment of nasal and upper airway resistance by RM in some children (8).

Acoustic rhinometry (AR), introduced a decade ago for assessment of the nasal airways of adults (9), has several attractive features relevant to application in a pediatric population (10). AR provides a graphic representation of nasal cross-sectional areas from the most anterior part of the nose and enables the nasal volume between two chosen points to be calculated (9).

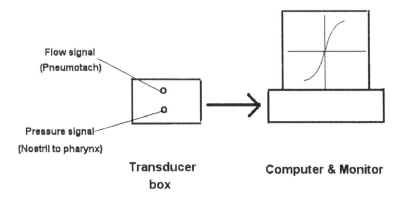

Figure 16.1 Setup of instrumentation. Differential pressures between nostril and pharynx and from the pneumotach are transduced to electrical signals which are processed by the computer to display a pressure/flow curve on a monitor screen in real time. Computed nasal resistance values are also displayed.

Technical details, useful applications and limitations of rhinomanometry and acoustic rhinometry with reference to young children are discussed below.

II. Rhinomanometry

Airflow resistance varies inversely and exponentially with cross-sectional dimensions of a conduit. Therefore, rhinomanometric assessments are very sensitive to the effects of structural and/or mucosal intrusions on the nasal lumen.

A. Technical Details

Airflow Measurement

In order to conduct respiratory air to a measuring device (usually a pneumotach) several techniques are available:

1.   Insertion of a nasal nozzle: Simple to use but sensitive to measurement error by distortion of the lumen of the compliant alar region which is the major site of nasal airflow resistance (11). Indeed, it is the major resistor of the respiratory airway from nostril to alveolus. It should be noted also that a small diameter nozzle can add resistance.

2.   Masking (Fig. 16.2): The commonest method, but a single mask cannot fit all faces. Anesthetic masks provide a wide range of sizes, CPAP masks are in three sizes and fit larger children, small fireman-type masks are unavailable and SCUBA mask results are unreliable. The poorer the fit of the mask, the greater the pressure against facial tissues is required to obtain a seal. Forceful pressure risks distortion of the compliant nasal alar region with consequent error in resistance measurement and it is disliked by young children.

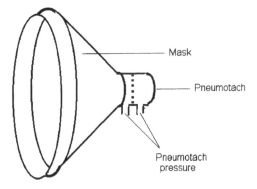

Figure 16.2 Mask with attached pneumotach. Differential pressures across the pneumotach resistor are transduced to electrical signals. See Fig. 16.4.

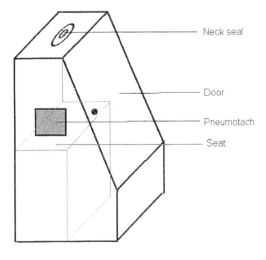

Plethysmograph

Figure 16.3 Head-out body plethysmograph with adjustable seat height. When the neck seal is in place the subject's body volume change with breathing displaces air through the pneumotach and flow is transduced to electrical signals. See Fig. 16.4.

3. Head-out plethysmograph (Fig. 16.3): Provides an indirect and reliable method that avoids the problems of masks and nozzles and is preferred by young children, in fact many find it fun. Contrary to much of the literature, success can be expected in children as young as 4 years in the hands of an experienced operator. The apparatus is bulky and may be unsuitable in some locations.

Pressure Measurement

Transnasal airflow is accompanied by a differential pressure between the atmosphere and the pharynx or, if a mask is used, between the mask interior and the pharynx. Several methods are in common use for pressure measurement.

1. An oral tube is held between closed lips to determine pharyngeal pressure (Fig. 16.4) while a mask or plethysmograph (see section "Airflow Measurement," items 2 and 3) is used to measure respiratory airflow. The subject is instructed to breathe quietly through the nose and to relax the throat (oropharyngeal aperture) in order to maintain a patent airway between nasopharynx and mouth. This method of assessment of nasal resistance to airflow is known as posterior RM and it requires patience and persistence from subject and investigator. As noted above, with an experienced investigator, failure to obtain reliable results is rare, indeed, some children achieve success more readily than adults do. The method is of particular value in young children because adenoid is included in the airway measurement.

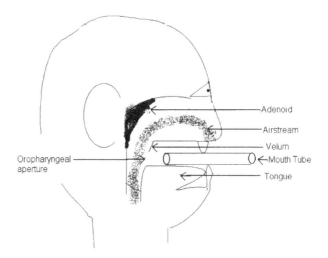

Figure 16.4 This diagram illustrates positioning of the mouth tube, the patent oropharyngeal aperture and the site of adenoid tissue.

2. A fine catheter is sealed in one nasal vestibule to register nasopharyngeal pressure while the subject breathes quietly through the opposite side. The vestibular pressure equals that in the nasopharynx. Airflow is measured by mask or plethysmograph. This method is known as anterior RM (Fig. 16.5), it does not require the patient to maintain oropharyngeal patency but it is a lengthy procedure and tedious for young children. Adenoid obstruction is not reliably assessed.

3. A fine catheter (8F gauge) is passed pernasally to the nasopharynx. It is a simple procedure if the catheter is inserted without hesitation along the insensitive floor of the nose and, in the absence of adenoid obstruction it is employed universally in our own laboratories for adults and teenagers. Airflow is measured with mask or plethysmograph.

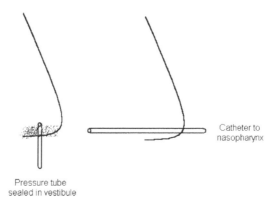

Figure 16.5 Position of nasal catheters for anterior and posterior rhinomanometry.

It should be noted that there are several methods in use for calculation of nasal airflow resistance. The Toronto method measures resistance to breathing of subjects at rest and resulting values may differ from those obtained at a fixed flow or pressure (6,7,12–17). The relatively small differences in resistance to breathing between children and adults (Table 16.2) results from differences in resting nasal airflow. As pediatric nasal airways grow over time, resting breathing flow also increases. By contrast, results of methods employing fixed pressure or flow relate to airway caliber.

Airflow and Pressure

These signals are processed electronically by transducers and, in modern RM, resistance, the ratio of pressure to flow (Rn = P/V) is computed and displayed numerically on a monitor screen (6,7) (Fig. 16.1). In addition, as the subject breathes, the signals are displayed in real time as a sigmoid P/V curve. Regular respiratory repetition of a smooth P/V curve, which can be observed by patient and operator, must be achieved to obtain meaningful resistance values. (*Note*: The V symbol stands for flow.)

Table 16.2 Guidelines for Nasal Resistances of Children and Adults Based on Clinical Experience and on Refs. 3,4, and 11.

	Nasal resistance	
	cm H_2O/L per second	Pa/cm^3 per second
Unobstructed children (age 4+)		
Average	2.5	0.25
Maximum	3.5	0.35
Decongested	1.5	0.15
Unobstructed adults		
Average	1.5	0.15
Maximum	2.5	0.25
Decongested	1.0	0.10

Note: The relatively small differences in resistance to breathing between young children and adults, as obtained by the Toronto system, results from differences in resting nasal breathing. As pediatric nasal airway caliber increases with age, resting breathing flows increase also. Results differ from those obtained at a fixed pressure of flow which are related to airway caliber rather than resting breathing. The International Committee on Standardization of Rhinomanometry recommends expression of nasal resistance in SI units as Pa/cm^3 per second. Guidance values for young children and adults.

B. Clinical Use

Assessment of nasal patency by symptomatology is unreliable, especially in young children. Rhinoscopy of the small nose has limitations, and a major source of rhinoscopic error results from alar retraction by the blades of a speculum. This procedure displaces anatomic relations of the alae on which the major portion of nasal resistance is dependent (11). RM offers an objective and quantitative alternative.

Since appraisal of an adenoid contribution to resistance is a common requirement in children, posterior RM is the method of choice (see sections titled "Airflow Measurement", items 2 and 3; "Pressure Measurement", item 1).

In the ENT Department of the Hospital for Sick Children, Toronto, more than 400 children are referred annually for posterior RM. Airflow is measured by head-out plethysmography (Fig. 16.3) which we prefer to the alternative of face masking (Fig. 16.2). It is the method of choice in more than 20 centers worldwide.

The oral pressure detecting tube is positioned by an experienced technician who persuades the patient to maintain oropharyngeal patency while breathing quietly and exclusively through the nose (Fig. 16.4). As this is achieved, a regular sigmoid curve is displayed in real time on the monitor screen and repeated with each consecutive breath. The screen is visible to patient and technician, and by feedback the patient is encouraged to maintain the pattern. When this regularly repeating pattern is established, a reading is taken and a numerical resistance value is computed and displayed. The procedure is repeated until a dependable average is obtained.

In centers where a mask is employed in the measurement of airflow, a suitable size should be chosen with care and strict caution must be exerted to minimize displacement of mobile facial tissues (e.g., the upper lip and the cheeks) that could otherwise obstruct the nostrils or displace compliant alar tissues. Displacement of facial tissues as far from the alar region as the zygoma can seriously affect nasal airflow resistance.

A usual pediatric routine following history and clinical examination is rhinomanometric measurement of the combined nasal cavities after clearing the nose of excess secretion. The mucosa is then decongested and 10 min following xylometazoline 0.1% spray, measurements of the combined nasal cavities and the left and right sides are obtained.

The results indicate (a) the presence or absence of nasal obstruction and, when the mucosa is decongested (11) (Table 16.2), (b) the degree of mucovascular contribution to resistance, (c) asymmetry of resistance between sides is consistent with structural obstruction and alar retraction will reveal its site, and (d) residual bilateral obstruction is consistent adenoid hypertrophy.

Mucovascular swelling is the commonest obstructive finding in children (Table 16.1). Response to therapy for this or other obstructive conditions (adenoid or structural obstruction) can be assessed objectively from rhinomanometric measurements posttherapy or at intervals over time. New treatments can be evaluated in a similar manner (18).

III. Acoustic Rhinometry

Audible acoustic signals generated in a wave tube are conducted via a nasal adapter to the nasal cavity under examination. The incident signal and its reflections from the nasal cavity are detected by a microphone within the sound wave tube. Resulting electrical signals are processed by analyzing software to provide a graphic display of cross-sectional area–distance relationships and a numeric description of minimum cross-sectional areas (MCA) and volumes between selected points in the nasal cavity (9,19) (Fig. 16.6).

A. Acoustic Rhinometry in Children

AR represents a quick and noninvasive method for objective assessment of the nasal airways and requires minimal cooperation from the child. In the early

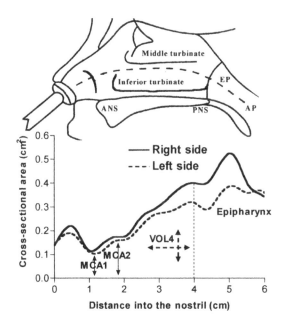

Figure 16.6 Result of reflection to area transform. Drawing illustrating the course of the acoustic pathway (AP) position of the inferior turbinate, middle turbinate, anterior and posterior nasal spine (ANS/PNS), epipharynx (EP) and their relationship to the features of an acoustic rhinogram from a 1-year-old infant. MCA1 is the cross-sectional area corresponding to the internal isthmus, MCA2 corresponds to the head of the inferior turbinate and VOL4 is the volume of the anterior 4 cm.

1990s, AR was applied to both infants (20,21) and preschool children (22), using modified adult probes. Although rhinological authorities debate the relative advantage of RM and AR in adults, few dispute the potentials of AR in very young children in whom RM is not an option. In fact, the smaller dimensions of the nasal airways in infants permit application of a higher maximum bandwidth frequency, thus significantly improving accuracy of acoustic measurements (10,23). However, in order to benefit from this unique feature and to achieve optimal results it is, essential that all components of the rhinometer are matched to the nasal airway dimensions of the age group in question (23). Unfortunately, these important factors are seldom recognized in studies addressing the accuracy and validity of AR. This point is illustrated by the significantly improved resolution obtained by means of a sound wave tube with a mechanical design (small and flexible) and technical properties optimised for infants (RhinoMetrics, Lynge, Denmark) (10) (Fig. 16.6). Furthermore, when the pulsed signal of traditional rhinometers is replaced by a continuous signal the time for data acqusition is reduced, permitting a higher rate of repeated measurements to be attained.

B. Advantages of Acoustic Rhinometry

Valid AR measurements can be obtained in a few seconds and require minimal patient cooperation. Time is of paramount importance to measurement in infants and children. Combined with its noninvasive nature, the mobility and small size of the equipment makes it well suited for repeated examination of infants and small children. If continuous movement and crying impedes data acquisition, measurements can, if necessary, easily be obtained during sleep and in a variety of body positions (10).

The acoustic rhinogram provides a description of the degree and location of obstruction, physiological changes and responses to various types of intervention. The high correlation between AR derived dimensions at the choanal aperture and dimensions obtained by direct *in vivo* and postmortem measurements (24,25), in models (20,26) and on CT-scans (24) indicates validity of the method in infants. The small size of the sinuses at birth and the moderate development childhood (24,25) prevent or reduce the potential artefacts due to loss to the sinuses in adults (27).

The sound wave tube optimised for infants is not suitable for those above the age of 1–2 years (10,28). When children reach an age of 6–10 years, the adult sound wave tubes seem appropriate. Currently, there is no sound wave tube on the market which is optimized for small children, but a new probe covering the age-span is likely to be commercialised fairly soon.

C. Limitation of Acoustic Rhinometry

The prime limitation of AR is its static nature. Ventilation in a dynamic process and ventilatory characteristics change rapidly with growth and maturation in childhood. Furthermore, the cross-sectional areas and volumes provided by AR do not describe the shape of cross-sectional areas. The aerodynamic properties of an orifice is strongly influenced by its shape, linear velocity of airflow, and the prevailing flow regime (29). Laminar, transitional, and turbulent flow can occur simultaneously in different parts to the nasal passage and complicate the interpretation of cross-sectional areas in terms of resistance. Finally, flexibility of the alae may be the source of dynamic collapse of the compliant part of the external nose induced by transmural respiratory pressures. This will not be detected by a static measurement (7,11). The respiratory induced pressure changes may represent a problem in small children (23,30). That will be solved in future versions of rhinometric sound wave tubes.

The basic algorithms used in AR assume negligible sound loss. Behind narrow constrictions this may not be true and result in underestimation (23). Studies employing adult probes in adult subjects refer to a lower limit for accurate determination of posterior dimensions ranging between 0.2 and 0.7 cm^2 (9,22), whereas validation of the infant probe in infants shows this value to be 0.05 cm^2 (23). In cases of mucosal inflammation, congestion in the posterior part of the nasal cavity reduces the risk of artifacts.

D. Sources of Error

In addition to the importance of awareness of the limitations above, attention must be drawn to further potential sources of error which can jeopardize results. Early studies used conical nosepieces which obviously risk expanding the anteriorly located valve area. Even anatomical adapters have been found to reduce the MCA by 10–15% (31), and a minor sound leakage between the rim of the nostril and the adapter may cause severe overestimation of posterior dimensions. Awareness and proper training is essential to avoid these errors. In addition, repeated reapplication of the sound wave tube until three independent curves with a CV% of <5% is obtained will reduce the risk of systematic error. Finally, external noise, pressure and temperature can also affect AR measurements (23,30,32) and appropriate action should be taken to avoid or reduce such influences.

E. Acoustic Rhinometry in Infants

The striking consistency of AR studies of healthy neonates in three studies published by independent groups and the agreement with CT-derived and directly measured choanal dimensions are strong indications of reliability in infants (10,28). The mean MCA in neonates of 0.1 cm is doubled by the age of 1 year (10). At birth, the MCA is located at the internal isthmus and its increase with growth was found to correlate significantly with circumference of the head (10). With age and in response to inflammation, the second constriction corresponding with the head of the inferior turbinate, becomes more evident and the rhinometric curve assumes a shape similar to that of adults (20,22) (Fig. 16.7).

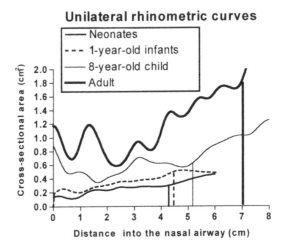

Figure 16.7 Graph showing the relative rhinometric dimensions at different ages. The curves for neonates and year-old infants represent the mean unilateral curves from the same 39 infants. The curve from the 8-year-old child and the adult are typical. The measurements of the infants were performed with the optimised infant sound wave tube, whereas the curves for the child and the adult were performed with an adult sound wave tube with anatomic nose adapters (RhinoMetrics A/S, Denmark). The large difference at the origin of the curves is partly due to the difference in sound wave tube dimension (infant sound wave tube: 0.13 cm^2; adult sound wave tube, 1.2 cm^2). The vertical lines indicate the transition to the epipharynx.

In year-old infants following recent URTI, the volumes posterior to the internal isthmus were significantly reduced to healthy controls after adjustment for gender and AR dimension at birth (10). The acoustically inferred depth of the nasal cavity in neonates of 4–5 cm, corresponds with dimensions measured on radiograms and CT scans (2) and its growth is very limited in the first years of life (10) (Fig. 16.7). These finding further support the validity and sensitivity of AR in infants.

AR can assist in the diagnosis of infants with acquired and congenital nasal obstruction (2) and craniofacial anomalies (33) and its potential role in diagnosis and follow-up of such conditions have been described. AR has proven useful in the evaluation of relationships between nasal dimensions and pulmonary function, both in healthy neonates (34) and in infants challenged with histamine (35).

The technique is promising as a method for evaluation of normal nasal physiology in infants. It may also assist in determining the role of nasal obstruction as a contributing factor in sudden infant death syndrome as measurements can performed repeatedly during both wakefulness and sleep. The infant sound wave tube has been found suitable also for examination of premature infants, but no systematic studies have not yet been published.

F. Acoustic Rhinometry in Older Children

The number of AR studies in older children is limited (22,36–38). One obvious reason is the lack of optimized equipment for children between 1 and 10 years of age. In 1993, Riechelmann et al. (22) published a study of 37 preschool children (3–6 years) using a modified adult probe. By comparing the rhinograms from infants (10), it is evident that the second constriction corresponding to the head of the turbinate gradually takes over as the flow-limiting segment (Fig. 16.1) in half of the 3–6-year-old children (22) and two-thirds of 6–11-year-old children (Djupesland, unpublished data). Repeated infections, allergies, and maturational changes in combination probably contribute to this development. This may explain the increasing incidence of mouth breathing and high nasal resistance in children in this age group (1,39). In a group of 20 older children (7–16 years) Zavras et al. (38) reported significantly reduced nasal volumes in the ten children with a history of chronic mouth breathing. Marchioro et al. (40) demonstrated by acoustic rhinometry that rapid maxillary expansion of palates in children significantly increased the nasal MCA.

G. Growth and Maturation of the Nasal Airway

Nasal dimensions in adults approximate those of neonates by a factor of 6 and of year-old infants by a factor of 3 (10,20,21). The mean acoustically derived dimension in a group of healthy children aged 6–10 years (TMCA = $0.77\,\mathrm{cm}^2$, TVOL0–5 = $6.0\,\mathrm{cm}^3$) (Djupesland, unpublished observations) examined with an adult sound wave tube and a small anatomic nose adapter, were approximately half of the mean adult dimensions obtained with adult anatomic nose adapters (TMCA = $1.3\,\mathrm{cm}^2$, TVOL0–5 = $12\,\mathrm{cm}^3$) (41,42). In the 6–10-year age group, configuration of the rhinogram was similar to that of adults (Fig. 16.7). The acoustically derived depth of the nasal cavity was 4–5 cm in infants (10), 6 cm in 6–10-year-olds (43), and 7–9 cm in adults (9) (Fig. 16.7).

Mean minute ventilation is doubled from $1.2\,\mathrm{L/min}$ at birth to $2.4\,\mathrm{L/min}$ at 1 year and is more than doubled again in adults (1,44). The changes in tidal volume, respiratory rate, and the described changes in position and location of the flow-limiting segment in the nose, make interpretation of dimensions in terms of resistance difficult. Thus, given the rapid maturational changes in both nasal dimensions and ventilatory characteristics in childhood, systematic studies establishing normative values for nasal airway dimensions in relation to age and body size, are required to augment the clinical and predicative value of AR.

H. Allergy and Environmental Exposure to Pollutants—Epidemiological Studies

The incidence of both allergic rhinitis and asthma is increasing in children. Simple and reliable objective methods for on-site evaluation of nasal patency, are essential to detect deleterious health effects of outdoor and indoor exposures and to justify expensive medical therapy and prophylactic interventions (45). Acoustic rhinometry has been applied succesfully to adults in such settings. Rigid stabilisation of the head and sound wave tube is not required if proper care is taken to avoid sound leaks and alar distortion (41). At present, only one manufacturer offers a portable lap-top version (RhinoMetrics A/S, Denmark) permitting measurements to be made on-site in a variety of environments. The mobility, simplicity and noninvasive nature of AR are important assets in epidemiological studies, particularly in children.

I. Future Directions and Perspectives

Adenoid hypertrophy is a common cause of significant airway obstruction in children (5) as are disturbances of the craniofacial and dentofacial development (46). Some studies claim that AR can detect absolute (47) and relative (48) changes in nasopharyngeal dimensions. However, the reliability of acoustic reflection technique in assessment of the nasopharynx, is disputed by other studies (2,36) and by inherent theoretical restrictions related to the algorithms currently used (9,41). Given the high prevalence of nasal and nasopharyngeal obstruction in children and its relation to sleep disturbances and otitis media, future research should be directed towards the development of algorithms permitting accurate determination of nasopharyngeal dimensions. AR may also prove useful in diagnosis, evaluation, and documentation of long-term healing and end-results of congenital and acquired septal deviations, in neonates and children. Prospective studies in infants and children are needed to detect such potential relationships.

AR also has potential in visualisation of dynamic processes in the airways. Due to the higher rate of repetition of measurements, the continuous wide-band noise technique has potential advantages in future visualization of dynamic processes compared to the traditional transient pulsed technique (23).

IV. Conclusions

The numerical value of airflow resistance obtained by RM provides a sensitive indicator of how hard it is for a subject to breathe through the nose. Objective assessment of nasal patency by RM is a practical procedure in children as young as 4 years. It is of particular value in children since assessment by symptomatology and rhinoscopy has serious limitations.

AR is an attractive method for assessment of the nasal airway patency and related pathologies in infants and children. It is, however, essential that the personnel performing and interpreting the AR are aware of the potential sources of error related to data acquisition and that the physician interpreting the rhinograms has sufficient knowledge of the aerodynamics of the nasal airways. This applies to all ages, but is particularly important when applied to infants and children due to the growth-related changes in dimensions as well as respiratory airflow characteristics. The technique is still young and further studies and development of the technique are required to improve its diagnostic and predicative value in pediatric research and clinical practice.

References

1. Cole P. The Respiratory Role of the Upper Airways: A Selective Clinical and Pathophysiological Review. Cleansing and Conditioning. St. Louis, MO: Mosby-Year Book Inc., 1993:1–158.
2. Djupesland PG, Kaastad E, Franzén G. Acoustic rhinometry in the evaluation of congenital choanal malformations. Int J Pediatr Otorhinolaryngol 1997; 41:319–337.
3. Parker LP. Diagnostic Rhinomanometry Using Head-out Volume Displacement Plethysmography on 1000 Consecutive Subjects. Thesis, University of Toronto, 1987.
4. Parker LP, Crysdale WS, Cole P, Woodside D. Rhinomanometry in children. Int J Pediatr Otorhinolaryngol 1989; 17(2):127–137.
5. Van Cauwenberge PB, Bellussi L, Maw AR, Paradise JL, Solow B. The adenoid as a key factor in upper airway infections. Int J Pediatr Otorhinolaryngol 1995; 32(suppl):S71–S80.
6. Cole P, Roithmann R, Roth Y. Measurement of airway patency. A manual for users of the Toronto systems and others interested in nasal airway patency measurement. Ann Otol Rhinol 1997; 171(suppl):1–23.
7. Roithmann R. Studies of Structure and Function of the Nasal Valve Area: The Contribution of Acoustic Rhinometry and Rhinomanometry. Ph.D. thesis, Federal University of Rio Grande do Sul, Brazil, 1997; 131.
8. Crysdale WS, Djupesland PG. Nasal obstruction in infants and children, evaluation and management. Adv Otorhinolaryngol 1998.
9. Hilberg O, Pedersen OF. Acoustic rhinometry: influence of paranasal sinuses. J Appl Physiol 1996; 80(5):1589–1594.
10. Djupesland PG, Lyholm B. Nasal airway dimensions in term neonates measured by continuous wide-band noise acoustic rhinometry. Acta Otolaryngol (Stockh) 1997; 117(3):424–432.
11. Cole P. Nasal airflow resistance: a survey of 2500 measurements. Am J Rhinol 1997; 11(6):415–420.
12. Hoshino T, Togawa K, Nishihira S. Statistical analysis of changes of pediatric nasal patency with growth. Laryngoscope 1988; 98(2):219–225.
13. Principato JJ, Wolf P. Pediatric nasal resistance. Laryngoscope 1985; 95:1067–1069.
14. Saito A, Nishihata S. Nasal airway resistance in children. Rhinology 1981; 19:149–154.
15. Stocks J, Godfrey S. Nasal resistance during infancy. Respir Physiol 1978; 34:233–246.
16. Van Cawenberge PB. Clinical use of rhinomanometry in children. Int J Pediatr Otorhinolaryngol 1984; 8(2):163–175.
17. Van Cawenberge PB. Variations in nasal resistance in young children. Acta Otorhinolaryngol Belg 1980; 34(2):145–156.

18. Hynes B, Cole P, Forte V, Corey P, Smith CR. The evaluation of intranasal topical beclomethasone spray in the treatment of children with non-purulent rhinitis using rhinometric, cytologic and symptomatologic assessment. J Otolaryngol 1989; 18(4):151–154.

19. Djupesland PG, Lyholm B. Changes in nasal airway dimensons in infancy. Acta Oto-laryngol (Stockh) 1998; 118(6):852–858.

20. Buenting JE, Dalston RM, Drake AF. Nasal cavity area in term infants determined by acoustic rhinometry. Laryngoscope 1994; 104(12):1439–1445.

21. Pedersen OF, Berkowitz R, Yamagiwa M, Hilberg O. Nasal cavity dimensions in the newborn measured by acoustic reflections. Laryngoscope 1994; 104 (8 Pt 1):1023–1028.

22. Riechelmann H, Reinheimer MC, Wolfensberger M. Acoustic rhinometry in pre-school children. Clin Otolaryngol 1993; 18:272–277.

23. Djupesland PG, Lyholm B. Technical abilities and limitations of acoustic rhinometry optimised for infants. Rhinology 1998; 36(3):104–113.

24. Corsten MJ, Bernard PA, Udjus K, Walker R. Nasal fossa dimensions in normal and nasally obstructed neonates and infants: preliminary study. Int J Pediatr Otorhinola-ryngol 1996; 36(1):23–30.

25. Wolf G, Anderhuber W, Kuhn F. Development of the paranasal sinuses in children: implications for paranasal sinus surgery. Ann Otol Rhinol Laryngol 1993; 102(9):705–711 (Review with 20 references).

26. Djupesland PG. Acoustic Rhinometry Optimised for Infants, Technical Properties and Clinical Applications. Ph.D. thesis, 1999.

27. Hilberg O, Jackson AC, Swift DL, Pedersen OF. Acoustic rhinometry: evaluation of nasal cavity geometry by acoustic reflection. J Appl Physiol 1989; 66(1):295–303.

28. Djupesland PG, Qian W, Furlott H, Cole P, Zamel N. Acoustic rhinometry: a study of transient and continuous noise techniques with nasal models. Am J Rhinol 1999; 13(4):323–329.

29. Hey EN, Price JF. Nasal conductance and effective airway diameter. J Physiol (Lond) 1982; 330:429–437.

30. Tomkinson A, Eccles R. Errors arising in cross-sectional area estimation by acoustic rhinometry produced by breathing during measurement. Rhinology 1995; 33(3):138–140.

31. Roithmann R, Cole P, Chapnik J, Shpirer I, Hoffstein V, Zamel N. Acoustic rhinometry in the evaluation of nasal obstruction. Laryngoscope 1995; 105(3 Pt 1):275–281.

32. Tomkinson A, Eccles R. The effect of changes in ambient temperature on the reliability of acoustic rhinometry data. Rhinology 1996; 34(2):75–77.

33. Kunkel M, Wahlmann U, Wagner W. Nasal airway in cleft-palate patients: acoustic rhinometric data. J Craniomaxillofac Surg 1997; 25:270–274.

34. Djupesland PG, Lodrup Carlsen KC. Nasal airway dimensions and lung function in healthy, awake neonates. Pediatr Pulmonol 1997; (25):99–106.

35. Kano S, Pedersen OF, Sly PD. Nasal response to inhaled histamine measured by acoustic rhinometry in infants. Pediatr Pulmonol 1994; 17(5):312–319.

36. Fisher EW, Palmer CR, Lund VJ. Monitoring fluctuations in nasal patency in children: acoustic rhinometry versus rhinohygrometry. J Laryngol Otol 1995; 109(6):503–508.

37. Fisher EW, Palmer CR, Daly NJ, Lund VJ. Acoustic rhinometry in the pre-operative assessment of adenoidectomy candidates. Acta Otolaryngol (Stockh) 1995; 115(6):815–822.

38. Zavras AI, White GE, Rich A, Jackson AC. Acoustic rhinometry in the evaluation of children with nasal or oral respiration. J Clin Pediatr Dent 1994; 18(3):203–210.

39. Warren DW, Hairfield WM, Dalston ET. Effect of age on nasal cross-sectional area and respiratory mode in children. Laryngoscope 1990; 100(1):89–93.

40. Marchioro EM, Rizatto SD, Roithmann R, Lubianca JF. O efeito da expansão rápida da maxila na geometria e função nasal. Ortodontia Gaúcha 1997; 1:3–7.

41. Djupesland PG, Qian W, Furlott H et al. Acoustic rhinometry in the diagnosis of nasal obstruction—practical aspects. Allergy 1999 (Abstract).

42. Roithmann R, Chapnik J, Zamel N, Barreto SM, Cole P. Acoustic rhinometric assessment of the nasal valve. Am J Otolaryngol 1997; 11(5):379–385.

43. Qian W, Djupesland PG, Chatkin JM et al. Aspiration flow optimized for nasal nitric oxide measurement. Rhinology 1999; 37:61–65.

44. ATS-ERS statement. Respiratory mechanics in infants: physiologic evaluation in health and disease. Eur Respir J 1993; (suppl 6):279–310.

45. Walinder R, Norback D, Wieslander G, Smedje G, Erwall C. Nasal congestion in relation to low air exchange rate in schools. Evaluation by acoustic rhinometry. Acta Otolaryngol (Stockh) 1997; 117(5):724–727.

46. Crysdale WS, Djupesland PG. Nasal obstruction in children with craniofacial malformations. Int J Pediatr Otorhinolaryngol 1998.

47. Mostafa BE. Detection of adenoidal hypertrophy using acoustic rhinomanometry. Eur Arch Otorhinolaryngol 1991; 16(1):84–86.

48. Elbrond O, Hilberg O, Felding JU, Blegvad Andersen O. Acoustic rhinometry, used as a method to demonstrate changes in the volume of the nasopharynx after adenoidectomy. Clin Otolaryngol 1991; 16(1):84–86.

17

Current Approach on Diagnosis of and Therapy for Sinusitis in Children

**BERNARDO EJZEMBERG and
TANIA MARIA SIH**

University of São Paulo,
São Paulo, Brazil

RAINER HAETINGER

Hospital Beneficência Portuguesa,
São Paulo, Brazil

I. Introduction

Sinusitis cases form a peculiar group among the upper airway diseases, which are difficult to confirm and to evaluate from the etiological and pathophysiological standpoints and, therefore, become a problem for adequate therapeutic intervention [1,2]. Differently from the mouth and middle ear, paranasal cavities cannot be directly seen at physical examination [3–5]. Although collecting material for exam is recommended in pharyngeal infections, it cannot be routinely done in sinusitis (4). Causes are also difficult to determine, as different chemicals (combustion particles, gases, pollen) and infectious agents can lead to sinus inflammation (6–8). These aspects very often occur simultaneously or sequentially, such as bacterial infections associated with allergic or viral rhino-sinusal inflammations (6). Besides these initial difficulties in the evaluation of sinusitis, others occur during evolution leading to limited possibilities of evaluation of resolution and increased severity of local inflammation and sterilization of cavity and mucosa; the same applies to recognition of cases of retained sinus secretions (ostium obstruction) (9–11). Thus, several interpretations have been proposed for the occurrence of sinusitis and the definition of diagnostic and therapeutic criteria (12–14).

As a result of all these factors, sinusitis has been discussed for several decades from the pediatric, otorhinolaryngological, and radiological perspectives (15–18). These discussions were recently revived because of the concern about progressive bacterial resistance to antibiotics and inadequate and excessive use of antibiotics is an important factor to be taken into account (19–21). Antimicrobials are frequently unnecessarily indicated to treat children that are assumed to have bacterial sinusitis and other airway infections (2,22–24), and this was the starting point for recent diagnostic and therapeutic new focus on sinusitis and other airway inflammations/infections (4,20,22,23). At the same time, a set of studies carried out in the USA in the last two decades established clinical parameters to recognize childhood sinusitis, as well as the basis to define standard therapy approaches (25–30). These measures were adopted by the International Consensus of American, European, and Japanese pediatricians and otorhinolaryngologists (31). The authors of the present article report these conclusions as well as a review of other relevant aspects of childhood sinusitis diagnosis and therapy, based on the experience of the medical services they represent.

II. Epidemiological Aspects

The incidence of respiratory diseases, including sinusitis, in children increased in the last decades (32–35). The increase was due to changes in lifestyle and living conditions of the population, directly or indirectly resulting in increased intensity and/or frequency of infectious, chemical and allergic factors that are aggressive to the sinus mucosa (see following section) (36,37).

As to the environment, progressive urbanization has worsened the quality of the inhaled air, both indoor and outdoors (6). At home, cigarette smoking and gas used for cooking (GLP) are factors that cause greater impact as rooms have progressively become smaller. Besides, there is often little sunlight exposure, which promotes humidity, and increases inhaled allergens (mites and fungi) (37). The contact with combustion residues from automobiles, gases, and particulate matter also increased the extra-home pollution (38). Although the environment is more preserved in rural areas, extensive use of fire in agriculture has resulted in high levels of pollutants that are markedly irritating for the airway (6).

As to lifestyle changes, female labor resulted in children going more often to daycare centers and earlier to school, greatly increasing respiratory infection rates (39,40). As viral transmission takes place more easily, these children have a fivefold increase in the prevalence of respiratory problems when compared to children staying at home (39,40). Swimming is frequently found in a large portion of the urban population. This practice can result in some advantages to children's health but it is also related to increased irritation of the rhinosinusal mucosa and occurrence of sinusitis (7,41).

Working mothers also had other implications, such as early weaning and use of cow milk and processed foods (with chemical additives), which can lead to food allergy and possible impact on respiratory problems (11,42).

Among respiratory diseases, the role of sinusitis is becoming progressively recognized in children with acute and chronic respiratory problems (43–46). In the last three or four decades, diagnosis of acute sinusitis showed more than a ten-fold increase among urgent cases. Three decades ago, the frequency of sinusitis diagnosis represented 0.2% of pediatric urgent cases, but it has reached levels between 0.5% and 5% in the present days (43–46). As a result of the real increase in the occurrence of sinusitis and the progressive attention given by pediatricians and otorhinolaryngologists, there has been a higher number of recognized cases (3,21,47). The involvement of paranasal cavities, however, is much more frequent than reported by the aforementioned figures mentioned (48–50). Frequent acute viral rhinopharyngitis could be recognized as rhinopharyngosinusitis in a significant number of cases (50). The paranasal cavities are contiguous, share the same epithelium, are in direct communication with the nasal fossa and get infected concurrently (14).

Diagnosis of chronic sinusitis (lasting for >3 months) has also been more often made (31,46,51). Particularly among patients with allergies, mucoviscidosis, and primary ciliary dyskinesia, as a result of attention focused on chronic rhinosinusal pathologies, it has increased the identification rates of complications in these sites (52,53).

There is also a great difference among the rates estimating incidence of acute problems and the prevalence of chronic problems in different population samples (54–56). This variation is often apparent and only reflects the use of different diagnostic criteria. We observed a distortion that has been found in many areas. It results from the high value given to plain radiographs of the paranasal cavities, taken in a large number of children who are misdiagnosed as having acute sinusitis (see Chapter 15, section "Diagnostic Confirmation") (3). To start with, we should only accept larger variations in sinusitis incidence and prevalence when there is a variation in age groups and the presence of other risk factors in the populations or samples being studied (57–61).

III. Physiology and Pathophysiology of the Paranasal Cavities

Despite the reduced dimensions, the maxillary and ethmoidal paranasal cavities are present at birth, and the frontal and sphenoidal sinuses start their development after 3 years of age (14,48,62). These bone cavities communicate with the nose and receive from it the inspired air to be warmed and filtered. The anatomic and functional integrity of the paranasal cavities depend on the immune system, as irritating gases, particles suspended in the air and organisms have access to these anatomic sites (63).

The immunoglobulins present in the secretion of the lining mucosa neutralize the bacteria and viruses that reach the sinus cavity coming from the nose. IgA class antibodies represent three-fourths of local immunoglobulins that are increased in the early stage of infections, as IgG only appears at a later stage (14,64). The mucociliary system aggregates and transports particles and organisms towards the nasal cavity, draining secretions through openings located close to the turbinates. The patency of these communication ostia with the nasal fossa is essential for the functioning of the paranasal cavity defense system. When drainage is obstructed and intrasinusal secretions accumulate, commensal organisms of the nose cavity, namely bacteria, multiply in the liquid collection and promote inflammation of the sinus wall (65,66). The main bacteria involved are the more pathogenic aerobes that usually colonize the nasal cavity: *Streptococcus pneumoniae, Haemophilus influenzae*, and *Moraxella catarrhalis* (7,40,66). In prolonged obstruction of the ostia, other organisms can be present, such as *Staphylococcus aureus* and other anaerobic bacteria. In diabetic and immunodeficient patients, infections caused by fungi can sometimes occur: *Aspergillus* sp., *Nocardia* sp. (67,68).

Pathophysiology of sinusitis is determined by child-related systemic and local factors and environment-related factors (55). As to the patient, inflammations are favored by lower immune competence as occurs in antibody deficiency, diabetes, mucoviscidosis (secretions become thicker), respiratory allergy, primary ciliary diskynesia, and AIDS (64,67). Different aspects specifically related to the paranasal cavity characteristics can determine if inflammations are more frequent and/or more severe. Figure 17.1 shows a normal coronal section computed tomography (CT) scan of the ostiomeatal complex. Progressive attention has been given to congenital or acquired anatomical deformities of the lateral nasal wall, septum, and juxtaostium structures, particularly of the ostiomeatal complex (OMC) (11,69–72). Anatomical variations are more important in older children (>7 years of age). In younger children (<7 years of age) an immature immune system is more frequently responsible for chronic rhinosinusitis. This anatomic site is located below the medial concha or turbinate and receives secretions from the anterior paranasal cavities. Alterations of the OMC are extremely important in the pathophysiology of recurrent and chronic sinusitis. Adenoid hypertrophy is another alteration of the

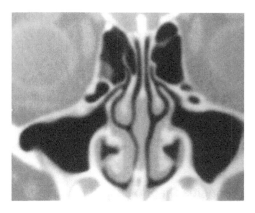

Figure 17.1 Coronal section CT scan showing the ostiomeatal complex: maxillary sinus (1), maxillary sinus drainage ostium (2), ethmoidal infundibulum (3), hiatus semilunaris (4), middle concha (5), middle meatus (6), and uncinate process (7).

anatomy that can cause secretion to accumulate in the nasal fossa, secondary ostium obstructions and sinusopathy (73).

In general, environmental factors such as viruses, bacteria, allergens and inhaled pollutants trigger sinus inflammation (27,62,74). Most often, sinusitis is triggered by viral infections (rhinovirus, adenovirus, syncytial respiratory virus, parainfluenza, and others) which affect the mucosa of one or more paranasal cavities (15,67,75). The process lasts for approximately 1 week. Sometimes, the sinus inflammation becomes more severe in children as a result of one or more of the following aspects: exacerbated pathogenicity of the viral agent, reduction of the child's immune system competence, alteration of the paranasal cavity structure, and interference of other concomitant environmental factors (6,76,77). In more severe cases of nasosinusal mucosa inflammation, ostium obstruction is a frequent result of intrasinusal secretion accumulation, a substrate for the development of secondary bacteria (71,72).

Primary bacterial infections are not frequent and in general result from diving into contaminated swimming pools (41,57). Under such circumstances, gram-negative enterobacteria cause intense local inflammations, with systemic effects.

Acute sinus inflammation caused by inhaled allergens follows a pathophysiological pattern that is slightly different from those previously described. In these cases, the triggering factor of allergy is generally persistent, acting both on the nose and sinuses, causing more long-lasting problems (78,79). As obstruction of sinus drainage persists longer, secondary bacterial infections tend to occur more often.

Recurrent and/or persistent inflammation of the paranasal cavities cause alterations of the mucous membrane (hypo- or hypertrophy) and sometimes can even cause bone erosion or calcification (70,80). Secondary impairment of local defenses leads to chronification of the process. This pathophysiological process is determined by repeated exposure to the triggering factors described earlier and/or the presence of predisposing factors (81,82). The first case includes children exposed to school and daycare center at younger ages (repeated viral infections) or to swimming (bacteria) (39). The second circumstance includes patients with rhinosinusal allergy or local anatomic alterations (causing obstruction of the drainage ostia) (74,81). Children with mucoviscidosis, diabetes and primary ciliary dyskinesia form a group that deserves special attention in relation to recurrent and chronic sinusitis (14,31,67).

IV. Acute Sinusitis Diagnosis and Management

In the International Consensus, the inflammation of paranasal cavities lasting less than three months was named acute sinusitis (31). Some authors, however, only consider acute the cases that last less than one month, and subacute cases are those with history between one and three months (23). As diagnosis and therapy are uniform for all cases lasting less than three months, we adopted in this article the classification of the International Consensus (23,31,47,82,83).

Acute sinusitis occurs at the same time as viral rhinopharyngitis, is self-limiting and very little symptomatic, lasting less than a week (21,51). In this clinical situation, fever, cough, and nasal secretion increase during a short period, with progressive reduction of symptoms until its end. Under these circumstances, the diagnostic confirmation of sinus inflammation is in general unnecessary as there are no clinical implications. But there are situations in which the benign evolution of rhinopharyngosinusitis as described above may not occur and the clinical signs become more severe or persistent (31). We call them complicated acute sinusitis, and they can have three clinical presentations that will be defined in this review as early extrasinusal complication, early sinusal complication and persistent complication (23,29,62).

The early sinusal complication (severe or nonsevere form) is recognized in an episode of acute rhinopharyngosinusitis as clinical symptoms become more severe after the third day of evolution, marked mainly by fever and sometimes facial pain. The purpose of having the clinical diagnosis of complicated acute sinusitis is to outline a subgroup of children in which the likelihood of having a secondary bacterial infection is already high. Using sinus puncture, studies conducted in this clinical situation concluded that bacterial infection occurs in 50% of the cases (40,66,84). It is interesting to observe that the other 50% remains intensely symptomatic, with pus in the sinus, but the culture results are often negative (sterile).

In such circumstances, the pediatrician and the otorhinolaryngologist are faced with a febrile patient, with maintained cough and nasal secretion, requiring concurrently evaluation of other anatomic sites—airway and middle ear (22,25). In this clinical presentation of complicated sinusitis, characteristics of the secretion (color, amount) and cough intensity are considered secondary (44,45,84).

These aspects related to symptoms are important. Erroneously, complicated sinusitis is suspected in children with pertussis-like cough or yellowish nasal secretion, both lasting <2 days, and with isolated headache (18,85). When they have a short duration and are isolated, these signs and symptoms do not indicate clinical diagnosis of complicated acute sinusitis (21).

Once a purely clinical diagnosis has been made, auxiliary exams have very little to offer (see diagnostic confirmation) (31). In all cases, management is based on the subgroup with secondary bacterial infection and antibiotic therapy is initiated (85). Several authors have indicated the prescription of amoxicillin, with a minimum dose of 40 mg/kg per day (19,66). With the objective of treating *S. pneumoniae* partially resistant to penicillin, we decided to use a higher dose—70 mg/kg per day (19,23,25). Even considering the resistance to amoxicillin of some *H. influenzae* strains and almost all *M. catarrhalis* strains, the treatment results were satisfactory in 90% of cases (23,25,86).

The use of amoxicillin clavulanate (30 mg/kg per day) or second generation cephalosporins, such as cefuroxime (30 mg/kg per day), should be reserved only for therapy failures. These drugs or others, such as third generation cephalosporins and macrolides, do not provide better results in complicated acute sinusitis (90% efficacy) (23,25,86), except for some amoxicillin-resistant bacteria (41,57). This is an interesting aspect, as some of the most recent antibiotics show better action profile in *in vitro* studies but the same results have not been obtained in comparative assays (22,23).

Clinical diagnosis of persistent nonsevere acute sinusitis is established for children who still have day and night cough and nasal secretion 10–14 days after the beginning of rhinopharyngosinusitis (23,83). Such cases have no or almost no fever. The clinical situation is very similar to that described for sinusal acute complication, but intensity is lower. The probability of being faced with bacterial sinusitis is very high and confirmation exams are not very useful (23,83). After the clinical picture has been recognized and other causes eliminated, the use of antibiotics is indicated. Amoxicillin is also the drug of choice under such circumstances, other antibiotics being reserved for therapeutic failures (10%) (23,83).

Early extrasinusal complication is defined by the dissemination of sinusal infection to other sites, whether adjoining or remote (87,88). It is recognized on the first days of rhinopharyngosinusitis in patients with involvement of the juxtasinusal subcutaneous cellular tissue, the orbit, intracranial or sepsis (82). There is fever, variable toxemia, and alterations detected at the physical examination are compatible with the infected sites. These cases are severe and patients have to be hospitalized to receive parenteral antibiotics in an attempt to cover the most probable bacteria—*S. pneumoniae* and *H. influenzae* (82,87,88).

Third generation cephalosporins are generally prescribed—ceftriazone or cefotaxime 50–100 mg/kg per day (87). Due to the peculiarities involved in these treatments and the likelihood of surgical intervention, readers are referred to reviews on meningitis, brain abscess, cavernous sinus thrombosis and intraorbitary abscess therapy (82,88). An intraorbitary abscess can be seen in Fig. 17.2.

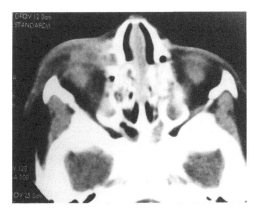

Figure 17.2   Axial section CT scan showing ethmoidal and sphenoidal sinusitis on the right side, complicated by extraconal liquid collection (abscess) close to the medial orbital wall.

The use of nonhormonal antiinflammatories, antihistamines, systemic deconge-stants, mucolytics, and nebulizations is unnecessary in the treatment of compli-cated acute sinusitis (89). Local washing with lukewarm saline solution is recommended to remove secretions (38). When congestion and turbinate edema are marked, causing pain and severe obstruction, a sympathomimetic decongestant can be topically used, but not for >5 days, so as not to cause rhinitis medicamentosa (38). Less frequently, topical corticoids can be indicated in patients with symptomatic allergy to reduce the OMC edema, resulting in better ventilation and drainage of paranasal cavities (90,91).

V.   Diagnosis and Management of Chronic and Recurrent Sinusitis

Chronic sinusitis classification is established for cases with ongoing clinical manifestations for >3 months (31) and, when the situation becomes more severe, it is named acute exacerbation of chronic rhinosinusitis. This picture is different from recurrent acute sinusitis, in which multiple acute episodes occur (at least three every 6 months) and there are no other signs and symptoms between them (31,38,71).

The clinical management of repeated or prolonged sinusitis episodes can differ from that adopted for acute situations, as will be seen below. Besides clinical suspicion (based on history and physical examination), diagnosis may demand a second stage—confirmation.

Clinical suspicion is essentially based on history and also on physical exam-ination (38). The history should cover a long period of time, characterizing the disease episodes and the intercritical periods. The differentiation between usual common cold episodes and recurrent/persistent rhinosinusal cases is not always simple, but should be carefully made (39). In some chronic sinusitis this can be more difficult when there are few symptoms (92). Nasal and oral breathing, diurnal and nocturnal, as well as unilateral airflow obstructions are important elements in the evaluation. Allergy manifestations should also be carefully evaluated, as they are an important factor of recurrence and sinusal chronification (93). This item should also record the detection of nasal/pharyngeal pruritus, sneezing, and respiratory reaction to environmental alterations. Questions about habits and housing conditions of the child should also be included here, as well as recent modifications (4,94,95). These aspects are fundamental in establishing the therapeutic and prophylactic schedule for chronic and recurrent rhinosinusitis cases. Some groups of children are particularly prone to having sinus pathologies and should be identified by their history—mucoviscidosis, immunodeficiency, ciliary motility disorders, and gastroesophageal reflux (67).

Similarly to acute sinusitis, chronic sinusitis clinical signs are in general more pronounced when the patient is presented to the physician (96). Cough, purulent nasal secretion, nasal obstruction, rhinopharynx drainage of nasal secretion and, sometimes, fever are common signs. Headache, facial pain, sinus pressure, localized edema, and sometimes pain in the maxillary teeth, can be observed in school-age children and preadolescents. Parents often complain about halitosis. This situation is easily recognized, but under some circumstances isolated signs and symptoms can occur, as will be seen in the subsequent text.

Cough can be practically the only manifestation of chronic sinus pathology (97). Diagnosis is suggested by the cough characteristics, starting when the child goes to bed and wakes up, which is due to the drainage of posterior secretion to the pharynx. Cough reported in lower airway allergy, on the other hand, usually starts in the early morning, a characteristic that is very helpful in establishing differential diagnosis (33).

In recurrent or chronic sinusitis, isolated nasal obstruction without secretion is rarely the complaint of the child/family (98,99). This isolated complaint is more frequent in situations such as turbinate hypertrophy (whether it has an allergic or infectious etiology), marked septal deviation, presence of polyps and foreign body (98,99).

The presence of persistent nasal secretion with different characteristics (aqueous, clear mucoid, purulent, or with blood traces) can be an isolated clinical manifestation of chronic sinusitis (66,84). The presence of persistent nasal secretion requires differential diagnosis with multiple sequential colds, isolated allergic rhinitis, foreign body (unilateral secretion) and dysfunction of the respiratory epithelium, as occurs in cystic fibrosis and primary ciliary dyskinesia (54,95).

Drainage of nasal secretion through the pharynx is often referred by school age children and can appear as an isolated complaint, but generally it also generates nocturnal cough that can be confirmed by other family members. In such cases, differential diagnosis should be made with adenoid hypertrophy, which often originates posterior nasal secretion (98,99).

Isolated halitosis is a rare presentation of chronic sinusitis as the odor produced by anaerobic infections also originates nasal secretion and obstruction.
More often, halitosis is determined by some other cause—caseum in the
tonsils and, sometimes, foreign bodies (49).

Headache is rarely an isolated manifestation of sinus pathology (85,100). It
can occur when there are points of contact between the lateral nose wall and the
septum and in OMC obstruction cases. In some chronic sphenoidal sinusitis
cases, headache can be the only symptom (100). In most complaints of isolated
headache, sinus pathology is not involved but misdiagnoses are frequent in this
situation. They can occur when plain radiographs of the paranasal cavities are
made, because this exam has low specificity for the diagnosis of chronic sinusitis
(see auxiliary exams) (3). Therefore, sinusitis is very often misdiagnosed in
patients with migraine, visual disorders and psychosomatic alterations.

Unexplained fever is a presentation of sinus pathology that is sometimes
mentioned (40,66), but the pathophysiology acceptance of this clinical picture
is not clear. It would require the occurrence of a major sinusal infection that
would not lead to any local manifestation (and then the fever would no longer
be unexplained). We believe that the reports of chronic sinus pathology as a
cause of unexplained fever are unlikely. As a result of the difficulties in microbiological exploration of such cases, the diagnosis is sometimes not adequately
confirmed and empirical therapy with antibiotics is provided (21,46).

When there is a suspicion of chronic/recurrent sinusitis, the physical examination should focus on the distortions of the craniofacial structure, particularly the
nose (96). Anatomic deformities can lead to sinus pathologies. Evidence of localized edema, uni- or bilateral nasal obstruction, as well as the presence of nasal
secretion, are suggestive aspects of the diagnosis and, surprisingly, they are not
usually reported in the history ("because it has always been like that"). The confirmation of localized pain over the paranasal cavities suggests chronic inflammation,
but sometimes it can originate misleading responses, depending on the child's
personality. The simplest way for the pediatrician to examine the vestibule of
the nose is by rising the nose tip with the index finger and using the light of the
otoscope (101). Under these conditions it is possible to observe the presence or
absence of secretion, its color, and the size of the head of the lower turbinate. If
the turbinate mucosa is pale, atopy is a possibility and if it is hyperemic, an infection may be present (101). Thus, at least a part of chronic or recurrent sinusitis
differential diagnosis can be based on the turbinates examination (98,99).

At the end of the clinical suspicion phase, with history and physical
examinations ready, diagnosis of most chronic or recurrent sinusitis cases can
be established (31,52). CT and nasal fiberscope are described under complementary methods (90,98,102). These exams are auxiliary, detect local pathophysiological factors and are fundamental in establishing the therapeutic schedule
for each case.

When underlying systemic diseases or other rhinosinusal diseases are being
suspected, auxiliary exams specific for the pathologies should be performed, such

as fasting glucose, chlorine in the sweat, immunity studies, HIV serology, etc. (67).

In planning the therapy for recurrent and chronic patients, pathophysiological mechanisms and factors should be addressed as well as the treatment of acute episodes/exacerbations (103).

Treatment of recurrent acute episodes and exacerbations of chronic rhinosinusitis (when there are complications of nonsevere acute sinusitis) are approached in the same manner as severe acute sinusitis (23,103). Thus, antibiotic therapy is indicated when fever appears and/or cough lasts for >10 days (see Section IV). Antibiotic therapy is used for 2–6 weeks, more often 2–3 weeks, and should be maintained for 1 week after clinical manifestations of sinusitis have disappeared (14,103). The antimicrobial agent should be selected for each case, based on recent previous treatment, trying to avoid using the same drugs to reduce therapeutic failures (14,38). When no antimicrobials were used in the two previous months, amoxicillin could be used at a 70 mg/kg per day dose, as in acute sinusitis (87). When there is no clinical response, fever is maintained for three days and/or cough for 1 week, amoxicillin/clavulanate can be used (30 mg/kg per day) or second generation cephalosporins (cefuroxime, 30 mg/kg per day), with the objective of acting against beta lactamase-producing strains (*Haemophilus* sp. *M. catarrhalis*, some anaerobes) (38,104). Cefalexine is another option in more refractory infections, with the objective of treating *S. aureus* (103). Metronidazole can eventually be associated to one of the antibiotics mentioned above for the treatment of mixed infections involving anaerobes (87).

In the rare cases in which there is no resolution of clinical manifestations or extrasinusal dissemination of the infection occurred, material should be collected from the sinus for microbiological evaluation (52,103,104).

Nasal washing (two times per day) is always recommended to remove secretions and crusts (105). Besides, cleaning provides a better area to receive adequate nasal application of other products that are necessary, such as topical corticosteroids (106). A buffered hypertonic saline solution (lukewarm) should be used in nasal washing with a syringe or dropper (105). It can be prepared at home, by diluting one teaspoon of sodium chloride and one of sodium bicarbonate in 250 mL of boiled water (105). A fresh solution should be made every week.

The objective of treating recurrent and chronic cases is to eliminate pathophysiological factors. Whenever possible, daycare centers and nurseries should be avoided as well as swimming pools (39). Allergic children should be identified by a specific approach, being recognized by the clinical and family history, nasal cytology, and IgE serum levels, if necessary (93,107). As a general measure, hygiene of the physical environment should always be recommended, as the respiratory mucosa is potentially sensitive to different substances present close to the child. House dust and mites should be reduced by removing carpets, curtains, mattresses, and plush toys. It is also advisable to use slip covers on mattresses and pillows, to boil bed sheets (and also the slip covers), and to use products to kill the mites and to denature pet hairs (tannic acid solution, benzyl benzoate powder) (59).

The more severe cases should be referred to an allergist, to perform skin sensitivity tests and RAST (radioallergosorbent test), as an attempt to identify the allergens (27,78,79). These evaluations can result in some specific prophylactic recommendations for inhaled or ingested allergens. The use of desensitizing vaccines in such cases is still controversial (27,78,79).

Nasal topical corticosteroids are recommended for chronic/recurrent sinusitis patients with symptomatic allergic rhinitis (8,108,109). As corticotherapy is immunosuppressant, the concomitant infection should already be under control. Thus, the corticosteroid is prescribed in clinical practice after antibiotic therapy, when nasal turbinates are hypertrophic, causing nasal obstruction, and secretion is no longer purulent. Mometasone furoate can be given in a single daily application. In clinical tolerance studies with this product, the evaluation of 3–12-year-old children with allergic rhinitis showed an incidence of side effects similar to that of placebo (108,110). Children tolerated better the aqueous formulation of some of these steroids (78,91,106,108). Another option of topical corticosteroid is budesonide that can be used by children aged between 2 and 4 years, as a puff in each nostril two times a day, during 1 month. Patients older than 5 years can receive three daily puffs for up to 3 months, followed by monitoring of signs and symptoms. Other topical corticosteroids are triamcinolone acetate, fluticasone propionate, beclomethasone dipropionate and flunisolide.

Nonsedating, second generation antihistamines (compete with histamine for the H1 receptor)—loratadine, cetirizine, mizolastine, ebastine, and fexofenadine—can also be used by oral administration in rhinosinusitis with a major allergic component (111). They are an efficient treatment for sneezing, pruritus and aqueous rhinorrhea, associated with allergic rhinitis, but have little or no action over nasal obstruction. The prolonged use, however, induces tolerance and occurrence of adverse effects, such as mood alterations and hyperphagia (37). Thus, the indication should be limited to short periods, especially during the seasons with more clinical manifestations—fall and spring. The nasal antihistamines have been used as spray in patients with seasonal rhinitis (hay fever) associated to sinusitis (91). This clinical picture is related to the pollen season and is uncommon in Brazil, except for some regions in the south of the country. The use of topical antihistamines anti-H1 have a limited use in children due to local irritation (burning) that can occur right after application (89), leading to low compliance rates in children.

Topical antihistamines block the symptoms depending on local histamine action (pruritus, sneezing, rhinorrhea), with low action on nasal obstruction.

Other adjuvant drugs used in the treatment to control nasal symptoms are ipratropium bromide (anticholinergic) that should have its use restricted to rhinitis with vasomotor component and major aqueous rhinorrhea, as it controls mucus production, and cromolyn sodium (prevents degranulation of sensitized mast cells) available at 2% and 4%. In a small number of patients there are reports of epistaxis, dryness, irritation, sneezing, and burning as side effects of the use of these two drugs.

In patients with strong clinical evidence of immunodeficiency (repeated infections in different sites and/or systemic infections) humoral immunity should be evaluated by determining serum immunoglobulins, IgG subclasses, antibodies against pneumoccocus (64). A minority in the group of children with chronic and recurrent sinusitis, the cases of immunodeficiency can eventually benefit from immunoglobulin replacement therapy or antibacterial active immunization.

Systemic decongestants, nonsteroidal antiinflammatory drugs, mucolytic, nebulizations and non-specific immunotherapy are not indicated in the treatment of children with chronic/recurrent sinusitis (89). Topical vasoconstrictors should also be firmly discouraged as they can cause rhinitis medicamentosa (rebound effect) and increase severity.

The surgical approach of chronic and recurrent sinusitis has precise and uncommon indications in the therapy schedule presently established by different authors (31,112,113). It is indicated in acute episodes with extrasinusal infectious spreading—except orbital cellulitis in an early phase—and in patients with anatomical anomalies (31,112,113).

Frequently used in the past, sinus puncture is presently considered to have no efficiency in treating sinusitis episodes in children (31,40,66). The objective of current surgical procedures is to restore paranasal cavity functions, allowing drainage of rhinosinusal secretions. Adenoidectomy is the surgery most often indicated for choanal obstruction, generally determined by adenoid hypertrophy (see section on physiology of paranasal cavities) (73,99). Another procedure, functional endoscopic surgery (mini functional endoscopic sinus surgery or mini-FEES) has obtained good results in selected ostiomeatal obstruction cases (31,112). It is performed by anterior ethmoidectomy removing the uncinate process, with or without maxillary antrostomy and opening the ethmoidal bulla.

Indications for sinus surgery were defined in the International Consensus on Management of Chronic Rhinosinusitis in Children (31). Absolute indications are: (1) complete nasal obstruction in cystic fibrosis due to massive polyposis or nose closure due to medial position of the lateral nasal wall; (2) antrochoanal polyp; (3) intracranial complications; (4) mucocele and mucopyocele; (5) orbital abscess; (6) traumatic lesion of the otic canal; (7) dacryocystitis refractory to drug treatment and secondary to sinusitis; and (8) fungal sinusitis. In chronic rhinosinusitis, surgery has a relative indication in therapy failure, in spite of adequate drug management, after an underlying pathology has been excluded.

In acute exacerbation episodes of chronic sinusitis, as well as in recurrent sinusitis, the therapeutic management, in our opinion, can be carried out by the general pediatrician. It is recommended that risk factors be removed as much as possible and that antibiotics are used for longer periods. This should resolve most of these episodes. However, long-term follow-up therapy schedule for these recurrent and chronic cases should be established by an otorhinolaryngologist. This choice is determined by the need of performing nasal fiberscopic examination in the diagnosis and follow-up of cases, as well as by the sequential evaluation when there is surgical indication. The frequency of evaluations in patient's follow-up will be individual, according to pathological manifestations of each child (114). To complement the information and provide consistency, multidisciplinary interaction involving the pediatrician, the otorhinolaryngologist, the specialized radiologist and often the immunologist is fundamental from diagnosis to follow-up.

VI. Complementary Exams

In relation to sinusitis, complementary exams have four objectives: to corroborate, to determine the pathophysiology of the process, to verify extrasinusal complications, and to establish etiology (42,66). The first three aspects can be approached at the same time by direct observation and by imaging; the fourth involves microbiological tests.

A. Direct Observation and Imaging Examinations

Several resources are used to recognize sinusitis and its complications. However, all of them have limitations in some aspects: precision, invasiveness, the need for special equipment and specialized professionals, and high cost. In this context, most (acute) cases are diagnosed only by the history and physical examination, as previously described (23). The uncertain, complicated, recurrent and chronic cases, however, need higher diagnostic precision and auxiliary resources are thus indicated.

An unquestionable confirmation of sinusitis is histology (10,14). Inflammation of the sinus mucosa can be established by cytological evaluation of the sinus contents, but it is not performed as the procedure to obtain the intrasinusal material is very invasive. Local puncture is only performed when there is an additional purpose, as will be explained later.

Rhinoscopy or rhinoscopic examination could be included as part of the physical examination, during the investigation stage when there is suspicion of chronic or recurrent sinusitis, as was mentioned before. Based on some technical details, it is recommended that it should be performed by the otorhinolaryngologist. The examination should only be performed with the aid of adequate size nasal speculum. It requires good frontal illumination (photophore) and use of special forceps (115). In case there is edema in the turbinates, rhinoscopy can be performed after the mucosa has been decongested with the local use of cotton soaked in a vasoconstrictor and topical anesthetic (87). It is possible to examine the medial (septum) and lateral (turbinates) walls of the nose and have partial view of the OMC. The limitation of this procedure in diagnosing maxillary, frontal and anterior ethmoidal sinusitis is related to the nasal anatomy (70), but it is useful in evaluating chronic and recurrent sinusitis.

Nasal fiber endoscopy or nasal fiberscopy can quite precisely corroborate the diagnosis of sinusitis in most cases, when it evidences passage of secretion through the sinus ostia (it is possible to see directly with the OMC), or intrasinusal observation (42,70,98). It is not always feasible either due to the difficult access to the paranasal cavity or to complete ostium obstruction, but it is clearly superior to plain rhinoscopy.

Besides, observation and anatomic and functional evaluation of rhinosinusal conditions are possible with this method. The possible pathophysiological mechanism of sinusitis can also be evaluated, and this examination is considered to be fundamental in chronic and recurrent cases (41,42). Evaluation includes turbinates size and status, polyps, septum deviation, OMC structure and edema, adenoid position and dimensions, and presence of mucocele (intrasinusal). The nasal fiberscope examination has another important aspect—the evaluation of permeability of the nasal air passage during the respiratory cycle. With this dynamic evaluation it is possible to recognize cyclic obstructions of the nasal fossae. The choanae can be occluded only during inspiration, caused by the inferior turbinate hypertrophy (70,99). Nasal collapse and the adenoid/choana ratio are also dynamically observed. The endoscopic examination often shows that small adenoids (seen in the cavum profile radiography) cause choanae obstruction during inspiration, by touching the turbinates tail or even by moving towards the choana. In other occasions, though, it does not occur with large adenoids (70,99).

Thus, with nasal fiberscopy it is possible to observe anatomic and/or functional rhinosinusal distortions that cannot be recognized even by CT scans (11,33,54). This aspect is really valuable in the treatment and prognosis of chronic or recurrent sinusitis cases. In cases with major function alterations, with poor prognosis, the examination can determine or accelerate the option for surgical treatment (97). Therefore, surgery of paranasal cavities should be preceded by nasal fiberscopy. The exam is often repeated in patients with chronic sinusitis submitted to surgery, evaluating the result and eventually indicating reinterventions (112,114,116). Due to the specificity of both equipment and technique, the procedure should only be performed by specialized professionals. It is necessary to have the skills and experience in dealing with children.

Transillumination has low sensitivity and specificity, and is only technically feasible in school children who have suspicion of maxillary sinusitis. The other paranasal cavities are not susceptible to this form of evaluation (117,118). This examination is no longer being used.

Plain radiographies detect most acute sinusitis, with good sensitivity for maxillary and frontal cavities. However, it is estimated that 5–30% of the cases cannot be recognized and the rate of false negative results in ethmoidal sinusitis can be as high as 40%. The radiological signs compatible with sinusitis include thickening of the mucosa lining (>4 mm), fluid level or total obliteration of one or more paranasal cavities (81,116).

In most cases where sinusitis is suspected, only Waters (mentonasal) and profile (lateral) planes are used, the former being favorable in the evaluation of maxillary and frontal cavities (36,80). The profile incidence is used to make Waters plane more conclusive and also to evaluate the sphenoidal paranasal cavities (as well as the cavum, as additional information). However, these incidences are not very adequate in the evaluation of ethmoidal sinusitis, the most frequent type. Although the specific incidence of Caldwell (frontonasal) has higher sensitivity, and still only partial, in general it underestimates the diagnosis of ethmoidal sinusitis (69,72,83). Hirtz's incidence (basal or axial) is used in the evaluation of sphenoidal cavities. It is indicated only for children above 6 years of age or adolescents, in the presence of specific clinical suspicion of sphenoidal sinusitis (persistent headache in the cranial vertex or intracranial abscess) (80).

The exam with plain radiographs has reduced specificity, it is not possible to make a distinction between recent or previous (scars) inflammation images, and even of anatomical variations such as paranasal cavity hypoplasia (42,77). In summary, due to limited specificity for children sinusitis, plain radiographs can be used as a preliminary method, but not for the diagnosis of sinus inflammation during the acute stage (77,102).

Age is another important aspect to be discussed. In the first 12 months of life, the radiological imaging has no sensitivity or specificity to diagnose sinusitis, as the paranasal cavities mucosa is thick or redundant, and very often it is not possible to distinguish between the normal aspect and the inflamed mucosa (38). However, there is an internationally accepted consensus that radiological examinations should not be performed during the first year of life, except in extrasinusal complications. Although the literature is not unanimous as to the indication or not of radiological studies between 12 and 18 months of age, we consider that they should also be avoided in this age range, as only maxillary cavities can be reasonably seen, and very often it is difficult to evaluate the degree of mucosa thickening. As the small child usually cries while the test is being performed, the result can be even further distorted due to the accumulation of rhinosinusal secretion. Frontal and sphenoidal cavities should not be evaluated radiographically in children younger than 3–4 years of age, as they are incipient (27,33,119).

CT is presently considered to be the best complementary examination for the diagnosis of sinusitis, as it has high sensitivity and specificity. Considering cost, access and radiation, however, the exam should be carefully indicated (31,54,119). Besides, the need for absolute immobilization during the exam should also be considered, as children younger than 3 years of age must be under sedation. These aspects restrict the use of CT in complicated acute cases, recurrent and chronic sinusitis, as well as in evaluations before endonasal surgeries (11,47,72,102,120). Besides evaluating paranasal cavities, this exam also allows an analysis of OMC, complementing the nasal fiberscopy results. This evaluation is fundamental to understand the pathophysiology of recurrent and chronic cases. Figures 17.3–17.5 show coronal sections computed

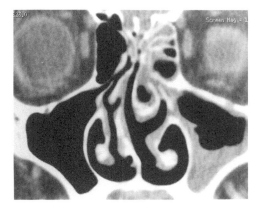

Figure 17.3 Coronal section CT scan shows bullous and large middle concha on the left side, causing middle meatus narrowing and leading to maxillary, frontal and anterior ethmoidal sinusitis.

tomography exams with anatomic alterations of OMC, showing a large concha bullosa (Fig. 17.3), a giant Haller cell (Fig. 17.4) and a protuberant ethmoidal bulla, leading to obstruction and chronic sinusitis (Fig. 17.5).

The right time to perform the CT scan depends on the clinical situation. In sinusitis cases where extra-sinusal infectious spreading can occur (see Fig. 17.2), CT scan should be immediately performed, but this is not recommended for chronic or recurrent cases (69,112). In such clinical circumstances, CT should be delayed four weeks, and during this period the therapy with antibiotics will

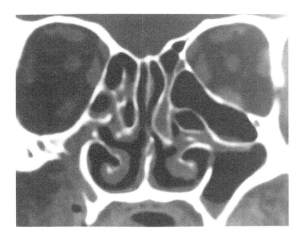

Figure 17.4 Coronal section CT scan shows a large Haller's cell causing stenosis in the left ethmoidal infundibulum.

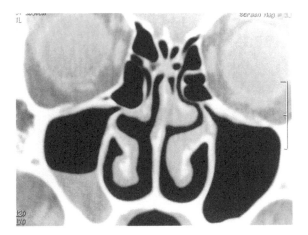

Figure 17.5 Coronal section CT scan shows a prominent ethmoidal bulla with caudal extension narrowing the ethmoidal infundibulum, preventing maxillary sinus drainage and causing sinusitis.

reduce local secretion and mucosa edema, so a more detailed evaluation of OMC will be possible (69).

When no extrasinusal complication is being suspected, the exam can be performed without intravenous contrast. However, in cases where there is suspicion of cellulitis or periorbitary abscess, as well as vascular thrombosis, the intravenous contrast is indispensable. Chronic or recurrent sinusitis cases may be an indication for contrast tomography (67,102). It is recommended when there is additional suspicion of nasal polyps or tumors, or even with unexplained severe or recurrent epistaxis for exclusion of the presence of vascular malformations (8).

Magnetic resonance imaging is a sensitive exam, but not much used in the diagnosis of childhood sinusitis. Absence of irradiation is an advantage in relation to CT scan, but it has low resolution for bone alterations and higher cost, as well as the need for general anesthesia in younger children. This method is only indicated when sinusitis complications are being suspected: periorbitary or intracranial abscess, meningoencephalitis [Figs. 17.6(a) and (b)], thrombosis of the ophthalmic vein or cavernous sinus. It is also indicated in the studies of concurrent tumor process and in the rare cases where fungal sinusitis is being suspected (13,120,121).

Ultrasonography has low sensitivity and specificity in the diagnosis of childhood sinusitis. Its use is not recommended in clinical applications (31,35,69).

B. Microbiological Examinations

Sinusitis is an inflammatory pathology, usually with infectious etiology. Although they are responsible for most acute cases, viruses are not studied in

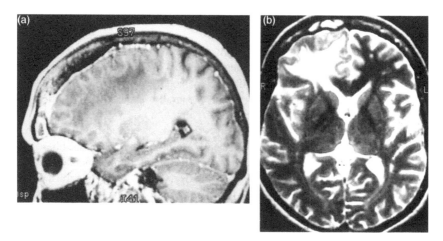

Figure 17.6 Magnetic resonance imaging shows frontal sinusitis and meningoencephalitis. (a) Corresponds to the post-gadolinium in T1-weighted sequence (sagittal section), showing the mucosa impregnation and secretion accumulated in the right frontal sinus, besides the impregnation of the meningeal section and brain edema (hypointense). (b) Corresponds to the T2-weighted sequence (axial section), where the brain edema is shown as hyperintense in the right frontal lobe.

pediatric and otorhinolaryngologic pediatric practices, mostly due to methodology difficulties and absence of specific therapy against these agents (1,21,51). Bacterial agents are always present in both healthy and unhealthy children and, in these cases, in subacute and chronic sinusitis (23). Recognizing the presence of bacteria in paranasal cavities has a therapeutic interest, but it is difficult to collect adequate clinical specimens for etiological identification (9,103). Although bacteria causing sinusitis come from the nasal fossa, the correlation between the flora of the nose and the paranasal cavity is not very good, but the correlation between the microbiology of the middle meatus and the nasal maxillary sinus is quite good. Precise identification of the bacterial agent can only be made by collecting intra-sinusal material, an invasive procedure that is difficult to perform in children, requiring general anesthesia (9,103). Thus, evaluation of the intra-sinusal material is reserved for the rare chronic and recurrent cases of therapeutic failure, in the presence of intraorbitary or intracranial suppuration and exceptionally in acute major toxemia episodes (25,31,82). Evaluation of sinus material by aspiration is sometimes indicated in risk groups for rare infections—patients with diabetes, AIDS, mucoviscidosis, and tumors (67).

Microbiological evaluation of bacteria is performed both in aerobic and anaerobic media, particularly in chronic sinusitis where anaerobes are associated with aerobes (including *Staphylococcus aureus*) (9,103). Smears and cultures in Saburaud medium can be made in cases where fungal infection is suspected in children with some kind of immunodeficiency (122).

VII. Conclusions

Recognition of complicated acute sinusitis is essentially clinical, based on history and physical examination. Complementary exams are reserved to be used only in extra-sinusal complications. Antibiotic management is based on the use of amoxicillin and more expensive drugs are generally not used. Other drugs are unnecessary in this clinical situation.

Chronic and recurrent sinusitis cases are also suspected based on clinical information, but they should be confirmed by tomography and nasal fiberscopy evaluation. In order to establish the therapy schedule, it is fundamental to determine the pathophysiological mechanism in every case. Only in rare cases is microbiological evaluation performed, the use of antibiotic being based on clinical characteristics, always individual and restricted to the periods with symptoms.

It is the opinion of the authors and of others that diagnosis and therapy standardization in childhood sinusitis, as focused in this review, leads to reduction in the number of unnecessary antibiotic treatments (21,23,26,28,31). Our objective is mainly to reduce the inadequate use of antimicrobial agents recently introduced in the pharmacopoeia. As a final result, iatrogeny, antibiotic bacterial resistance and treatment costs would be equally reduced.

References

1. Arruda LK, Mimica IM, Sole D. Abnormal maxillary sinus radiographs in children: do they represent bacterial infection? Pediatrics 1990; 85:553–558.
2. Barden LS, Dowell SF, Schwartz B, Lackey C. Current attitudes regarding use of antimicrobial agents: results from physicians and parents focus group discussions. Clin Pediatr (Phila) 1998; 37:665–671.
3. Ejzenberg B. Epidemia radiológica de sinusites. Pediatr (S. Paulo) 1998; 20:4.
4. Ejzenberg B, Nascimento SL, Gilio AE, Lotufo JP, Okay Y. Faringoamigdalites episódicas e recorrentes. Pediatria (S. Paulo) 1998; 20:191–210.
5. Sih T, Caldas S, Schwartz S. Prophylaxis for recurrent acute otitis media: a Brazilian study. Int J Pediatr Otorhinolaryngol 1993; 25:19–24.
6. Sih T. The role of air pollution-induced allergy in otitis media pathogenesis in children. In: Tos M, Thomsen J, Balle V, eds. Otitis Media Today. The Hague: Kugler, 1999:75–80.
7. Wald E. Epidemiology, pathophysiology and etiology of sinusitis. Pediatr Infect Dis J 1985; 4(S):51–53.
8. Wüthrich B, Schindler C, Leuenberger P, Ackerman-Liebrich U. Prevalence of atopy and pollinosis in Switzerland (Sapaldia Study). Int Arch Allergy Immunol 1995; 106:149–156.
9. Bacteriologic features of chronic sinusitis in children. J Am Med Assoc 1981; 246:967–970.
10. Diament M. The diagnosis of sinusitis in infants and children: X-ray, computed tomography, and magnetic resonance imaging. J Allergy Clin Immunol 1992; 90:442–444.

11. Haetinger RG. Avaliação por Imagem dos Seios Paranasais na Correlação com Endoscopia e Cirurgia Endoscópica Endonasal. Rev Bras Otorrinol 1998; 64(S):17–29.
12. Aitken M, Taylor JA. Prevalence of clinical sinusitis in young children followed up by primary care pediatricians. Arch Pediatr Adolesc Med 1998; 152:244–248.
13. Evans KL. Recognition and management of sinusitis. Drugs 1998; 56:59–71.
14. Giebink GS. Childhood sinusitis: pathophysiology, diagnosis and treatment. Pediatr Infect Dis J 1994; 13(S):55–65.
15. Gohd R. The common cold. N Engl J Med 1954; 250:687–691.
16. Hays GC, Mullard JE. Can nasal bacterial flora be predicted from clinical findings? Pediatrics 1972; 49:596–599.
17. Monto AS, Ullman BM. Acute respiratory illness in an American community. J Am Med Assoc 1974; 227:164–169.
18. Wynder EJ, Lemon FR, Mantel N. Epidemiology of persistent cough. Am Rev Respir Dis 1965; 91:679–700.
19. Dowell SF, Schwartz B. Outcome of infections caused by penicillin-non susceptible pneumoccoci. Pediatr Infect Dis J 1996; 15:554–556.
20. Dowell SF. Principles of judicious use of antimicrobial agents for pediatric upper respiratory tract infections. Pediatrics (S) 1998; 101:161–184.
21. Schwartz B, Mainous AG, Marcy SM. Why do physicians prescribe antibiotics for children with upper respiratory tract infections? J Am Med Assoc 1998; 279:881–882.
22. Dowelll SF, Schwartz B, Phillips WR. Appropriate use of antibiotics for URIs in children: Part II. Cough, pharyngitis and the common cold. The Pediatric URI Consensus Team. Am Pham Phys 1998; 58:1335–1342.
23. Dowelll SF, Schwartz B, Phillips WR. Appropriate use of antibiotics for URIs in children: Part I. Otitis media and acute sinusitis. The Pediatric URI Consensus Team. Am Pham Phys 1998; 58:1313–1318.
24. Williams JW, Holleman DR, Samsa GP, Simel DL. Randomized controlled trial of 3 vs 10 days of trimethoprim/sulfametoxazole for acute maxillary sinusitis. J Am Med Assoc 1995; 273:1015–1021.
25. Cohen R. The antibiotic treatment of acute otitis media and sinusitis in children. Diagn Microbiol Infect Dis 1997; 27:35–39.
26. Incaudo GA, Wooding LG. Diagnosis and treatment of acute and subacute sinusitis in children and adults. Clin Rev Allergy Clin Immunol 1998; 16:157–204.
27. Isaacson G. Sinusitis in childhood. Pediatr Clin North Am 1996; 43:1297–1318.
28. Lund VJ, Kennedy DW. Quantification for staging sinusitis. The staging and therapy group. Ann Otol Rhinol Laryngol 1995; 167(S):17–21.
29. Manning SC, Biavati MJ, Phillips DL. Correlation of clinical sinusitis signs and symptoms to imaging findings in pediatric patients. Int J Pediatr Otorhinolaryngol 1996; 37:65–74.
30. O'Brien KL, Dowell SF, Schwartz B, Marcy SM, Phillips WR, Gerber MA. Acute sinusitis—principles of judicious use of antimicrobial agents. In: Dowell SF, ed. Principles of judicious use of antimicrobial agents for pediatric upper respiratory tract infections. Pediatrics (S) 1998; 101:174–177.
31. Clement PAR, Bluestone CD, Gordts F, Lusk RP, Otten FWA, Goossens H, Scadding GK, Taskahashi H, Van Buchem L, Van Cauwenberge P, Wald ER. Management of rhinosinusitis in children. Consensus Meeting, Brussels, Belgium. Arch Otolaryngol Head Neck Surg 1998; 124:31–34.

32. Gwaltney JM. Acute community acquired sinusitis. Clin Infect Dis 1996; 23:1209–1225.
33. Havas TE, Motbey JA, Gullane PJ. Prevalence of incidence abnormalities on computed tomographic scans of the paranasal sinuses. Arch Otolaryngol Head Neck Surg 1988; 114:45–50.
34. Healy GB. Acute sinusitis in childhood. N Engl J Med 1981; 304:779–781.
35. Newton DA. Sinusitis in Children and Adolescents. Primary Care 1996; 23:701–717.
36. Quackenboss JJ, Krzyzanowsky M, Lebowitz MD. Exposure assessment to environmental approaches to evaluate respiratory health effects of particulate matter and nitrogen dioxide. J Exp Anal Environ Epidemiol 1991; 1:83–107.
37. Sibbald B. Epidemiology of allergic rhinitis. In: Burr ML, ed. Epidemiology in Clinical Allergy. Basel: Karger, 1993:61–79.
38. Pereira MBR. Sinusitis. In: Sih T, ed. Pediatric Otorhinolaryngology Manual. São Paulo: International Federation of Oto-Rhino-Laryngological Societies, 1998:90–99.
39. Schwartz B, Giebink GS, Henderson FW, Reichler MR, Jereb J, Collet JP. Respiratory infections in day care. Pediatrics 1994; 94:1018–1020.
40. Wald ER. Sinusitis in children. Pediatr Infect Dis J 1988; 7(S):150–153.
41. Sayfield DL, Fraser DJ. Persistence of *Pseudomonas aeruginosa* in chlorinated swimming pools. Can J Microbiol 1980; 76:350–355.
42. Wagner W. Changing diagnostic and treatment strategies for chronic sinusitis. Cleve Clin J Med 1996; 63:396–405.
43. Wald E, Milmoe G, Bowen A, Ledesma-Medina J, Salamon N, Bluestone C. Acute maxillary sinusitis in children. N Engl J Med 1981; 304:749–754.
44. Wald E, Reilly J, Casselbrant M. Treatment of acute maxillary sinusitis in childhood: a comparative study of amoxicillin and cefaclor. J Pediatr 1984; 104:297–302.
45. Wald E, Guerra N, Byers C. Upper respiratory tract infections in young children: duration of and frequency of complications. Pediatrics 1991; 87:129–133.
46. Wald ER. The microbiology of chronic sinusitis in children. A review. Acta Otorhinolaryngol Belg 1997; 51:51–54.
47. Weinberg EA, Brodsky L, Brody A, Pizzuto M, Stiner H. Clinical classification as a guide to treatment of sinusitis in children. Laryngoscope 1997; 107:241–246.
48. Glasier CM, Ascher DP, Williams KD. Incidental paranasal sinus abnormalities on CT of children. Clinical correlations. Am J Neuroradiol 1986; 7:861–864.
49. Glasier CM, Mallory GB, Steele R. Significance of opacification of the maxillary and ethmoid sinuses in infants. J Pediatr 1989; 114:45–50.
50. Gwaltney J, Phillips C, Miller R, Riker D. Computed tomographic study of the common cold. N Engl J Med 1994; 330:25–30.
51. Ramadan HH, Farr RW, Wetmore SJ. Adenovirus and Respiratory Syncytial Virus in chronic sinusitis using polymerase chain reaction. Laryngoscope 1997; 107:923–925.
52. Mellis CM. Evaluation and treatment of chronic cough in children. Pediatr Clin North Am 1979; 26:553–564.
53. Muntz HR. Allergic fungal sinusitis in children. Otolaryngol Clin North Am 1996; 29:169–183.
54. Kronemer KA, McAlister WH. Sinusitis and its imaging in the pediatric population. Pediatr Radiol 1997; 27:837–846.

55. Lombardi E, Stein RT, Wright AL, Morgan WJ, Martinez FD. The relation between physical diagnosed sinusitis, asthma, and skin test reactivity to allergens in 8 year old children. Pediatr Pulmonol 1996; 22:141–146.

56. McCaig LF, Hughes JM. Trends in antimicrobial drug prescribing among office-based physicians in the United States. J Am Med Assoc 1995; 273:214–219.

57. Calderon R, Mood EW. An epidemiological assessment of water quality and swimmer's ear. Arch Environ Health 1982; 37:300–305.

58. Gunney E, Tayeri Y, Kanderi B, Yalcin S. The effect of wood dust on the nasal cavity and paranasal sinuses. Rhinology 1987; 25:273–277.

59. Institut of Allergy Chemin du Foriest. European Allergy White Paper: Allergic Diseases as a Public Health Problem in Europe. Brussels: UCB, 1997.

60. Krzyzanowsky M, Quackenboss JJ, Lebowitz MD. Chronic respiratory effects of indoor formaldehyde exposure. Environ Res 1990; 52:117–125.

61. Lesserson JA, Kiesrman SP, Finn DG. The radiographic incidence of chronic sinus disease in the pediatric population. Laryngoscope 1994; 104:159–166.

62. DeBock GH, Kievit J, Mulder JD. Acute maxillary sinusitis in general practice: a decision problem. Scand J Prim Health Care 1994; 12:9–14.

63. Environmental Protection Agency. Environmental Tobacco Smoke and Respiratory Diseases. Washington, DC: EPA, 1992.

64. Herrod HG. Immunologic considerations in the child with recurrent or persistent sinusitis. Allergy Asthma Proc 1997; 18:145–148.

65. Gwaltney JM. The common cold. In: Mandel GL, Douglas R, Bennet JE, eds. Principles and Practice of Infectious Diseases. 4th ed. New York: Churchill Livingstone, 1995:561–566.

66. Wald E. Sinusitis in children. N Engl J Med 1992; 326:319–323.

67. Brihaye P, Jorissen M, Clement PA. Chronic rhinosinusitis in cystic fibrosis (mucoviscidosis). Acta Otorhinolaryngol Belg 1997; 51:323–337.

68. Lebeda MD, Haller JR, Graham SM, Hoffman HT. Evaluation of maxillary sinus aspiration in patients with fever of unknown origin. Laryngoscope 1995; 105:683–685.

69. Lusk RP. Pediatric Sinus Pathology. Syllabus 32nd Annual Scientific Conference & Post Graduate Course in Head & Neck Imaging, Phoenix, Az, April. Phoenix: ARS, 1998:353–355.

70. Willner A, Choi SS, Vezina LG, Lazar RH. Intranasal anatomic variations in pediatric sinusitis. Am J Rhinol 1997; 11:355–360.

71. Yousen DM. Imaging of sinonasal inflammatory disease. Radiology 1993; 188:303–314.

72. Zinreich J. Imaging of inflammatory sinus disease. Otol Clin North Am 1993; 26:535–547.

73. Takahashi H, Fujita A, Honjo I. Effect of adenoidectomy on otitis media with effusion, tubal function, and sinusitis. Am J Otolaryngol 1989; 10:208–213.

74. Gungor A, Corey JP. Pediatric sinusitis: a literature review with emphasis on the role of allergy. Otolaryngol Head Neck Surg 1997; 116:4–15.

75. Gwaltney JM. Rhinovirus. In: Mandel GL, Douglas R, Bennet JE, eds. Principles and Practice of Infectious Diseases. 4th ed. New York: Churchill Livingstone, 1995:1656–1662.

76. Shapiro GG. Allergic Rhinitis. In: Cotton RT, Myer CM, eds. Practical Pediatric Otolaryngology. Philadelphia: Lippincott-Raven, 1999:379–394.

77. Som PM, Curtin HD. Sinonasal Cavities: Anatomy, Physiology and Plain Film Normal Anatomy. Head and Neck Imaging. 3rd ed. Boston: Mosby, 1996:79–96.
78. Waldner DL, Falciglia M, Willging JP, Myer CM 3rd. The role of second-look nasal endoscopic after pediatric functional endoscopic surgery. Arch Otolaryngol Head Neck Surg 1998; 124:425–428.
79. Wang DY, Clement P, DeWaele M, Derde MP. Study of nasal cytology in atopic patients after nasal allergen challenge. Rhinology 1995; 33:78–81.
80. Valvassori GE, Potter GD, Hanafee WN, Carter BL, Buckingham RA. Radiology of the Ear, Nose and Throat. Saunders: Philadelphia, 1984:130–142.
81. Shankar L, Evans K, Hawke M, Stammberger H. The role of anatomic variants of the ostiomeatal complex and paranasal sinuses. In: Shankar L, Evans K, Hawke M, Stammberger H, eds. An Atlas of Imaging of the Paranasal Sinuses. London: Martin Dunitz, 1994:73–81.
82. Uzcategui N, Warman R, Smith A, Howard CM. Clinical practice guidelines for the management of orbital cellulitis. J Pediatr Ophthalmol Strabismus 1998; 35:73–79.
83. Ueda D, Yoto Y. The ten day mark as a practical diagnosis approach for acute paranasal sinusitis in children. Pediatr Infect Dis J 1996; 15:576–579.
84. Wald ER. Purulent nasal discharge. Pediart Infect Dis J 1991; 10:329–333.
85. Burton LJ, Quinn B, Pratt Chenney JL, Pourani M. Headache etiology in a pediatric emergency department. Pediatr Emerg Care 1997; 13:1–4.
86. Wald E, Chiponis D, Ledesma- Medina J. Comparative effectiveness of amoxicillin-clavulanate potassium in acute paranasal sinus infections in children: a double-blind, placebo-controlled trial. Pediatrics 1986; 77:795–800.
87. Kluka EA. Medical treatment of rhinosinusitis in children. In: Cotton RT, Myer CM, eds. Practical Pediatric Otolaryngology. Philadelphia: Lippincott-Raven, 1999:395–404.
88. Singh B, Van-Dellen J, Ramjettan S, Maharaj TJ. Sinogenic intracranial complications. J Laryngol Otol 1995; 109:945–950.
89. Bricks LF, Sih T. Medicamentos controversos em Otorrinolaringologia. J Pediatr 1999; 75:11–22.
90. Wang DY, Clement P, Smitz J, DeWaele M. The activity of recent anti-allergic drugs in the treatment of seasonal allergic rhinitis. Acta Otorhinolaryngol Belg 1996; 50:25–32.
91. Wang D, Smitz J, DeWaele M, Clement P. Effect of topical applications of budesonide and azelastine on nasal allergen challenge during the pollen season. Int Arch Allergy Immunol 1997; 114:185–192.
92. Som PM, Lidov M. The significance of sinonasal radiodensities: ossification, calcification, or residual bone? Am J Radiol 1994; 15:917–922.
93. Bergman KE, Bergman RL, Bauer CP, Dorch W, Foster J, Schmidt E, Schulz J, Whan U. Atopie in Deutschland. Deutsches Ärzteblatt 1993; 190:1341–1347.
94. Chilmonczyk BA, Salmun LM, Megathlin KN. Association between exposure to environmental tobacco smoke and exacerbations of asthma in children. N Engl J Med 1993; 328:1665–1669.
95. Saldiva PHN, King M, Delmonte VLC, MachIone M, Parada MAC, Daliberto ML et al. Respiratory alterations due to urban air pollution: an experimental study in rats. Environ Res 1992; 57:19–33.

96. Parsons DS, Van Leewen N. Sinusite em Pediatria. In: Chinski A, Sih TS, eds. II Manual de Otorrinolaringologia da IAPO (Interamerican Association of Pediatric Otorhinolaryngology). São Paulo: Ateliê, 1999:185–200.
97. Parsons DS. Chronic sinusitis: a medical or surgical disease? Otolaryngol Clin North Am 1996; 29:1–9.
98. Wang DY, Clement P, Kaufman L, Derde MP. Fiberoptic examination of the nasal cavity and nasopharynx in children. Int J Pediatr Otorhinolaryngol 1992; 24:35–44.
99. Wang DY, Bernheim N, Kaufman L, Clement P. Assessment of adenoid size in children by fiberoptic examination. Clin Otolaryngol 1997; 22:172–177.
100. Lew D, Southwick FS, Montomery WW. Sphenoid sinusitis. A review of 30 cases. N Engl J Med 1983; 309:1149–1154.
101. Handler SD, Myer CM. Atlas of Ear, Nose and Throat Disorders in Children. Hamilton: BC Decker, 1998:44–64.
102. Gomes ACP, Mendonça RA, Haetinger RG. Tomografia Computadorizada do Nariz, Seios Paranasais e Estruturas Correlatas. In: Stamm A, ed. Microcirurgia Naso-Sinusal. Rio de Janeiro: Revinter, 1995:79–89.
103. Brook I, Yocum P. Antimicrobial management of chronic sinusitis in children. J Laryngol Otol 1995; 109:1159–1162.
104. Jiang RS, Hsu CY. Bacteriology of chronic sinusitis after ampicillin therapy. Am J Rhinol 1997; 11:467–471.
105. Shoseyov D, Bibi H, Shai P, Shoseyov N, Shasaberg G, Hurvitz H. Treatment with hypertonic saline versus normal saline nasal wash of pediatric chronic sinusitis. J Allergy Clin Immunol 1998; 101:602–605.
106. Barlan IB, Erkan E, Bakir M, Berrak S, Basaran MM. Intranasal budesonide spray as an adjunct to oral antibiotic therapy for acute sinusitis in children. Ann Allergy Asthma Immnol 1997; 78:598–601.
107. Jirapongsanaruruk O, Vichyanond P. Nasal cytology in the diagnosis of allergic rhinitis in children. Ann Allergy Asthma Immunol 1998; 80:165–170.
108. Meltzer E, Nolop K, Mesarina-Wicki B. A dose-ranging study mometasone furoate aqueous spray in children with seasonal allergic rhinitis. Allergy Suppl 1997; 37:136.
109. Pelikan Z. The role of allergy in sinus disease of children and adults. Clin Rev Allergy Clin Immunol 1998; 16:55–156.
110. Brannan MD, Herron JM, Affrime MB. Safety and tolerability of once-daily mometasone furoate aqueous nasal spray in children. Clin Ther 1997; 19:1330–1339.
111. McCormick DP, John SD, Swischuk LE, Uchida T. A double-blind placebo-controlled trial of decongestant-antihistamine for the treatment of sinusitis in children. Clin Pediatr (Phila) 1996; 35:457–460.
112. Lusk RP. The surgical management of chronic sinusitis in children. Pediatr Ann 1998; 27:820–827.
113. Poole MD. Pediatric endoscopic sinus surgery: the conservative view. Ear Nose Throat J 1994; 73:221–227.
114. Wang D, Duyck F, Smitz J, Clement P. Efficacy and onset of action of fluticasone propionate aqueous nasal spray on nasal symptoms, eosinophil count, and mediator release after nasal allergen challenge in patients with seasonal allergic rhinitis. Allergy 1998; 53:375–382.

115. Freitas EB, Lessa HA. Exame otorrinolaringológico da criança. In: Sih T, ed. Otorrinolaringologia Pediátrica. Rio de Janeiro: Revinter, 1998:14–16.
116. Hebert RL, Bent JP. Meta-analysis of outcome of pediatric functional endoscopic sinus surgery. Laryngoscope 1998; 108:796–799.
117. Rohr AS, Spector SL, Siegel SC. Correlation between A mode ultra sound and radiography in diagnosis of maxillary sinusitis. J Allergy Clin Immunol 1986; 2:58–61.
118. Shapiro GG, Furukawa CT, Plerson WE. Blinded comparison of maxillary sinus radiography and ultrasound for diagnosis of sinusitis. J Allergy Clin Immunol. 1986; 77:59–64.
119. McAlister WH, Lusk R, Muntz HR. Comparison of plain radiographs and coronal CT scans in infants and children with recurrent sinusitis. AJR Am J Roentgenol 1989; 153:1259–1264.
120. Som PM, Shapiro MD, Biller HF. Sinonasal tumors and inflammatory tissues: differentiation with MR imaging. Radiology 1988; 167:803–808.
121. Mendonça RA, Haetinger RG, Gomes ACP. Ressonância Magnética do Nariz, Seios Paranasais e Estruturas Correlatas. In: Stamm A, ed. Microcirurgia Naso-Sinusal. Rio de Janeiro: Revinter, 1995:90–100.
122. Gillespie MB, O'Malley BW Jr, Francis HW. An approach to fulminant invasive fungal rhinosinusitis in the immunocompromised host. Arch Otolaryngol Head Neck Surg 1998; 124:520–526.

18

Chronic Rhinosinusitis—A Medical or Surgical Disease?

DAVID S. PARSONS

Pediatric Otolaryngology and Sinus Care, Greenville, South Carolina, USA

MARCELLA BOTHWELL

University of Missouri, Columbia, Missouri, USA

Today's progressive pediatric community asks a popular question, "What is the best *state of the art* therapy for rhinosinusitis?" Currently, children are taken to the operating room for pediatric functional endoscopic sinus (FES) surgery when "maximal medical therapy has failed." A fair question to ask a surgeon is "What is maximal medical therapy?" After this chapter defines the mechanism of pediatric chronic rhinosinusitis, it will challenge the reader to find a more thoughtfully considered definition of rhinosinusitis and its treatment. The next pertinent question to be considered, "Is rhinosinusitis a medical or surgical disease?"

In the mid-1980s, the senior author concluded that chronic rhinosinusitis was clearly a surgical disease. This conclusion was made after having dealt with a worldwide patient population of military dependents. Large numbers of cases were referred for FES surgery and the waiting line for surgery was upwards of 2 years. For these waiting children, a plan of action had to be made. A medical treatment plan was developed in the interim before scheduled FES surgery. Despite long-term broad-spectrum antibiotic therapy offered as either chronic courses of full dose or prophylactic schedules, continuous two to four times per day nasal steroids, and nasal irrigation with various solutions, these children met nearly everyone's criteria for failed maximal medical therapy. To the author, this clearly was a sign for surgical intervention and substantiated the idea that chronic rhinosinusitis was a surgical disease (1).

Based on the described pathophysiology of rhinosinusitis, sinus disease was at that time, considered primarily an infectious disease. However, given the authors' *further* experience, it has been determined that rhinosinusitis is *not* a primary bacteriologic infection. The primary etiology is nasal mucosal edema with the resultant bacterial infection being a secondary factor.

Many articles regarding acute, subacute, and chronic sinusitis have shown multiple different pathogens. The articles' basic premise is that rhinosinusitis is an infectious disease. However, cultures of chronic rhinosinusitis do not show the same well-defined pure growth patterns of pathogens as do acute and subacute sinus infection cultures (2,3). Anaerobic cultures have shown a variability of 2–100% (3–8). One otolaryngic surgeon found an enormous assortment of bacterial isolates in his prospective study. He was so discouraged about not getting any well-defined trends that he thought his work would not be accepted for publication (A. Lenis, personal communication, 1995). The inconsistent isolation of bacterial isolates further questions bacterial infection as the primary etiology of rhinosinusitis. Many studies considering the microbiology of sinus disease with samples collected endoscopically have not been quantitated and are difficult to interpret. Variation could be attributed to the method of collection or laboratory technique. It also may show that the initiating etiology of rhinosinusitis, in fact, may not be infectious but rather the primary underlying cause may be investigated as some other etiology of sinonasal mucosal edema. Antibiotic regiments may be directed at a secondary infection, an opportunistic infection, or no infection at all, ignoring the inciting cause or causes of the child's chronic disease.

I. The Work-up

The similarity of work-up of children with significant recurrent or chronic ear disease and recurrent or chronic rhinosinusitis is remarkable (9). The singular common cause is mucosal edema. The two most common etiologies are upper respiratory viral infection (URI) and allergy. While eliminating URI exposure from daycare centers when one or both parents work is unpractical, families should be directed toward smaller daycare facilities, whenever possible.

Allergies persist as a common problematic cause of sinonasal edema. Parsons and Phillips (10) reported that 80% of their pediatric FES operative cases had positive skin testing to inhalant allergy. Yeoh (11) reported similar results with 77% of children presenting for evaluation of chronic rhinosinusitis having a positive study to inhalant allergies, while 97% of the same patients had positive evaluations for food allergy. Intradermal provocation food tests were used to test food allergy prevalence. While the contribution of food allergy to ear or sinus disease has not been proven, toddlers with either recurrent otitis media or otitis media with effusion and milk allergy often show significant improvement with simple elimination diet. Given the allergic contribution to chronic and recurrent ear and sinus disease, the authors routinely test for inhalant and food allergy and offer appropriate management with follow-up before consideration of surgical intervention.

Parsons and Phillips (10) also showed that 13% of the children they evaluated had a negative allergy history but the skin testing was positive. Because of the high occurrence of allergic disease in sinus patients, an allergy evaluation should be obtained on every patient, who is unresponsive to initial medical management, regardless if the history is positive for allergy.

Anyone who has done skin testing on children would recognize its difficulty. While intradermal testing is felt to be the most sensitive, Pharmacia CAP (ImmunoCAP), an *in vitro* blood study is accurate to within 5–8% of the intradermal tests (12,13). The ImmunoCAP is an effective screen for both food and inhalant allergies.

Environmental irritants such as smoke exposure, either primary or second hand, should be evaluated in children with recurrent or recalcitrant ear or sinus disease. While the "smoking habit" is recognized as difficult to stop, families must understand the damaging effect of environmental secondary smoke on their children. Products of the tobacco settle into caregiver's clothing and hair, and into couches, carpets, carseats, etc. The playful child stirs up these products and inhales them even when the smokers are not present. Preadolescent and teen patients should be questioned if they are smoking or if their friends smoke around them. In daycare facilities, workers should be regarded as potential sources of second-hand smoke and should be asked regarding their smoking habits. Improved environment has had a profound positive effect on many of our young patients.

The differential diagnosis must also include primary or secondary immunodeficiency in a child with recurrent or chronic sinus disease. Initial testing can include total immunoglobulins (IgA, IgM, and IgG). IgG subclass deficiency is identified with more frequency but also may show inconsistent results. Many allergists no longer recommend obtaining this study because the therapy may be worse than the deficiency (14,15).

Gastroesophageal reflux disease (GERD) or extra esophageal reflux (EER) has been found to be a common important cause for sinus disease in children and is under investigation regarding its contribution to ear disease (16,17). The startling discovery of reflux as a cause of sinusitis in both children and adults has led to increased interest in how to diagnose and treat this problem. While the idea of refluxed acids reaching into the nose without the patient's awareness seems improbable, studies have demonstrated that this regularly occurs in GERD patients. Most children have silent reflux and do not have symptoms directly attributable to GERD such as heartburn, frequent emesis, or regurgitation and may present with such nonspecific signs as stomach upset. Silent reflux is a well-described condition in children and its manifestations are generally found in the upper and lower airway (18).

The acid results in nasal edema, which closes sinus ostia. The secondary growth of bacterial flora in the sinuses gives the illusion of a primary disease. However, long-term therapy must address the reflux of acids.

Chronic illnesses, such as cystic fibrosis (CF) and primary ciliary dyskinesia, must always be considered and evaluated if appropriate. Not all children with CF have significant malabsorption problems. Some CF children may not be thin, and may even be overweight as to confuse the investigator!

The presence of a large adenoid pad should be investigated if the work-up is negative, or evaluations are found to be positive but directed therapy is still inadequate. The signs and symptoms of nasal obstruction due to adenoid hypertrophy can often mimic the presenting symptoms of rhinosinusitis, especially if allergies are also present. Adenoidectomy is always considered as a separate surgical step *prior* to consideration of FES surgery in young children. If adenoidectomy fails to resolve sinus complaints, the child is observed while remaining on all appropriate medical therapies. If sinus symptoms persist an evaluation for FES surgery may be indicated.

II. Radiographic Evaluation

Generations of physicians have used plain X-rays to demonstrate mastoiditis or sinusitis. Many children with acute otitis media show mucosal edema in the mastoid air cells on plain mastoid films. However, radiographically precise anatomic landmarks often cannot be read. The ostiomeatal complex (OMC) which is a discrete drainage site of the paranasal sinuses is also not visible on routine four-view sinus series X-rays (Waters, Caldwell, lateral, submental, vertex). Obstructive locations are masked because of the bony overlay of the nasal bones in the Waters view and the petrous apex in the Caldwell view. Consequently, sinus series, particularly in children, are frequently misread. They are inconsistent, unreliable and often misleading (19,20).

The gold standard radiographic study is the computed tomography (CT) for determining the presence of mucosal inflammation or bony abnormalities of the mastoids, middle ear, or paranasal sinuses. A CT scan will even demonstrate the presence of minor mucosal edema, which occurs frequently as an isolated finding in the OMC or other paranasal sinuses. The clinical significance of this finding must be correlated with the patient's symptoms and whether or not there has been a recent URI (21). The physician and surgeon should remember that the CT scan is simply a snapshot of the patient at the particular moment. Sinus membranes are dynamic and constantly changing except in three situations: (1) fungal sinusitis, (2) mucopyoceles, and (3) CF. Remember the nasal cycle, which decongests and swells, cycles with the turbinates multiple times each day. In a patient with GERD, allergies, or a URI, the nasal cycle will appear more intense, improperly suggesting "sinus disease" when in fact the primary problems are multifactorial and not bacterial disease.

Caution should also be used when interpreting CTs, as >60% of all pediatric CTs will, in children, show a "surgically correctable" problem. More recently, CT scans of children scheduled for FES surgery vs. CT scans of children with no obvious rhinosinusitis symptoms were compared. Authors report that Lund-MacKay scores greater than 5 has an excellent predictive value of "true disease" (22). A Lund-MacKay score less than or equal to 2 had an excellent negative predictive value of "true disease." However, children should not be subjected to multiple CT scans for only diagnosis. History of signs and symptoms should dictate timing of CT scan in planning for FES surgery.

The extent of surgery also should not be determined based of the CT scan except in the three static situations listed above. In the vast majority of children needing sinus mini FES surgery will be adequate and effective.

Two major types of anatomic abnormalities are found on the CT scan in patients with recurrent acute or chronic paranasal sinus disease: bony and/or mucosal. Bony abnormalities include structural defects that may block of the infundibulum or other sites. These are listed in Table 18.1. Specifically directed surgery toward these bony anatomic variations in the paranasal sinuses often can be treated effectively with specifically directed functional sinus surgery (not aggressive total sphenoethmoidectomies). However, such abnormalities may actually be coincidental and not be the problem.

Mucosal abnormalities may coexist with any bony abnormalities. Causes of mucosal edema are listed in Table 18.2. Without proper management of the primary etiology of sinonasal mucosal edema, even optimal FES surgery can fail. The goal of sinus treatment should be to control sinus symptoms to a reasonable level without subjecting the child to unnecessary morbidity.

CT should be obtained after the child has had maximal medical management. Medical management is determined based on history and physical exam

Table 18.1 Anatomic Abnormalities Found in Patients with Recurrent Acute or Chronic Paranasal Sinus Disease

Air cell within the turbinate (concha bulla)
Air cell within the uncinate process (uncinate bulla)
Paradoxical curve to the middle turbinate compressing the infundibulum
Hypoplasia of the uncinate process
Hypoplasia of the maxillary sinus
Enlarged infraorbital cell obstructing maxillary sinus drainage
Enlarged supraorbital or frontal cell obstructing frontal sinus drainage
Enlarged agger nasi cell producing impairment of drainage of the frontal sinus
Deviated nasal septum
Craniofacial abnormality affecting the paranasal sinuses

Table 18.2 Causes of Mucosal Edema

Recurrent URI
Nasal or systemic allergies (inhalant/food)
Gastroesophageal reflux disease
Vasomotor rhinitis
Cystic fibrosis
Environmental irritants (secondary smoke,
  rhinitis medicamentosa including nasal
  cocaine abuse, etc.)
Primary or secondary immunodeficiency
Primary ciliary dyskinesia
Adenoid hypertrophy

findings. The CT is used as a road map for surgery and should not be obtained if the child responds to medical management (23). If the child fails to respond to 4 weeks of maximal medical management, then CT should be obtained. CT is generally obtained while the child is still in the last week of therapy. An obvious exception would be signs of acute orbital or central nervous system complications for which a CT should be obtained immediately. Even if significant signs of subacute or chronic rhinosinusitis are observed, it is not necessarily an absolute indication for FES surgery.

III. Medical Management

All the previous medical evaluations are considered essential for the maximal medical work-up. Rhinosinusitis is demonstrated to be a complex multifactorial disease. The key to effective treatment of pediatric chronic rhinosinusitis is to diagnose and treat all the possible etiologies of rhinosinusitis (14,24). Rarely does a child present with only one apparent etiology.

While initial therapy includes a broad-spectrum antibiotic, this should not be the only treatment. The sinonasal edema must be addressed. Buffered hypertonic nasal saline used several times per day has been shown to be effective in reducing sinonasal edema (25). Buffered hypertonic nasal saline has been used by thousands of patients over the world and has been shown to be safe and effective. (see Tables 18.3–18.5)

Children start using a small spray bottle, and irrigation should be attempted a minimum of twice a day. Children are slowly conditioned to nasal irrigation by initiating nasal cleansing with a simple nasal spray. Do not be aggressive. As the child becomes more tolerant of the nasal spray, then advance to irrigation. The hypertonicity should be increased over a few weeks from 1–1.5 M to 2–3 M saline. One heaping teaspoon per liter equals approximately 140 mEq or 1 M saline. The irrigation physically cleans the nose and the hypertonicity of the solution actually decongests the sinonasal membranes.

Table 18.3 Salt Water Rinse for the Nose (Buffered Hypertonic Saline Nasal Irrigation)

The benefits
When you rinse your nose with this salt water and baking soda mixture, it washes crusts and other debris from your nose
Salty water pulls fluid out of the swollen membranes of your nose. This decongests the nose and improves airflow. Not only does this make breathing easier, but it also helps open the sinus passages
Studies show that this mixture of concentrated salt water and baking soda (bicarbonate) helps the nose work better and moves mucus out of the nose faster

Mucociliary transport is also enhanced. Studies by Meyer et al. (R. Meyer, personal communication, 1994) demonstrate that mucociliary transport is enhanced 12-fold after irrigation of *in vitro* tracheal mucosa with such a solution. Talbot et al. (25) have shown with saccharin testing that the mucociliary transport is indeed enhanced significantly with this irrigation. The effectiveness of nasal steroids is also improved when sprayed into a nose that has been cleansed and decongested. Commercial preparation and irrigation devices are available in the USA (Bradley Pharmaceuticals, Fairfield, New Jersey).

IV. Surgical Management

When all the previously discussed etiologies of chronic rhinosinusitis have been investigated and appropriate treatments have failed, FES surgery may be indicated. Other indications for FES surgery include resistant organisms in the sinonasal tract. As more bacterial resistance is discovered, FES surgery and

Table 18.4 Salt Water Rinse for the Nose (Buffered Hypertonic Saline Nasal Irrigation)

The recipe
Carefully clean and rinse a $\frac{1}{4}$ of a glass jar (250 cm^3). Fill the clean jar with tap water or bottled water. You do not have to boil the water, unless you live in a place where the water is not adequately treated
Add one heaping teaspoon of "pickling/canning" salt. *Do not* use table salt. Table salt has unwanted additives. You can ask for pickling salt at the grocery store or, in some countries, marine pure salt (no additive)
Add one level teaspoon of baking soda (pure bicarbonate)
Stir or shake before each use. Store at room temperature, in a closed receptacle. After a week, pour out any mixture that is left over and make a new recipe
If the mixture seems *too strong, use less salt*—try $\frac{1}{2}$ teaspoon of salt
For children, it is best to start with a weaker salt water mixture: try $\frac{1}{4}$ to $\frac{1}{3}$ teaspoon of salt. Gradually increase to $\frac{1}{2}$–1 teaspoons of salt, or whatever your child will accept

Table 18.5 How to Rinse the Nose with Salt Water (Buffered Hypertonic Saline Nasal Irrigation)

The instructions

Plan to rinse the nose with the salt–water mixture two to three times each day. Make the salt water and baking soda mixture according to the recipe. You will need a bulb/ear syringe, or a large medical syringe (30 cm³), or a water pik

Pour some salt–water mixture into a clean bowl. Many people like to warm the salt water in a microwave oven to about body temperature. Be sure that the salt water is *not hot*

Fill the syringe with salt water from the bowl. *Do not* put your used syringe back into the jar, because that will contaminate your salt water

Stand over the sink or in the shower and squirt the salt water into each side of your nose. Aim the stream toward the back of your head, *not* the top of your head. This lets you spit some of the salt water out of your mouth. It will not hurt if you swallow a little

Most people notice a mild burning feeling the first few times they use the salt water mixture. This usually goes away in a few days. Please consult your doctor if you have any problems or questions

For young children

You can put the salt water into a small spray container, like an Ocean® spray or nasal steroid spray bottle. Squirt it *many* times into each side of the nose. *Do not force* your child to lie down. It is easier to do when sitting or standing

If you use a nasal steroid: You should *always* use the salt water mixture first, *then* use your nasal steroid spray. The steroid works better when it is sprayed onto nasal membranes that have been cleaned and decongested by the salt water. Then the steroid medicine will reach deeper into the nose and sinuses

---

drainage procedures may be required more often. With frequent use of antibiotics, a growing number of children are developing adverse reactions or allergy to specific antibiotics. Both resistance and antibiotic allergy may become a major problem in the near future and may obligate the need for FES surgery more often. When antibiotic prophylaxis is used it should be a narrow spectrum antibiotic to prevent broad-spectrum coverage resistance (26). If breakthroughs occur, a minimally invasive procedure may be all that is required (27).

Reactive airway disease or asthma may be an additional indication for FES surgery. Despite comprehensive asthma therapy, these children and adults have incapacitating lifestyle limitations. Remember that both asthma and sinusitis may be caused by GERD (16,17).

Contact point headaches can also be incapacitating. If a CT obtained at the end of maximal medical therapy shows contact points, FES surgery with contact point release may be indicated. The point of contact is usually between the turbinates and the septum and should be released endoscopically (28).

The most common indication in these authors' experience for FES surgery in children is revision or failure of one or more previous inadequately preformed sinus operations (29). Either the child's symptoms are no better, or in some cases worse from previous FES surgery. The most common reason for revision is the missed ostium sequence. Facial growth after pediatric FES surgery has not been shown to be significantly affected even ten years after surgery. However, FES surgery has been shown to be safe and effective therapy in many children with recalcitrant rhinosinusitis symptoms (30,31).

In previous years, the authors readily admit to performing FES surgery without the adequate work-up as described previously. Surgical results seemed acceptable. Only after multiple FES surgical failures, did the authors investigate other possible etiologies contributing to surgical failure. After having adopted the thorough medical investigation described, the number of sinus procedures has dramatically been reduced. Almost 90% of our children have avoided FES surgery simply with maximal medical management including acid reflux therapy. The question is again asked, "Is chronic sinusitis a medical or surgical disease?" The authors feel strongly that it is a medical disease. A complete medical evaluation and adequate medical therapy must be offered for each positive finding before FES surgery is considered. However, when a good systematic approach to the child with rhinosinusitis is done and medical therapy has failed, FES surgery is safe and effective.

References

1. Parsons DS. Preface: pediatric sinusitis. Otolaryngol Clin North Am 1996; 29(1):11–25.
2. Wald ER, Milmoe J, Bowen A et al. Acute maxillary sinusitis in children. N Engl J Med 1981; 304:749–754.
3. Wald ER. Diagnosis and management of sinusitis in children. Adv Pediatr Infect Dis 1996; 12:1–20.
4. Brook I. Bacteriologic features of chronic sinusitis in children. J Am Med Assoc 1981; 246:967–969.
5. Carenfelt C, Lundberg C, Nord CE et al. Bacteriology of maxillary sinusitis in relation to quality of the retained secretion. Acta Otolaryngol 1978; 86:298.
6. Frederick J, Braude A. Anaerobic/infection of the paranasal sinuses. N Engl J Med 1974; 290:135–137.
7. Lundberg C, Carenfelt C, Engquist S et al. Anaerobic bacteria in maxillary sinusitis. Scand J Infect Dis 1979; 19(suppl):74–76.
8. Muntz HR, Lusk RP. Bacteriology of the ethmoid bullae in children with chronic sinusitis. Arch Otolaryngol Head Neck Surg 1991; 117:179–181.
9. Parsons DS, Wald E. Otitis media and sinusitis: similar diseases. Otolaryngol Clin North Am 1996; 29(1):11–25.
10. Parsons DS, Phillips SE. Functional endoscopic surgery in children. A retrospective analysis of results. Laryngoscope 1993; 103:889–903.
11. Yeoh HKH. Allergic disease as an etiology of sinusitis. Presented at the International Pediatric Otolaryngology, Head and Neck Surgery Meeting, Singapore, November, 1994.
12. Cook PR. In vivo testing and immunotherapy. Curr Opin Otolaryngol Head Neck Surg 1994; 2:118–127.

13. Williams PB, Dolen WK, Koepke JW et al. Comparison of skin testing and three in vitro assays for specific IgE in the clinical evaluation of immediate hypersensitivity. Ann Allergy 1992; 68:34–45.

14. Cook PR, Nishoika GJ. Allergic rhinosinusitis in the pediatric population. Otolaryngol Clin North Am 1996; 29(1):39–56.

15. King WP, Notes JM. The intracutaneous progressive dilution multi-foot test. Otolaryngol Head Neck Surg 1991; 104:235–323.

16. Barbero GJ. Gastroesophageal reflux and upper airway disease: a comentary. Otolaryngol Clin North Am 1996; 29(1):27–38.

17. Bothwell MR, Parsons DS, Barbero GJ, Talbot A, Wilder B. Outcome of gastroesophageal reflux on pediatric sinusitis. Otolaryngol Head Neck Surg 1999; 121(3):255-262.

18. Burton DM, Pransky SM, Katz RM et al. Pediatric airway manifestations of gastroesophageal reflux. Ann Otol Rhinol Laryngol 1992; 101:742–749.

19. Diament MJ, Senac MO Jr, Gilsanz V et al. Prevalence of incidental paranasal sinus opacification in pediatric patients: a CY study. J Comput Assist Tomogr 1987; 11:426–431.

20. McAllister WH, Lusk R, Muntz H. Comparison of plain radiographs and coronal CT scans in infants and children with recurrent sinusitis. AJR Am J Roentgenol 1989; 153:1259–1264.

21. Gwaltney JM Jr, Phillips CD, Miller RD et al. Computed tomographic study of the common cold. N Engl J Med 1994; 330:25–30.

22. Bhattacharya N, Jones DT, Hill M, Shapiro NL. The diagnostic accuracy of computed tomography in pediatric chronic rhinosinusitis. Arch Otolaryngol Head Neck Surg 2004; 130(9):1029–1032.

23. Havas TE, Motbey JA, Gullane PJ. Prevalence of incidental abnormalities on computed tomographic scans of the paranasal sinuses. Arch Otolarynol Head Neck Surg 1998; 114:856–859.

24. Clement PAR, Bluestone CD, Gordts F, Lusk RP, Otten FWA, Goossens H, Scadding GK, Takahashi H, Louk van Buchem F, Van Couwenberge P. Management of rhinosinusitis in children. Arch Otolaryngol Head Neck Surg 1998; 124.

25. Talbot AR, Parsons DS. The effect on intranasal mucocilary transit times following buffered hypertonic irrigation. Submitted for publication.

26. Gandhi A, Brodsky L, Ballow M. Benefits of antibiotic prophylaxis in children with chronic sinusitis: assessment of outcome predictors. Allergy Proc 1993; 14:37–43.

27. Setliff RC. Minimally invasive sinus surgery. The rational and the technique. Otolaryngol Clin North Am 1996; 29(1):115–130.

28. Parson DS, Batra PS. Functional endoscopic sinus surgical outcomes for contact point headaches. Laryngoscope 1998; 108.

29. Parsons DS, Setliff RC III, Chambers D. Special considerations in pediatric functional endoscopic sinus surgery. Oper Tech Otolaryngol Head Neck Surg 1994; 5(1):40–42.

30. Lusk RP, Muntz HR. Endoscopic sinus surgery in children with chronic sinusitis: a pilot study. Laryngoscope 1990; 100:654–658.

31. Talbot AR. Frontal sinus surgery in children. Otolaryngol Clin North Am 1996; 29(1):143–158.

32. Parsons DS. Chronic sinusitis: a medical or surgical disease? Otolaryngol Clin North Am 1996; 29(1):1–9.

19

Rhinosinusitis in Immunodeficient Children

PAOLA MARCHISIO and NICOLA PRINCIPI

University of Milan,
Milan, Italy

I. Primary Immunodeficiency

Despite technological advances in prenatal and early postnatal diagnosis for genetically inherited immunodeficient diseases, most primary or congenital immunodeficiencies continue to be clinically detected because of recurrent, or unusually chronic infections. Among these, rhinosinusitis, which has been recognized as a source of infection in healthy children, plays a major role. Children with cystic fibrosis, ciliary dyskinesia syndrome (which includes Kartagener's syndrome), and immunoglobulin deficiencies frequently present with radiographic evidence of chronic sinus disease (1,2).

In most of these patients the types of organisms cultured from the sinuses are similar to those associated with acute and subacute sinusitis in normal children, such as *Streptococcus pneumoniae*, nontypable *Haemophilus influenzae*, and *Moraxella catarrhalis*. Moreover, viruses such as parainfluenzae and adenovirus may be co-responsible for the disease.

In particular, in children with cystic fibrosis, in whom prevalence of sinusitis approaches 100%, two distinct patterns of sinus disease have been recently described: chronic sinusitis and polyposis. Children with chronic sinusitis present with headache as major complaint, while those with polyposis suffer nasal obstruction alone unless a mucocele is associated. After surgical treatment a significant and long-term improvement in symptoms can be observed.

II. Secondary Immunodeficiency Syndromes

Among children with secondary immunodeficiency syndromes, those with human immunodeficiency virus (HIV) infection are quantitatively the most important and qualitatively the best studied. HIV infection has become a progressively severe problem in the last 15 years and nowadays affects millions of people.

In the last few years attention has been given not only to the main problems related with HIV infection, such as wasting syndrome and opportunistic infections, but also to minor manifestations of the disease, such as sinusitis. Recurrent sinusitis has been described in adults infected with HIV. In prospective studies 25–30% of HIV infected outpatients presented with at least one episode of sinusitis. In HIV infected adults sinusitis appears to be severe, to involve multiple sinuses, to respond only incompletely to antibiotic therapy and to be associated with a worsening of the immunodeficiency, characterized by a decline of CD4+ lymphocyte counts. However, recently Belafsky et al. (3) have demonstrated that sinusistis is not associated with an increased hazard of death; this may have implications for treatment, because a diagnosis of sinusitis does not portend a poor prognosis in individuals infected with HIV. Moreover, sinusitis in adult AIDS patients may involve less common organisms, such as *Pseudomonas aeruginosa*, in addition to common pathogens.

In HIV infected children, contrarily to what happens in adults, infections with bacteria that are serious and recurrent occur frequently and are one of the most common manifestations and complications of the complex syndrome related to HIV. While infections such as otitis media and pneumonia have been quite extensively studied, little attention has been given for a long time to sinusitis. The lack of information has been recently solved by a work conducted during a multicenter clinical trial on intravenous immunoglobulin carried out by the National Institute of Child Health in the USA. This study, while monitoring a cohort of hundreds of children, was aimed to get data on the clinical presentation, radiological, laboratory and treatment characteristics of sinusitis in HIV infected children (4).

To face the problem of sinusitis in these subjects, we have to answer a lot of questions. The first question concerns the frequency of the disease. In normal children sinusitis complicates 5–10% of upper respiratory infections (which occur six to eight times annually) (5). In the already quoted cohort of HIV infected children 16% of subjects had sinusitis at some time during the study. In one-third of the patients sinusitis was a recurrent problem: 67% of the children had a single episode, 20% had two episodes, 13% had between three and five episodes. Sinusitis was the fourth most frequent infection described in this cohort, exceeded only by otitis, pneumonia, and skin infections.

The second question regards the possibility to predict sinusitis in HIV infected children on the basis of clinical characteristics. The characteristics at study entry of the children who had one or more sinusitis episodes were generally similar to those of the children who did not have sinusitis. Children with sinusitis were slightly older than those who did not have sinusitis and in the vast majority had full blown disease (only 13% were asymptomatic but with some degree of immunosuppression) although the CD4+ cell counts were similar in the two groups.

The diagnosis was based on the combination of clinical symptoms and diagnostic roentgenograms. In HIV infected children the most commonly reported symptoms were persistent (>7 days) nasal discharge (67.4%) and nocturnal and persistent (>7 days) cough (54.7%). The mean duration of nasal discharge and cough before diagnosis were 17 days (range from 3 to 90 days) and 19 days (range from 3 to 90 days). Symptoms were thus more frequent than those recently reported in a cohort of normal children, in whom nasal discharge was reported in about 40% of the cases. It is important to focus on the fact that most children did not present fever and that symptoms more specific for acute sinusitis, such as facial pain and periorbital swelling, were reported less frequently.

Laboratory markers of infections were not altered in most of the cases: most episodes were not associated with leukocytosis (total WBC counts of <10,000/mmc and <15,000/mmc in 73% and 91% of the episodes). In addition, most episodes were not associated with granulocytosis.

In this study CT scanning was performed only in less than 10% of the episodes. In about two-thirds of the patients sinusitis involved only a single sinus, while in one-third it involved two sinuses. The maxillary and ethmoidal sinuses, which are the most aerated in young children, were the most frequently involved. However, the radiological aspect was identical to what is found in normal children.

The overall clinical impression of the observed sinusitis episodes was that of a more chronic indolent process rather than an acute bacterial infection accompanied by systemic toxicity. The most commonly reported symptoms were nonspecific and subacute, often being present for more than 1 month before diagnosis. This would suggest that sinusitis should be looked for in HIV infected children and that radiographs should be performed more frequently.

Another question concerns the etiology of sinusitis. Invasive diagnostic procedures (such as sinus aspiration) are only rarely performed. No systematic studies documenting the microbiology of sinusitis in children or adults infected with HIV are available. However, it is likely that, as documented for acute otitis media, HIV infected children become infected with the same organisms that usually infect immunocompetent hosts (6).

As a consequence, treatment is usually recommended taking into account the known pathogens of sinusitis. In the study of Mofenson et al. (4) most children received a single antibiotic (70%) and about three-fourths were administered orally. Multiple antibiotics (most of which were orally administered) were required for treatment of 29% of the episodes, with 6% of episodes requiring three of more medications. As the response to the treatment was relatively good and substantially similar to that reported for normal children, this supports the hypothesis of a similar etiology of sinusitis.

However, it must be remembered that other, uncommon, organisms have been documented to cause (rarely) sinusitis in HIV infected patients: *S. aureus*, *S. epidermidis*, fungi (in particular *C. albicans*), and Mycobacteria (including *M. avium-intracellulare* and *Kansasii*). Thus, in the presence of an immunodeficient host it is rational to administer initially the same antibiotic which would be chosen for an immunocompetent child, being aware of the possibility of another etiology if the response to treatment is not prompt. Amoxicillin (90 mg/kg per day in two doses) is recommended for most initial and uncomplicated cases of sinusitis. If improvement is not evident within 48–72 h, if the sinusitis is complicated (e.g., episodes associated with development of high fever or periorbital swelling), a broader-spectrum oral antimicrobial should be given. No large comparative studies of broad-spectrum antibiotics in immunocompromised children have been performed. When treating patients who have presented with long-standing symptoms (months rather than weeks) antimicrobial selection should include agents active against *S. aureus* and respiratory anaerobes. It is recommended that therapy be extended for at least 1 week beyond the resolution of all respiratory symptoms, thus 4 weeks of antimicrobial therapy may be required.

No specific suggestions have been made regarding ancillary treatments for immunodeficient children: the same treatments recommended for immunocompetent children can be applied.

When fungal sinusitis is suspected or documented, treatment with amphotericin B is the first choice, remembering that therapy should be instituted in an accelerated schedule to quickly achieve a daily dose of 1 mg/kg. Liposomal amphotericin has been effective in some cases unresponsive to conventional amphotericin B or when the latter has been complicated by deteriorating renal function. The utility of the newer marketed antifungal agents such as fluconazole and itraconazole has yet to be defined (7).

In conclusion, frequently, sinusitis is there in HIV infected children if you look for it. Its good response to treatment can improve the clinical condition of the children.

References

1. Gentile VG, Issacson G. Patterns of sinusitis in cystic fibrosis. Laryngoscope 1996; 106:1005–1009.
2. Marchisio P, Principi N, Sorella S, Sala E, Tornaghi R. Etiology of acute otitis media in human immunodeficiency virius-infected children. Pediatr Infect Dis J 1996; 15:58–61.

3. Belafsky PC, Amedee R, Moore B, Kissinger PJ. The association between sinusitis and survival among individuals affected with the human immunodeficiency virus. Am J Rhinol 2001; 15:343–345.

4. Mofenson LM, Korelitz J, Pelton S, Moye J, Nugent R, Bethel J. Sinusitis in children infected with human immunodeficiency virus: clinical characteristics, risk factors and prophyalxis. Clin Infect Dis 1995; 21:1175–1181.

5. Stokes DC, Bozeman PM. Sinopulmonary infections in immunocompromised infants and children. In: Patrick CC, ed. Infections in Immunocompromised Infants and Children. Churchill Livingstone Inc., 1992:357–375.

6. Wald ER. Diagnosis and management of sinusitis in children. Adv Pediatr Infect Dis 1996; 12:1–20.

7. Wald ER, Dashefsky B. Otitis media and sinusitis in patients with HIV infection. In: Pizzo PA, Wilfert CM, eds. Pediatric AIDS. 3rd ed. Williams & Wilkins, 1998:127–137.

20

Chronic Cough in Children

ELIZABETH ARAÚJO

Brazilian Society of Rhinology,
Porto Alegre, Brazil

BRUNO CARLOS PALOMBINI

Federal University of Rio Grande do Sul,
Porto Alegre, Brazil

**MARIA CAROLINA GOUVEIA MIORIM,
DAYSE CARNEIRO ALT, and CARLOS OLIVEIRA PALOMBINI**

Federal University of Rio Grande do Sul,
Porto Alegre, Brazil

Cough accounts for 2.5% of the total number of annual medical visits in the USA, and persistence of cough is the main reason for seeing the doctor (1,2). Asthma, upper and lower respiratory tract infections, and gastroesophageal reflux (GER) are the most common causes of acute and chronic cough in children (3–13).

The definition of chronic cough is arbitrary, but it is usually described as a persistent cough or a cough that recurs for over 3 weeks. This duration excludes mostly self-limiting and uncomplicated viral respiratory tract infections. Physicians and patients become very anxious because cough is almost always an unspecific manifestation of different diseases, with variable severity.

Therefore, chronic cough becomes a diagnostic challenge due to the absence of specific, easily performed tests. However, a complete rational assessment is required to investigate this complaint, in order to avoid expensive and needless tests (1,7).

I. Pathophysiology

Cough is not an autonomous disease, but represents an important manifestation of upper or lower airway diseases (1).

As a voluntary act or an involuntary one, it can remove secretions or any other irritant materials existing in the airways. It is frequently set off by the irritation of receptors located between the pharynx and the terminal bronchioli. It should be recalled that cough receptors are also found in the external ear canal, pharynx, and stomach, because foreign bodies lodged within these structures may cause coughing.

There are several sites where the cough stimulus is located throughout the airways. Psychogenic cough may begin in the central nervous system; other situations causing cough are irritative processes of the pleura, diaphragm, pericardium, and esophagus and the stimulation of Arnold's nerve, that is, the ramus auricularis of vagus nerve (foreign body or cerumen in the external ear) (14).

The afferent impulses pass through the branches of the vagus and glossopharyngeal nerves until the center command of the cough. Later, through the efferent path, the impulses are brought from the cough center, through the vagus, phrenic, and motor nerves located in the medulla to the larynx, chest wall, abdomen, and pelvic floor (1,15). Control to begin or suppress voluntary cough depends on cortical participation (Fig. 20.1).

Coughing can be divided into three stages: (1) deep inspiration; (2) glottal closure, diaphragm relaxation, and contraction of the expiratory muscles; and (3) sudden glottal opening. The pressure and speed of airflow in coughing are very high: the intrathoracic pressure during the second stage gets as high as 300 mmHg and the airflow speed may attain three-fourths of the speed of sound (14,15).

It should be remembered that children with glottal dysfunction or who have undergone tracheostomy present less effective cough.

II. Differential Diagnosis

In most cases, cough presents a self-limited course, but if chronic, it is usually a frustrating problem. The most common causes of chronic cough are viral infections of the upper respiratory tract or hyperreactivity of the airways and gastroesophageal reflux (1,4–6,8,9,11,13). In a retrospective study of 72 children and adolescents above the age of 16, with normal chest X-ray, referred to the

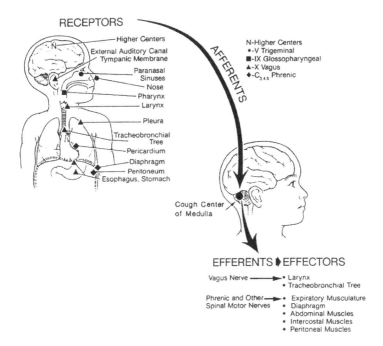

Figure 20.1 Anatomy of the cough reflex arc. The afferent structures include receptors and afferent paths. The cough center is the coordinating locus of the cough. The efferent path carries impulses to the muscles that effect the cough. [Adapted from Ref. (2).]

otorhinolaryngologist due to clinical picture of cough for over 3 weeks, asthma was the most common cause (39%), followed by sinusitis (23%), GER (15%), presence of aberrant innominate artery (12%), psychogenic mechanisms (10%), and subglottal stenosis (7%) (1,4,16). The main causes of chronic cough are summarized in Table 20.1 (1).

Children have an average of six to eight respiratory infections a year. This frequency increases depending on exposure at home and at school. Due to colds that occur in winter, some symptoms may persist for over 2 weeks, resulting in more severe infections and producing chronic cough. Infections of the upper respiratory tract are usually caused by respiratory syncytial virus, parainfluenza virus, rhinovirus, or adenovirus (1).

Although cough may be associated with wheezing and respiratory dysfunction, it should be recalled that chronic cough could be the only manifestation of airway hyperreactivity. The mechanism by which airway reactivity produces cough has not yet been well explained (1,16,17).

It is estimated that approximately 1–5% of the upper respiratory tract infections are complicated by acute infections of the paranasal sinuses (PNS). Postnasal dripping (PND) and chronic cough are prominent clinical findings in

Table 20.1 Causes of Chronic Cough

Most common	
Viral infection of the upper respiratory tract	Chronicity may be caused by recurrent infection
Airway hyperreactivity	Almost always begins due to viral infections
Common	
Allergy	Usually associated with upper airway hyperreactivity
Sinusitis	Postnasal dripping and cough
Irritative	Usually initiated by viral infection or secondary to smoking
Psychogenic	Disappears during sleep
Infections (Chlamydia, pertussis, tuberculosis)	Diagnosis performed by clinical suspicion and specific laboratory tests
Least common	
Foreign body	Most common in children but may occur at all ages
Congenital abnormalities	Tracheoesophageal fistulae, or any structure which could compress the airways

this situation. The PNS most commonly involved during the first year of life are the ethmoidal and maxillary sinuses, followed by the frontal and sphenoid sinuses in the following years (1,18).

Allergic and infectious processes produce obstruction of the PNS ostia and sometimes cause secondary infection. The constant drainage of the sinuses stimulates the receptors and begins the cough process. The microorganisms most commonly responsible for bacterial sinus diseases are *Streptococcus pneumoniae*, *Moraxella catarrhalis*, and *Haemophilus influenza* (1,18).

Obstructive adenoids may cause obliteration at the level of the auditory tube, resulting in otitis; they may also cause secretion stasis, leading to mucosal edema and consequent obstruction of the PNS, and then sinusitis. Sometimes, the PND itself, as well as the allergic status of the patient, can cause adenoiditis. Nasal obstruction and nocturnal snoring also provide additional signs of this clinical picture (19).

Other less common causes may trigger chronic cough. In children aged 1–3 months with cough, tachypnea, and conjunctivitis, the diagnosis of pneumonia due to *Chlamydia* organisms must be considered. Tuberculosis and fungal infections (hystoplasmosis and paracoccidioidomycosis) may produce dry, hoarse cough, because of compression or widening of perihilar nodules. Whooping cough may begin with soft cough and rhinorrhea, progressing to paroxysmal cough (1).

Although more usual in small children, foreign body aspiration may occur at any age and it should always be taken into account when evaluating causes of chronic cough. The presence of a foreign body may also produce dysphagia and airway obstruction, although there have been reports of asymptomatic children. The presence of the foreign body in the lower airway can produce emphysema, atelectasis, and recurring pneumonia. Foreign body mobility can produce paroxysmal cough associated with episodes of cyanosis and stridor, secondary to migration of the foreign body. In some patients, it may lead to airway obstruction with risk of death. The presence of cough with a history of foreign body aspiration requires diagnosis and treatment by rigid bronchoscopy (1,20).

The diseases with involvement of the immune defense of the respiratory tract present with repeated pneumonia and persistent respiratory symptoms. The first manifestation of an immune disorder is often a respiratory infection that persists or recurs immediately after discontinuation of the antibiotic therapy. This may result in the formation of bronchiectasis and infection (1).

The clinical presentation of lymphocytic interstitial pneumonia as a complication of HIV infection is unproductive chronic cough, respiratory dysfunction, pulmonary infiltration, and failure to thrive (1).

Other causes of chronic cough are secondary to a reduction in the clearing mechanism of secretions and foreign bodies located in the respiratory tract. Patients with cystic fibrosis could present cough, delayed growth, and recurring pneumonias. Thick mucus is produced, which is difficult to eliminate from the airway. Respiratory infection by *Pseudomonas* sp. normally accompanies cystic fibrosis. In ciliary dyskinesia, there is an involvement of the mucociliary system, which also results in frequent pulmonary infections. Structural and functional abnormalities of the cilia are observed in primary ciliary dyskinesia, and also in the Kartagener syndrome, an association of sinusitis, bronchiectasis, and "situs inversus" (1).

Congenital abnormalities of the aortic arch and pulmonary artery that compress the trachea and the bronchi may result in cough associated or not with stridor and wheezing (1,4).

Tracheobronchomalacia, alone or associated with aberrant vessels, may cause recurrent cough, which worsens in the presence of lower respiratory tract infections (1,4).

Other congenital lesions, from lung sequestration to bronchogenic cysts, may be asymptomatic or lead to persistent cough due to infection or airway compression. Congenital mediastinal tumors may produce cough and if there is rapid growth or malignant transformation, they may be associated with the compression of other mediastinal structures, causing vocal cord dysfunction or upper vena cava syndrome (4).

It should be borne in mind that acyanotic congenital cardiac diseases can produce chronic cough in children, resulting from bronchial compression by hypertension of the pulmonary artery, widening of the left atrium, or narrowing of the peripheral airway due to pulmonary edema (4,21).

Cardiac lesions which may cause chronic cough associated with wheezing or respiratory distress include ventricular septal defects, patent ductus arteriosus, pulmonary stenosis, and tetralogy of Fallot (4,21).

III. Clinical Presentation and Diagnosis

The assessment of chronic cough in children is similar to the process in adults (7). The precise etiology of the chronic cough can be determined using a diagnostic protocol based on the anatomy of cough receptors and afferent nerves (2,5,6,9,11,13).

A. Diagnostic Protocol (2)

A. History

   Age, characteristics, duration of symptoms, immunizations

B. Physical examination

   Nose, pharynx, larynx, paranasal sinuses, cervical region, chest, ears

C. X-ray

   Chest X-ray (posteroanterior and lateral views)

   Assessment of soft tissues of the cervical region

   Assessment of paranasal sinuses; computed tomography; barium eso-
      phagogram/assessment of the gastrointestinal tract

D. Esophageal scintigraphy

   Assessment of GER

E. Pulmonary function studies (with bronchoprovocation test)

F. Laboratory tests

   Total leukocyte count in blood with differential

   Nasal secretion smear

   Titration of fluorescent antibodies for whooping cough

   Titration for fungi and virus

   Quantitative assessment of immunoglobulins

   Alpha-1-antitripsin dosage

G. Skin tests

   Dosage of electrolytes in the perspiration

   Allergy tests

   PPD

H. Assessments

   Allergist

   Pneumologist

   Infectologist

   Cardiologist

 I. Endoscopy

   Indications

   Severity of symptoms

   Duration of symptoms (over 6–8 weeks)

   History or physical examination suggesting aspiration of foreign body
      or obstructive lesion

   Failure of diagnosing by other methods

J. Complementary studies
    Cultures: bacteria, fungi, virus, *Chlamydia* sp.
    Cytology: eosinophils, macrophages
    Smears: Gram, Giemsa
    Biopsies: H & E, electron microscopy
K. Procedures
    Nasopharyngoscopy: nasal examination
    Laryngoscopy: direct examination, flexible fiberlaryngoscope
    Bronchoscopy: general anesthesia, spontaneous breathing, rigid
        bronchoscope, biopsy, aspiration of secretions
    Esophagoscopy: biopsy

In the clinical history, it is important to identify the duration and nature of the cough, seasonal and circadian variation, and presentation alone or in paroxysms, whether it is nocturnal or diurnal, unproductive or productive. Look for associated symptoms such as a temperature, loss of weight, dyspnea, wheezing, and others (1).

The origin of the cough should be meticulously assessed, including the difference between wheezing and hoarse cough, and the aspect of expectoration. If the child has purulent expectoration, this does not always mean acute infection, since it may be the result of chronic diseases such as sinusitis. The child's position should also be looked at (if the cough appears when in decubitus, or when the child gets up in the morning), the sign of PND, or whether there is a clinical suggestion of GER.

The onset is also an important indication for the identification of its origin, and also associations with the patient's routine. Coughing after eating may occur due to aspiration secondary to gastroesophageal reflux or tracheoesophageal fistula, and night cough may be due to asthma, PND (usually sinusitis), or also GER (1,10). If the cough is productive and occurs in the morning, it may be caused by bronchiectasis or sinusitis. If it occurs after exercises, or in the presence of cold air, it indicates bronchial or pharyngeal hyperreactivity (16,17). The association of cough and wheezing must be investigated, as well as exposure to allergens in the child's daily life: feather pillows, rooms with curtains or carpeting, cats and dogs in the home, etc. Active or passive exposure to smoking should be taken note of (1,4,10).

Research must also be done regarding foreign body aspiration, allergies, sleep disorders (snoring and apnea), and history of medications (1,10).

Other essential data pertaining to the history are those that refer to the child's immunizations (especially for whooping cough) and family history of cystic fibrosis, tuberculosis, allergy, asthma, bronchitis, and chronic cough (1,4,10).

Some types of cough are also characteristic of certain diseases, such as a barking cough, indicating whooping cough or viral croup. Through family members, the child's daily activities should be assessed, and whether coughing occurs during mealtimes. Intense coughing secondary to pneumothorax and cough syncope should be considered, and also headaches, visual disorders, paresthesias, and tremors in the case of neurological disorders (10).

At physical examination, growth and signs of general wellness may be important indications of severity or chronicity of the cough. Other aspects of the examination are also similar to those of the adult, but attention must be given to the presence of chest deformity, increased anteroposterior diameter, pectus excavatum or *P. carinatum*, Harrison's groove, and digital hippocratism (10).

Before the request for new laboratory tests, all results of previous tests should be reviewed, in order to avoid unnecessary repetitions. For instance, in a child with a history of chronic cough provoked by the usual precipitants of asthma crisis, or with a history compatible with asthma without other symptoms, in the presence of normal physical examination, a laboratory assessment may be considered dispensable (4,10,16,17).

The chest X-ray will yield more information when performed in stabilized patients. If there is suspicion of the presence of a foreign body, inspiratory, expiratory, and decubitus X-ray studies could be useful in younger children. Fluoroscopy will be helpful if the foreign body occludes a larger-caliber respiratory pathway. Fiberbronchoscopy provides more information in highly suspected cases, although rigid bronchoscopy is essential as a therapeutic maneuver when there is a history compatible with foreign body aspiration. This examination is also useful when specimens are desired for a microbiological examination of secretions or studies of cilia structure and motility. A barium swallow study helps detect GER, foreign body in the esophagus, tracheoesophageal fistula, chronic aspiration, vascular abnormalities or masses which lead to extrinsic compression of the airways (1,4–6,10,11).

The relationship between PND and sinusitis is not so clear in children, as compared with adults. Changes in the PNS X-rays are often seen in banal infections of the upper respiratory tract, and it frequently shows changes in individuals with no history and physical examination compatible with sinusitis. On the other hand, a normal X-ray does not exclude PNS disorders, therefore its use presents limitations. Other techniques, such as computed tomography of the paranasal sinuses, fiberoptic rhinoscopy, or MRI could also be useful to help the diagnosis (1,4,18,22).

Posterior rhinoscopy, nasopharyngoscopy, and profile X-rays of the nasopharynx confirm the diagnosis of adenoiditis or hyperplasia of the adenoids (19).

The history of sinusitis and recurring pneumonias should lead to nasal biopsy in order to exclude primary ciliary dyskinesia (1).

Pulmonary function tests can be performed in most children from the age of 7 and, occasionally, in smaller children. Spirometry with pharmacodynamic tests using a bronchodilator could help in the diagnosis of variant cough in bronchial asthma. In younger children, an alternative to spirometry is the institution of a therapeutic test using a (β-adrenergic) bronchodilator associated with cromoglycate or an inhaled steroid, followed by clinical observation. Pulmonary function tests are often normal in children with chronic cough as a manifestation of asthma (4,10,12,16,17).

If there is suspicion of infection of the lower airways, a sputum specimen, if possible, should be obtained for direct examination and culture tests, including the study of alcohol-acid fast bacillus and staining for fungi, if indicated. A nasal swab could help diagnose of *Mycoplasma*, whooping cough, or *Chlamydia*. The tuberculin test must be requested when there is chronic cough in a child who did not receive BCG vaccine and without another established diagnosis. Complete blood counts are rarely useful. Serum immunoglobulin dosage could be helpful when there is recurrent pneumonia. The sweat test for cystic fibrosis should be requested even when the diagnosis is remotely considered (4,10). See the algorithm for evaluation of chronic cough (1) (Fig. 20.2).

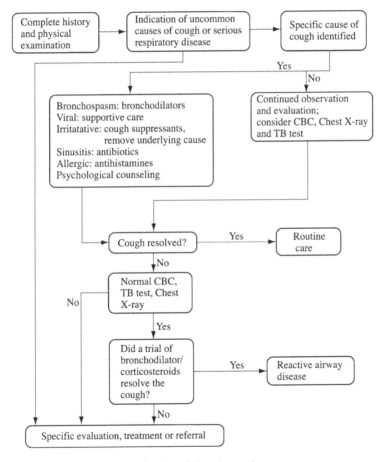

Figure 20.2 Algorithm for evaluation of chronic cough.

IV. Treatment

Chronic cough in infants and children is best managed when its precise etiology can be determined and the specific treatment instituted, a management similar to that employed for adults (2,10). When the performed treatment is not effective, it means that the cough is being undertreated, the family or the patient did not comply with the treatment, the diagnosis or therapy incorrect, or there is more than one cause involved (2,9,12,13).

The treatment of symptoms of chronic cough is rarely necessary when its specific cause is treated (2).

The role of empirical treatment in the differential diagnosis of chronic cough has not been strictly studied. Even so, it is reasonable to consider it when PND or bronchial hyperreactivity (BHR) or GER is very likely, and if tests considered gold standard (paranasal sinuses CT scan, bronchial and pharyngeal provocation tests, and 24-h esophageal pH-monitoring) are not available or cannot be performed. Empirical treatment, appropriately chosen for PND or BHR, should begin to produce a favorable response in 1 week, whereas for GER this period may be extended to 2–3 months (10,22).

As previously mentioned, a favorable response to specific therapy for PND with resolution of the cough is a crucial stage to confirm its etiological participation in the cough. The combination of first-generation antihistamines and decongestants is considered the single most effective form of treatment in most patients with PND unrelated to sinusitis (4).

The diagnosis of sinusitis is usually made from the persistence of nonspecific findings already described. If the history and physical examination are compatible with this diagnosis, antibiotic therapy can be instituted. The first choice for uncomplicated cases is amoxicillin, although second-generation cephalosporins and combined agents such as amoxicillin–potassium clavulanate could be considered when there is a high prevalence of β-lactam-resistant microorganisms.

In cases of GER, general measures should be taken (raising the head of the bed by 12–15 cm, abstaining from fatty meals, coffee, tea, tea mate, chocolate, etc.), and in children who are malnourished due to excessive regurgitation of food, caloric density and frequency of meals should be increased, reducing their volume (23). If esophagitis and chest pain are the main symptoms, aggressive treatment by omeprazole or H2 blocker prevent esophageal lesions caused by acid, allowing them to heal. In less intense cases, H2 receptor blockers can be used in association with prokynetics, such as metochlopramide, cisapride, and domperidone (10,13).

In patients with GER associated with tracheoesophageal fistula and esophageal atresia, clinical experience has shown significant improvement after anti-reflux surgery (23).

The treatment of asthma (and also the cough variant of asthma) is better achieved using systemic corticosteroids initially (if the symptoms are more severe), followed by an inhaled agent, or only inhaling in association with β-2-agonists (oral or inhaled) to relieve acute symptoms. Maximum therapeutic response is achieved after 6–8 weeks of inhaled corticoids. The time between discontinuation of treatment and the recurrence of cough is variable, which may not occur (4,16,17).

If the medication prescribed is to be given using nebulizers, care must be taken with the application technique. It is frequently not adequate and the drug remains in the pharynx or is swallowed. The joint use of spacers is mandatory in small children, and must also be considered in older children and adolescents (1,16,17).

Allergic symptoms can be treated with antihistamines, sodium cromoglycate or corticosteroids (1).

Many studies have shown improvement in the cardiopulmonary capacity of asthmatic children after aerobic exercise programs, with or without change in the BHR. Therefore, one must encourage regular physical exercises in these children, and not allow asthma to limit its practice in all cases (15).

Generally speaking, cough induced by viral infection must not be suppressed due to its significant role in removing secretions from the respiratory tree. However, in cases of irritative cough, this only has the function of constantly stimulating the receptors, keeping the child and its parents awake during the night. In these circumstances, the patient can benefit from cough inhibitors. The anticough drugs most widely used with proven efficacy in adults are codeine and dextrometorfane. However, there are no studies that have tested the efficacy and safety of these drugs in children. Expectorants and mucolytics act to modify the composition of respiratory secretion and, therefore, reduce cough, but their efficacy is questionable (1).

In cases of bronchiectasis, respiratory physiotherapy must be associated with drugs that stimulate mucociliary clearance and systemic antibiotics. Inhaled antibiotics are recommended only in cases of cystic fibrosis (4). The use of bronchodilators in patients with bronchiectasis or cystic fibrosis must be reserved for cases with a positive response shown by spirometry (15).

In cases of cystic fibrosis, recent findings have shown that the combination of regular exercise with the elimination of secretion from the airways contributes to increase survival, reduce mortality, and enhance the patients' quality of life (15).

As mentioned previously, when there is suspicion of foreign body aspiration, rigid bronchoscopy is indicated for diagnosis and therapy (1,25).

Postinfection cough must be an exclusion diagnosis, considered when the patient mentions cough only after an episode of respiratory infection, with normal chest X-ray. Although this cough resolves spontaneously, oral or inhaled corticoid or ipratropium bromide may attenuate it (4).

In tracheomalacia, if the patients are highly symptomatic, tracheostomy can be indicated until the cartilages harden, taking on sufficient rigidity to maintain pervious airways during inspiration and expiration. Vascular anomalies, as well as mediastinal masses, almost always require surgical treatment (23).

Cough due to passive exposure to smoking tends to cease when the child is removed from this environmental stimulation (4).

After the exclusion of other causes, psychogenic cough must also be considered. This can be treated with psychotherapy and anticough therapy for a short period of time (1,4).

References

1. Kamei RK. Chronic cough in children. Pediatr Clin North Am 1991; 38(3):593–605.
2. Holinger LD, Sanders AD. Chronic cough in infants and children: an update. Laryngoscope 1991; 101:596–605.
3. Braman SS. Common causes of chronic unexplained cough. Pulm Perspect 1995; 95:4–6.
4. Irwin RS, Boulet LP, Cloutier MM et al. Managing cough as a defense mechanism and as a symptom: a consensus panel report of the American College of Chest Physicians. Chest 1998; (suppl 114):133–181.
5. Irwin RS, Curley FJ, French CL. The spectrum and frequency of causes, key components of the diagnostic evaluation and outcome of specific therapy. Am Rev Respir Dis 1990; 141:640–647.
6. Irwin RS. Cough. In: Irwin RS, Curley FJ, Grossman RF, eds. Diagnosis and Treatment of Symptoms of the Respiratory Tract. 1st ed. New York: Futura Publishing Co., 1997:1–54.
7. Menon MA, Fiss E. Roteiro diagnóstico da tosse na infância. Pediatr Mod 1995; 31:456–466.
8. Palombini BC, Villanova CAC, Gastal OL et al. Chronic cough quantification of the different probabilities of association as regards the most common causal factors. Am J Respir Crit Care Med 1997; 4:A174.
9. Palombini BC, Villanova CAC, Gastal OL et al. Introducing the concept of a "causal triad of chronic cough": its components are able to explain three fourths of the cases. Am J Respir Crit Care Med 1996; 153:A516.
10. Palombini BC et al. I Consenso Brasileiro sobre Tosse. J Pneumol 1998; 24(suppl 1):S2–S10.
11. Poe RH, Harder RV, Israel RH, Kallay MC. Chronic persistent cough. Experience in diagnosis and outcome using an anatomic diagnostic protocol. Chest 1989; 95:723–728.
12. Stolz DP, Palombini BC, Villanova CAC et al. When you treat bronchial hyperreactivity for the control of chronic cough you may fail in more than 85% of the cases if you do not recognize associated comorbidities. Am J Respir Crit Care Med 1996; 153:A516.
13. Villanova CAC. Tosse crônica: diagnóstico diferencial. Análise de 78 casos. Tese de conclusão do curso de Doutorado, Universidade Federal do Rio Grande do Sul, Porto Alegre, Brazil, 1996.
14. Widdicombe I. Cough: methods and mechanisms. Pulm Pharmacol 1996; 6:259–260.
15. Paterkamp H. The history and physical examination. In: Chernick V, Kendig EL, eds. Disorders of the Respiratory Tract in Children. 5th ed. Philadelphia, PA: WB Saunders Company, 1990:56–77.

16. Cloutier MM, Loughlin GM. Chronic cough in children. A manifestation of airway hyperreactivity. Pediatrics 1981; 67:6–12.
17. Hannaway PJ, Hopper DK. Cough variant asthma in children. J Am Med Assoc 1982; 247:206–208.
18. Pereira EA. Sinusobronquite: estudos com ênfase no componente otorrinolaringológico. Dissertação de conclusão do curso de Mestrado, Universidade Federal do Rio Grande do Sul, Porto Alegre, Brazil, 1991.
19. Palombini BC. Tosse e expectoração. J Pneumol 1984; 10:175–194.
20. Brown TCK, Clark CM. Inhaled foreign bodies in children. Med J Aust 1983; 2:322–326.
21. Stranger P, Lucas RV, Edward JE. Anatomic factors causing respiratory distress in acyanotic congenital cardiac disease. Pediatrics 1969; 43:760–766.
22. Palombini BC, Villanova CAC, Pereira EA et al. Differential diagnosis of chronic cough: the obligation to perform CT scanning of paranasal sinuses, test for airway hyperresponsiveness to carbachol and 24-h esophageal pH monitoring. Chest 1994; 106:2.
23. Myer CM, Cotton RT, Shott SR. The Pediatric Airway—An Interdisciplinary Approach. 1st ed. Philadelphia, PA: JB Lippincott Company, 1995.

21

Gastroesophageal Reflux and Upper Airways

TANIA QUINTELLA

Pediatric Society of São Paulo,
São Paulo, Brazil

Respiratory manifestations of gastroesophageal reflux disease (GERD) have been more and more often recognized. Lower airway disorders called aspiration pneumopathy are well known to physicians and surgeons, but upper airways reflux-induced diseases have only recently caught the attention of specialists and researchers. It was probably due to the great difficulty in treating recurrent and refractory otolaryngologic diseases, cases where GERD is not an uncommon etiology. The aim of this chapter is to review the main concepts related to gastroesophageal reflux (GER), revising the clinical manifestations and injury mechanisms to the upper airways, besides discussing the diagnostic methods and medical and surgical therapies.

I. Introduction

The term "reflux" comes from Latin *re* (going back) and *fleure* (flux). GER is the retrograde transit of gastric material into the esophagus; it is a physiological event that occurs in humans at any age, in the postprandrial period, without causing damage. Sometimes GER becomes pathologic, and gives origin to various clinical manifestations. GER can reach the mouth, characterizing vomiting or regurgitation (symptomatic GER) or can be limited to the esophagus and constitutes the so-called occult or silent reflux.

GER can be defined as a kind of dysphagia—disorder of deglutition in its esophageal phase. Esophageal diseases, inclusive GERD, can cause swallowing dysfunction, including impairment of the other phases in a retrograde manner (1–3).

II. Classification

Boyle (4) proposed the classification below:

Physiological GER—Low frequency of brief refluxes, limited to the distal third of the esophagus, which occur after meals, in the upright position, with no more than 1 h of esophageal acidification during a day; it never causes the disease.

Functional GER—Implies a greater frequency of reflux episodes than the physiological one, children have no underlying morbid condition, and there is no primary mechanical, biochemical, or inflammatory cause to explain it. Thus, it was assumed to be a developmental disorder of the gastrointestinal motility, similar to infant cramps. The majority of infants with this type of GER have daily emesis, but it can be occult, diagnosed only by pH monitoring. These infants have no disease, but at any time in the follow-up, functional GER can become pathogenic, requiring treatment to avoid complications.

Pathogenic GER—Besides pathological signs observed in the diagnostic tests, this GER causes the disease: esophagitis, stricture, Barret's esophagus, apnea, respiratory disease, failure to thrive.

Secondary GER—Occurs in patients with specific morbid conditions that predispose to reflux: severe neurological or physical impairment, hiatal hernia, esophageal atresia, dysautonomia. Commonly, the most affected group is that of children with cerebral palsy, mainly anoxic encephalopathy survivors. This kind of GER is often pathogenic and resistant to medical treatment.

Note: It must be clear that cow's milk protein allergy is not an etiology of GER, but a distinct morbid condition to be suspected when associated with diarrhea and family history of atopy.

III. Physiopathology of GERD

The esophagus is a muscular tube composed of an inner circular and an outer longitudinal layer; it is designed to conduct food and saliva from the pharynx to the stomach. It is bounded above by the upper esophageal sphincter (UES) and below by the lower esophageal sphincter (LES), which was thought to be only functional—now, it is known as a set of muscular fibers with special features of length and tension.

The UES is basically formed by the cricopharyngeal muscle, and its resting pressure has the contribution of the thyropharyngeal muscle, cricoid lamina, and upper esophagus muscles. When at rest, it is closed in tonic contraction and relaxes during deglutition of food or saliva. Its function is to prevent air ingestion during respiration and the reflux of gastric material to upper airways and to the lungs. UES pressure is significantly diminished during sleep, which causes a greater risk of aspiration. On the other hand, acid perfusion of distal esophagus augments UES pressure, the same way it does during a reflux episode.

Pathogenic GER results when the antireflux barrier is overcome. The most important component of this barrier is the LES—the main mechanisms causing GER are related to its dysfunction, though other factors are implicated:

- LES diminished resting pressure (hypotonia)
- augmented frequency of transient LES relaxation
- transient increases of abdominal pressure
- delayed gastric emptying
- presence of esophagitis

Basal hypotonia of LES and *increases in abdominal pressure* (which occur in physiological situations such as crying, defecation, coughing, etc.) are only contributing factors since some studies showed that a considerable amount of patients have normal LES resting pressure. Additionally, increases in abdominal pressure need simultaneous LES relaxation to cause GER.

On the other hand, LES relaxations occur associated to deglutition; but relaxations were also verified after meals, when they are called *spontaneous transient relaxations*—probably because food distends gastric walls, stimulating a vago-vagal reflex and inducing LES opening. In patients, frequency and duration of these transient relaxations are considerably greater than in healthy subjects, resulting in higher proportion of refluxes. Recently, this has been considered the main physiopathologic mechanism to explain GER.

Delayed gastric emptying is observed in almost 50% of the patients and could favor the increase in transient spontaneous relaxations because it causes distension on the gastric walls.

It was observed that patients who have *esophagitis* show LES resting pressure lower than individuals with GER without esophagitis. The esophagitis releases inflammatory mediators, especially prostaglandin E3, which provokes motor disorders of the esophagus, decreasing LES pressure, favoring GER and, consequently, causing more esophagitis. This vicious circle must be broken with treatment to avoid GER complications.

Esophagitis is found in 60–83% of the children presenting GER and it can be documented through endoscopy and/or biopsy. Microscopic esophagitis is more frequent than the macroscopic type. The onset of esophagitis depends on:

- the potential injury of the refluxate
- the contact time of the refluxate with the esophageal mucosa
- efficiency of esophageal clearance
- spontaneous swallowing frequency and the volume and buffering power of saliva
- presence of associated alkaline duodenal gastric reflux
- the sensitivity and resistance of the esophageal mucosa

IV. Mechanisms of GER-Induced Respiratory Disease

Digestive manifestations of GER (symptomatic or occult GER) are easily understood, but pulmonary and otolaryngologic manifestations require some explanations. GER-induced respiratory disease will occur if there is:

1. pathologic GER, and
2. failure of the defense mechanisms against aspiration: closure of nasopharynx, laryngeal elevation, glottic closure reflex, and opening of the UES at the right moment (1,2,5), or
3. low threshold of airway response to the stimulation of esophageal receptors by GER.

GER can cause respiratory disease by direct contact of the refluxate with the lower and upper airway mucosa (*aspirative mechanism*) or because reflux stimulates receptors in the esophageal mucosa (*reflex mechanism*) or in the airway mucosa (after microaspiration), triggering reflex responses (*mixed mechanism*).

- aspiration and microaspiration—causing chemical bronchitis and pneumonitis with secondary infection or not, pulmonary fibrosis, reflux laryngitis or posterior acid laryngitis, contact ulcer of the larynx, tracheal and laryngeal stenosis, postintubation subglottic stenosis, vocal cord granuloma and laryngeal cancer. Gastropharyngeal reflux can cause chronic pharyngitis, adenoiditis, and rhinitis, provoking Eustachian tube dysfunction (6–14). Otitis could also appear, like recurrent otitis and intractable sinusitis, which could result if the refluxed material gets access to the middle ear through the Eustachian tube (6,7,9,13,15–17).
- microaspiration with stimulation of receptors in the airways—causing reflex bronchospasm, reflex laryngospasm, and obstructive apnea, and also central reflex apnea. Clinical manifestations include cough, dyspnea, wheezing, stridor, apparent life-threatening event (ALTE), and sudden infant death syndrome (1,4–8,18).
- stimulation of esophageal mucosal receptors—leading to persistent cough, reflex bronchospasm, laryngospasm, central reflex apnea, ALTE, and sudden infant death syndrome (4,5,14).

V. Epidemiology and Natural History of GERD

Estimates of GERD in infancy vary from the denial of its existence to the mere affirmative that every child refluxes (19). The majority of texts and articles state that GER is very common in childhood, so that there was a reluctance to accept it as a cause of clinical problems (20). Ivo Carrè, one of the first researchers on this theme, estimated the incidence of GER as 1 in 300 living births, but his sample was composed of patients with symptomatic and severe GER and does not reflect general GER incidence, in addition to omitting the incidence of occult GER (21). Vandenplas (20) reported that the incidence of GER assessed by prolonged pH monitoring among unselected children is about 8%.

However, there has recently been a clear increase in the frequency of children presenting GER—how can this be explained?

Herbst (19) suggested that the question is more related to better recognition and diagnosis than properly increased incidence. On the other hand, Sutphen (22) considered that modern practices of infant care are to a great extent responsible for the development of infantile GER. Primitive tribes breastfed their infants every 13 min, for about 2 min and between feedings the baby was kept upright in a sling. In contrast, we increased the bolus size to obtain an interfeeding interval of 3–4 h, while the infant stays recumbent in a crib; in addition, a diaper change is often performed after a meal, involving elevation of the legs above the stomach—the author concluded that it is a miracle that not all infants have chronic GER.

Kibel (4) reported the follow-up of infants at a welfare clinic and observed that, at two months of age, 47% of them presented regurgitation after meals; at 6 months, this was verified in only 4%.

The natural history of GERD is benign. Carrè (*apud* Orenstein, 1991) (21) reported the follow-up of untreated severe cases, showing that the majority improved by 9 months of age, and 65% were asymptomatic at 2 years of age; 35% had clinical symptoms up to 4 years, among which 8% had pulmonary sequelae and 5% had developed esophageal stricture. The remaining 5% died from GER complications.

Boix-Ochoa (23) treated 2045 infants: 4% required antireflux surgery before 1 year of age, while in the group over 1 year, the surgical treatment was necessary in 20% of the cases.

These considerations show that GERD has good prognosis as time goes on, probably because involved structures grow and mature with time.

VI. Clinical Manifestations of GER

Digestive manifestations: Frequent emesis or regurgitation, rumination, hypersalivation, bad breath, dental erosions, water-brash, retrosternal pain, pyrosis, abnormal crying in infants, excessive hiccups, belching, oropharyngeal dysphagia, painful deglutition (6,15,19–21,24–28).

Note: Dysphagia present in patients with GER was classically described as obstructive, caused by peptic stenosis of the esophagus. However, it has been recently verified that *non-obstructive dysphagia* can occur in up to 46.8% of the patients presenting reflux esophagitis, even when esophageal dysmotility is absent, in adults (28) and children (25).

Pulmonary manifestations: Asthma bronchitis, wheezy-baby syndrome (2,4,5,14,19,22,24,27,29–32), repeated pneumonias (4,5,15,22,26,27,29–33), chronic bronchitis, pulmonary fibrosis, lung abscess, bronchiectasis, hemoptysis (4,5,14,21,23,34).

Otolaryngologic manifestations: Oral burning, persistent nocturnal cough, chronic cough, lateral cervical pain, recurrent stridor, dysphonia, hoarseness, chronic throat clearing, chronic sore throat, *globus pharyngeus*, chronic rhinitis, recurrent otitis media, laryngospasm, recurrent laryngitis, posterior laryngitis, contact ulcer of the larynx, subglottic stenosis, vocal process granulomas, and finally pharyngeal and laryngeal cancer (2,5,7,8,10,12–15,17–19,26,27,34–37).

Other manifestations: Low weight gain, anorexia, noncardiac chest pain, bradycardia reflex, abnormal head and neck posturing, choking, infant obstructive apnea, awake apnea syndrome, sudden infant death syndrome (5,6,14,20,21,26,27,29,34,38), some special and rare manifestations and neuropsychiatric syndromes (15,19,21,24,26).

Excellent reviews confirming the importance of the association between GER and respiratory disease have been published (5,14,34) and in 1968, the otolaryngologic literature presented one of the first articles considering GER as an etiologic factor of contact ulcer of the larynx, vocal cord granuloma and *globus pharyngeus* (12).

Koufman (12) studied the relationships between otolaryngologic disease and GER in 225 adults whose most common symptoms were: hoarseness (71%), chronic cough (51%), *globus* sensation (47%), and chronic throat clearing (42%). It must be noted that only 43% of the patients had gastrointestinal symptoms of GERD. The clinical and laboratory investigation, including 24 h esophageal pH-monitoring, led to the following diagnoses:

- laryngeal carcinoma in 31 patients, 71% of them presenting GER on pH-monitoring;
- tracheal and laryngeal stenosis in 33 cases, 78% of them with GER;
- reflux laryngitis in 61 patients, 60% of them showing GER;
- *globus pharyngeus* in 27 cases, 58% presenting GER on pH-monitoring;
- chronic cough in 30 patients, 52% with GER; and
- dysphagia in 25 cases, 45% of them associated with GER.

This author also documented *esophagopharyngeal refluxes*, placing a second pH-probe in the hypopharynx and he verified that the frequency of GERs reaching the pharynx varied from 10% in the dysphagia group to 58% among laryngeal carcinoma victims or tracheal/laryngeal stenosis patients. Koufman (12) did more—he tested hydrochloric acid, pepsin, and saline infusion on the larynx of animals and showed that *pepsin* is the main noxious agent causing damage.

Hanson et al. (33) studied 223 adults with *chronic laryngitis*, presenting symptoms for at least 3 months: chronic/recurrent sore throat, hoarseness, post-nasal drip sensation, throat clearing, chronic cough, and *globus*. A few patients had digestive GER-related complaints and 182 received antireflux treatment—96% had their acid posterior laryngitis cure documented through laryngoscopy, including 7% with ulcerations and 3% with vocal cord granuloma.

Chronic cough is a very important manifestation of GER. Smyrnios et al. (39) prospectively investigated 30 adults, finding 40 causes of chronic cough. Post-nasal drip, GERD, and asthma were the most frequent. Ing et al. (18) studied healthy controls and adult patients presenting cough for more than 2 months, and documented GERD as the etiology of the cough using 24 h pH-monitoring. Irwin et al. (36) found chronic cough as the only manifestation of GERD in adults.

Contencin and Narcy (7) studied children with *recurrent laryngotracheitis* compared to healthy children, finding GER in all of them. These authors also did nasal–pharyngeal pH-monitoring in children presenting *chronic rhinopharyngitis*, showing the importance of GER in this disease. Other authors found similar results in children (2) and also in adults (15,17).

Contencin et al. (8) studied 22 children with *chronic dysphonia* using laryngoscopy and esophageal pH-monitoring, and found that 64% of them presented pathologic GER.

Giannoni et al. (16) diagnosed GER in 64% of 27 children presenting *laryngomalacia* and they observed that there was a statistically significant association between GER and severe symptoms and a complicated clinical course.

Barbero (2) studied 22 children with *chronic sinusitis* according to Parsons and Phillips criteria, submitting them to endoscopy and 24 h esophageal pH-monitoring. There was a clear relation between the results of endoscopy and pH-monitoring which was positive in 16 patients. It is noteworthy that 13 cases definitely improved their otolaryngologic disease with GER treatment.

GER-induced *apnea* generally occurs in neonates and infants before 6 months of life. It usually occurs after regurgitation or emesis, and even after occult GER, and is one of the most serious effects of GER, being responsible for part of ALTE cases and sudden infant death (14,19,21). This apnea can be obstructive (laryngospasm) or central (cessation of respiratory movements), which is more common in preterm babies and associated to suction and swallowing.

Andze et al. (29) studied more than one 1000 children suspected of having GER, and noted 500 with respiratory disease—36% had apneic spells, cyanosis, pallor, and hypotonia.

Spitzer et al. (38) described the *awake apnea syndrome* observing 15 infants that, after meals, became rigid with staring, fixed eyes, plethoric and soon cyanotic—the apnea was polygraphically documented and GER was diagnosed by esophageal pH-monitoring in all patients.

VII. Diagnostic Methods

GER can be documented by upper gastrointestinal series, ultrasonography, scintigraphy, and prolonged esophageal pH-monitoring. Other tests can be performed in order to evaluate its severity and consequences: lung aspiration test, esophago-gastroduodenoscopy, Bernstein's test, esophago-gastric manometry, gastric emptying evaluation and swallowing study.

It is evident that not all patients must be investigated. In the majority of cases, a *positive therapeutic test* is sufficient and considered solid evidence of GERD (20,21). Tests will be necessary to stop treatment or to indicate surgery.

Upper gastrointestinal series—This exam is very useful in infancy because it can show congenital or acquired defects of gastrointestinal tract such as pyloric hypertrophic stenosis, esophageal compression, antral or duodenal webs, hiatal hernia, and gastrointestinal malrotation. Dysmotility and stricture of the esophagus can also be identified, but *radiology often fails to separate physiological from pathogenic reflux* and so it has a great rate of false-positive results. Otherwise, common causes of false-negative results are crying during the test or insufficient gastric filling (14,19,20,21,24).

Esophagogastric scintigraphy—Radiation exposure is much less than on barium series, so the observation time can be extended and children take their usual meals. Its sensitivity is reported to be 59–90% and it also allows the evaluation of gastric emptying (Fig. 21.1). The disadvantages are: costs, children must be contained, regurgitant reflux is frequently missed (14) and scintigraphy does

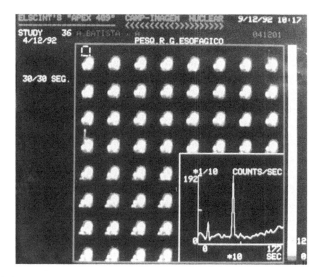

Figure 21.1 Esophagogastric scintiscan showing two GER episodes.

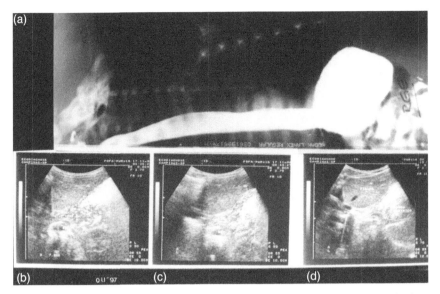

Figure 21.2 Ultrasonography (b–d) presenting GER grade 3 as it is seen on barium radiography (a).

not easily distinguish physiological from pathologic reflux, but it diagnoses neutral refluxes that are missed in pH-monitoring. Besides these, an accepted normal standard for children is still missing (14,21,27).

Abdominal ultrasonography—This is a very helpful screening test for GER and has many advantages: it is noninvasive, has no radiation, is inexpensive and uses children's habitual meals (Fig. 21.2). It can also identify some congenital gastrointestinal malformations, permit the evaluation of His angle, calculation of abdominal esophagus length, and LES opening size, and the counting of reflux episodes (20,27,35,37). Finally, it has a normal standard reference determined with more than 300 children (35,37), is very sensitive, and has high specificity (27).

Prolonged esophageal pH-monitoring—This is considered the "gold standard" test to diagnose reflux. GER is documented with a probe in the distal esophagus during 15–24 h. (Fig. 21.3). The test can verify temporal relation between GER and clinical manifestation and is particularly useful in children presenting respiratory diseases because typical pH patterns have already been described:

- *Discontinuous pattern*: Jolley et al. noted that, in normal children, reflux frequency diminishes 2 h after a meal; in patients with respiratory disease it diminishes by the end of the third hour.
- *Mean duration of GER during sleep (ZMD)*: This is greater than 3.8 in children with respiratory GER-induced disease, as found in a controlled study with 388 patients by Halpern et al. (40).

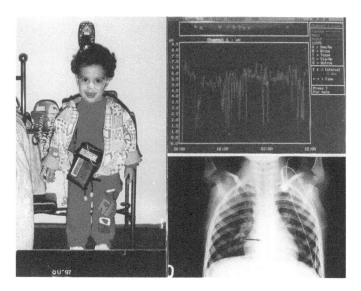

Figure 21.3 Prolonged pH-monitoring in a child with obstructive bronchitis and recurrent otitis.

- Mean pH at night is 1.0–2.3 units below the mean pH during daytime, as found by Vandenplas (20).

It is worth mentioning that these signs occur even when the whole pH-monitoring is normal, considering commonly used parameters, which were determined by gastroenterologists in order to estimate the risk of esophageal peptic disease. It is not known if these are valid criteria to diagnose GER causing respiratory disease (20,21). The parameters usually taken into account are (4):

1. Fraction of time with pH below 4—normal up to 6%, for children >1 year of age.
2. Frequency of GER episodes—normal up to 1.5 per hour.
3. Number and duration of refluxes during the night.
4. Number of refluxes longer than 5 min—0.3 per hour monitored.
5. Mean esophageal clearance—normal up to 4 min per reflux.
6. Duration of the longest reflux—if greater than 20 min, indicates abnormal clearance.

On the other hand, pH-monitoring has some disadvantages, such as costs, duration, sophisticated equipment, and difficulties in choosing normal scores for each pediatric range. In addition, it is very important to remember that pH-metry does not diagnose neutral refluxes, which can be aspirated and cause respiratory disease.

In otolaryngologic patients, pH-monitoring is indicated when therapeutic testing is negative, in cases of apnea when other etiologies were ruled out, and before antireflux surgery.

Double-probe esophageal pH-monitoring—Many authors used distal and proximal pH-monitoring of the esophagus in an attempt to define parameters for respiratory disease (Fig. 21.4). In adults, Koufman (12) could demonstrate a very strong correlation between high GER and otolaryngologic disease. In children, a noncontrolled study could not show significant difference between patients with and without wheezing, as related to distal and proximal reflux index (41). Another small casuistic study suggested that double-probe pH-metry is useful in children with otolaryngological diseases (7).

Aspiration diagnosis—Tests were designed to confirm aspirative mechanisms of lower airways, although some authors have documented the presence of barium in the Eustachian tube and middle ear of vomiting infants (13) and we, personally, have verified barium on the adenoids of a toddler presenting repeated sinusitis and nocturnal bronchospasm. Aspiration is usually investigated through scintigraphy, 2–24 h after gastric scintiscan, when the child returns to the gamma camera to detect the radiotracer in the lungs. The sensitivity is very low because aspiration is an intermittent event. Others methods include the determination of lactose or dyes in the tracheobronchial lavage and, recently, the direct sampling of tracheobronchial secretions for quantitative detection of lipid-laden macrophages—the quantification is an attempt to diminish the high rate of false-positives. One must be aware that these methods do not distinguish oral aspiration from that of stomach contents.

Laryngeal and upper digestive endoscopy—These procedures diagnose GER complications such as esophagitis, esophageal stricture, and associated disease like hiatal hernia, gastritis, and duodenitis (Fig. 21.5). Laryngoscopy allows one to verify the presence of acid posterior laryngitis and to make

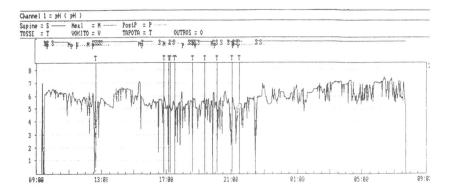

Figure 21.4 "Normal" pH-metry tracing showing coincidence between GER (pH < 4) and cough (T).

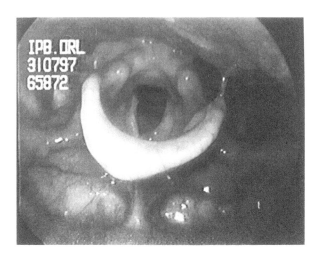

Figure 21.5   Laryngoscopy showing acid posterior laryngitis. (Courtesy of Dr. Ariovaldo Armando Silva.)

differential diagnosis with other laryngeal lesions. It is formally indicated in patients presenting recurrent abdominal pain, haematemesis, or noncardiac chest pain. It must be noted that normal endoscopy does not exclude esophagitis in a biopsy, and the latter is more sensitive (21,24) (Fig. 21.5).

Esophageal histopathology—Although a Quinton tube provides suction biopsies of better size and quality, grasp biopsies obtained endoscopically are largely employed to diagnose esophagitis, according to the following criteria:

- Basal layer hyperplasia occupying in at least 50% of the epithelium thickness
- Presence of intraepithelial eosinophil leukocytes
- Presence of intraepithelial polymorphonuclear neutrophils

Bernstein acid perfusion test—It is not very useful in pediatric patients, except perhaps in teenagers. Alternatively, saline and chloridic acid are instilled on the distal esophagus to try to elicit the clinical manifestation referred by the patient, mainly noncardiac chest pain. It can be associated to pulmonary function tests and also to bronchial hyper-reactivity tests.

Esophagogastric manometry—This method documents esophageal dysmotility and gives information about the UES and LES. It does not diagnose GER but it is indicated in cases of *globus* or noncardiac chest pain, and is very useful to evaluate oropharyngeal dysphagia. It is very useful in preoperative patients suspected of having esophageal dysmotility, since peristaltic dysfunction of distal esophagus originates several complications after tight fundoplication (1,20,21).

Swallowing studies—It is mandatory in neurologically affected children with secondary GER, since they have a high incidence of dysphagia, sometimes without specific signs, manifested only by respiratory disease (1,6). The evaluation includes specific anamnesis and clinical examination, barium swallow, ultrasonography, videofluoroscopy, and manometry:

- Modified barium swallow has been used with success in adults (3) but its applicability is unknown in children. The common barium swallow is used with limitations (1).
- Upper airway fibroscopy can evaluate competency and sufficiency of palatoglossal sphincter, the presence of residual food in the pyriform sinuses, allowing the diagnosis of reflux laryngitis and the collection of tracheal secretion samples to confirm aspiration (1,12).
- Videofluoroscopy is considered the best method to study swallowing disorders, using the deglutition of solid and liquids mixed with barium to localize the compromised phase. The process is filmed for posterior analysis (1,3).

Sensitivity and specificity determine how much a test is reliable; in a perfect test, both must be elevated and specificity has to be greater than 85% (20,21). Among the tests to diagnose GER, only prolonged esophageal pH-monitoring has such high specificity. The *quantified* scintigraphy presented adequate rates in adults and a few studies stated that ultrasonography has specificity >85%. On the other hand, the sensitivity is high for all methods, as long as they are executed within the correct recommendations. The most important point is that, except for pH-metry, none of these methods easily distinguishes physiological from pathologic GER (19–21,24,31).

VIII. Medical Treatment

The aim of therapy is to control reflux and to avoid its digestive and respiratory complications, until the age when the esophagogastric junction dysfunctions are solved. Medical treatment is often successful in infants and in patients with respiratory manifestations. GER therapy has prolonged effect on respiratory disease.

This does not occur in typical GER disease with esophagitis; patients present a relapse rate of around 70–90%, mainly older children. Patients older than 1 year of age with difficult to control disease can require surgery in 20% of the cases (23).

Who, when, and how to treat is a decision based on the physician's professional experience. Infants with very frequent regurgitation, without other manifestation, can receive just postural treatment and thicker diet. Infants with recurrent otitis can have a trial period with prokinetic and acid suppression drugs.

Duration of therapy depends on the natural history of the disease, the child's age, and clinical manifestation. An infant can be medically controlled beyond 1 year, while a toddler requires at least 3 months to evaluate the response to therapy. Relapses are frequent after 4 years of age and the responsibility of a surgical decision, mainly in less severe cases, should be shared with the family.

Severe manifestations, regardless of age, must be rapidly investigated and surgery can be considered after 1–3 months of clinical intervention.

Medical treatment of GERD requires postural and feeding measures, plus drug therapy.

Postural treatment—Is a basic procedure, since 25% of infants have their reflux controlled just with posturing (4,20,21,24). The prone position, 30° elevated, showed fewer GER episodes, quicker gastric emptying, fewer risks of pulmonary aspiration, and better esophageal clearance (20,21) (Figs. 21.6 and 21.7) when compared to flat supine posture. This posturing is in apparent conflict with that of studies about the increase in sudden death of infants that slept in prone position, but the former were sleeping on flat and soft bedding, and not on 30° elevated hard surfaces as recommended.

Dietary management—We recommend thickened diet because it increases caloric intake, decreases emesis and crying time, and increases sleeping time, although pH-monitoring studies showed it does not decrease GER (19,20). Infants must not be fed during the night, and children must stop eating 2 h

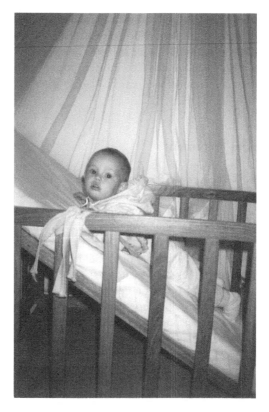

Figure 21.6   Postural treatment: the prone position 30° elevated.

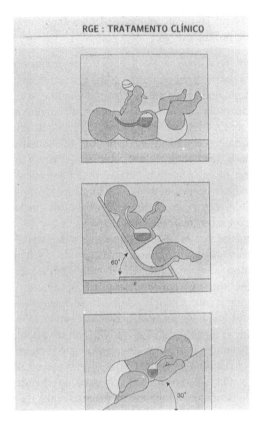

Figure 21.7 Food image in the stomach of an infant in different postures.

before going to bed. Foods containing a high fat and acid content and carbonated beverages must be avoided because they affect LES pressure or delay gastric emptying.

Similarly, the treatment of associated diseases must avoid drugs that can favor GER or cause damage to gastrointestinal mucosa like nonsteroid anti-inflammatory drugs and some antibiotics (21). Bronchospasm must be controlled with inhalatory drugs and theophylline cannot be used.

Deglutition disorders, namely oropharyngeal dysphagia, and intestinal constipation, if present, must be carefully treated, and the treatment of obesity is indispensable.

Pharmacological therapy—Must be indicated in patients with pathogenic GER, secondary GER, or functional GER with exaggerated emesis. Clinical esophagitis or esophagitis confirmed with endoscopy/biopsy must be treated, since there is the possibility of a vicious circle GER–esophagitis, as discussed before.

Prokinetic agents—Until now, no drug is able to diminish the frequency of inappropriate spontaneous transient relaxation of LES, but prokinetic drugs can increase LES pressure, stimulate esophageal clearance, and accelerate gastric emptying (20). The prokinetics are:

- Betanecol is a cholinergic agent; it can induce bronchospasm and increases gastric acid secretion, so its use is limited.
- Metochlopramide is an antagonist of dopamine, which is an inhibitory neurotransmitter, and so metochlopramide improves esophagogastric motility and increases LES pressure. Side effects related to intracerebral dopamine antagonism occur in 20% of the patients; the most frequent ones are: somnolence, agitation, extrapyramidal symptoms, gynecomastia, galactorrhea, amenorrhea (dependent on hyperprolactinemia, which occurs with all dopamine antagonists), headache, and irreversible *dyskinesia tardive.* Nevertheless, metochlopramide is a very inexpensive and useful drug.
- Domperidone is a peripheral dopamine antagonist, so it causes fewer side effects related to the central nervous system, around 7%. Its main action is to accelerate gastric emptying; it seems not to improve esophageal motility, nor to increase LES pressure.
- Bromopride is also a peripheral dopamine antagonist and has few references in the literature. Its mode of action is similar to that of domperidone.
- Alizapride is an antiemetic agent with selective central action, derived from benzamide. It presents few neuroleptic properties and its primary ability is to cause a prolonged pylorus relaxation. Like bromopride, alizapride is relatively unstudied in children, so other drugs are preferable.
- Cisapride is unique among the prokinetics since it is a noncholinergic, non-antidopaminergic agent that enhances acetylcholine release from postganglionic nerve endings of the myenteric plexus, leading to improved propulsive motor activity of the esophagus, stomach, small bowel, and large bowel. European studies showed the ability of cisapride to improve esophageal peristalsis, to increase LES pressure and to stimulate gastric emptying (20). Unfortunately, cisapride recently became unavailable in account of its side effects on cardiac muscle, although they are rare in children.

Acid-reducing agents—These are used to relieve symptoms such retrosternal pain and heartburn, and to treat peptic esophagitis. There are two groups of drugs:

- Antacids were suggested to be efficient to treat esophagitis, but the adherence to neutralizing therapy is impaired as it is necessary to administrate seven to eight doses per day. Preparations of aluminum and magnesium salts are available and the ones containing little dimeticone are preferable. The association with *alginic acid* is useful because it is a foaming agent that makes the antacid fluctuate and so it will be the first component of the refluxate to contact the esophageal mucosa during a reflux episode.

- Antisecretory drugs the *H2-histamine receptor antagonists* reduce considerably the gastric acid secretion and have to be used during at least 2 months in cases of esophagitis. Cimetidine was successfully used but the good experience with ranitidine, its administration only twice a day and fewer side effects made it become the first choice. Famotidine and nizatidine have been more recently tested. *Proton pump blockers* are agents that exert deep suppression of the acid secretion from parietal cells of the gastric mucosa. Omeprazole has been used in adults and children presenting esophagitis refractory to H2-blockers, with good results. Other compounds are available (lanzoprazole, pantoprazole, etc.) but have not been tested in children yet.

Other drugs

- Cytoprotective agents—*Sulcrafate* is an octasulfated complex of carbohydrate and aluminum that has the property of binding to exposed protein on the mucosal layer of gastrointestinal tract, the so-called "band-aid effect." It is a very safe and inexpensive drug to treat reflux esophagitis and is presently underused (42).
- Erythromycin—This macrolide antibiotic has similar effects to motilin on the gastrointestinal motor activity and it seems to be a motilin agonist. There are experimental studies on animals and trials on GER refractory to classical treatment and also in diabetic gastroparesis but, at present, it is not used to treat GER (43).

Note: The association of GERD and oropharyngeal dysphagia occurs in 10–20% of cases and must be efficiently treated. The typical cases are children with cerebral palsy and babies younger than 6 months presenting cricopharyngeal lack of coordination. It must be kept in mind that feeding problems and respiratory diseases are similarly caused by both diseases and the disappointment with the results of GER therapy in children with untreated oropharyngeal dysphagia is common. Surgical management of adult dysphagia is routine practice but it is not yet well established for children (33).

IX. Surgical Treatment

Surgery must be postponed to the second year of life whenever possible, since evolution usually is satisfactory at this time. Surgery has an efficacy of 90–95% and mortality rate is less than 1%, including severe cases. Surgery indications of GER are (24):

- *Independent of medical treatment*—Esophageal stricture, life-threatening apnea, massive aspiration, Barret's esophagus, secondary GER (operated esophageal atresia, large hiatal hernia, severe neurological impairment).

- *GERD refractory to therapy or repeated recurrence on withdrawal of treatment*—Failure to thrive, severe esophagitis, recurrent pneumonia, apnea, refractory bronchospasm, brochopulmonary dysplasia, refractory heartburn, or regurgitation in older children (especially with sliding hiatal hernia).
- *Prophylaxis*—Patients requiring feeding gastrostomy (children with cerebral palsy, intractable oropharyngeal dysphagia, severe mental retardation, or physical handicap).

There are various types of antireflux surgery, but surgeons prefer Nissen's transabdominal fundoplication, where gastric fundus is wrapped 360° around 2–3 cm of distal esophagus, which is pulled into the abdomen, following a hiatoplasty. Nowadays the laparoscopic modified Nissen surgery is routine (44). Other techniques recommend wraps of 240° (partial fundoplications of Lind, Toupet, Hill, Thal, etc.). Recently, Boix-Ochoa (23) proposed his "physiological approach" to the antireflux surgery in which he performs a 180° fundoplication.

The controversy around the most adequate surgery is the result of 32% postoperative morbidity and the most common clinical complications are: gas bloat (manifested as nausea, retching, gagging, and abdominal fullness), dysphagia, slow eating, inability to burp or vomit, and dumping. Surgical complications occur in 7–10% of the cases; herniation of the wrap and small-bowel obstruction due to adhesions are the most frequent ones (19,20,21,24).

Surgical failure to control reflux happens in up to 10% of the cases and is often seen in the neurologically impaired, which seems to be independent of the surgical technique employed.

References

1. Arvedson JC, Brodsky L, eds. Pediatric Swallowing and Feeding. Assessment and Management. San Diego, CA: Singular Publishing Group Inc, 1992.
2. Bauman NM, Sandler AD, Smith RJH. Respiratory manifestations of gastroesophageal reflux disease in pediatric patients. Ann Otol Rhinol Laryngol 1996; 105:23–32.
3. Mendelsohn M. New concepts in dysphagia. J Otolaryngol 1993; 22(suppl 1):2–24.
4. Boyle JT, Tuchman DN, Altschuler SM, Nixon TE, Pack AI, Cohen S. Mechanisms for the association of gastroesophageal reflux and bronchospasm. Am Rev Respir Dis 1985; 131(suppl):S16–S20.
5. Rudolph C. Gastroesophageal reflux and airway disorders. In: Myer CM III, ed. The Pediatric Airway. Philadelphia: JB Lippincott Company, 1995:327–357.
6. Barbero GJ. Gastroesophageal reflux and upper airway disease. Otolaryngol Clin N Am 1996; 29:27–38.
7. Contencin P, Narcy P. Gastropharyngeal reflux in infants and children. A pharyngeal pH monitoring study. Arch Otolaryngol Head Neck Surg 1992; 118:1028–1030.
8. Contencin P, Gumpert L, Kalach N, Dogliotti MP, DuPont C. Gastroesophageal reflux and dysphonia in children. Rev Laryngol Otol Rhinol Bord 1997; 118:253–257.

9. Contencin P, Viala P, Narcy P. Nasopharyngeal pH monitoring in infants and children with rhinopharyngitis. Int J Pediatr Otorhinolaryngol 1991; 22:249–256.
10. Deschner KW, Benjamin SB. Extraesophageal manifestations of gastroesophageal reflux disease. Am J Gastroenterol 1989; 84:1–5.
11. Eizaguirre I, Tovar JA. Predicting preoperatively the outcome of respiratory symptoms of gastroesophageal reflux. J Pediatr Surg 1992; 27:848–851.
12. Koufman JÁ. The otolaryngologic manifestations of gastroesophageal reflux disease (GERD): a clinical investigation of 225 patients using ambulatory 24-hour pH monitoring and an experimental investigation of the role of acid and pepsin in the development of laryngeal injury. Laryngoscope 1991; 101(suppl 53):1–78.
13. Pincney LE, Currarino G. Reflux of barium into the middle ear during upper gastrointestinal series. Radiology 1980; 135:653–654.
14. Platzker ACG. Gastroesophageal Reflux and Respiratory Illness. In: Chernic V, Kendig EL Jr, eds. Disorders of the Respiratory Tract in Children. 5th ed. WB Saunders Comp., 1990:466–475.
15. Bain WM, Harrington JW, Thomas LE, Schaefer SD. Head and neck manifestations of gastroesophageal reflux. Laryngoscope 1983; 93:175–179.
16. Giannoni C, Sulek M, Friedman EM, Duncan III NO. Gastroesophageal reflux association with laryngomalacia: a prospective study. Int J Pediatr Otorhinolaryngol 1998; 43:11–20.
17. Kambic V, Radsel Z. Acid posterior laryngitis. Aetiology, diagnosis and treatment. J Laryngol Otol 1984; 98:1237–1240.
18. Ing AJ, Ngu MC, Breslin ABX. Chronic persistent cough and gastroesophageal reflux. Thorax 1991; 46:479–483.
19. Herbst JJ. Gastroesophageal reflux. J Pediatr 1981; 98:859–870.
20. Vandenplas Y. Oesophageal pH Monitoring for Gastroesophageal Reflux in Infants and Children. West Sussex, UK: John Wiley and Sons, 1992.
21. Orenstein SR. Gastroesophageal reflux. Curr Probl Pediatr 1991; 21:193–241.
22. Sutphen JL. Pediatric gastroesophageal reflux disease. Gastroenterol Clin North Am 1990; 19:617–630.
23. Boix-Ochoa J. The physiologic approach to the management of gastroesophageal reflux. J Pediatr Surg 1986; 12:1032–1039.
24. Boyle JT. Gastroesophageal reflux in the pediatric patient. Gastroenterol Clin North Am 1989; 18:315–337.
25. Catto-Smith AG, Machida H, Butzner JD, Gall DG, Scott RB. The role of gastroesophageal reflux in pediatric dysphagia. J Pediatr Gastroenterol Nutr 1991; 12:159–165.
26. Pearlman NW, Stiegmann GV, Teter A. Primary upper aerodigestive tract manifestations of gastroesophageal reflux. Am J Gastroenterol 1988; 83:22–25.
27. Quintella T. Evaluation of gastroesophageal reflux in the morbidity of atopic and non-atopic wheezy infants. Ph.D. Thesis, State University of Campinas, São Paulo, Brazil, 1997.
28. Triadafilopoulos G. Non-obstructive dysphagia in reflux esophagitis. Am J Gastroenterol 1989; 84:614–618.
29. Andze GO, Brandt ML, St. Vil D, Bensoussan AL, Blanchard H. Diagnosis and treatment of gastroesophageal reflux in 500 children with respiratory symptoms. The value of pH monitoring. J Pediatr Surg 1991; 26:295–300.

30. Gunasekaran TS, Hassal EG. Efficacy and safety of omeprazole for severe gastroesophageal reflux in children. J Pediatr 1993; 123:148–154.

31. Meyers W, Roberts CC, Johnson DG, Herbst JJ. Value of tests for evaluation of gastroesophageal reflux in children. J Pediatr Surg 1985; 20:515–520.

32. Quintella T, Espin-Neto J. Respiratory disease and gastroesophageal reflux: study with 230 atopic and non-atopic children. J Pneumol 1997; (suppl 2):S19.

33. Hanson DG, Kamel PL, Kahrilas PJ. Outcomes of antireflux therapy for the treatment of chronic laryngitis. Ann Otol Rhinol Laryngol 1995; 104:550–555.

34. Orenstein SR, Orenstein DM. Gastroesophageal reflux and respiratory disease in children. J Pediatr 1988; 112:847–858.

35. Gomes H, Lallemand PH. Infant apnea and gastroesophageal reflux. Pediatr Radiol 1992; 22:8–11.

36. Irwin RS, Zawacki JK, Curley FJ, French CL, Hoffman PJ. Chronic cough as the sole presenting manifestation of gastroesophageal reflux. Am Rev Respir Dis 1989; 140:1294–1300.

37. Riccabona M, Maurer U, Lackner H et al. The role of sonography in the evaluation of gastroesophageal reflux to pH-metry. Eur J Pediatr 1992; 151:655–657.

38. Spitzer AR, Boyle JT, Tuchman DN, Willian WF. Awake apnea associated with gastro-esophageal reflux: a specific clinical syndrome. J Pediatr 1984; 104:200–205.

39. Smyrnios NA, Irwin RS, Curley FJ, French CL. From a prospective study of chronic cough: diagnostic and therapeutic aspects in older adults. Arch Intern Med 1998; 158:1222–1228.

40. Halpern LM, Jolley SG, Tunell WP, Johnson DJ, Sterling CE. The mean duration of gastroesophageal reflux during sleep as an indicator of respiratory symptoms from RGE in children. J Pediatr Surg 1991; 26:686–690.

41. Cucchiara S, Santa Maria F, Minella R, Alfieri E et al. Simultaneous prolonged recordings of proximal and distal intraesophageal pH in children with gastroesophageal reflux disease and respiratory symptoms. Am J Gastroenterol 1995; 90:1791–1796.

42. Argelles-Margin F, Gonsales-Fernandes F, Gentles MG. Sucralfate versus cimetidine in the treatment of reflux esophagitis in children. Am J Med 1989; 86(suppl 6A):73–76.

43. Stacher G, Peeters TL, Bergmann S et al. Erythromycin effects on gastric emptying, antral motility and plasma motilin and pancreatic polypeptide concentrations in anorexia nervosa. Gut 1993; 34:166–172.

44. Lobe TE, Schropp P, Lunsford K. Laparoscopic Nissen fundoplication in children. J Pediatr Surg 1993; 28:358–361.

C. Medical Management

22

Management of the Common Cold

LUCIA FERRO BRICKS

University of São Paulo,
São Paulo, Brazil

I. Introduction

The common cold, also known as acute viral nasopharyngitis or acute viral rhinosinusitis, is the most common illness in humans. Although it is a mild respiratory infection, it is a major cause of morbidity and is responsible for enormous economic losses due to lost productivity and expenditure on medicines (1–9). It is estimated that in the USA, every year, about 25 million people visit their family doctors with uncomplicated upper respiratory infections and the common cold is responsible for 20 million days of absence from work and 22 million days of absence from school (6,8). Recently, a nationwide telephone survey of US households ($n = 4051$) revealed that 67% of adults and 87% of American children experienced at least one non-influenza-related viral respiratory tract infection in the last year. The average adult experienced 2.2 episodes per year, while children less than 18 years old experienced an average of 3.0 annually. The annual expenditure by Americans on over-the-counter (OTC) drugs for treatment of coughs or common colds was substantial; 69% of those survey respondents that had colds self-medicate with an OTC product, 8.2% received prescriptions for antibiotics and 3% for symptomatic therapies. If these data could be extrapolated to the US population, non-influenza-related viral respiratory tract infections were responsible for 500 million episodes annually, and the estimated total cost in the USA approaches \$40 billion annually (5). In Brazil, there are no precise statistics regarding the economic impact of acute respiratory infections of viral etiology; however, the medications used for common cold therapy are among the most frequently sold, with or without medical prescription, and the abusive use of antibiotics is very common (1,2).

The incidence of acute viral rhinosinusitis is greater in children than in adults; these infections are responsible for over 30% of pediatric visits. Furthermore, over half of the children presenting a common cold who are taken to see a physician receive an antibiotic prescription. The medicines used to treat common cold symptoms are sold without medical prescriptions and are amply used by both doctors and the public, who consider them safe and free from adverse effects (1,2,10,11). However, these medications can cause serious adverse reactions in young children. Besides, in Brazil and other countries, indiscriminate use of antibiotics to treat acute respiratory infections of viral etiology is considered to be one of the principal causes of the increase in bacterial resistance (1–5,9–17).

II. Etiology

Common cold is a complex acute catarrhal syndrome, caused by over 200 immunologically distinct types of virus, which present different patterns of seasonal variation and can cause other clinical syndromes. Confirming the diagnosis of a viral infection is a clinical challenge. Results from cultures are not available in a clinically useful time frame and rapid antigen testing is not available for rhinovirus infection. The development of sensitive reverse-transcription poly-merase chain reaction assays has helped to increase the yield of viral pathogens identified and thereby clarify the role of viruses, rhinovirus in particular, in respiratory infections and their complications (14). Rhinoviruses are the most common cause of viral respiratory infections in all age groups, but many other viruses, such as coronaviruses, parainfluenza viruses, influenza viruses, respiratory syncytial viruses (RSV), adenoviruses, enteroviruses, metapneumovirus can cause the same clinical presentation (8).

The relative proportions of different viruses in the cause of common cold vary dependent on age, season, and other factors (Table 22.1) (3,4,7,8,18–20).

Rhinoviruses are the principal agents of acute nasopharyngitis and acute rhinosinusitis; although they generally cause localized disease in the upper respiratory tract, they frequently induce bronchial hyperresponsiveness in young infants and people with chronic respiratory disease (6,14). The systemic manifestations of the common cold are generally less intense than the picture caused by the influenza virus and respiratory syncytial virus; these agents also compromise the lower respiratory tract with greater frequency. In approximately one-third of the cases of acute viral rhinosinusitis it is not possible to identify the etiologic agent, probably due to lack of sensitivity of diagnostic methods currently used to detect viral infections. Although the clinical and epidemiological indications suggest the common cold agent, in the majority of cases the symptoms of the infections caused by different viruses are not specific and, without the aid of laboratory tests, it is impossible to identify the causal agent of acute rhinopharyngitis. Furthermore, in 5–10% of the cases one cannot distinguish rhinopharyngitis of viral etiology from mild rhinopharyngitis caused by group A beta-hemolytic streptococci (2–5,7,9,12–14,16,17,19–21).

III. Epidemiology

The viruses which cause the common cold are found throughout the world and can cause the disease in people regardless of their race, gender, age, or social status. However, the incidence of infections is affected by age, immunological status, exposure, nutritional situation, time of the year, and factors related to personal and environmental hygiene. On average, children aged under 5 have five to eight common cold episodes per year, while adults present only two or three. In the first months of life, the maternal antibodies are transmitted transplacentally and breast feeding provides protection against viral infections. The greatest incidence of viral rhinopharyngitis occurs between 6 and 24 months of age and the children within this age group who live in promiscuous or crowded environments (nurseries, day care centers, large families, institutions) often present up to 10 to 12 common cold episodes per year. Infants also present a greater number of symptoms (fever, bronchospasm) and complications due to bacterial superinfection. Exposure to cigarette smoke and other pollutants aggravates common cold

Table 22.1 Characteristics of the Main Common Cold Agents

Agent	Rhinovirus	Coronavirus	Influenza	SRV[a]	Adenovirus
Immunologic types	100 one subtype	3 or more	3 (A, B, C) several subtypes	2 (A, B)	47
Acute rhinosinusitis (%)	30–50	10–15	5–15	<10	<10
Infection of lower respiratory tract	Rare	Occasional	Common	Common	Common
Season	Autumn and spring	Winter	Winter	Winter	Late winter, spring, and early summer
Incubation period (day)	2–3 days	2–4 days	1–3 days	1–3 days	—
Contagious period (day)	7–10, (up to 3 weeks)	?	7	3–8, (up to 4 weeks)	—

[a]SRV, syncytial respiratory virus.

symptoms and predisposes to complications. There is evidence that some genetic factors, psychological stress and heavy physical training increase the risk of respiratory infections (1–9,12–14,17–20,22).

Children are the main reservoir of respiratory viruses. In general, they are infected in the day care center or school and then transmit the infection to the rest of their family. Direct and prolonged contact with infected individuals is the most efficient means of transmission of respiratory viruses; generally, infections are transmitted by respiratory droplets, but rhinoviruses are most easily acquired via self-inoculation. Experimental studies have demonstrated that 40–90% of the rhinovirus-infected volunteers presented contamination of the hands; the viruses are then passed from person to person through brief hand contact and self-inoculation occurrs when susceptible individuals place their contaminated fingers in direct contact with the nasal or conjunctival mucosa. Transmission of the rhinoviruses and the risk of contracting a common cold are directly related to the presence of high titers of virus in the nasal secretions, contamination of the hands by nasal secretion, and duration of contact with infected individuals. The rhinoviruses, adenoviruses, and respiratory syncytial viruses can be isolated from objects (such as door handles, toys, cups, and glasses) and since they can survive for hours and even days on contaminated surfaces they can also be transmitted by fomites (3–5,7–9,13,16,17,19,20).

The common cold is at its most contagious peak on the second or third day of the disease, a period which coincides with the greatest viral shedding and intensity of symptoms. The majority of the respiratory viruses are shed for a period of less than 7 days; however, in 10–15% of the cases, the rhinoviruses can be isolated from nasal secretions up to 2–3 weeks after the infection and some viruses can be shed for more prolonged periods (Table 22.1) (3,7,8,13,14,16,17).

IV. Clinical Features

The main common cold symptoms are nasal obstruction, watery rhinorrhea, and sneezing, which tend to be most aggravated on the second and third day of the disease. In infants, nasal obstruction frequently interferes with feeding and sleep, besides causing respiratory discomfort. Fever, which occurs in 10–20% of individuals suffering from a common cold, is generally of low grade; however, children aged between 6 months and 3 years tend to present elevated temperature, accompanied by malaise, anorexia, and myalgia. One to three days after the disease onset, nasal secretions which were initially aqueous, become thicker and more purulent. Complaints of throat irritation or soreness, mucupurulent rhinorrhea, and cough are very frequent, occurring in over 30% of the cases; there can also be occasional complaints of earache and hoarseness. Upon physical examination, besides nasal congestion, the physician can also detect hyperemia of the oropharynx, the presence of secretions in the nasopharynx, and, eventually, alterations of the tympanic membrane and discreet enlargement of the ganglions within the cervical region. The common cold symptoms generally disappear spontaneously after 2–7 days, but in 35% of the cases mucupurulent rhinitis and cough can persist for up to 2 weeks. Cough tends to be more intense when there is a great increase in secretions or bronchospasm; it is important to bear in mind that viruses which cause common cold frequently trigger asthmatic attacks and wheezing in infants and individuals with chronic pulmonary disease (3,4,6–8,14–17,19,20).

V. Complications

Sinusitis of viral etiology is 20–200 times more frequent than bacterial sinusitis; however, bacterial superinfection is observed in 0.5–2% of viral rhinosinusitis (1,6,7). It should be remembered that the purulent aspect of rhinorrhea is part of the common cold picture and that bacterial sinusitis must only be diagnosed if cough and mucupurulent rhinorrhea persist for more than 10–14 days (2–5,8,9,13,18–20).

Acute otitis media (AOM) occurs in less than 2% of adults with common cold, but it is very frequent in infants (up to 25%). Although AOM is generally considered a bacterial disease because bacteria are isolated from middle ear fluid in two-thirds of the cases, AOM often occurs concurrently with viral respiratory tract infections (2,4,14–16). Recent studies have shown concomitant respiratory virus infection in 26–42% of the patients with AOM. Rhinovirus, respiratory syncytial virus, parainfluenza viruses, and influenza viruses are most frequently isolated. Some studies have shown that the presence of viruses in middle ear fluid interferes with the bacteriologic response to antibiotic and can significantly worsen the clinical course of bacterial AOM (6,7,18).

The rhinoviruses rarely cause lower respiratory tract infections; however, over 20% of the infants present wheezing during infection by rhinovirus and up to 70% manifest it after infection by RSV. Individuals with chronic respiratory disease not only present worsening of the pulmonary function due to the viral infections but also present a greater rate of bacterial complications especially following infection by the influenza virus (7,9,14,16,19).

VI. Pathogenesis

The respiratory infections begin with local invasion of the epithelial cells, but tissue lesions vary according to the infectious agent and viral burden. Rhinoviruses are the cause of more than 50% of respiratory tract infections (6), and the majority of information regarding the pathogenesis of the common cold has been obtained from studies based on rhinovirus-infected volunteers (3,7).

The cells infected by the rhinovirus include the ciliated and nonciliated nasal epithelial cells. The virus particles have an affinity for the intracellular adhesion molecule 1 (ICAM-1) surface receptors of the epithelial cells and use these sites to attach to and subsequently infect the cell (16,17). Rhinoviruses primarily infect the epithelial cells of the nasopharynx, present low virulence, and cause few histological alterations to the mucosa. Examination of nasal mucosa biopsy specimens shows only edema and vasodilatation in the submucosa, with small infiltration by inflammatory cells. Although the infection causes desquamation of the nasopharynx epithelial cells, the rhinoviruses are isolated from a small number of cells; however, there seems to be a direct correlation between the titers of the virus found in the nasal secretions and the occurrence and severity of the disease. Since the rhinoviruses do not cause major cytopathic effects, it is believed that the pathological alterations are related to the host's inflammatory response. Several studies have shown that experimental infection by rhinovirus is associated with increase in the concentration of different chemical mediators in the nasal secretions (bradykinin, interferon, and interleukins 1β, 2, 6, and 8) and that increase in these cytokines is directly related to the presence and severity of nasal obstruction, coryza, and sore throat (3,6,7,14,16,17,19,20,23). However, since the use of nonsteroidal antiinflammatory drugs and oral steroid therapy does not alleviate the symptoms of nasopharyngitis (2,7,19,24), the role of these chemical mediators in the pathogenesis of the common cold has yet to be established (16,17,19,20,25). Following infection by rhinovirus, no increase in histamine has been observed nor in the other mediators derived from mast cells in nasal secretions (6) and the use of antihistamines does not alleviate nasal symptoms, although it can reduce sneezing (19).

Recent studies have shown that rhinoviruses stimulate the proliferation of lymphocytes Th1-CD4, which produce interferon and IL-2 and that cellular response could have a relevant role in the genesis of common cold symptoms. It has been observed that 3–4 days after infection by rhinovirus there is an increase in lymphocytes and neutrophils in the nasal secretion; in individuals with bronchial hyperresponsiveness, an increase in lymphocytes in biopsy tissue from the bronchial mucosa has been verified. These alterations appear to be associated with the recruiting of lymphocytes from the blood as they coincide with the lymphopenia which accompanies the infection and with the increase in the number of lymphocytes Th1-CD4 in the bronchial mucosa (26). The increase in the local production of interferon-γ contributes to viral clearance, but aggravates common cold symptoms, and since the exogenous administration of interferon-γ does not protect against infection by rhinovirus, some authors have suggested that the pathogenesis of the common cold is due to inappropriate stimulation of the local inflammatory response (19).

The inflammation of the mucosa of the upper respiratory tract, associated with reduction in the mucociliary clearance and the accumulation of secretions, frequently causes an obstruction of the drainage orifices of the paranasal sinuses together with alterations in the functioning of the eustachian tube. These alterations favor growth and penetration of bacteria in the middle ear and paranasal sinuses and are responsible for bacterial complications. The prevalence of otitis media with effusion in autumn, winter, and spring coincides with the period marked by the greatest circulation of rhinovirus, suggesting that these agents are in some way related to this pathology. The influenza viruses and the respiratory syncytial virus, which predominantly circulate during winter, are clearly related to increase in the incidence of AOM of bacterial etiology. Over 70% of the otitis media with effusion and ~93% of AOM begin after acute viral nasopharyngitis, thus common cold prevention can reduce the prevalence of otitis media (6–8,14–17).

Upper respiratory infections caused by rhinoviruses are commonly linked to asthma exacerbations in children and adults (14). There is sample evidences that rhinovirus upper respiratory infections may affect the lower airway by various mechanisms: promoting distal influx of inflammatory cells, stimulating the production of a wide range of inflammatory mediators and the releasing of allergic mediators, stimulating the cholinergic nervous fibers of the respiratory tract, increasing the bronchial hyperresponsiveness, and direct infection of the lower airways (14,17,19,27).

VII. Medicines Used in the Treatment of Common Cold

Different medications with a viricidal action have been tested as common cold treatments; however, whereas many drugs are capable of inactivating some viruses *in vitro*, there are various difficulties involved in the developing of medications with a broad spectrum of action that do not cause an increase in viral resistance. At present, specific antiviral treatments for respiratory viruses are commercially available only for influenza viruses and no viricidal medicine has proven to be effective in the prevention of common colds (2,8,13,15,17,20,28,29).

In the absence of a specific treatment, common cold therapy is directed toward relieving the principal symptoms: nasal congestion, rhinorrhea, cough and irritation, and sore throat. Discharge of nasal secretions not only relieves the discomfort caused by an accumulation of secretions but also reduces the number of bacteria, which is one of the main factors of virulence, decreasing the risk of complications. Nasal hygiene should be performed using saline solution (NaCl 0.9%) and with the child's head tilted back to facilitate the penetration of the solution into the paranasal cavities, increasing the efficacy of the procedure (2,7,16,30). The saline solution can be prepared at home by adding a level tablespoon of salt into boiled water; to avoid contamination, the solution should be kept in a sterilized bottle with a stopper and stored in a refrigerator. The saline solution should be warmed before use. Inhalation of water vapor heated to 40°C alleviates nasal symptoms by increasing the ciliary clearance and reduces the nasal shedding of rhinovirus (1). Humidifying the environment and keeping the child well hydrated also aids in the elimination of mucus and bacteria (2,16,25,30).

While the majority of medicines used in the therapy of common cold symptoms cause few reactions in adults, they can cause serious adverse events when administered to children. Therefore, risks and benefits should be considered with caution (1,2,4,7–9,12–17,19,21,25,29,30).

A. Intranasal Decongestants

Intranasal decongestants can produce vasoconstriction and relieve nasal congestion within 5–10 min; however, they are easily absorbed by the mucosa and may cause vasodilatation rebound. Small children are very sensitive to these medicines and their use should be avoided in infants whenever possible; however, if the nasal obstruction interferes with alimentation or sleep, then nasal instillation of phenylephrine (0.125–0.25%) is recommended, by applying a two-drop dose in each nostril 15–20 min before breast or bottle feeding for 4 or 5 days. The intranasal use of prolonged action vasoconstrictors (naphazoline, tetrahydrazoline, and oxymetazoline) is not recommended for infants, since these medicines frequently cause adverse events such as increased arterial pressure, bradycardia, and neurological alterations (depression or excitation of the central nervous system). Older children present less sensitivity to these medications; nevertheless, topical decongestants should not be used for periods of over 5–10 days in order to avoid irritation of the mucosa and rebound effect (1,2,8,12,13,15–17,19–21,29,30).

B. Combinations Containing Decongestant and Antihistamine (Oral Decongestant) for Systemic Use

The majority of oral decongestants used in the treatment of the common cold are associated with a first-generation antihistamine. In adults, the isolated or associated action of these drugs appears to cause a slight improvement in nasal congestion, rhinorrhea, and cough, without provoking the vasodilatation rebound effect (2,4,7,12,13,23). Since histamine does not play an important role in the pathogenesis of common cold, it is believed that the action of the first-generation antihistamine drugs is due to their anticholinergic effects (2,14–17,19,20,25,29–31). Although these combinations may provide relief for some of the common cold symptoms in adults, there are no well-controlled studies demonstrating the effectiveness of these medicines in children; besides, children aged under 6 years present great susceptibility to the anticholinergic effects of antihistamines and the vasopressor effects of the sympathomimetic amines, which may lead to insomnia, irritability, tachycardia, hypertension, fever, and, more rarely, psychomotor agitation and hallucinations (1,2,4,12,14–17,19,20,25,29–33).

Every year in Brazil, hundreds of children are admitted to hospitals due to adverse events caused by intranasal or oral decongestants (1,2). It is not uncommon for children treated with these medicines to present fever, irritability, or somnolence. They are then submitted to invasive procedures, such as analysis of cerebrospinal fluid, to exclude clinical picture of bacterial meningitis. Thus, the risk/benefit ratio weighs against the use of these medicines in small children (1,2,8,12,14–17,19,20,25,29–32).

The evidence for the efficacy of phenylpropanolamine (D,L-norephedrine) as a nasal decongestant and as an appetite-supressant is very limited, and on November 6, 2000, the US Food and Drug Administration (FDA) removed this drug from OTC status in the USA because of an increased risk of haemorrhagic stroke. Many other regulatory authorities from the main Latin American countries withdrew the drug or implemented similar restrictive actions (32).

C. Topical Anticholinergic Agents

Studies conducted in adults have demonstrated that the topical use of ipratropium bromide (a quaternary derivative of atropine) causes a significant reduction in aqueous hypersecretion. This medicine is barely absorbed by the nasal mucosa and does not cause systemic effects or rebound congestion. Its adverse effects are discreet and less than 10% of the treated individuals need to interrupt the use of this medicine due to the occurrence of epistaxis or dryness of the mucosas. Although it reduces rhinorrhea, ipratropium bromide does not offer relief for other common cold symptoms (congestion and sneezing) (1,2,4,8,12, 13,15–17).

D. Expectorants and Mucolytic Agents

Some expectorants, such as potassium iodine, have a mucolytic action *in vitro*; however, there are no controlled studies which demonstrated the clinical efficacy of these medicines in the treatment of common colds and coughs. The benefits attributed to them are probably due to placebo effect or lack of knowledge regarding the natural history of the common cold. Those cough syrups which contain iodine are contraindicated for children due to the high frequency of hypersensitivity reactions; besides, they may suppress the thyroid activity and cause hypothyroidism. Bromexin is one of the most frequently used mucolytics for the treatment of children, but in addition to failing to improve common cold symptoms, it hinders the resolution of otitis media with effusion (1,2,4,8,12, 13,15–17).

E. Antitussives

Cough is one of the most frequent cold symptoms and is present in 60–80% of all acute viral rhinosinusitis cases. Although this symptom disturbs the child and the family, in the majority of cases it is a protective respiratory reflex triggered in order to remove secretions from the tracheobronchial tree and, thus, should not be suppressed by the use of drugs. At the normally used dose, the majority of antitussives have no efficacy beyond that of a placebo; it is believed that the action of these drugs owes more to the syrups' high sugar content than to any pharmacological effect, since solutions sweetened with sugar or honey also alleviate cough. The mechanism by which sugar reduces cough is notknown, but it may be related to an increase in saliva production and the stimulation of swallowing or the formation of a protective barrier over the nerve fiber endings. To avoid unnecessary expenditure on potentially toxic medicines with questionable efficacy, it is preferable to try to alleviate cough by offering homemade solutions sweetened with sugar or honey. The use of antitussives, preferably nonopioid (dextromethorphan), may be recommended for children with irritative dry cough, provided that there has been no improvement after the use of home-made syrups. However, it is important to note that very young children are highly sensitive to these medicines and may present somnolence and sometimes neurological and respiratory depression, even at weight-adjusted doses. The cough of asthmatic infants and young children is frequently associated with bronchial hyper-responsiveness and, in this situation, the use of bronchodilators (preferably, given by inhalation) may alleviate the symptom (2,4,8,15–17,20,29).

F. Nonsteroidal Anti-inflammatory Drugs

The use of acetaminophen can alleviate the symptoms of irritation or soreness of the throat, as well as other systemic manifestations caused by common cold (fever, malaise, and myalgia). Although some recent studies have demonstrated that the use of naproxen, sulindac, and indometacin may alleviate cough in adults with rhinovirus common cold, the majority of the nonsteroidal anti-inflammatory drugs (NSAIDs) are not approved for use in children. They do not reduce the inflammatory process located on the mucosas and have a narrower safety margin than acetaminophen, due to the risks of digestive bleeding and hypersensitivity reactions. Aspirin, although very much used by adults, is formally contraindicated in children presenting diseases of viral etiology, since even when used in low doses, aspirin increases the risk of Reye's syndrome (2,4,12,16).

G. Antibiotics

The abusive use of antibiotics to treat rhinosinusitis and nasopharyngitis of viral etiology is observed throughout the world. This use of antibiotics is due to lack of knowledge regarding the natural history of the common cold or the belief that these medicines can reduce the incidence of bacterial complications; however, meta-analysis studies have indicated that the prophylactic use of antibiotics does not prevent the occurrence of these complications. The excessive use of antibiotics leads to a series of problems, for both the child and the community: the adverse reactions to antibiotics are not rare and in some cases can be particularly serious (hematological, allergic or pseudoallergic reactions such as serum sickness and Stevens Johnson's syndrome). Furthermore, they interfere with the diagnosis of potentially serious bacterial diseases by preventing the growth of agents in cultures, in addition to increasing the cost of medical treatment and favoring the growth and spread of antibiotic-resistant bacterial strains. It is important to emphasize that mucupurulent rhinitis frequently accompanies common cold, but its presence is not an indication for the use of antibiotics unless it persists without improvement for over 10–14 days (1–5,7–13, 16,17,19,29).

H. Nontraditional Treatments

Recently, the immunomodulating properties of herbal medicines have been studied, because *Echinacea* (herbs, roots, or whole plant) has gained popularity as a treatment for colds (17). Some studies have suggested that some preparations of *Echinacea* could have a possible role in the treatment or prevention of cold, but there is insufficient evidence on the efficacy of these products. It should be emphasized that there are more than 200 different preparations based on different plants and different methods of extraction. Recently, a randomized, double-blind, placebo-controlled study failed to demonstrate any possible benefit in reducing the rate of infection (34) and besides, anaphylaxis has been reported after *Echinacea* use (8,16,34).

VIII.   Common Cold Prevention

A great number of viral strains, each one with its own distinct immunological characteristics, are capable of causing cold, which prevents the development of vaccines. The vaccines against influenza virus can be recommended for children aged over 6 months; however influenza viruses are only responsible for 15% of common colds (9,13–17,19,21,35).

Many medicines have been used in an attempt to prevent infections by rhinovirus or stop their replication in the nasal mucosa.

A.   Vitamin C

The role of vitamin C in the prevention of acute respiratory infection has been the subject of heated debates in the literature. Analysis of six major placebo-controlled studies has shown that daily use of vitamin C in doses above 1.0 g neither prevents nor reduces common cold symptoms. However, some authors have suggested that the use of high doses of vitamin C can reduce the incidence of common cold among certain groups of individuals, but it is possible that these beneficial results can be explained by publication bias (4,36). It should be emphasized that the possible benefits from high doses of vitamin C are minimal when compared to the risks that this therapy entails, such as the formation of renal calculus and the appearance of signs and symptoms of scurvy if the treatment is abruptly interrupted (2).

B.   Zinc Salt Lozenges and Intranasal Zinc

At the beginning of the 1970s, several studies demonstrated that zinc salt lozenges could inhibit *in vitro* replication of rhinoviruses; however, recent meta-analysis of the studies that investigated the effect of zinc salt lozenges in adults with common cold demonstrated that, *in vivo*, these medicines are not effective. Furthermore, zinc salt lozenges have a very disagreeable taste and cause side effects (nausea, altered taste, dry mouth, abdominal pain and headache) in over 40% of the individuals receiving this treatment (2,4,28).

C. Interferons

In adults, the topical use of interferon-α 2 prevents experimental inoculation by rhinovirus. Furthermore, the topical application of interferon and ipratropium bromide, together with the oral use of naproxen, are capable of reducing nasal shedding of rhinovirus and alleviate the disease's symptoms. However, these drugs are expensive and frequently cause irritation and ulceration to the nasal mucosa and have not been tested in children yet (16,17,19,20).

D. New Antiviral Agents

1. *Monoclonal antibody anti-ICAM-1 (tremacamra)*: Attachment of most rhinovirus subtypes to cells depends on a cellular receptor, ICAM-1 (25). This discovery led to attempts to block the attachment of the virus to the receptor, using an anti-ICAM-1 monoclonal antibody (tremacamra) to block receptor sites (4,8,25). Tremacamra or placebo was given beginning 7 h before inoculation with rhinovirus type 39 or 12 h after, in four randomized, double-blind, placebo-controlled trials to 177 volunteers (18–60 years). This drug reduced the severity of experimental rhinovirus colds and was not associated with adverse effects or evidence of absorption through the nasal mucosa (25). Although the drug could give some benefit in the treatment groups, there is a necessity for other studies to evaluate the effect of this drug on symptom severity when given after symptoms have begun (4,8,25).

2. Pleconaril: This is a new drug that can inhibit selectively the replication of picornaviruses and appears to have a good safety profile. The benefits with the use of pleconaril have been demonstrated only when this drug is started within 24 h of symptom onset (8,20).

3. AG7088: This is a 3C protease-inhibitor that can disrupt the function of the rhinoviruses. AG7088 can inhibit cytokine production in the rhinovirus-infected nasal mucosa, but until now there are insufficient data on whether it could be useful and secure to prevent or treat the common cold (8,17).

Many studies have shown that frequent hand washing reduces the transmission of rhinovirus by over 60% and without doubt this procedure is the most effective means of preventing common cold. Training programs for children and the staff of day care centers regarding the importance of hand washing and strict environmental hygiene have proven to be very effective in reducing the rate of common cold transmission (9,35). Families need to be advised against the risks associated with acute respiratory infections and informed about the importance of a well-balanced diet (including exclusive breast feeding for the first 4–6 months) and personal and environmental hygiene. Children should not remain in closed, promiscuous, or polluted environments and, above all, should not be exposed to cigarette smoke. Families should also be instructed regarding the natural evolution of the common cold and also the risks of self-medication with OTC cold remedies, which should be used with parsimony and stored safely out of the reach of children in order to prevent accidental ingestion (2,14–17,20,29).

References

1. Bricks LF, Leone C. Terapêutica das infecções respiratórias agudas: problemas e desafios na melhoria das prescrições médicas. In: Benguigui Y, ed. Investigações operacionais sobre o controle das infecções respiratórias agudas (IRA). Washington, DC: OPAS, c1997:101–108.
2. Bricks LF, Sih T. Controversial drugs in otorhinolaryngology. In: Sih T, Chinski A, Eavey R, eds. II Manual of Pediatric Otorhinolaryngology, IAPO/IFOS. Brazil:Interamerican Association of Pediatric Otorhinolaryngology, 2001:68–87.
3. Couch RB. Rhinoviruses. In: Fields BN, Kniper DM, Howley PM, eds. Fields Virology. 3rd ed. Philadelphia, PA: Lippincott-Raven Publishers, 1996:713–732.
4. Del Mar CB, Glasziou P. Upper respiratory tract infection. Am Fam Physician 2002; 66:2143–2144.
5. Frendrick Am, Monto AS, Nightengale B, Sarnes M. The economic burden of non-influenza related viral respiratory tract infection in the United States. Arch Intern Med 2003; 163:487–494.
6. Greenberg SB. Respiratory consequences of rhinovirus infection. Arch Intern Med 2003; 163:278–284.
7. Gwaltney JM Jr. The common cold. In: Mandel GL, Bennet JE, Dolin R, eds. Mandell, Douglas and Bennett's Principles and Practice of Infectious Diseases. 4th ed. New York: Churchill Livingstone, 1995:561–566.
8. Heikkinen T, Jarvinen A. The common cold. Lancet 2003; 361:51–59.
9. Monto AS, Lehmann D. Acute respiratory infections (ARI) in children: prospects for prevention. Vaccine 1998; 16:1582–1589.
10. Arrow B, Kenealy T. Antibiotics for the common cold (Cochrane review). In: The Cochrane Library. Issue 4 Oxford: Update Software, 2000.
11. Arrow B, Kenealy T, Kerse N. Do delayed prescriptions reduce the use of antibiotics for the common cold? A single-blind controlled trial. J Fam Pract 2002; 51:324–328.
12. Meltzer EO, Tyrell RJ, Rich D, Wood CC. A pharmacological continuum in the treatment of rhinorrhea: the clinician as economist. J Allergy Clin Immunol 1995; 95:1147–1152.
13. Mossad SB. Treatment of the common cold. Br Med J 1998; 317:33–36.
14. Osur SL. Viral respiratory infections in association with asthma and sinusitis: a review. Ann Allergy Asthma Immunol 2002; 89:533–560.
15. Schroeder K, Fahey T. Over the counter medications for acute cough in children and adults in ambulatory settings. Cochrane Database Syst Rev 2001; 4, CD 001831 (latest version May 25, 2001).
16. Snell NJC. New treatments for viral respiratory tract infections—opportunities and problems. J Antimicrob Chem 2002; 47:251–259.

17. Tami TA, Chung SJ. Advances in treating the common cold: an update for otolaryngologists. Curr Opin Otolaryngol Head Neck Surg 2002; 10:179–183.
18. Heikkinen T, Thint M, Chonmaitree T. Prevalence of various respiratory viruses in the middle ear during acute otitis media. N Engl J Med 1999; 340:160–264.
19. Turner RB. Epidemiology, pathogenesis, and treatment of the common cold. Ann Allergy Asthma Immunol 1997; 78:531–540.
20. Turner RB. The treatment of rhinovirus infections: progress and potential. Antiviral Res 2001; 49:1–14.
21. Nairn SJ, Diaz JE. Cold-syrup induced movement disorder. Pediatr Emerg Care 2001; 17:191–192.
22. Cohen S, Doyle WJ, Skoner DP, Rabin BS, Gwaltney JM Jr. Social ties and susceptibility to common cold. J Am Med Assoc 1997; 277:1940–1944.
23. Gwaltney JM, Winther B, Patrie JT, Hendley JO. Combined antiviral-antimediator treatment for the common cold. J Infect Dis 2002; 186:147–154.
24. Gustfson LM, Proud D, Hendley O, Hayden FG, Gwaltney JM. Oral prednisone therapy in experimental rhinovirus infections. J Allergy Clin Immunol 1996; 97:1009–1014.
25. Turner RB, Wecker MR, Pohol G, Witeck TJ, McNally E, St George RMS, Winther B, Hayden FG. Efficacy of tremacamra, a soluble intercellular adhesion molecule 1, for experimental rhinovirus infection: a randomized clinical trial. J Am Med Assoc 1999; 281:1797–1804.
26. Wimalasundera SS, Katz DR, Chain BM Characterization of the T cell response to human rhinovirus in children: implications for understanding the immunopathology of the common cold. J Infect Dis 1997; 176:755–759.
27. Weiner J, Abramson MJ, Puy RM. Intranasal corticoesteroids versus oral H1 receptor antagonists in allergic rhinitis: systematic review of randomised controlled trials. Br Med J 1998; 317:1624–1629.
28. Jackson JL, Lesho E, Peterson C. Zinc and the common cold: a meta-analysis revisited. J Nutr 2000; 130(suppl):1512S–1515S.
29. Taverner D, Bickford L, Draper M. Nasal decongestants for the common cold (Cochrane Review). In: The Cochrane Library. Issue 3 Oxford: Update Software, 2001.
30. Tomooka LT, Murphy C, Davidson T. Clinical study and literature review of nasal irrigation. Laryngocopy 2000; 110:1189–1193.
31. Walsh GM. Second-generation antihistamines in asthma therapy. Is there a protective effect? Am J Respir Med 2002; 1:27–34.
32. Figueras A, Laporte JR. Regulatory decisions in a globalised World: the domino effect of phenylpropanolamine withdrawal in Latin America. Drug Saf 2002; 25:689–693.
33. Wellington K, Jarvis B. Cetirizine/pseudoephedrine. Drugs 2001; 61:2231–2240.
34. Barrett B, Brown RL, Locken KBA, Maberry RBA, Bobula JA, D'Alessio D. Treatment of the common cold with unrefined Echinacea: a randomized, double-blind placebo-controlled trial. Ann Intern Med 2002; 137:939–946.
35. Niffnegger JP. Proper handwashing promotes wellness in child care. J Pediatr Health Care 1997; 11:26–31.
36. Hemila H. Vitamin C intake and susceptibility to the common cold. Br J Nutr 1997; 77:59–72.

23

Allergic Rhinitis and Its Impact on Asthma

PAUL VAN CAUWENBERGE and HELEN VAN HCECKE

University Hospital Ghent,
Ghent, Belgium

JEAN BOUSQUET

University of Montpellier,
Montpellier, France

I. Introduction

Many guidelines have been published nowadays. Some say too many guidelines. I believe that guidelines are extremely useful, especially for the general practitioner, and also for the specialist.

The general practitioner and other primary care health workers are overwhelmed with new, and sometimes conflicting data, so that it is impossible for them to distil the most important data from this multitude of data and to translate them into something useful for their practice. But the specialist also wants to posses a document that summarizes and critically reviews all the data available.

We believe that the time of only opinion-based guidelines is over. Only evidence-based guidelines are acceptable in our era. But we should always bear in mind that guidelines are based on the cross-sectional patient and that every patient is unique! Guidelines should be known by the practitioner, so that he or she can provide the best actual diagnosis and treatment for their patient, but modulation of these guidelines is often necessary in the individual patient because of specific personal or circumstantial reasons. A guideline is not a dictate but a warm suggestion.

Until now there were no global guidelines for allergic rhinitis, although some national or continental position papers and guidelines were produced.

Besides providing an extensive information about what is known about the epidemiology and basic pathophysiological mechanisms, the ARIA working group produced guidelines for the diagnosis and management of allergic rhinitis. It is also the first time that an international evidence-based document is produced about the impact of allergic rhinitis on asthma. For the layperson it is difficult to believe that more than 80% of allergic asthma patients have allergic rhinitis and that about 30% of patients with allergic rhinitis have asthma, but those are the real figures. It also became evident that an appropriate management of allergic rhinitis has a beneficial effect on asthma, and it is essential that this news should be spread to all physicians and health workers concerned.

II. Preface

- Allergic rhinitis is *clinically defined* as a symptomatic disorder of the nose, induced after allergen exposure, by an IgE-mediated inflammation of the nasal membranes.
- Allergic rhinitis represents a *global health problem*. It is a common disease worldwide, affecting at least 10% to 25% of the population, and its prevalence is increasing. Although allergic rhinitis is not usually a severe disease, it alters the social life of patients and affects school performance and work productivity. Moreover, the costs incurred by rhinitis are substantial.
- *Asthma and rhinitis* are common comorbidities, suggesting the concept of "one airway, one disease."
- New knowledge about the mechanisms underlying allergic inflammation of the airways has resulted in better therapeutic strategies. New routes of administration, dosages, and schedules have also been studied and validated.
- Guidelines for the diagnosis and treatment of allergic rhinitis have already been published. However, they have not been evidence-based with a formal assessment of the evidence for recommendations, and have not considered the recommendations in terms of patient comorbidities.
- The Allergic Rhinitis and its Impact on Asthma (ARIA) initiative has been developed in collaboration with the World Health Organization (WHO). This document is intended to be a state-of-the-art pocket guide for the specialist as well as for the general practitioner. It aims to
  — update clinicians' knowledge of allergic rhinitis;
  — highlight the impact of allergic rhinitis on asthma;
  — provide an evidence-based approach to diagnosis;
  — provide an evidence-based approach to treatment;
  — provide a stepwise approach to the management of the disease.

III. Recommendations

1. Classification of allergic rhinitis as a major chronic respiratory disease due to its
   - prevalence;
   - impact on quality of life;
   - impact on work/school performance and productivity;
   - economic burden;
   - links with asthma;
   - association with sinusitis and other comorbidities such as conjunctivitis.
2. Along with other known risk factors, allergic rhinitis should be considered as a risk factor for asthma.

3. A new classification of allergic rhinitis has been made into:
   - intermittent;
   - persistent.
4. The severity of allergic rhinitis is classified as "mild" or "moderate/ severe," depending on the severity of symptoms and quality of life outcomes.
5. Depending on the subdivision and severity of allergic rhinitis, a stepwise therapeutic approach is outlined.
6. The treatment of allergic rhinitis should combine the following:
   - allergen avoidance (when possible);
   - pharmacotherapy;
   - immunotherapy.
7. Environmental and social factors should be optimized to allow the patient to lead a normal life.
8. Patients with persistent allergic rhinitis should be evaluated for asthma by history, by chest examination, and, if possible, by assessment of airflow obstruction before and after a bronchodilator.
9. Patients with asthma should be appropriately evaluated (history and physical examination) for rhinitis.
10. A combined strategy should ideally be used to treat coexistent upper and lower airway diseases in terms of efficacy and safety.
11. In developing countries, a specific strategy may be needed, depending on available treatments and interventions, and their cost.

IV. Classification of Allergic Rhinitis

- *Allergic rhinitis* is clinically defined as a symptomatic disorder of the nose, induced by an IgE-mediated inflammation after allergen exposure of the membranes of the nose.
- *Symptoms* of allergic rhinitis include the following:
  - rhinorrhea;
  - nasal obstruction;
  - nasal itching;
  - sneezing.
- Allergic rhinitis was previously subdivided, based on time of exposure, into seasonal, perennial, and occupational. This subdivision is not entirely satisfactory.
  The following is the new classification of allergic rhinitis:
  - uses symptoms and quality of life parameters;
  - is based on duration and is subdivided into "intermittent" or "persistent" disease;
  - is based on severity and is subdivided into "mild" or "moderate–severe," depending on the symptoms and quality of life (Fig. 23.1).

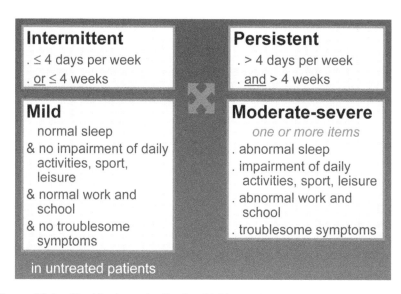

Figure 23.1 Classification of allergic rhinitis. [Adapted from Bousquet J, van Cauwenberge P, Khaltaer N. World Health Organization. Allergic rhinitis and its impact on asthma. Executive summary of the workshop report. Allergy 2002; 57(1):841–855.]

V. Triggers of Allergic Rhinitis

A. Allergens

- *Aeroallergens* are often involved in allergic rhinitis.
    - The increase in domestic allergens is partly responsible for the increase in the prevalence of rhinitis, asthma, and allergies.
    - The allergens present in the home are principally from mites, domestic animals, or insects or are derived from plants.
    - Common outdoor allergens include pollens and molds.
- *Occupational rhinitis* is less well documented than occupational asthma, but nasal and bronchial symptoms often coexist in the same patient.
- *Latex allergy* has become an increasing concern to patients and health professionals. Health professionals should be aware of this problem and develop strategies for treatment and prevention.

B. Pollutants

- Epidemiological evidence suggests that pollutants exacerbate rhinitis.
- The mechanisms by which pollutants cause or exacerbate rhinitis are now better understood.
- *Indoor air pollution* is of great importance since subjects in industrialized countries spend over 80% of their time indoors. Indoor pollution

includes domestic allergens and indoor gas pollutants, among which *tobacco smoke* is the major source.

- In many countries, *urban-type pollution* is primarily of automobile origin and the principal atmospheric pollutants include ozone, oxides of nitrogen and sulfur dioxide. These may be involved in aggravation of nasal symptoms in patients with allergic rhinitis or in nonallergic subjects.
- Diesel exhaust may enhance the formation of IgE and allergic inflammation.

C. Aspirin

Aspirin and other nonsteroidal anti-inflammatory drugs (NSAIDs) commonly induce rhinitis and asthma.

VI. Mechanisms of Allergic Rhinitis

- Allergic rhinitis is classically considered to result from an IgE-mediated response associated with nasal inflammation.
- Allergic rhinitis is characterized by an inflammatory infiltrate made up of different cells. This cellular response includes the following:
  - chemotaxis, selective recruitment, and transendothelial migration of cells;
  - release of cytokines and chemokines;
  - activation and differentiation of various cell types including eosinophils, T-cells, mast cells, and epithelial cells;
  - prolongation of their survival;
  - release of mediators by these activated cells. Among these, histamine and cysteinyl-leukotrienes (CystLT) are the major mediators;
  - communication with the immune system and the bone marrow.
- Nonspecific nasal hyperreactivity is an important feature of allergic rhinitis. It is defined as an increased nasal response to normal stimuli resulting in sneezing, nasal congestion, and/or secretion.
- Intermittent rhinitis can be mimicked by nasal challenge with pollen allergens, and it has been shown that an inflammatory response occurs during the late-phase reaction.
- In persistent allergic rhinitis, allergic triggers interact with an ongoing inflammatory reaction. Symptoms are due to this complex interaction.
- "Minimal persistent inflammation" is a new and important concept. In patients with persistent allergic rhinitis, allergen exposure varies throughout the year and there are periods in which there is little exposure. Even though these patients are symptom-free, they still present with inflammation of the nose.

- The understanding of the mechanisms of disease generation provides a framework for rational therapy in this disorder based on the complex inflammatory reaction rather than on the symptoms alone.

VII. Comorbidities

Allergic inflammation does not limit itself to the nasal airway. Multiple comorbidities have been associated with rhinitis.

A. Asthma

- The nasal and bronchial mucosa have many similarities.
- Epidemiological studies have consistently shown that asthma and rhinitis often coexist in the same patients.
- Most patients with allergic and nonallergic asthma have rhinitis.
- Many patients with rhinitis have asthma.
- Allergic rhinitis is associated with and also constitutes a risk factor for asthma.
- Many patients with allergic rhinitis have increased nonspecific bronchial hyperreactivity.
- Pathophysiological studies suggest that a strong relationship exists between rhinitis and asthma. Although differences exist between rhinitis and asthma, the upper and lower airways are considered to be affected by a common, and probably evolving, inflammatory process, which may be sustained and amplified by interconnected mechanisms.
- Allergic diseases may be systemic. Bronchial challenge leads to nasal inflammation, and nasal challenge leads to bronchial inflammation.
- When considering a diagnosis of rhinitis or asthma, an evaluation of both the lower and upper airways should be made.

B. Other comorbidities

- These include sinusitis and conjunctivitis.
- The associations between allergic rhinitis, nasal polyposis, and otitis media are less well understood.

VIII. Symptoms of Allergic Rhinitis

- Clinical history is essential for an accurate diagnosis of rhinitis and assessment of its severity and likely response to treatment.
- In patients with mild intermittent allergic rhinitis, a nasal examination is optimal. All patients with persistent allergic rhinitis need a nasal examination. Anterior rhinoscopy, using a speculum and mirror,

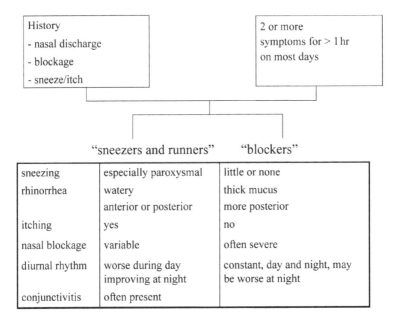

Figure 23.2 Clinical assessment and classification of rhinitis. [Adapted from Lund VJ et al. International Consensus Report on the Diagnosis and Management of Rhinitis. International Rhinitis Management Working Group. Allergy 1994; 49(suppl 19):1–34.]

gives limited information. Nasal endoscopy, usually performed by specialists, is more useful (Fig. 23.2).

IX. Diagnosing Allergic Rhinitis

- *A diagnosis of allergic rhinitis* is based on the following:
  - A typical history of allergic symptoms.
  - Allergic symptoms are those of "sneezers and runners." However, these symptoms are not necessarily of allergic origin.
  - Diagnostic tests.
    — *In vivo* and *in vitro* tests used to diagnose allergic diseases are directed towards the detection of free or cell-bound IgE. The diagnosis of allergy has been improved by allergen standardization, providing satisfactory diagnostic vaccines for most inhalant allergens.
    — *Immediate hypersensitivity skin tests* are widely used to demonstrate an IgE-mediated allergic reaction. These represent a major diagnostic tool in the field of allergy. If properly performed, they yield useful confirmatory evidence for the

diagnosis of a specific allergy. As there are many complexities in their performance and interpretation, it is recommended that they should be carried out by trained health professionals.

— *The measurement of allergen-specific IgE* in serum is of importance and is of similar value as skin tests.

— *Nasal challenge tests* with allergens are used in research and, to a lesser extent, in clinical practice. They may be useful, especially in the diagnosis of occupational rhinitis.

— *Imaging* is not usually necessary.

- *Diagnosis of asthma*
  - Due to the transient nature of the disease and the reversibility of the airflow obstruction (spontaneously or with treatment), a *diagnosis of concomitant asthma* may be difficult.
  - Guidelines for recognizing and diagnosing asthma have been published by the Global Initiative for Asthma (GINA) and are recommended by ARIA.
  - Measurement of lung function and confirmation of the reversibility of airflow obstruction are essential steps in diagnosis of asthma.

X. Management

- The nasal and bronchial mucosa have many similarities.
- The management of allergic rhinitis includes the following:
  - *Allergen avoidance*
    - Most allergen avoidance studies have dealt with asthma symptoms and very few have studied rhinitis symptoms. A single intervention may be insufficient to control symptoms of rhinitis or asthma.
    - However, allergen avoidance, including house mites, should be an integral part of a management strategy.
    - More data are needed to fully appreciate the value of allergen avoidance.
  - *Medications (pharmacological treatment)*;
  - *Specific immunotherapy*;
  - *Education*;
  - *Surgery* may be used as an adjunctive intervention in a few highly selected patients.
- These recommendations provide a strategy that combines the treatment of both upper and lower airway disease in terms of efficacy and safety.
- Follow-up is required in patients with persistent rhinitis and severe intermittent rhinitis (Fig. 23.3).

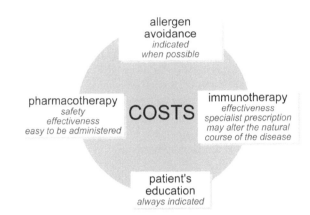

Figure 23.3   Therapeutic considerations. [Adapted from *idem* Fig. 23.1]

XI.   Recommendations Are Evidence-based

- *Recommendations are evidence-based*
  They are based on randomized-controlled trials (RCT) carried out on
  studies performed with the previous classification of rhinitis:
  - seasonal allergic rhinitis (SAR);
  - perennial allergic rhinitis (PAR).
- *The strength of recommendation is*
  - A: recommendation based on RCT or meta-analysis;
  - D: recommendation based on the clinical experience of experts.

For sublingual and nasal SIT, the recommendation is only for very high
dose treatment.

Intervention	Seasonal		Perennial	
	Adult	Children	Adult	Children
Oral H1-antihistamines	A	A	A	A
Intrasanal H1-antihistamines	A	A	A	A
Intrasanal corticosteroids	A	A	A	A
Intrasanal chromones	A	A	A	
Antileukotrienes	A			
Subcutaneous SIT[a]	A	A	A	A
Sublingual SIT	A	A	A	
Nasal SIT	A	A	A	
Allergen avoidance	D	D	D	D

[a]SIT: specific immunotherapy.
Source: Adapted from *idem* Fig. 23.1.

XII. Select Medications

- Medications have no long-lasting effect following discontinuation. Therefore, in persistent disease, maintenance treatment is required.
- Tachyphylaxis does not usually occur with prolonged treatment.
- Medications used for rhinitis are most commonly administered either intranasally or orally.
- Some studies have compared the relative efficacy of these medications, demonstrating that intranasal corticosteroids are the most effective. However, the choice of treatment also depends on many other criteria.
- The use of alternative therapy (e.g., homeopathy, herbalism, acupuncture) for the treatment of rhinitis is increasing. There is an urgent need for large, randomized, and controlled clinical trials for alternative therapies of allergic diseases and rhinitis. Scientific and clinical evidence are lacking for these therapies.
- Intramuscular injection of glucocorticosteroids is not usually recommended due to the possible occurrence of systemic side effects.
- Intranasal injection of glucocorticosteroids is not usually recommended due to the possible occurrence of severe side effects.

Table 23.1   Pharmacological Management of Allergic Rhinitis

	Effect of therapies on rhinitis symptoms				
	Sneezing	Rhinorrhea	Nasal obstruction	Nasal itch	Eye symptoms
H1-antihistamines					
Oral	++	++	+	+++	++
Intranasal	++	++	+	++	0
Intraocular	0	0	0	0	+++
Corticosteroids					
Intranasal	+++	+++	+++	++	++
Chromones					
Intranasal	+	+	+	+	0
Intraocular	0	0	0	0	++
Decongestants					
Intranasal	0	0	++++	0	0
Oral	0	0	+	0	0
Anticholinergics	0	++	0	0	0
Antileukotrienes	0	+	++	0	++

Source: Adapted from van Cauwenberge P, Bachert C, Panalacqua G, Bousquet J, Canonica GW, Durham SR, Fakkens WJ, Howarth PH, Lund V, Malling HJ, Mygind N, Passale D, Scadding GK, Wang DY. Consensus statement on the treatment of allergic rhinitis. European Academy of Allergology and Clinical Immunology. Allergy 2000; 55(2):116–134.

Table 23.2 Glossary of Rhinitis Medications

Generic name	Mechanism of action	Side effects	Comments
		Oral H1-antihistamines	
Second generation	Blockage of H1 receptor	Second generation	New generation oral H1-antihistamines are preferred for their favourable efficacy/safety ratio and pharmacokinetics
Cetirizine	Some antiallergic activity	No sedation for most drugs	Rapidly effective (<1 h) on nasal and ocular symptoms
Ebastine	New generation drugs can be used once daily	Some anticholinergic effect	Poorly effective on nasal congestion
Fexofenadine	No development of tachyphylaxis	No cardiotoxicity	Cardiotoxic drugs should be avoided
Loratadine		Acrivatisne has sedative effects	
Mizolastine		Oral azelastine may induce sedation and a bitter taste	
Acrivastine		First generation	
Azelastine		Sedation is common	
New products		And/or anticholinergic effect	
Desloratadine			
Levocetirizine			
First generation			
Chlorpheniramine			
Clemastine			
Hydroxyzine			
Ketotifen			
Mequitazine			
Oxatomide			
Cardiotoxic			
Astemizole			
Terfenadine			

Local H1-antihistamines (intranasal, intraocular)			
Azelastine Levocabastine	Blockage of H1 receptor Some antiallergic activity for azelastine	Minor local side effects Azelastine: bitter taste in some patients	Rapidly effective (<30 min) for nasal or ocular symptoms
Intranasal corticosteroids			
Beclomethasone Budesonide Flunisolide Fluticasone Mometasone Triamcinolone	Reduce nasal hyperreactivity Potently reduce nasal inflammation	Minor local side effects Wide margin for systemic side effects Growth concerns with some molecules only (*see pediatric section*) In young children consider the combination of intranasal and inhaled drugs	The most effective pharmacological treatment of allergic rhinitis Effective on nasal congestion Effect on smell Effect observed after 6–12 h but maximal effect after a few days
Oral/IM corticosteroids			
Dexamethasone Hydrocortisone Methylpredisolone Prednisolone Prednisone Triamcinolone Betamethasone Deflazacort	Potently reduce nasal inflammation Reduce nasal hyperreactivity	Systemic side effects common in particular for IM drugs Depot injections may cause local tissue atrophy	When possible, intranasal corticosteroids should replace oral or IM drugs However, a short course of oral corticosteroids may be needed with severe symptoms

(continued)

Table 23.2 *Continued*

Generic name	Mechanism of action	Side effects	Comments
Local chromones (intranasal, intraocular)			
Cromoglycate	Mechanism of	Minor local	Intraocular chromones are very
Nedocromil	action poorly known	side effects	effective
			Intranasal chromones
			are less effective and their effect is
			short lasting
			Overall excellent
			safety
Oral decongestants			
Ephedrine	Sympathomimetic drug	Hypertension	Use oral decongestants with caution
Phenylephrine	Relieve symptoms	Palpitations	in patients with heart disease
Pseudoephedrine	of nasal congestion	Restlessness	Oral H1-antihistamine
Others		Agitation	decongestant combination
		Tremor	products may be more effective
		Insomnia	than either product alone, but side
		Headache	effects are combined
		Dry mucous membranes	
		Urinary retention	
		Exacerbation of	
		glaucoma or thyrotoxicosis	

		Intranasal decongestants
Epinephrine Naphtazoline Oxymethazoline Phenylephrine Tetrahydrozoline Xylometazoline	Sympathomimetic drug Relieve symptoms of nasal congestion	Act more rapidly and more effectively than oral decongestants Limit duration of treatment to less than 10 days to avoid rhinitis medicamentosa Same side effects as oral decongestants but less intense Rhinitis medicamentosa (a rebound phenomenon occurring with prolonged use over 10 days)
Others		*Intranasal anticholinergics*
Ipratropium	Anticholinergic block almost exclusively rhinorrhea	Minor local side effects Almost no systemic anticholinergic activity Effective in allergic and nonallergic patients with rhinorrhea
		Antileukotrienes
Montelukast Pranlukast Zafirlukast	Block CystLT receptor	Well tolerated Promising drugs used alone or in combination with oral H1-antihistamines, but more data are needed to position these drugs

Source: Adapted from *idem* Fig. 23.1.

XIII. Consider Immunotherapy

- Specific immunotherapy is effective when optimally administered.
- Standardized therapeutic vaccines are favored when available.
- Subcutaneous immunotherapy raises conflicting efficacy and safety issues. Thus, the use of optimal doses of vaccines labeled either in biological units or in mass of major allergens has been proposed. Doses of 5–20 μg of the major allergen are optimal doses for most allergen vaccines.
- Subcutaneous immunotherapy alters the natural course of allergic diseases.
- Subcutaneous immunotherapy should be performed by trained personnel and patients should be monitored for 20 min after injection.

A. Subcutaneous Specific Immunotherapy Is Indicated

- In patients insufficiently controlled by conventional pharmacotherapy.
- In patients in whom oral H1-antihistamines and intranasal pharmacotherapy control symptoms insufficiently.
- In patients who do not wish to be on pharmacotherapy.
- In patients in whom pharmacotherapy produces undesirable side effects.
- In patients who do not want to receive long-term pharmacotherapy treatment.

B. High-Dose Nasal and Sublingual-Swallow Specific Immunotherapy

- May be used with doses at least 50–100 times greater than those used for subcutaneous immunotherapy.
- In patients who had side effects or refused subcutaneous immunotherapy.
- The indications follow those of subcutaneous injections.

In children, specific immunotherapy is effective. However, it is not recommended to commence immunotherapy in children under 5 years of age.

XIV. Treat in a Stepwise Approach (Adolescents and Adults)

See figure on next page.

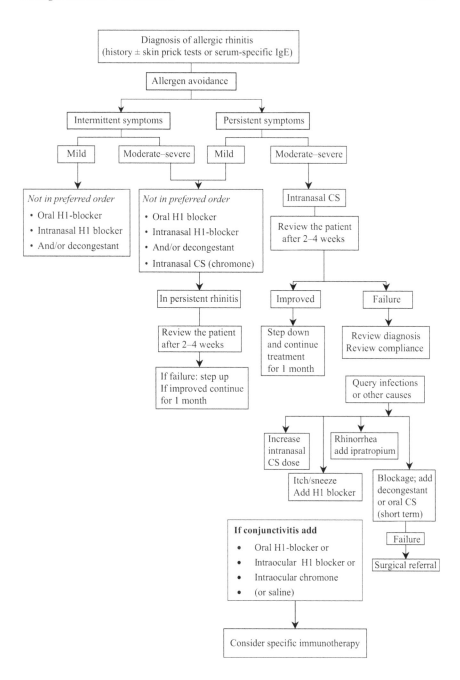

In case of improvement step down. In case of worsening step up. [Adapted from *idem* Fig. 23.1.]

XV. Treatment of Concomitant Rhinitis and Asthma

Treatment of asthma should follow the GINA guidelines

- Some drugs are effective in the treatment of both rhinitis and asthma (e.g., glucocorticosteroids and antileukotrienes).
- However, others are only effective in the treatment of either rhinitis or asthma (e.g., α- and β-adrenergic agonists, respectively).
- Some drugs are more effective in rhinitis than in asthma (e.g., H1-antihistamines).
- Optimal management of rhinitis may improve coexisting asthma.
- Drugs administered by oral route may affect both nasal and bronchial symptoms.
- The safety of intranasal glucocorticosteroids is well established. However, large doses of inhaled (intrabronchial) glucocorticosteroids can induce side effects. One of the problems of dual administration is the possibility of additive side effects.
- It has been proposed that the prevention or early treatment of allergic rhinitis may help to prevent the occurrence of asthma or the severity of bronchial symptoms, but more data are needed.

XVI. Pediatric Aspects

- Allergic rhinitis is part of the "allergic march" during childhood. Intermittent allergic rhinitis is unusual before 2 years of age. Allergic rhinitis is most prevalent during school age years.
- Allergy tests can be done at any age and may yield important information.
- The principles of treatment for children are the same as for adults, but special care has to be taken to avoid the side effects typical in this age group.
- Doses of medication have to be adjusted and special considerations followed. Few medications have been tested in children under the age of 2 years.
- In children, symptoms of allergic rhinitis can impair cognitive functioning and school performance, which can be further impaired by the use of sedating oral H1-antihistamines.
- Oral and intramuscular glucocorticosteroids should be avoided in the treatment of rhinitis in young children.
- Intranasal glucocorticosteroids are an effective treatment for allergic rhinitis. However, the possible effect on growth of some, but not all, intranasal glucocorticosteroids is of concern. It has been shown that

the recommended doses of intranasal mometasone and fluticasone did not affect growth in children with allergic rhinoconjunctivitis.

- Disodium cromoglycate is commonly used to treat allergic rhinocon-junctivitis in children because of the safety of the drug.

XVII. Adapting Guidelines for Use in Low-income Countries

- In developing countries, the management of rhinitis is based on medi-cation affordability and availability.
- The rationale for treatment choice in developing countries is based upon the following:
  - level of efficacy;
  - low drug cost affordable for the majority of patients;
  - inclusion in the WHO essential list of drugs (only chlorpheniramine and beclomethasone are listed);
  - it is hoped that new drugs will shortly be included in this list.
- Immunotherapy is not usually recommended in developing countries for the following reasons:
  - many allergens in developing countries are not well identified;
  - specialists must prescribe desensitization.
- Stepwise treatment proposed:
  - *Mild intermittent rhinitis*—oral H1-antihistamines.
  - *Moderate–Severe intermittent rhinitis*—intranasal beclometha-sone (300–400 μg daily). If needed, after a week of treatment, oral H1-antihistamines and/or a short-term course of oral cortico-steroids will be added.
  - *Mild persistent rhinitis*—treatment with oral H1-antihistamines or a low dose (100–200 μg) of intranasal beclomethasone will be sufficient.
  - *Moderate–severe persistent rhinitis*—intranasal beclomethasone (300–400 μg daily). If symptoms are severe, add oral H1-antihistamines and/or a short course of oral corticosteroids at the beginning of the treatment.
- *Asthma management* for developing countries is included in the IUATLD Asthma Guide. The affordability of inhaled steroids is usually low in developing countries. If the patient can afford to be treated for the both manifestations of the disease, it is recom-mended to add the treatment of allergic rhinitis to the asthma management plan.

ALLERGIC RHINITIS AND ITS IMPACT ON ASTHMA (ARIA)
WORKSHOP REPORT—2001
(J Allergy Clin Immunol 2001; 108:148–336)
In collaboration with the World Health Organization

Members of the Workshop Allergic Rhinitis and Its Impact on Asthma (ARIA)

Expert Panel

Jean Bousquet, Chair
Paul van Cauwenberge, Co-Chair
Nikolai Khaltaev

Nadia Aït-Khaled
Isabella Annesi-Maesano
Claus Bachert
Carlos Baena-Cagnani
Eric Bateman
Sergio Bonini
Giorgio Walter Canonica
Kai-Hakon Carlsen
Pascal Demolí
Stephen R. Durham
Donald Enarson
Wytske J. Fokkens
Roy Gerth van Wijk
Peter Howarth
Nathalia A. Ivanova
James P. Kemp
Jean-Michel Klassek

Richard F. Lockey
Valerie Lund
Ian MacKay
Jans-Jörgen Malling
Eli O. Meltzer
Niels Mygind
Minoru Okuda
Ruby Pawankar
David Price
Glenis K. Scadding
F. Estelle R. Simons
Andrzej Szczeklik
Erkka Valovirta
Antonio M. Vignola
De-Yun Wang
John O. Warner
Kevin B. Weiss

24

Microbiology and Antimicrobial Treatment of Sinusitis in Children

ELLEN R. WALD

University of Pittsburgh,
Pittsburgh, Pennsylvania, USA

Sinusitis is a common complication of viral upper respiratory infection and allergic inflammation. Although the paranasal sinuses are believed to be sterile under normal circumstances, the upper respiratory tract—specifically the nose and oral cavity—are heavily colonized with normal flora.

To determine the microbiology of sinusitis, a sample of sinus secretions must be obtained from one of the paranasal sinuses without contamination by normal respiratory or oral flora (1). The maxillary sinus is the most accessible of the paranasal sinuses. A transnasal approach affords the easiest and safest route of sinus aspiration in patients. A trocar is passed beneath the inferior nasal turbinate across the lateral nasal wall; because the nasal vestibule is so heavily colonized it is essential to attempt to sterilize the area of the nose beneath the inferior turbinate through which the trocar is passed. If this is not done, contaminating nasal flora isolated in the sinus aspirate may be misconstrued as pathogens. Sterilization can be easily accomplished with a topical solution of 4% cocaine. The advantage of cocaine vs. povidine–iodine is that it provides both topical antisepsis and anesthesia and does not irritate the mucosa. Furthermore, to avoid misinterpretation of culture results, infection is defined as the recovery of a bacterial species in high density, that is, a colony count of at least 10^4 colony forming units per milliliter (CFU/mL). This quantitative definition increases the probability that organisms recovered from the maxillary sinus aspirate truly represent *in situ* infection and not contamination. In fact, most sinus aspirates from infected sinuses are associated with colony counts in excess of 10^4 CFU/mL. If quantitative cultures cannot be performed, Gram stain of aspirated specimens affords semiquantitative data. If bacteria are readily apparent on a Gram stain, the approximate bacterial density is 10^5 CFU/mL. The Gram stain is also helpful if bacteria seen on the smear of the specimen fail to grow using standard aerobic culture techniques; anaerobic organisms or other fastidious bacteria should be suspected.

Some authorities recommend performing cultures of the middle meatus instead of aspiration of the maxillary sinus to determine the cause of the bacterial sinusitis (2). However, there are no data in children that correlate cultures of the middle meatus with cultures of the maxillary sinus aspirate (3). Furthermore, unlike the situation in adults, the middle meatus of healthy children is frequently colonized by sinus pathogens (4).

I. Microbiology of Acute Sinusitis in Children

Despite the substantial prevalence and clinical importance of sinusitis in childhood, there has been relatively limited study of the microbiology of sinusitis in pediatric patients. Using a study design similar to the one described by investigators at the University of Virginia, we undertook an investigation of the microbiology of acute sinusitis in pediatric patients in 1979. Patients were eligible for this study if they were between the ages of 2 and 16 years and presented with one of two clinical pictures: onset with either persistent or severe respiratory symptoms. The majority of subjects presented with persistent symptoms, that is, symptoms which lasted more than 10, but less than 30, days and had not yet begun to improve. A minimal duration of 10 days was used to separate simple upper respiratory infection (URI) from acute sinusitis and the maximum duration of 29 days was used to distinguish acute from subacute or chronic sinusitis. The time course of most simple URIs is 5–7 days. Although a patient with a URI may not be completely asymptomatic by the 10th day, usually their symptoms have peaked in intensity and begun to improve. Therefore, persistence of respiratory symptoms beyond 10 days without improvement suggests the presence of a bacterial complication, that is, sinusitis. The respiratory symptoms of acute sinusitis consist of nasal discharge of any quality (thick or thin, serous, mucoid, or purulent) or daytime cough or both. A smaller subset of subjects with acute sinusitis presented with severe respiratory symptoms. Severity was defined as high fever (temperature of at least 102°F) and purulent (thick, colored, and opaque) nasal discharge concurrently for at least three to four consecutive days. This clinical dyad is thought to signify sinus infection when contrasted with the course of the usual URI. Most simple URIs begin with clear nasal discharge, which may become purulent after a few days, but then reverts to a clear quality again before finally resolving. If fever is present at all during an uncomplicated URI, it usually occurs at the beginning of the viral syndrome. By the time the nasal discharge becomes purulent, most children with simple URIs are afebrile. Accordingly, the combination of purulent nasal discharge and fever for several days is suggestive of a bacterial complication, that is, acute sinusitis (5).

Eligible children with either of these two presentations had sinus radiographs performed. The sinus films were considered to be abnormal if they showed diffuse opacification, mucosal thickening of greater than 4 mm, or an air–fluid level. If the sinus films were abnormal and informed consent was provided by the parent, then a sinus puncture was performed, using a transnasal approach.

When a maxillary sinus aspirate was performed on children presenting with either persistent or severe symptoms and significantly abnormal sinus radiographs, bacteria in high density were recovered from 70%. Table 24.1 shows the bacterial species cultured from 79 sinus aspirates obtained from 50 children in their relative order of prevalence.

Streptococcus pneumoniae was the most common, followed closely by *Moraxella catarrhalis* and *Haemophilus influenzae*. Both *M. catarrhalis* and *H. influenzae* may be beta-lactamase producing and thereby amoxicillin resistant. The *H. influenzae* found in sinus aspirates, like those found in infected middle ear cavities, are almost always the nontypeable organisms, reflecting their frequent colonization of the nasopharynx, in contrast to *H. influenzae* type b. Only a single anaerobic bacterial species, a peptostreptococcus, was isolated. No staphylococci were recovered. Mixed infection with heavy growth of two bacterial species was

Table 24.1 Bacterial Species Cultured from 79 Sinus Aspirates in 50 Children

	Single isolates	Multiple isolates	Total
S. pneumoniae	14	8	22
M. catarrhalis	13	2	15
H. influenzae	10	5	15
Eikenella corrodens	1	0	1
Group A *Streptococcus*	1	0	1
Group C *Streptococcus*	0	1	1
α-*Streptococcus*	1	1	2
Peptostreptococcus	0	1	1
Moraxella spp.	1	0	1

occasionally found. In 25% of patients with bilateral maxillary sinusitis, there were discordant bacterial culture results. In some cases, one sinus aspirate was positive, while the other was negative. In the remaining cases, different bacterial species were recovered from each.

Viral cultures were also performed on the maxillary sinus aspirates. Since many children were evaluated after 10 or more days of symptoms, viruses were recovered infrequently. Adenovirus as the only isolate was grown from the aspirate of one subject; parainfluenza virus in combination with a bacterial isolate was recovered from a second. In studies of adults with acute sinusitis other viruses including influenza and rhinovirus have been recovered from ∼10% of sinus aspirates.

II. Microbiology of Subacute Sinusitis in Children

The signs and symptoms of children with subacute sinusitis were described in 1989. These youngsters were evaluated in the context of several different comparative trials of antimicrobial therapy. All children had persistent respiratory symptoms—nasal discharge or cough, or both, lasting between 30 and 120 days. These children were generally well (with minimal constitutional complaints) except for their respiratory symptoms. Intermittent fever was a complaint in 25% of patients but was rarely documented at the time of presentation. Some of these children had previously received one or more courses of antimicrobial agents. In each case they either failed to respond to the antimicrobial or only improved slightly and experienced symptomatic recurrence following cessation of antibiotics. Table 24.2 shows the bacterial species cultured from 52 sinus aspirates from 40 children. Again, the three predominant organisms were *S. pneumoniae*, *H. influenzae*, and *M. catarrhalis*.

III. Microbiology of Chronic Sinusitis in Children

Assessing the microbiology of chronic sinusitis has been particularly difficult. Aspirates are frequently performed immediately after or during a course of

Table 24.2 Bacterial Species Cultured from 52 Sinus Aspirates in 40 Children

Species	Single isolates	Multiple isolates	Total
S. pneumoniae	9	3	12
H. influenzae	9	2	11
M. catarrhalis	6	2	8
Streptococcus pyogenes	2	0	2
Streptococcus viridans	0	1	1
Moraxella species	0	1	1

antimicrobials, which has failed to eliminate the patient's symptoms. Furthermore, sterilization of the mucosa and quantitation of isolates are infrequently performed. The frequent recovery of coagulase-negative staphylococci, viridans streptococci, and diphtheriods is a good example of the dilemma. Often, patients are evaluated during acute exacerbations of chronic sinusitis, which explains the frequent recovery of *S. pneumoniae, H. influenzae,* and *M. catarrhalis.* Three recent series of chronic sinusitis in pediatric patients have been reported (6–8). Methods of obtaining material for culture were either an aspirate of the maxillary sinus (6,7) or an irrigation of the sinus cavity (8). The microbiology of this disorder was described to include primarily *H. influenzae, S. pneumoniae, M. catarrhalis,* coagulase-negative staphylococci, and alpha hemolytic streptococci (9). Anaerobes were recovered from 40% and 13% of the specimens in two of these studies (6,7).

IV. Acute, Subacute, and Chronic Sinusitis in Children

Review of the available data for children permits two summary statements. In patients with acute exacerbations of chronic sinusitis (characterized by persistent or intermittent episodes of purulent nasal discharge), the usual microorganisms associated with acute sinusitis are causative, that is, *S. pneumoniae, M. catarrhalis,* and *H. influenzae.* However, in patients with chronic persistent sinusitis (nasal congestion or rhinorrhea or cough, alone or in combination), the role of bacterial agents is less clear. Most organisms have been recovered in low density, after inadequate sterilization of the contiguous mucosa, and frequently from patients receiving antibiotics to which these organisms are susceptible. The persistence of symptoms despite multiple courses of appropriate antimicrobials is counter to the notion that bacterial infection is a significant component of chronic sinusitis. All of these observations support the hypothesis that bacterial infection has a minor role, if any, in many patients with chronic sinusitis.

In a sense, the very definition of chronic sinusitis, respiratory symptoms that have lasted more than 3 months, implies a failure to respond to antibiotics. At least in the USA, 3 months of respiratory symptoms would almost certainly result in the prescription of several courses of antibiotics. The persistence of symptoms despite the courses of antibiotics is what allows a duration of symptoms long enough to qualify as chronic. The failure to respond to multiple antibiotics, given the tremendous availability of a wide variety of broad-spectrum antimicrobial agents, is less likely a failure to prescribe the correct agent than a reflection of the fact that the process causing the chronic symptoms is not caused by bacterial agents.

V. Microbiology of Sinusitis in Children with Asthma

There have been several very small studies of children with asthma who have sinusitis (10). Many of these patients were experiencing an acute exacerbation of a chronic mucosal process. One such study of eight patients was reported in 1984 by Friedman et al. (10). Sinus puncture and quantitation were performed as described. In this small study, half of the children had positive maxillary sinus aspirates. The bacterial species recovered included *M. catarrhalis, H. influenzae,* and *S. pneumoniae.* A more recent investigation evaluating 12 children between 3 and 11 years of age with asthma was reported by Goldenhersh et al. In this study all subjects had documented respiratory allergy and chronic respiratory symptoms of at least 30 days' duration. All patients had opacification of one or both maxillary sinuses. When maxillary sinus aspiration was performed, *M. catarrhalis* was recovered from six patients and mixed cultures of streptococci were recovered from three patients. Only one patient had anaerobic streptococci mixed with aerobic streptococci.

VI. Medical Treatment

The prescription of antimicrobials is the backbone of the medical management of sinusitis. Table 24.3 shows a list of antimicrobials that have been used to treat patients with acute sinusitis. Amoxicillin at 60 mg/kg per day in two divided doses is acceptable and desirable for the treatment of many cases of bacterial sinusitis in children (11). This is especially true if the episode of acute bacterial sinusitis is uncomplicated, mild to moderate in degree of severity, and if the

Table 24.3 Antimicrobials and Dosage Schedules for the Treatment of Sinusitis in Children

Antimicrobial	Dosage
Amoxicillin	45–90 mg/kg per day in two divided doses
Amoxicillin plus	90 mg/kg per day (of amoxicillin) in two divided doses
Amoxicillin–potassium clavulanate	6.4 mg/kg per day (clavulanate) in two divided doses
Erythromycin– sulfisoxazole	50/150 mg/kg per day in four divided doses
Sulfamethoxazole– trimethoprim	40/8 mg/kg per day in two divided doses
Cefuroxime axetil	30 mg/kg per day in two divided doses
Cefprozil	30 mg/kg per day in two divided doses
Cefixime	8 mg/kg per day in a single daily dose
Cefpodoxime proxetil	10 mg/kg per day in two divided doses
Cefdinir	14 mg/kg per day in a single daily dose
Azithromycin	10 mg/kg per day on day 1; 5 mg/kg per day on days 2–5 in a single daily dose
Clarithromycin	15 mg/kg per day in two divided doses

patient has not recently (<1 month) been treated with antimicrobial agents. Amoxicillin is effective most of the time, inexpensive, and safe.

The emerging problem in the management of acute or recurrent sinusitis is infection caused by *S. pneumoniae* that are resistant to penicillins and cephalosporins (12). The frequency of pneumococci that are resistant to penicillin varies geographically and many isolates of pneumococci are resistant to other commonly used antimicrobials such as erythromycin and trimethoprim–sulfamethoxazole. Therapeutic options include high dose amoxicillin (80–90 mg/kg per day), clindamycin, and rifampin. The increase in the usual dose of amoxicillin from 45 to 90 mg/kg per day represents an attempt to exceed the minimum inhibitory concentration of most *S. pneumoniae* that are resistant to penicillin. The optimal therapy for these infections is not known; antibiotic selection should be guided by susceptibility results when available.

While amoxicillin is preferred in most cases, there are several clinical situations in which a broader-spectrum regimen is appropriate (Table 24.4). These include (1) failure to improve while being treated with amoxicillin, (2) recent treatment with amoxicillin (<1 month), (3) residence in a geographic area with a high prevalence of beta-lactamase producing *H. influenzae*, (4) the occurrence of frontal or sphenoidal sinusitis, (5) the occurrence of complicated ethmoidal sinusitis, and (6) presentation with very protracted (more than 30 days) symptoms.

Antimicrobials with the most comprehensive coverage for patients with sinusitis are the combination of amoxicillin and amoxicillin–potassium clavulanate, amoxicillin–potassium clavulanate alone, cefuroxime axetil, and cefpodoxime proxetil. For patients with chronic sinusitis, amoxicillin–potassium clavulanate is especially attractive because the mechanism for resistance of most pathogens in patients with chronic sinusitis is beta-lactamase production. Eight new antimicrobial agents are available for management of respiratory infections but have not been evaluated in published studies of acute bacterial sinusitis in children: cefixime, ceftibuten, cefprozil, cefpodoxime, cefdinir,

Table 24.4 Indications for Choosing an Alternative Antimicrobial to Amoxicillin for Children with Acute Bacterial Sinusitis

---

Allergy to amoxicillin
Failure to improve while receiving amoxicillin
Recent treatment (<1 month) with amoxicillin
Residence in a geographic area with a high prevalence
    of beta-lactamase producing *Haemophilus influenzae*
    and *Moraxella catarrhalis*
Frontal or sphenoidal sinusitis
Complicated ethmoidal sinusitis
Presentation with very protracted (>30 days) symptoms

---

loracarbef, clarithromycin, and azithromycin. Each of these antibiotics has been investigated in adults with acute sinusitis and found to be satisfactory.

Patients with acute sinusitis may require hospitalization because of systemic toxicity or inability to take oral antimicrobials. These patients may be treated with cefotaxime at a dosage of 200 mg/kg per day, intravenously, in four divided doses or ampicillin–sulbactam at a dose of 200 mg/kg per day, intravenously in four divided doses. These doses of antimicrobials can be expected to be effective in treating virtually all the likely pathogenic bacterial species that cause sinusitis in immunocompetent children.

Clinical improvement is prompt in nearly all children treated with an appropriate antimicrobial agent. Patients febrile at the initial encounter will become afebrile, and there is a remarkable reduction of nasal discharge and cough within 48 h. If the patient does not improve, or worsens, in 48 h, clinical re-evaluation is appropriate. If the diagnosis is unchanged, sinus aspiration may be considered for precise bacteriologic information.

The appropriate duration of antimicrobial therapy for patients with sinusitis has not been systematically investigated. Many patients have a brisk response to antimicrobial intervention and experience dramatic improvement in respiratory symptoms in 3–4 days. For these patients 10 days of treatment is adequate. For patients who respond more slowly, a reasonable recommendation is to treat until the patient is asymptomatic and then for an additional 7 days. A short-course regimen of sulfamethoxazole–trimethoprim (3 days) has been compared to a standard 10-day course in adults with presumed bacterial sinusitis. Although the authors concluded that 3 days of antibiotics were as effective as 10 days, many of their patients may have had viral rhinosinusitis rather than acute bacterial sinusitis.

Adjuvant therapies such as antihistamines, decongestants, and anti-inflammatory agents have received little evaluation. Limited study of systemic decongestants has shown their effect to be an increase in the patency (but not the diameter) of the maxillary sinus ostium and a decrease in nasal airway resistance. Their overall impact on the clinical course of episodes of acute bacterial sinusitis has not been reported. Furthermore, sequential CT scans have shown that decongestants have little or no effect in promptly draining the sinuses. This may in part be due to the viscous quality of sinus secretions in patients with rhinosinusitis. Antihistamines have not been routinely recommended in the treatment of either viral rhinosinusitis or acute bacterial sinusitis. However, recent data generated during experimentally induced rhinovirus infections showed a reduction of sneezing and rhinorrhea in volunteers receiving an antihistamine.

The potential role of topical intranasal steroids as an adjunct to antibiotics in the treatment of acute bacterial sinusitis has recently been evaluated in children and adults. The availability of agents with a rapid onset of activity prompts consideration of these agents for the management of acute symptoms. These agents may exert a modest beneficial effect during the second week of treatment. Further prospective studies will be necessary to fully evaluate the role of these agents in acute bacterial sinusitis.

References

1. Sinus and Allergy Health Partnership. Antimicrobial treatment guidelines for acute bacterial rhinosinusitis. Otolaryngol Head Neck Surg 2000; 123:1–31.
2. Gold SM, Tami TA. Role of middle meatus aspiration culture in the diagnosis of chronic sinusitis. Laryngoscope 1997; 107:1586–1589.
3. Gordts F, Abu Nasser I, Clement PA, Pierad D, Kaufman L. Bacteriology of the middle meatus in children. Int J Pediatr Otorhinolaryngol 1999; 48:163–167.
4. Gordts F, Harlewyck S, Pierard D, Kaufman L, Clement PA. Microbiology of the middle meatus: a comparison between normal adults and children. J Laryngol Otol 2000; 114:184–188.
5. Nash D, Wald ER. Sinusitis. Pediatr Rev 2001; 22:111–116.
6. Brook I, Yocum P, Shah K. Aerobic and anaerobic bacteriology of concurrent chronic otitis media with effusion and chronic sinusitis in children. Arch Otolaryngol Head Neck Surg 2000; 126:174–176.
7. Don D, Yellon RF, Casselbrant M, Bluestone CD. Efficacy of stepwise protocol that includes intravenous antibiotic treatment for the management of chronic sinusitis in children and adolescents. Otolaryngol Head Neck Surg 2001; 127:1093–1098.
8. Slack CL, Dahn KA, Abzug MJ, Chan KH. Antibiotic-resistant bacteria in pediatric chronic sinusitis. Pediatr Infect Dis J 2001; 247–250.
9. Goldenhersh MJ, Rachelefsky GS, Dudley J et al. The bacteriology of chronic maxillary sinusitis in children with respiratory allergy. J Allergy Clin Immunol 1990; 85:1030–1039.
10. Friedman R, Ackerman W, Wald E, Casselbrant M, Friday G, Fireman P. Asthma and bacterial sinusitis in children. J Allergy Clin Immunol 1984; 74:185–189.
11. American Academy of Pediatrics. Subcommittee on Management of Sinusitis and Committee on Quality Improvement. Clinical practice guideline: management of sinusitis. Pediatrics 2001; 108:798–808.
12. Austrian R. The Pneumococcus at the millenium: not down, not out. J Infect Dis 1999; 179(suppl 2):S338–S341.

25

Controversies about Drugs Used Frequently in Respiratory Infections and Allergy in Children

LUCIA FERRO BRICKS and TANIA MARIA SIH

University of São Paulo,
São Paulo, Brazil

I. Introduction

Otorhinolaryngological problems are extremely common in children, especially acute respiratory infections (ARIs) in general associated with fever. In many countries, excessive use of drugs considered as unnecessary and harmful to children is observed in the treatment of these pathologies, as well as abuse of antibiotics, as most ARIs have a viral etiology and cure spontaneously (1,2).

It is estimated that two-thirds of all drugs used in children can have little or no therapeutic value, which results in huge wasting of resources. Besides, the exposure of children to drugs during the period of intensive growth and development is a matter of great concern, as children are more sensitive to the toxic effects of drugs than adults. This question is even more critical when recently launched drugs are being used, as the safety data on new drugs are very limited, especially in relation to its use in children. Unfortunately, little attention has been given to the risk/benefit ratio after marketing release. Few physicians know that adverse effects that occur in less than 1/2000 exposures to drugs cannot be evaluated before drugs are released, as the tests involving drugs before they are marketed are seldom carried out with more than 2000 patients or take more than 3 years. Therefore, the detection of rare events will often occur only after the drug has been marketed, and will depend upon the quality of postmarketing surveillance and the rate of suspicion that physicians have about the possibility of adverse reactions to the drugs. In general, only adults are involved in pharmacological tests and some groups are excluded: children, pregnant women, the elderly, or patients with complex diseases, using a large number of drugs, which can interfere with the drug being tested (1).

Similarly to many other pharmaceutical products, most drugs used in children for ARI treatment have been tested only in adults, often without adequate scientific control. This is a matter for concern, as literature data indicate that physicians are not aware of these problems in practice and use drugs without comprehensive knowledge about the cost/benefit ratio that this approach will bring to the child. Another fact to be considered is that the detection of rare adverse reactions to drugs relies basically on the suspicion of a relationship between the symptom and the use of a drug and on reported cases, which will be studied later on. In a research held in the USA, involving 1121 physicians, on the detection and report of adverse reactions to drugs, 37% had detected at least one adverse effect to drugs in the previous year but only 5% had reported their suspicions to the Food and Drug Administration (FDA). Therefore, it is concluded that knowledge on adverse effects is still very incomplete (1–10).

Despite underreporting, it is known that adverse reactions to drugs are not rare and can result in potential life risk. During a 4-year period (1985–1989), poison-control centers in the USA received ~670,000 consultations related to toxicity in children <6 years of age involving analgesics/antipyretics, cough/cold preparations, or gastrointestinal drugs (5). In Brazil, a research carried out in the two poison-control centers in the city of São Paulo revealed that the drugs with action on the respiratory tract and analgesics, antipyretics, and nonsteroidal antiinflammatory drugs were responsible for 21 and 14% of adverse reactions to drugs in children <10 years of age. It was also verified that more than 80% of adverse reactions were found in children <5 years of age (1).

It is known that many drugs are harmful to children, especially infants, and that drugs recently launched should be prescribed judiciously and under special circumstances. Children are much more sensitive than adults to the side effects of many drugs used in the treatment of ARIs (decongestants, antitussives, topical vasoconstrictors). Even so, treatments with over-the-counter drugs are a common health care management practice in many countries and account for up to 70% of all treatments. In the USA, there are more than 800 over-the-counter drugs for the treatment of cough and/or cold and the estimated expenditure with these drugs is almost $2 billion per year (5,11).

The three groups of drugs most often used in children in most countries, with or without prescription, are analgesic, antipyretic, and nonsteroidal antiinflammatory drugs, antibiotics, and drugs with action on the respiratory system. Although regional variations are found in the selection of the drugs most often used in children, most treatments have no efficacy for ARIs and, unfortunately, abusive use of antibiotics has been observed in the treatment of viral diseases, with risks for the child and the community. In the present chapter, the authors discuss the use of controversial drugs in the treatment of the most frequent otorhinolaryngological allergies and infections in children, emphasizing the respiratory infections (1,4–7,12).

II. Drugs Used as Analgesic, Antipyretic, and Nonsteroidal Antiinflammatory

Analgesic, antipyretic, and nonsteroidal antiinflammatory drugs (NSAIDs) are among the most widely used drugs in children, with or without prescription and, most often, their use is indicated for the treatment of fever and pain that occur in ARI (1).

NSAIDs are a group of substances with similar mode of action, acting on the metabolism of arachidonic acid. Arachidonic acid is normally stored in cell membranes and released under the action of several inflammation and trauma stimuli, and it is metabolized by two metabolic reactions:

1. the cyclooxygenase pathway, leading to the production of several prostaglandins and thromboxane;
2. the lipooxygenase pathway, resulting in the production of leukotrienes.

NSAIDs inhibit the action of cyclooxygenases, blocking the synthesis of prostaglandins and thromboxane, but do not inhibit the lipoxygenase pathway. They can alter the metabolism of the arachidonic acid and promote an increase in leukotrienes, substances that also take part in the inflammatory response.

In the USA, only aspirin, acetaminophen, and ibuprofen have their use approved for the treatment of pain and fever in children younger than 12 years of age. As they have not been adequately tested, the other NSAIDs are not approved by the FDA for use in children without medical supervision; their use is reserved for the treatment of chronic problems, when there is no response with the use of aspirin or ibuprofen (13).

In Brazil, however, most NSAIDs are sold over the counter as pediatric preparations and widely used (with and without prescription) in the treatment of pain and fever in the ARI caused by viruses and bacteria. In São Paulo, 40% of the analgesics used in children younger than 7 years of age have not received the approval of FDA to be used in children. In 1996, 14% of adverse reactions associated with the use of drugs by children living in the city of São Paulo were related to the administration of NSAIDs and, in 40% of the cases, the adverse reactions were related to the use of diclofenac, benzidamine, and piroxicam, drugs that have not been approved for use in children (1).

There is a general agreement in the literature considering acetaminophen as the safest analgesic and antipyretic drug for use in children. Although widely studied, aspirin is formally contraindicated when there is suspicion of viral disease, namely influenza and varicella, as there is an increased risk of Reye's syndrome, even with low doses (1,13).

Besides, aspirin and other NSAIDs cause toxic reactions associated with the inhibition of the enzymatic action of the cyclooxygenase (responsible for the synthesis of prostaglandins). It is important to remember that except for red blood cells, all cells are capable of producing prostaglandins and thromboxane and, besides taking part in the inflammatory response, these substances also participate in several physiological actions.

There are two forms of cyclooxygenase: cyclooxygenase-1 (COX-1), widely distributed in several organs and tissues, and cyclooxygenase-2 (COX-2), the enzyme related to inflammatory processes. Unfortunately, most NSAIDs do not inhibit COX-2 selectively and they act by also inhibiting COX-1, present in the digestive system, platelets, kidneys, and other organs.

Although the toxicity of different NSAIDs can vary, these drugs cause a series of adverse events related to the inhibition of COX-1. The most common adverse reactions occur in the gastrointestinal (GI) tract, skin, platelets, and kidneys. Although most adverse reactions to these drugs are mild, all NSAIDs can cause severe systemic reactions and threat the life of the patient.

Adverse effects on the GI tract can be a result of local irritative and inhibitory action over cyclooxygenase-1. More severe reactions, such as gastric and peptic ulcer that can perforate and bleed and pose a risk on life, are more related to the use of aspirin, diclofenac, fenoprofen, and piroxicam. Although these deleterious effect are more related to the chronic use of NSAIDs (specially in people with history of peptic ulcer), it is important to remember that most of these drugs are not studied in children, and that even ibuprofen (already approved for use in children in the USA) can cause GI bleeding. Another fundamental aspect is that digestive hemorrhage associated with use of NSAIDs can occur without any previous symptom and it has already been proved that NSAIDs can cause severe reactions (hypersensitivity and digestive bleeding), even when used topically (1,13).

The mechanism by which NSAIDs promote analgesia is still unknown, but the analgesic effect of the different NSAIDs is essentially the same. Acetaminophen has analgesic and antipyretic activity comparable to other NSAIDs, but its antiinflammatory activity is low. This fact, however, does not justify the use of other NSAIDs in children, as there are very few studies on the benefits of NSAID to alleviate pain and discomfort associated with ARI in children.

Besides, there is no evidence that NSAIDs reduce the inflammatory process of acute respiratory infections. There is evidence that the use of NSAIDs can compromise the immune response, as it has already been demonstrated that their use is associated with increased shedding of respiratory viruses and the decrease in antibody titers against rhinovirus.

Several studies have emphasized the danger of using NSAIDs. Aspirin and other NSAIDs are involved in 14–27% of drug-related adverse reactions and, in the UK, in 1986, 25% of all drug-related adverse reactions were due to the use of NSAIDs, although these drugs comprised only 5% of all prescribed drugs in that country. It is estimated that in Great Britain there are 12,000 hospitalizations and 2000 deaths per year as a consequence of digestive bleeding associated with the use of NSAIDs (1,13).

Besides digestive manifestations with or without bleeding, NSAIDs can cause anaphylactoid reactions with manifestations such as edema, hives, rhinitis, bronchospasm and, in very severe cases, shock and death. Although these reactions are mediated by nonimmune mechanisms, it is known that atopics are very sensitive to aspirin toxicity and, when there is a reaction to aspirin, it is recommended that other NSAIDs should be discouraged in this group due to the risk of cross reaction.

Thus, acetaminophen is the most indicated analgesic/antipyretic drug for the treatment of pain and fever associated with ARI. In spite of its safety, several cases of severe toxicity have been reported in the USA and UK after accidental ingestion or administration of multiple doses or doses above the recommended for children, as an attempt to reduce the fever in children with ARI.

In São Paulo, NSAIDs were responsible for 14% of the acute toxicity cases in children <10 years of age, and in more than 80% of the cases the child was younger than 5 years and ingested the drug accidentally. In the USA there have been legal requirements since 1970 (Poison Packaging Act of 1970) demanding the use of safe packages for drugs. The use of containers with child-resistant locks reduced from 40% to 55% the number of cases with accidental ingestion of aspirin which, in the 1970s, represented one of the main causes of accidental toxicity and death of children in that country. However, the use of safe packages is not enough to reduce the dangers of adverse reactions to drugs, and parents should be warned as to the excessive use of NSAIDs. The population should be educated, reminding anxious parents that fever plays an important role in immune defense and that there is no need for an aggressive therapy with antipyretic drugs to reduce the child's temperature. Antipyretics should be given with caution and kept out of reach of children to avoid accidental ingestion (1).

III. Drugs Used in the Treatment of Common Cold

ARIs are very frequent and several studies have shown that children younger than 5 years of age have between 4 and 14 episodes of ARI per year, with peak incidence between 6 and 24 months of age. These infections are responsible for >30% of the children <5 years of age who were seen both in emergency pediatric services and in outpatient clinics (10,11).

Most ARIs have a viral cause and common cold is undoubtedly the most frequent ARI in children. Although common cold is a benign and self-limiting disease, its symptoms are annoying and interfere in daily usual activities (school and work), and treatment attempts with several types of drugs are very common (1,5,11). Hutton et al. (4) found that ~25% of the pharmaceutical preparations prescribed for children include drugs for the treatment of common cold. The common cold and bronchitis were the most common reasons for using drugs in 1382 children younger than 7 years of age who attended day care centers in the city of São Paulo. Over half of the children with colds were treated with antibiotics and oral or intranasal decongestants, mucolytics, antitussives, and other cough syrups represented >10% of the all drugs used by the children (1). These data are cause for concern as until today there has been no specific or efficient treatment for the common cold, in spite of its high prevalence (1,12).

Over-the-counter drugs for the treatment of common cold are widely accepted, both by physicians and laypersons, but there is no conclusive evidence as to their clinical efficacy in improving the symptoms of upper airway infections in children. The beliefs that motivated their wide acceptance are based on non-controlled studies or tests with adults.

Drugs used to treat the common cold are:

1. *Vasoconstrictors for nasal use (intranasal decongestants)*—There is no need to use any pharmacological preparation in most acute rhinopharyngitis cases. However, when there is a major obstruction of the upper airways, the nasal instillation of imidazole, 15–20 min before meals can alleviate the symptoms. Phenylephrine is not a good decongestant and has more rebound than imidazole derivatives, which are more potent decongestants (act longer, less rebound, fewer side effects, and better therapeutic index). This procedure must be carried out with care and never for more than 5–10 days, due to the risks of causing mucosal lesions, rebound vasodilation and *rhinitis medicamentosa*. Intranasal decongestants are easily absorbed by the nasal mucosa but can lead to mucosal damages and rebound vasodilation can be seen after their use is interrupted. These drugs are frequent cause of neurological depression in infants. In 1996, in a 6-month period, these drugs caused toxicity in 59 children (1/3 were young than 1 year of age) and all of them had to be hospitalized. Examples of intranasal decongestants' generic names: epinephrine, naphazoline, oxymethazoline, phenylephrine, tetrahydrozoline, and others. Young infants are very sensitive to the effect of these drugs and, whenever possible, their use should be avoided in children younger than 1 year of age (1,12,14).

2. *Associations containing decongestants and antihistamine drugs (oral or systemic decongestants)*—The associations most commonly used in influenza

and colds include a decongestant and an antihistamine. It is less likely that oral decongestants will cause rebound congestion than intranasal decongestants. Most studies carried out in adults on isolated or associated action of these drugs have demonstrated an improvement in nasal symptoms (congestion and rhinorrhea) and decrease of coughing. Although oral decongestants can alleviate nasal congestion and the discomfort caused by colds and influenza, causing few reactions in adults, it is known that there is increased susceptibility to the anticholinergic effects of antihistamine and to the vasopressor effects of sympathomimetic amines in children. Major adverse effects in children include insomnia, irritability, tachycardia, hypertension, and fever. In several cases, the use of these drugs in infants leads to hospitalization and invasive exams (such as cerebrospinal fluid collection), as it is very difficult to differentiate toxicity and meningitis in an infant with irritability and fever. Cases with psychiatric alterations are not uncommon in children treated with products containing phenylpropanolamine, and it is advisable to avoid the use of these drugs in children younger than 6 years of age. Examples of oral decongestants' generic names: ephedrine, phenylephrine, pseudoephedrine, and others. Oral H1-antihistamine–decongestant combination products may be more effective than either product alone, but side effects are combined.

In 1990, one of every 15 cases taken to the poison-control center in Maryland (USA) was related to products used against colds and influenza. In a 6-month period, 149 children (<5 years of age) had adverse events associated with these medications in the city of São Paulo (Brazil), and 34% of them needed hospitalization for several hours. These facts demonstrate that the drugs are not risk-free (1).

In a wide review on the drugs used for treating common cold including studies published between 1950 and 1991, Smith and Feldman (10) concluded that there were no controlled studies demonstrating the efficacy of these drugs in treating common cold. More recently, the results of other studies demonstrated that literature offers very little support for the use of antihistamines in common cold. In 2000, the FDA prohibited, in the USA, the use of phenylpropanolamine due to side effects (1,8,9,12,15).

3. *Antitussives*—Cough is one of the most common cold symptoms and even if it disturbs the child and the family, it is important to remember that in most cases cough is a protective respiratory reflex triggered to remove secretions from the tracheobronchial tree and, thus, should not be suppressed with antitussives.

Most antitussives (codeine and dextromethorphan) only suppress cough when very high doses are given, close to the toxic dose. For most antitussives, the doses normally used in the treatment of cough do not have better effect than placebo. Korppi et al. (6) evaluated the response of children with ARI associated with cough when submitted to three different treatments: dextromethorphan (D), dextromethorphan/salbutamol (DS), and placebo (P), and no differences were found in the evolution of the three groups. In each group, more than half of the children improved with treatment (D = 66%, DS = 56%, and P = 73%), demonstrating that cough associated with ARI is a self-limiting condition.

The self-limiting character of most coughs associated with influenza and common cold has reinforced the popular concept that antitussives are excellent tools for the treatment of these problems and can explain their wide use. Although non-opioid antitussives such as dextromethorphan are considered as being very less toxic, it is known that these drugs are not free from side effects, and can cause drowsiness, nausea and, depending on the dose, even depression of the central nervous system (1).

In the 1990s, it was stated that the sugar content of cough syrups, expectorants, and antitussives have more effect in suppressing cough than the active pharmacological principles. The mechanisms by which sugar reduces cough are unknown, but it is well established that sugar increases saliva production and stimulates swallowing, interfering with the cough reflex. Sugar can also recover nerve endings, acting as a protective barrier against their stimulation. In view of this, it is safer to use household cough preparations or honey with lemon in treating cough associated with ARI than industrial products that contain potentially toxic substances and several additives besides sugar (1,12).

Prescription of antitussives (preferably dextromethorphan) is an exception, and should be restricted to situations where cough is irritative (dry) and interferes in the child's sleep. In these situations, it is important to remember that children younger than 1 year of age are very susceptible to respiratory depression caused by opiates, even when doses are adjusted to their weight. Therefore, whenever possible, drugs containing codeine or dextromethorphan should be avoided in this age group (1).

4. *Expectorants and mucolytics*—In spite of the low toxicity of expectorants and mucolytic agents, there are no controlled studies demonstrating their effectiveness in improving symptoms in children or adults and their action can possibly be related to their sugar content and placebo effect. It should be stressed that, similarly to other drugs, expectorants can cause adverse reactions (nausea, vomiting, and hypersensitivity reactions) (1).

The American Academy of Pediatrics has contraindicated the use of potassium iodide for children since 1976, due to evidence that this drug can suppress thyroid function. Expectorants containing iodine (potassium iodide) have their action proven *in vitro*, but the use of >1 mg/day is not considered to be safe, and can lead to hypothyroidism. Besides, there is large variation in relation to individual sensitivity to the toxic effects of these drugs, which can result in hypersensitivity reactions besides gastric irritation. Drugs containing potassium iodide are still largely used in Brazil, in spite of their restricted use in other countries.

The efficacy of expectorants and mucolytics in modifying the composition of respiratory secretions and decreasing cough is at least doubtful. As they can cause adverse effects and increase the cost of treatment, the use of these drugs in children is contraindicated.

5. *Vitamin C*—The use of vitamin C megadoses against cold and influenza is still the subject of heated debates in the literature. However, there has been no scientific evidence until now that the use of vitamin C is efficient in reducing the symptoms associated with these diseases. Some authors have advocated the use of high doses of vitamin C (up to 6 g/day) to prevent influenza, but it is important to stress that the possible benefits of using high doses of vitamin C are minimal when compared to the risks involved, such as the formation of kidney stones (due to excessive excretion of oxalates), presence of scurvy in fetuses of mothers ingesting high doses of vitamin C and occurrence of scurvy signs and symptoms when the use of vitamin C is suddenly interrupted (rebound scurvy) (1).

IV. Drugs Used in the Treatment of Allergic Rhinitis

It is estimated that 15% of the population is affected by allergic rhinitis and the incidence peak of this pathology is seen among school children, adolescents, and young adults. The major symptoms of allergic rhinitis are nasal congestion, rhinorrhea, sneezing, nasal itching, and tearing. Approximately half of the individuals with allergic rhinitis have perennial symptoms and, due to the presence of congestion and rhinorrhea, very often it cannot be differentiated from common cold.

Although the nasal symptoms associated with allergic rhinitis are not considered to be severe, millions of children and adults suffer because of this problem. Meltzer (16) referred that allergic rhinitis is a frequent cause of school absenteeism (loss of 2 million days/year) and work (loss of 10 million days/year), and that in the USA, in 1990, the total direct cost of allergic rhinitis treatment was $1.16 billion and the indirect cost (productivity loss) was $639 millions. Thus, it becomes extremely important for doctors to be familiar with the drugs used in treating allergic rhinitis.

1. *Antihistamines*—Antihistamines, also known as oral H_1-antihistamines, are a group of various drugs that differ as to their pharmacokinetics, pharmacodynamics, and potency to alleviate symptoms and capacity to produce adverse effects. First generation antihistamines were developed to reduce patient's complaints following the release of histamine from the mast cells in the respiratory tract. Histamine stimulation of blood vessels results in vasodilation and increased vascular permeability, which then results in edema formation and stimulation of sensory nerve endings in the nose, results in sneezing, itching and increased rhinorrhea (1,12).

Oral H_1-antihistamines relieve nasal itching, decrease sneezing and rhinorrhea, but their effect on nasal congestion is negligible. As to their toxicity, first generation antihistamines are lipophilic and can cross the blood–brain barrier, causing several undesirable reactions. Both central nervous system (CNS) stimulation and neurological depression can be observed. The adverse effects more commonly associated with first generation antihistamines are sleepiness, fatigue, weakness, attention deficit, and disturbance of functions requiring attention or use of cognitive skills. These effects are generally dose related. It is not rare, however, to observe an opposite effect, with increased irritability, insomnia, nervousness, tremors, and tachycardia. These reactions are common in children younger than 6 years of age and as they are not always related to the dose, prescription of these drugs for this age group should always be very carefully made.

The second generation antihistamines (nonsedating) do not cross the blood–brain barrier and are less associated with these adverse effects over the CNS. However, it should be stressed that there is less knowledge about these new drugs in relation to children. It was shown that terfenadine and astemizole can cause heart arrhythmia. Terfenadine has already caused the death of more than 100 people and sales have been discontinued in several countries (France, UK, Greece, Luxembourg). Most last long and all, except astemizole, have rapid onset of action. Second generation antihistamines are well absorbed when taken orally and most are metabolized in the liver, in addition to the fact that they are lipophobic (caution is indicated if the patient has decreased liver function). New generation oral H_1-antihistamines are preferred for their favorable efficacy/safety ratio and pharmacokinetics—rapidly effective (<1 h) on nasal and ocular symptoms. However, kidney function should be considered when cetirizine is administered, since its excretion is almost exclusively renal. Nonsedating antihistamines are indicated when the desired effect needs to be obtained without altering daily life activities of the patient. Desloratadine is a new antihistamine which is the orally active metabolite of the nonsedating H_1-antihistamine loratadine. Desloratadine 5 mg once daily in patients with seasonal allergic rhinitis reduce nasal (including congestion) and non-nasal symptoms and improve health-related quality of life. No clinically significant interactions have been reported between desloratadine and drugs that inhibit the cytochrome P450 system, nor the drug potentiate the adverse psychomotor effects of alcohol (in adults).

Some oral H_1-antihistamines, such as ketotifen and astemizole, can increase the appetite and weight gain, and they should always be used with great care (1,12,14,16–18). Examples of generic names of oral H_1-antihistamines:

> second generation—cetirizine, ebastine, fexofenadine, loratadine, mizolastine, acrivastine, azelastine;
> new products—desloratadine, levocetirizine;
> first generation—chlorpheniramine, clemastine, hydroxyzine, ketotifen, mequitazine, oxatomide, others;
> cardiotoxic—astemizole, terfenadine.

Nasal antihistamines, like azelastine, inhibit the release of chemical mediators, including leukotrienes and platelet-activating factor. Its use is safe and effective for seasonal allergic rhinitis. There is little information about the kinetics of azelastine, but the concentrations of its active metabolite, *N*-demillazolastine are 10–20% those of the primary drug. It is use in nasal sprays since it presents adverse reactions if administered through a different route. Levocabastine is a selective antagonist of H_1 receptors and it is applied topically. Levocabastine is structurally unrelated to any currently available antihistamine and appears to be one of the most potent H_1 antagonist yet developed. It has a very rapid onset of action and prolonged activity in both the nose and the eye. It significantly decreases sneezing, itching, rhinorrhea, and tearing, but not congestion. As burning is a frequent complaint among nasal antihistamine users, compliance is a real problem in the pediatric group (14,16,18,19).

2. *Intranasal and Oral Decongestants*—The nasal vasoconstrictors (pseudoephedrine, phenylpropanolamine, epinephrine, phenylephrine, naphazoline, tetyrahydrozoline, or oxymetazoline, xylometazoline) are effective nasal decongestants promoting vasoconstriction within 5–10 min after application. The vasoconstriction effect, however, does not alleviate itching, rhinorrhea, and sneezing symptoms.

The most common adverse effects are sensation of burning and dry mucosa; use for a prolonged time (>1 week) leads to rebound effect (rebound congestion) and *rhinitis medicamentosa*. The use of nasal decongestant can lead to stimulation of the CNS and, in children younger than 1 year of age, severe toxicity cases caused by these drugs are not uncommon, with increased blood pressure, bradycardia, and depression of the CNS.

Thus, nasal decongestants can only be used for short periods of time (5–10 days). If nasal obstruction is a major symptom, the use of oral decongestant is recommended. The use of phenylephrine, phenylpropanolamine, and pseudoephedrine by oral route does not involve rebound risk, but stimulation of the CNS can occur, with tremors, irritability, tachycardia, and insomnia (1,12).

3. *Anticholinergics*—The use of anticholinergic drugs reduces rhinorrhea and promotes a certain degree of vasoconstriction, but most anticholinergics have wide toxicity margin (dry mouth, urinary retention, visual problems, and tachycardia). Recently, several studies have shown that ipratropium bromide, a quaternary derivative of atropine that is little absorbed by the nasal mucosa and does not cross the blood–brain barrier, significantly reduces watery rhinorrhea. However, ipratropium bromide does not alleviate congestion and sneezing.

It is not much absorbed and does not cause systemic effects. Besides, the nasal administration of this drug does not cause rebound congestion. Most of the adverse effects are mild, and <10% of treated individuals need to interrupt the use of this drug due to epistaxis or drying of the mucosa. This seems to be a very promising drug in the management of rhinitis in children, but most efficacy studies involved adults (1,12).

4. *Sodium cromoglycate*—The 4% sodium cromoglycate nasal solution is used in the prophylactic treatment of allergic rhinitis. The drug has been approved in the USA since 1983. The benefits of treatment with this drug are

observed only after 1 week of use and sodium cromoglycate has little effect on nasal obstruction symptoms and is more useful in reducing nasal itching, rhinorrhea, and sneezing. This drug should be indicated when rhinorrhea is important, and its regular use is recommended even in the absence of crisis, with one or two applications in each nostril, four to six times a day. There are very few adverse effects, generally local, and less than 10% of treated individuals need to interrupt the use of this drug as a result of mucosal irritation, sneezing or unpleasant taste in the mouth (1,12,14,16).

5. *Corticosteroids*—Corticosteroids inhibit the inflammatory response in a very efficient manner, regardless of the stimulus (immune, infectious, or chemical). Their effect, however, is palliative and the systemic use of these drugs is associated with many adverse effects (sodium and water retention, arterial hypertension, growth stunting, immunosuppression, etc.), and their use should be reserved for the more severe cases. Corticosteroids developed for nasal use are free from these systemic effects and their potency in alleviating allergic rhinitis symptoms is superior to antihistamines and sodium cromoglycate. But, if there is marked nasal obstruction, a nasal decongestant should be used before the nasal corticosteroid (maximum for 5 days). Nasal corticosteroids are also effective in reducing sinunasal edema. They are more effective when used immediately after the nose has been cleansed and decongested with buffered hypertonic saline irrigation (described in this chapter). Nasal corticosteroids are able of reducing all phases of the allergic response including sneezing, nasal itching, nasal blockage, and rhinorrhea. They have proven to be more efficacious than antihistamines in controlled trials (1,12,17,20).

The nasal corticosteroids (like mometasone furoate, flunisolide, dexamethasone, beclomethasone, triamcinolone, budesonide, fluticasone propionate) are indicated for the treatment and prophylaxis of perennial and seasonal allergic rhinitis, especially when the obstructive component is predominant. Two applications should be made in each nostril (one directed upwards and the other to the lower part of the nasal fossa), twice a day, and preference should be given to water-based formulation. It is fundamental to remember that the effect of these drugs is not immediate (it takes 24–72 h) and some patients have local reactions such as mucosa irritation, burning sensation or pain, and epistaxis. The use of corticosteroid injections in the nasal turbinates is not recommended, as blindness has been reported in more than 10 cases as a consequence of this procedure (1,12,17,20).

V.   Buffered Hypertonic Saline Nasal Irrigation

The fluid trapped in the nose and paranasal sinuses provides an ideal culture medium for the growth of bacteria and high number of bacteria is unquestionably an important factor for virulence. Thus, the topical use of saline nasal washing (preferably at warm temperature), keeping the child well hydrated and in an environment with humidified air to favor the elimination of secretions, are the best approaches in treating cold and influenza. The use of buffered hypertonic saline nasal irrigation should always be encouraged for nasal hygiene in children with rhinitis and sinusitis. It has been used in thousand of patients worldwide and it appears to be safe and effective.

The benefits
- When rinsing the nose with salt water and baking soda mixture, crusts and other debris from the nose are washed from it.
- Salty water pulls fluid out of swollen tissue, which decongests the nose and improves air flow. This makes breathing easier and helps open the sinus passage.

The recipe
- Carefully clean and rinse a $\frac{1}{4}$ of a glass jar (250 cm^3). Fill the clean jar with tap water or bottled water. You do not have to boil the water, unless you live in a place where the water is not adequately treated.
- Add 1 heaping teaspoon of "pickling/canning" salt. *Do not* use table salt. Table salt has unwanted additives. You can ask for pickling salt at the grocery store or, in some countries, marine pure salt (no additive).
- Add one level teaspoon of baking soda (pure bicarbonate).
- Stir or shake before each use. Store at room temperature, in a closed recipient. After a week, pour out any mixture that is left over and make a new recipe.
- If the mixture seems *too strong, use less salt*—try $\frac{1}{2}$ teaspoon of salt.
- For children, it is best to start with a weaker salt water mixture: try $\frac{1}{4}$ to $\frac{1}{3}$ teaspoon of salt. Gradually increase to $\frac{1}{2}$–1 teaspoon of salt, or whatever your child will accept.

How to rinse the nose
- Make the salt water and baking soda mixture according to the recipe described earlier.
- Rinse your nose two to three times a day.
- You may wish to use a bulb or a syringe (about 20 cm^3), or a water pick.

Instructions
- Pour some of the mixture into a clean bowl. Many people like to warm it to about body temperature in a microwave oven. Make sure it is *not hot*.
- Fill the syringe or water pick with the mixture from the jar. *Do not* put the used syringe into the jar with the mixture, because it will contaminate your weekly supply.
- Stand over the sink or in the shower. Squirt the mixture into each side of your nose. Aim the stream toward the back of your head,

not the top of your head. This lets you spit some of the salt water. Swallowing a little will not hurt you.

- Most people notice a mild burning feeling the first few times they use the mixture. This feeling usually goes away in a few days.

For young children

- You can put the mixture in a small spray or aerosol container, like a saline spray or nasal steroid spray bottle.
- Squirt into each side of the nose, several times.
- *Do not* force your child to lie down. Rinsing the nose is easier when sitting or standing.

If you are using a nasal spray

- Always use the salt water mixture first, then use your nasal spray. The nasal corticosteroid (for instance) reaches deeper into the nose and sinuses when it is sprayed onto clean, decongested nasal tissues. Many children, once they started on irrigation and steroid spray, feel such a relief of symptoms that they readily allow the treatment.
- Irrigation should be performed at least twice a day. The initial goal for treatment is not aggressive irrigation, but rather to condition the child to use nasal washings. The washing has two actions: first, it washes debris, irritants, allergens, and excess mucus from the nose; second, the hypertonicity decongests the swollen mucosa. The buffering with sodium bicarbonate (baking soda) makes the solution more tolerable (1).

VI. Antibiotics

A worldwide abusive use of antibiotics in treating ARIs caused by viruses has been observed. In many areas, unfortunately, there is an increased use of antibiotics that should be reserved for the treatment of severe infections in children with acute otitis media or bacterial tonsillitis.

From 1990 to 1992, one in every six children seen by physicians in the USA received an antibiotic prescription, and more than 17 million antibiotic prescriptions were given for nonspecific infections of the upper airways, 16 million for bronchitis, and 13 million for pharyngitis (21). In São Paulo, a research carried out with more than 1000 children, <7 years old, demonstrated that 68% of antibiotics prescribed for children with ARIs were inadequate, most being given for the treatment of common cold (associated or not with wheezing episodes). The major problems found in otitis and tonsillitis cases were the choice of expensive antibiotics (second generation cephalosporins, macrolides), short treatments, and errors in the interval between doses or prescription of antibiotics that are inadequate for streptococci eradication from the oropharynx (sulfamethoxazole/ trimethoprim) (1).

The excessive use of antibiotics and inadequate treatment result in a number of problems for the child and for the community: adverse reactions to antibiotics are not uncommon and in some cases can be very serious (hematological, allergic or pseudoallergic reactions such as the serum sickness, Stevens Johnson's syndrome). In addition, the abusive use of antibiotics interferes in the diagnosis of potentially severe bacterial diseases by precluding growth in bacterial cultures, increases the cost of medical treatment, and favors the growth and spreading of antibiotic-resistant bacterial strains. Many times, the prescription of antibiotics for children with viral infections is an attempt to prevent bacterial complications, such as acute otitis media, sinusitis or pneumonia. However, this practice is totally inefficient in most cases. The prophylactic use of antibiotics should be reserved for specific situations, such as very young children with recurrent otitis media or with rheumatic fever.

Whether appropriate or not, the use of antibiotics has contributed to the emergence and spreading of bacterial resistance and, as already proven, the recent use of antibiotics is a risk factor for the invasive infection by pneumococci resistant to multiple antibiotics. Although physicians report being under pressure by patients and/or relatives to prescribe antibiotics, most parents are not aware of exerting such pressure on physicians. On the other hand, it has already been shown that the level of satisfaction in relation to the medical appointment does not depend on the prescription of drugs, and the decrease in antibiotic prescription can reduce the levels of bacterial resistance. Thus, it is fundamental to avoid the unnecessary use of these drugs both by physicians and laypersons.

The most recent recommendations on the use of antibiotics in ARIs are:

1. *Acute otitis media*—Acute otitis media (AOM) is one of the most frequent diagnosis in pediatrics, affecting 50% of children up to 1 year of age, 65% up to 2 years, and 70% up to 3 years. Otitis media with effusion (OME), however, has a prevalence estimated as 15% and AOM should be clearly differentiated from OME, as AOM can be treated with antibiotics but OME should not. AOM is defined as the presence of fluid in the middle ear, associated with signs and symptoms of acute local or systemic disease (fever, otalgia, otorrhea), while OME is defined as the presence of middle ear fluid, without signs and symptoms of acute ear infection. It is important to remember that after an AOM episode, and in spite of appropriate treatment, fluid can persist in the middle ear of 70% of the children for a 2-week period, 40–50% for 1 month, 20% for 2 months, and 10% for 3 months. Although 86–92% of children with AOM treated with placebo have spontaneous resolution, it is not possible to anticipate which children will have complications, and the use of antibiotics will result in much faster relief of symptoms (12,14,22). There has been an increase in mastoiditis incidence in countries where antibiotics are no longer used for AOM; thus, antibiotics are indicated in treating children with well documented AOM (1).

Children ≥2 years of age, with uncomplicated AOM can be treated for 5–7 days (1). Children ≤2 years, however, are under a higher risk of treatment failure

and should be treated for 10 days. Aggressive treatment of AOM with wide spectrum antibiotics reflects an unreal expectation in relation to their efficacy, both by
physicians and laypersons, as 70–90% of children with AOM improve without
antibiotics. Amoxicillin remains as the first therapeutic option for AOM, and
antibiotics with wider spectrum (amoxicillin-clavulanate, second and third generation cephalosporins) should be reserved for therapeutic failures. Antibiotics
should not be indicated for children with OME, as 80–90% of middle ear
effusions disappear spontaneously, without any treatment. When the middle
ear effusion persists for >3 months, the use of antibiotics can be considered,
although there is high chance of spontaneous cure even in such a situation.
The prophylactic use of antibiotics should be individualized and reserved for
the control of some recurrent AOM cases, due to the increase of microorganisms
resistance, before considering surgery (tympanostomy tube placement) (1,2,22).

    2. *Acute pharyngitis*—The use of antibiotics for children with acute
pharyngitis should be reserved for cases where, based on clinical, epidemiological and laboratory data, infection is considered to be caused by Group A
Streptococcus pyogenes (GAS). Before antibiotics are prescribed for all children
with sore throats, an attempt should be made to isolate the streptococcus from the
oropharynx. If, however, it is not possible to identify the agent and the situation is
not severe (low fever, low intensity pain, and absence of adenopathies), the child
with a sore throat complaint should be reevaluated every 24–48 h, as most
pharyngitis have a viral origin; even in the case of bacterial etiology, the use
of antibiotics can prevent late complications (glomerulonephritis and rheumatic
fever) up to 9 days after the process started. Signs and symptoms of streptococcal
pharyngitis are not specific but suggest bacterial etiology: acute onset, malaise,
abdominal pain, vomiting, presence of exudate, painful adenopathy, petechiae,
and palate edema. Presence of rhinorrhea, cough, hoarseness, conjunctivitis
and diarrhea suggest viral etiology and, therefore, antibiotics should not be
prescribed with such symptoms. Penicillin (penicillin benzathine, oral penicillin,
or amoxicillin) remains as the drug of choice for the treatment of pharyngitis
caused by GAS. Macrolides and cephalosporins are more expensive and due to
their wider spectrum exert more selective pressure over the bacteria, generating
higher bacterial resistance rates. Macrolides can be used in cases of allergy to
penicillin (1,23).

    3. *Sinusitis*—Sinusitis are complications of acute respiratory infections in
0.5–5% of the children. However, before sinusitis is diagnosed it is important to
consider the natural evolution of viral diseases: sore throat and rhinorrhea are in
general present from 3 to 6 days; fever, malaise and myalgia, from 6 to 8 days;
and in 25% of the children with ARI, cough and nasal discharge can be present up
to 14 days later. Due to the lack of specificity (false positives), cost and
irradiation, it is not necessary to take an X-ray of the sinuses in order to diagnose
sinusitis. The diagnosis of sinusitis should be based on the physical examination
and is considered when symptoms (cough, nasal/retropharyngeal secretion) are
persistent from 10 to 14 days after ARI. In spite of the emergence of β-lactamase

producing bacteria, amoxicillin is still the drug of choice for sinusitis and the treatment should be maintained for 10–14 days (7 days after improvement of symptoms), when the child has uncomplicated sinusitis and no underlying pathology (1,19).

4. *Common cold, cough, or bronchitis*—If cough has persisted for <10 days, children do not require antibiotics as most often the etiology is viral and/or allergic and the use of antibiotics does not prevent complications. Children with sinusitis (cough with mucopurulent secretion for >10–14 days), pertussis or infection by *Mycoplasma pneumoniae* should be treated with antibiotics. Before prescribing antibiotics for a child with persistent cough (>30 days), the physician should make differential diagnosis with pneumonia, aspiration of foreign body, cystic fibrosis, and tuberculosis. It should be emphasized that in spite of the increasing prevalence of aminopenicillin-resistant *Streptococcus pneumoniae* and *Haemophilus influenzae* strains, amoxicillin is still considered as the first choice antibiotic for the treatment of otitis and sinusitis in children, due to its lower cost, low incidence of side effects, excellent penetration in the middle ear and ability to eradicate pneumococci with partial resistance to penicillin. When compared to penicillin or amoxicillin, the association amoxicillin/clavulanate and new cephalosporins are less active against totally or partially sensitive pneumococci, and they should be prescribed for cases that failed to respond to treatment with amoxicillin, or when it has been determined that the agents are resistant to this antibiotic (1,2,11,15).

VII. Conclusions

Many drugs of controversial use are sold without medical prescription and most have been used in children, although their clinical efficacy had not been clearly established by well-controlled scientific studies. The possible explanations for the use of these drugs are that efficacy is known through "personal experience," or the belief that these drugs are as safe as the placebos, and can be prescribed as a response to parents' expectations, without major concerns. Although many physicians believe that parents taking their children to the pediatrician will only be satisfied after receiving a prescription, it has already been demonstrated that most families take their children with influenza symptoms to be evaluated in order to eliminate the possibility of more severe health problems. As to satisfaction with medical attention, no differences are seen between parents of children receiving a prescription and those that did not get a prescription. It has also been shown that good medical care is much more efficient than any placebo.

It is important to emphasize that the most recommended treatment for common cold is to alleviate the symptoms, provide relief from pain and fever, and to use saline nasal washing and humidified air to help eliminate secretions. Before prescribing drugs with doubtful action, the pediatrician should educate families as to the self-limiting nature of acute nasopharyngitis. It is known that the use of drugs, whether prescribed or not, is much higher when the mother's perception about the disease is increased. Therefore, it is very important that the families receive all the information about the evolution of the disease. Better communication between physicians and patients, detecting and providing information about their expectations and doubts on how to deal with ARI will certainly improve the quality of medical care provided to the population, and will also prevent huge wasting of resources. Besides the lack of well-controlled studies in children on the efficacy of the drugs most often used to treat influenza and cold, and the apparent low morbidity caused by these drugs, it is important to consider the cost, a common cause of their accidental or intentional ingestion by children <6 years of age. Although the mortality by accidental or intentional ingestion of these drugs is low, physicians prescribing drugs of doubtful efficacy should be prepared to justify their choice and be sure that their use will not cause their patients any harm. It should be remembered that children with poisoning caused by drugs should be treated with gastric lavage, activated charcoal and have to stay in the hospital for several hours.

It is fundamental that physicians make early diagnosis and provide adequate treatment for bacterial diseases in order to avoid their suppurative and non-suppurative complications. However, it should always be remembered that the adequate use of antibiotics is essential to prevent and control bacterial resistance. Another critical aspect is that no drug can replace preventive measures to avoid infectious and allergic diseases, such as good nutrition (including breast feeding for 4–6 months), vaccination, avoiding promiscuous environments, avoiding taking the child to daycare centers during the first year of life, avoiding polluted environments, specially with cigarette smoke and other pollutants that can trigger rhinitis crisis (household dust, mold, hairs and feathers from animals, cockroaches, insecticides, manufactured products containing coloring or preservative additives and other products with strong odor) (1,12).

References

1. Bricks LF, Sih, T. Controversial drugs in otorhinolaryngology. In: Sih T, Chinski A, Eavey R II, eds. Manual of Pediatric Otorhinolaryngology, IAPO/IFOS, Brazil, Interamerican Association of Pediatric Otorhinolaryngology, 2001:68–87.
2. Dowell SF, Marcy M, Phillips WR, Phillips W, Gerber MA. Principles of judicious use of antimicrobial agents for pediatric upper respiratory tract infections. Pediatrics 1998; 101:163–165.
3. Gadomski AM. Rational use of over-the-counter medications in young children. J Am Med Assoc 1994; 272:1063–1064.
4. Hutton N, Wilson MM, Mellitis E. Effectiveness of an antihistamine-decongestant combination for young children with the common cold: a randomized controlled trial. J Pediatr 1991; 118:125–130.
5. Kogan MD, Pappas G, Yu SM, Kotelchuck M. Over-the-counter medications use among US preschool-age children. J Am Med Assoc 1994; 272:1025–1030.

6. Korppi M, Laurikainen K, Pietikäinen M, Silvasti M. Antitussives in the treatment of acute transient cough in children. Acta Paediatr Scand 1991; 80:969–971.

7. Lester MR, Schneider LC. Atopic diseases and upper respiratory infections. Curr Opin Pediatr 2000; 12:511–519.

8. Schroeder K, Fahey T. Over the counter medications for acute cough in children and adults in ambulatory settings. Cochrane Databse Syst Rev, 2001; (4) CD 001831 (latest version 25 May 2001).

9. Schroeder K, Fahey T. Should we advise parents to administer over the counter cough medicines for acute cough? Systematic review of randomised controlled trials. Arch Dis Child 2002; 86:170–175.

10. Smith MBH, Feldman W. Over-the-counter cold medications. A critical review of clinical trials between 1950 and 1991. J Am Med Assoc 1993; 269:2258–2263.

11. Spector SL. The common cold: current therapy and natural history. J Allergy Clin Immunol 1995; 95:1133–1138.

12. Bousquet J. Allergic rhinitis and itis impact on asthma (ARIA). J Allergy Clin Immunol 2001; 108:S147–S336.

13. Litalien C, Jacqz-Aigrain E. Risks and benefits of nonsteroidal anti-inflammatory drugs in children. Pediatr Drugs 2001; 3(11):817–858.

14. Meltzer EO, Tyrell RJ, Rich D, Wood CC. A pharmacological continuum in the treatment of rhinorrhea: the clinician as economist. J Allergy Clin Immunol 1995; 95:1147–1152.

15. Snell HJC. New treatments for viral respiratory infections—opportunities and problems. J Antimicrob Chemother 2001; 47:251–259.

16. Meltzer EO, Prenner BM, Nayak A. Efficacy and tolerability of once-daily 5 mg Desloratadine, an H_1-receptor antagonist, in patients with seasonal allergic rhinitis. An overview of current pharmacotherapy in perennial rhinitis. Clin Drug Invest 2001; 21(1):789–796.

17. Yanez A, Rodrigo G. Intranasal corticoestroids versus topical H1 receptor antagonist for the treatment of allergic rhinitis: a systematic review with meta-analysis. Ann Allergy Asthma Immunol 2002; 89:479–484.

18. Wellington K, Jarvis B. Cetirizine/pseudoephedrine. Drugs 2001; 61:2231–2240.

19. American Academy of Pediatrics. Clinical practice guideline: management of sinusits. Pediatrics 2001; 108:798–808.

20. Weiner J, Abramson MJ, Puy RM. Intranasal corticoesteroids versus oral H1 receptor antagonists in allergic rhinitis: systematic review of randomised controlled trials. Br Med J 1998; 317:1624–1629.

21. O'Brien KL, Dowell SF, Schwartz B, Marcy M, Phillipis WR, Gerber MA. Cough illness/bronchitis—principles of judicious use of antimicrobial agents. Pediatrics 1998; 101:178–181.

22. Dagan R, McCracken GH. Flaws in design and conduct of clinical trials in acute otitis media. Pediatr Infect Dis J 2002; 21:894–902.

23. Schwartz B, Marcy M, Phillips WR, Gerber MA, Dowell SF. Pharyngitis—principles of judicious use of antimicrobial agents. Pediatrics 1998; 101:171–174.

26

Acute Sinusitis in Children: The Importance of Judicious Use of Antimicrobial Agents

FRANCISCO GIMÉNEZ SÁNCHEZ* and **SCOTT F. DOWELL**

Centers for Disease Control and Prevention (CDC),
Atlanta, Georgia, USA

I. Background

Acute sinusitis is defined as an inflammatory reaction of the mucosal lining of the sinuses that is present for <30 days. Such a reaction can be infectious or noninfectious and suppurative or nonsuppurative. Frontal, ethmoid, maxillary, or sphenoid sinuses may be involved. Although the development of ethmoidal and maxillary sinuses begins in the fetus and continues through late adolescence, they are difficult to detect by X-ray before the second year of life. The sphenoid sinuses are developed by the third year; the frontal sinuses are rarely a site of infections until 6 years of age (1,2). Viral rhinosinusitis is at least 20–200 times more common than bacterial sinusitis (3,4). Therefore, the diagnosis of

---

*Unidad de Investigación en Medicina Tropical y Salud Internacional, Instituto de Salud Carlos III, Madrid, Spain.

bacterial sinusitis should be limited to those children with clinical signs and or symptoms that most likely reflect true bacterial disease. In addition, as with cases of acute otitis media, ~60% of sinusitis episodes will resolve or improve spontaneously without antimicrobial therapy (5,6). Ensuring judicious antimicrobial therapy for bacterial sinusitis requires that the use of antimicrobial agents be limited to children most likely to benefit from treatment (7,8). The use of appropriate diagnostic criteria to accurately identify the small subgroup of patients who may have a bacterial infection of the sinuses is a primary goal in promoting the judicious use of antimicrobial agents (9–11).

II. Pathophysiology

Estimates show that most preschool and school-aged children have three to eight acute viral upper respiratory tract illnesses (URIs) a year (12). The typical duration of this acute illness is 7–14 days with subsequent total resolution (13). Recent evidence indicates that uncomplicated viral URIs properly referred to as rhinosinusitis and routinely produce congestion and inflammation of both the nasal and sinus mucosa (3,4,14). The inflammation may result in obstruction of the sinus ostia and in trapping of fluid in the sinus cavities. During an acute URI, the respiratory epithelium of the sinus ostia, of the ostiomeatal complex, and of the sinuses suffers an acute inflammatory response with altered ciliary function and increased secretory activity. Without proper drainage, bacteria that are part of the normal upper respiratory tract flora can be trapped and proliferate in this space. The precise mechanism by which bacterial seeding develops is not fully understood (15,16).

III. Diagnosis

The clinical diagnosis of bacterial sinusitis is generally based either on the duration of signs and symptoms of upper respiratory tract infection or on the presence of exaggerated symptoms and signs in the early period, such as fever of at least 39°C, facial swelling, or facial pain (1,9,17). Acute sinusitis among older children and adults occasionally can be diagnosed by the presence of classic signs and symptoms, such as sinus tenderness, tooth pain, headache, and high fever (18). However, these sign and symptoms are rare in young children. For diagnosis of young children, prolonged duration of the disease for >10–14 days without improvement, rather than simply the presence of any specific sign or symptom, is most discriminatory in differentiating between uncomplicated URIs and bacterial sinusitis (19).

   Studies both of experimentally induced infections with adult volunteers, and of patients with documented community-acquired rhinovirus causing URI have revealed the natural history of uncomplicated URIs (20–24). Most uncomplicated URIs improve within 5–7 days, although 20% of patients have persisting cough or nasal discharge at 14 days. Estimates show that 5–10% of URIs in early childhood are complicated by acute sinusitis (25). Although many clinicians believe that mucopurulent rhinitis (thick, opaque, or discolored nasal discharge) is a sign of bacterial sinusitis, studies of experimental rhinovirus colds have shown that nasal discharge changes from clear to purulent during the first few days of illness as part of the natural history of the disease (26). In addition, the color and characteristics of the discharge do not explain the etiology of the infection; these changes should be recognized as part of the natural course of an uncomplicated URI and not as a bacterial complication of the paranasal sinuses.

Although no radiographic images of sinuses alone can confirm a diagnosis of bacterial sinusitis, such images can sometimes support the clinical impression. Abnormal images depict inflammation, but do not indicate whether the inflammation is viral, bacterial, or allergic in origin. Conventional Waters views can show changes in acute sinusitis such as diffuse opacification, mucosal thickening of at least 4 mm, or fluid level (27). Because, the sinuses of children may not be fully developed, radiologic findings can be difficult to interpret and can lead to overdiagnosis of sinusitis (28–30). Therefore, more complicated radiologic investigation should be reserved for confirmation of clinical diagnoses of recurrent sinus infections; for evaluation of children with persistent, complicated, or severe infections; and for situations that potentially require surgical intervention.

IV. Microbiology

Most microbiologic data are derived from samples obtained directly from the maxillary sinus through the transnasal route. The maxillary sinus is the most accessible of the paranasal sinuses. Maxillary sinus puncture is the only reliable method of gathering material for bacterial culture because swab cultures do not correlate well with cultures of sinus aspirates. However, sinus puncture is not initially necessary for a diagnosis of children. Indications for sinus aspiration include unresponsiveness to therapy, sinus disease in immunocompromised hosts, or life-threatening complications.

Acute sinusitis is usually caused by the same bacterial pathogens that cause acute otitis media [i.e., *Streptococcus pneumoniae*, *Haemophilus influenzae* (usually nontypable), and *Moraxella catarrhalis*] (Table 26.1).

These bacteria are found in approximately three-quarters of maxillary sinus aspirates of patients with acute sinusitis, and are identified by strict criteria (31–33). Of 30 children with clinical and radiographic signs of maxillary sinusitis in one study, bacteria were cultured from maxillary sinus fluid of 77%, and viruses were cultured from fluid of 7% (32). Group A *Streptococci* are occasionally isolated from the sinus specimens of children. Of the isolates identified by culture of sinus aspirates of children and adults, *S. pneumoniae* accounts for 30–66%, *H. influenzae*, and *M. catarrhalis* each account for 20% and viral pathogens alone account for ~10% (5,32,34–36). *Staphylococcus aureus* is

Table 26.1 Bacteria Associated with Acute
Maxillary Sinusitis

Bacteria	% Associated
Negative bacterial culture	23–42
S. pneumoniae	13–36
H. influenzae	13–30
M. catarrhalis	4–19
S. aureus	4–12
Group A Streptococcus	1–2
Group C Streptococcus	1–4
S. viridans	0–2
Eikenella corrodens	0–1
Peptostreptococcus	0–1

rarely implicated in acute sinusitis among either children or adults (31). Several families of viruses have been directly implicated in the pathogenesis of acute sinusitis. In experimental rhinovirus infection, Turner et al. (37) found, through magnetic resonance scanning, mucosal thickening or fluid accumulation in the sinuses of one third of volunteers. Other viruses involved in acute sinus disease may be influenzae, parainfluenzae, respiratory syncytial (RSV), and on occasion, adenovirus (32). Fungal infection is a rare but serious cause of sinusitis, especially in older children. A diagnosis of fungal infection should be considered if routine antimicrobial treatments fail, in patients with nasogastric tubes or other foreign bodies, or in immunocompromised patients (38).

V. Treatment

Expert disagree on the treatment of acute sinusitis, including the indications for antimicrobial therapy and timing of intervention. Acute sinusitis will resolve without antimicrobial therapy in more than half of cases. In a trial among adults with acute maxillary sinusitis, 77% of patients taking placebo improved after 2 weeks (39). In another contemporary, randomized, double-blind trial, 52% of patients taking placebo recovered (40). Among children, Wald and colleagues (6) found a 60% clinical response rate among placebo-treated patients and a 77% rate among antibiotic-treated patients by day 10. A meta-analysis of 27 randomized clinical trials showed that in two-thirds of the cases of sinusitis either improved or resolved spontaneously without antibiotic treatment (41). However, treatment with any antibiotic reduced the rate of clinical failures by half, justifying antibiotics as the mainstay of sinusitis treatment.

Treatment should be directed toward *S. pneumoniae*, *H. influenzae*, and *M. catarrhalis*. Both the frequency of β-lactamase-producing *M. catarrhalis* and *H. influenzae* and the increasing prevalence of antibiotic resistance among

S. pneumoniae and other bacteria have prompted many physicians to use more expensive and broader-spectrum antibiotics. However, two recently published meta-analyses found that amoxicillin was as effective as more expensive antibiotics for the initial treatment of uncomplicated acute sinusitis (41,42). Despite β-lactamase production by some isolates, therapy with amoxicillin still is successful for the initial treatment of acute uncomplicated sinusitis among most children (15,16). Tetracyclines and erythromycin when are used alone, miss a large percentage of *H. influenzae* and *S. pneumoniae*. Cotrimoxazole might be another option; however, it is ineffective against group A *Streptococcus*, and *S. pneumoniae* is commonly resistant to it (43) and can induce very severe side effects.

The widespread use of antimicrobial agents, whether appropriate or inappropriate, has driven the emergence and spread of resistant organisms. The association of resistance with the use of antibiotics is well documented (44,45). For this reason, the use of broader-spectrum antibiotics should be reserved for patients who show no clinical response within 48–72 h of initial antibiotic treatment, patients with recurrent infections, or patients with history of frequent courses of multiple antibiotics. For treatment of these patients, a β-lactamase-stable agent, such as amoxicillin–clavulanate, or a second generation cephalosporin that is also active against penicillin-resistant pneumococci should be considered (46). When treating resistant bacterial infections, a new formulation of amoxicillin–clavulanate with 14:1 proportion might be used (90 mg/kg per day) to improve efficacy against pneumococci (47). The first-generation cephalosporins (e.g., cefadroxil, cephalexin) are not appropriate for treating sinusitis unless *S. aureus* or other *Streptococcus* infection has been confirmed (48). Whereas some second- and third-generation cephalosporins, such as cefprozil, cefuroxime, and cefpodoxime, are effective against *H. influenzae*, *M. catarrhalis*, and *S. pneumoniae*, other second- and third-generation cephalosporins, such loracarbef, cefaclor, cefixime, and ceftibufen have poor activity against *S. pneumoniae* (47,49–52). Among adults, shortened course antibiotic treatment with azithromycin (5 days) showed similar outcomes and side effects as treatment with amoxicillin (10 days) (53). Trials involving children with acute otitis media have demonstrated no differences between 3 and 5-day treatments with azithromycin and 10-day treatments with amoxicillin–clavulanate (54,55). Clarithromycin was reported to be as effective as amoxicillin in the treatment of acute maxillary sinusitis; however, this study did not independently evaluate effectiveness in patients with β-lactamase-producing organisms or resistant *S. pneumoniae* (56). The fluoroquinolones are active against a wide range of bacteria; newer members of this class have improved activity against *S. pneumoniae*. Levofloxacin has been evaluated in adults and appears to be an effective and safe treatment against the most common pathogens causing sinusitis (57). However, because of concern about cartilage toxicity seen in all juvenile animal models examined, fluoroquinolones remain generally contraindicated for children younger than 18 years.

The duration of antibiotic treatment for acute sinusitis is not clearly established by comparative studies. Most experts suggest that duration should be limited to seven days beyond the point of substantial improvement or resolution of signs and symptoms, making the total course of treatment 10–14 days. Several studies have found that shortened courses of cephalosporin treatment have similar results as 10-day courses (58). Other studies recommend prolonging therapy to a minimum of two weeks of antibiotic treatment (1). Nevertheless, more prolonged therapy (i.e., 3–4 weeks) is not necessary unless improvement in signs and symptoms is delayed.

References

1.   Incaudo G, Wooding LG. Diagnosis and treatment of acute and subacute sinusitis in children and adults. Clin Rev Allergy Immunol 1998; 16:157–204.
2.   Maltinski G. Nasal disorders and sinusitis. Prim Care 1998; 25:663–683.
3.   Gwaltney JM. Acute community-acquired sinusitis. Clin Infect Dis 1996; 23:1209–1225.
4.   Gwaltney J, Phillips C, Miller R, Riker D. Computed tomographic study of the common cold. N Engl J Med 1994; 330:25–30.
5.   Axelsson A, Chidekel N, Grebelius N, Jensen C. Treatment of acute maxillary sinusitis. Acta Otolaryngol 1970; 70:71–76.
6.   Wald E, Chiponis D, Ledesma-Medina J. Comparative effectiveness of amoxicillin and amoxicillin–clavulanate in acute paranasal sinus infections in children: a double-blind, placebo-controlled trial. Pediatrics 1986; 77:795–800.
7.   Morris P, Leach A. Antibiotics for persistent nasal discharge (rhinosinusitis) in children. Cochrane Database Syst Rev 2002:CD001094.
8.   McCaig LF, Besser RE, Hughes JM. Trends in antimicrobial prescribing rates for children and adolescents. J Am Med Assoc 2002; 287:3096–4027.
9.   O'Brien KL, Dowell SF, Schwartz B, Marcy M, Phillips WR, Gerber MA. Acute sinusitis—principles of judicious use of antimicrobial agents. Pediatrics 1998; (suppl 101):174–177.
10. Steinman MA, Landefeld CS, Gonzales R. Predictors of broad-spectrum antibiotic prescribing for acute respiratory tract infections in adult primary care. J Am Med Assoc 2003; 289:719–725.
11. Contopoulos-Ioannidis DG, Ioannidis JP, Lau J. Acute sinusitis in children: current treatment strategies. Paediatr Drugs 2003; 5:71–80.
12. Monto AS, Ullman BM. Acute respiratory illness in an American community. J Am Med Assoc 1974; 227:164–169.
13. Wald E, Guerra N, Byers C. Upper respiratory tract infections in young children: duration of and frequency of complications. Pediatrics 1991; 87:129–133.
14. Puhakka T, Mäkelä MJ, Alanen A, Kallio T, Korsoff L, Arstila P, Leinonen M, Pulkkinen M, Suonpää J, Mertsola J, Ruuskanen O. Sinusitis in the common cold. J Allergy Clin Immunol 1998; 102:403–408.
15. Giebink GS. Childhood sinusitis: pathophysiology, diagnosis and treatment. Pediatr Infect Dis J 1994; 13:S55–S65.

16. Glasier CM, Mallory GB, Steele RW. Significance of opacification of the maxillary and ethmoid sinuses in infants. J Pediatr 1989; 114:45–50.
17. Wald ER. Management of sinusitis in infants and children. Pediatr Infect Dis J 1988; 7:449–452.
18. Williams JW, Sinel DL, Roberts L, Samsa GP. Clinical evaluation for sinusitis. Making the diagnosis by history and physical examination. Ann Intern Med 1992; 117:705–710.
19. Ueda D, Yoto Y. The ten-day mark as a practical diagnosis approach for acute paranasal sinusitis in children. Pediatr Infect Dis J 1996; 15:576–579.
20. Farr BM, Conner EM, Betts RF, Oleske J, Minnefor A, Gwaltney JM. Two randomized controlled trials of zinc gluconate lozenge therapy of experimentally induced colds. Antimicrob Agents Chemother 1987; 31:1183–1187.
21. Gohd R. The common cold. N Engl J Med 1954; 250:687–691.
22. Gwaltney JM, Hendley JO, Jordan WS. Rhinovirus infections in an industrial population. J Am Med Assoc 1967; 202:158–164.
23. Anzueto A, Niederman MS. Diagnosis and treatment of rhinovirus respiratory infections. Chest 2003; 123:1664–1672.
24. Varonen H, Savolainen S, Kunnamo I, Heikkinen R, Revonta M. Acute rhinosinusitis in primary care: a comparison of symptoms, signs, ultrasound, and radiography. Rhinology 2003; 41:37–43.
25. Wald ER. Sinusitis in children. Isr J Med Sci 1994; 30:4032–4107.
26. Hays GC, Mullard JE. Can nasal bacterial flora be predicted from clinical findings? Pediatrics 1972; 49:596–599.
27. Kogutt MS, Swischuk LE. Diagnosis of sinusitis in infants and children. Pediatrics 1973; 52:121–124.
28. Glasier CM, Mallory GB, Steele RW. Significance of opacification of the maxillary and ethmoid sinuses in infants. J Pediatr 1989; 114:45–50.
29. McAlister WH, Lusk R, Muntz HR. Comparison of plain radiographs and coronal CT scans in infants and children with recurrent sinusitis. AJR Am J Roentgenol 1989; 153:1259–1264.
30. Dykewicz MS. 7. Rhinitis and sinusitis. J Allergy Clin Immunol 2003; 111:S520–S529.
31. Penttila M, Savolainen S, Kiukaanniemi H, Forsblom B, Jousimies-Somer H. Bacterial findings in acute maxillary sinusitis—European study. Acta Otolaryngol (Stockh) (suppl 529):165–168.
32. Wald ER, Milmoe GJ, Bowen A, Ledesma-Medina J, Salamon N, Bluestone CD. Acute maxillary sinusitis in children. N Engl J Med 1981; 304:749–754.
33. Wald ER. Microbiology of acute and chronic sinusitis in children. J Allergy Clin Immunol 1992; 90:452–460.
34. Arruda LK, Mimiça IM, Solé D, Schoettler J, Heiner DC, Naspitz CK. Abnormal maxillary sinus radiographs in children: do they represent bacterial infection? Pediatrics 1990; 85:553–558.
35. Gwaltney J, Sydnor A, Sande M. Etiology and antimicrobial treatment of acute sinusitis. Ann Otol Rhinol Laryngol 1981; 90:68–71.
36. Murphy TF. Respiratory infections caused by non-typeable *Haemophilus influenzae*. Curr Opin Infect Dis 2003; 16:129–134.
37. Turner BW, Cail WS, Hendley JO, Hayden FG, Doyle WJ. Physiologic abnormalities in the paranasal sinuses during experimental rhinovirus colds. J Allergy Clin Immunol 1992; 90:474–478.

38. Morpeth JF, Rupp NT, Dolen WK, Bent JP, Kuhn FA. Fungal sinusitis: an update. Ann Allergy 1996; 76:128–139.

39. Van Buchem FL, Knotterus JA, Schrijnemaekers VJJ, Peeters MF. Primary-care-based randomised placebo-controlled trial of antibiotic treatment in acute maxillary sinusitis. Lancet 1997; 349:683–687.

40. Lindbaek M, Hjortdahl P, Johnsen ULH. Antibiotic treatment in acute bacterial sinusitis. Lancet 1997; 349:1476.

41. De Ferranti SD, Ioannidis JPA, Lau J, Anninger WV, Barza M. Are amoxycillin and folate inhibitors as effective as other antibiotics for acute sinusitis? A meta-analysis. Br Med J 1998; 317:632–642.

42. de Bock GH, Dekker FW, Stolk J, Springer MP, Kievit J, Van Howelingen JC. Antimicrobial treatment in acute maxillary sinusitis: a meta-analysis. J Clin Epidemiol 1997; 50:881–890.

43. Hopp R, Cooperstock M. Medical management of sinusitis in pediatric patients. Curr Probl Pediatr 1997; 27:178–186.

44. Baquero F, Martinez-Beltran J, Loza E. A review of antibiotic resistance patterns of *Streptococcus pneumoniae* in Europe. J Antimicrob Chemother 1991; 28(suppl C): 31–38.

45. McGowan JE Jr. Antimicrobial resistance in hospital organisms and its relation to antibiotic use. Rev Infect Dis 1983; 5:1033–1048.

46. Poole M. Antimicrobial therapy for sinusitis. Otolaryngol Clin North Am 1997; 30:331–339.

47. Dowell SF, Butler JC, Giebink S, Jacobs MR, Jernigan D, Musher DM, Rakowsky A, Schwartz B. Acute otitis media: management and surveillance in an era of pneumococal resistance—a report from the drug-resistant *Streptococcus pneumoniae* Therapeutic Working Group. Pediatr Infect Dis J 1999; 18:1–9.

48. Schaefer SD, Ronis ML. Cephalexin in the treatment of acute and chronic maxillary sinusitis. South Med J 1985; 78:45–48.

49. Gehanno P, Depondt J, Barry B, Simonet M, Dewer H. Comparison of cefpodoxime proxetil with cefaclor in the treatment of sinusitis. J Antimicrob Chemother 1990; 26(suppl E):87–91.

50. Howie VM, Owen MJ. Bacteriologic and clinical efficacy of cefixime compared with amoxicillin in acute otitis media. Pediatr Infect Dis J 1987; 6:989–991.

51. Wald ER, Reilly JS, Casselbrant C, Chiponis DM. Treatment of acute sinusitis in children: Augmentin vs cefaclor. Postgrad Med 1984; (Augmentin Sym Suppl Sept–Oct):133–136.

52. Gwaltney JM Jr. Management update of acute bacterial rhinosinusitis and the use of cefdinir. Otolaryngol Head Neck Surg 2002; 127:S24–S29.

53. Casiano RR. Azithromycin and amoxicillin in the treatment of acute maxillary sinusitis. Am J Med 1991; 91(suppl 3A):27S–30S.

54. Aronovitz G. A multicentre, open label trial of azithromycin vs amoxicillin/clavulanate for the management of the acute otitis media in children. Pediatr Infect Dis J 1996; 15:S24–S29.

55. Principi N. Multicentre comparative study of the efficacy and safety of azithromycin compared with amoxicillin/clavulanic acid in the treatment of paediatric patients with otitis media. Eur J Clin Microbiol Infect Dis 1995; 14:669–676.

56. Karma P, Pukander J, Pentila M, Ylikoski J. The comparative efficacy and safety of clarithromycin and amoxicillin in the treatment of outpatients with acute maxillary sinusitis. J Antimicrob Chemother 1991; 27(suppl A):83–90.

57. Sydnor TA, Kopp EJ, Anthony KE, LoCoco JM, Kim SS, Fowler CL. Open-label assessment of levofloxacin for the treatment of acute bacterial sinusitis in adults. Ann Allergy Asthma Immunol 1998; 80:357–362.

58. Pichichero ME, Cohen R. Shortened course of antibiotic therapy for acute otitis media, sinusitis and tonsillopharyngitis. Pediatr Infect Dis J 1997; 16:680–695.

27

Antimicrobial Agents Most Often Used in the Main Otorhinolaryngological Infections in Children: Emphasis on Sinusitis

TANIA MARIA SIH

University of São Paulo,
São Paulo, Brazil

ITZHAK BROOK

Georgetown University,
Washington, D.C., USA

I. Introduction

Antimicrobial agents are substances that inhibit the growth or kill microorganisms. If of natural origin, they are called antibiotics, whereas if the origin is synthetic, they are called chemotherapic agents. Bacteriostatics are agents that inhibit bacterial growth. Bactericidal agents are those that destroy the bacteria. In some clinical situations, a therapeutic response may be reached with the use of any of the two types. In other situations, it is preferable to use a bactericide agent. This is the case, for example, in meningitis and endocarditis.

A. General Concepts About Antimicrobial Agents

Antimicrobial agents should ideally present the following characteristics:

- low toxicity and acceptale side effects;
- *in vivo* efficacy against the pathogen;
- appropriate spectrum according to the clinical indications;
- low incidence of development microbial resistance;
- low cost;
- ease of administration;
- sufficient concentration at the site of infection;
- adequate pharmacokinetics and pharmacodynamics.

Antimicrobial agent possess various mechanisms of action:

1. Agents that inhibit the synthesis of bacterial cell membrane, including: penicillin, cephalosporin, vancomycin, bacitracin, cycloserine, imidazole antimycotic agents (miconazole, clotrimazole, ketoconazole).

2. Agents that modify the microorganism cell membrane permeability. These include: polymyxin B, colistin (polymyxin E), polyene antimycotic agents, such as amphotericin B and nystatin.
3. Agents that affect the ribosome subunits 30S and 50S causing reversible inhibition of protein synthesis. These bacteriostatic agents include: chloramphenicol, tetracycline, clindamycin and macrolides (erythromycin, azithromycin, and clarithromycin).
4. Agents that bind to the ribosome subunit 30S and modify the protein synthesis, eventually leading to cell death. This group includes the aminoglycosides.
5. Agents that affect the metabolism of nucleic acid. This group includes the quinolones and rifampin.
6. Agents that block specific and essential microorganism metabolic pathways. This group comprises sulfonamides and trimethoprim.
7. Nucleic acid-analog agents that inhibit viral enzymes essential to DNA synthesis. This group includes acyclovir, zidovudine, gancyclovir, and vidarabine.

Specific action mechanisms of some antimicrobial agents are unkown.

The factors that affect clinical response are the following:

- patients' immunocompetence (immunodepressed patients respond poorly to antimicrobial therapy);
- site and of infection (i.e., deep infections, such as endocarditis or osteo-myelitis respond more slowly to antiinfectious agents);
- underlying medical condition (i.e., diabetes);
- virulence of the pathogen (more virulent species tend to present the worst therapeutic response);
- species of microorganisms (fungi or viruses generally have poorer responses to antimicrobial agents than bacteria);
- natural history of the disease (it is important to know the natural course of the disease, anticipating the clinical response, thus avoiding premature and inappropriate changes in the antimicrobial agents).

Failure in clinical responses to antimicrobial agents can also be caused by other reasons:

- inappropriate choice of antimicrobial agent, dosage or administration route;
- incorrect diagnosis of the microbial etiology;
- failure in the drug diffusing into the infected site;
- failure in draining purulent collections or removal of a foreign body;
- superinfection by other organism(s) common after prolonged chemotherapy;

- appearance of strains resistant to the antimicrobial agent(s) used;
- participation of two or more microorganisms in the infectious processes, when therapy is directed only against some of the causative
  organisms.

The objective of antimicrobial therapy is to achieve eradication of the
pathogen(s) from the specific infected site(s). The concepts of pharmacokinetics,
pharmacodynamics, and bioavailability provide information that is essential in
achieving optimal clinical efficacy and minimizes toxicity.

Pharmacodynamics correlates the drug concentration with its clinical or
pharmacological effect. In the case of an antibiotic, the correlation refers to the
drug's ability to kill or inhibit the growth of the microorganism involved. The
drug concentration is measured in relation to time in the serum,body fluid, or
in the tissues, using the concentrations that are necessary to determine the
minimum inhibitory concentration (MIC) of the antibiotic for the organism(s).
The drug concentration in blood (plasma or serum) has been correlated with
bacterial eradication *in vivo*.

Pharmacokinetic/pharmacodynamic (PK/PD) parameters, such as the
ratio of peak to minimum inhibitory concentration (peak/MIC ratio), ratio of
24-h area under the curve to MIC (24-h AUC/MIC ratio), and the time
above MIC, are good indicators of the drug dose–organism interaction.
Time above the MIC is the important determinant of the activity of
β-lactams, macrolides, clindamycin, and linezolid. Free drug serum levels of
these drugs should be above the MIC for at least 40–50% of the dosing interval to produce adequate clinical and microbiological efficacy. Peak/MIC and
24-h AUC/MIC ratios are major determinants of the activity of aminoglycosides and fluoroquinolones. In general, peak/MIC ratios should exceed 8 and
24-h AUC/MIC values should be >100 to successfully treat Gram-negative
bacillary infections and to prevent the emergence of resistant organisms
during therapy. The successful treatment of pneumococcal infections with
fluoroquinolones and azithromycin appear to require 24-h AUC/MIC ratios
of only 25–35. Mutation prevention concentrations are being reported for
various fluoroquinolones with different pathogens, but their clinical significance has not yet been established.

The physician must be well informed about pharmacodynamic aspects, as it
will allow him/her to integrate the drug microbiology with its pharmacokinetic
properties. Pharmacokinetics and pharmacodynamics of new antibiotics will
not be discussed in this brief summary, and readers are encouraged to consult
specialized textbooks.

We will initially present the main antimicrobial groups prescribed for children with upper airway infections. We will also discuss the appropriate antibiotic
therapy for children with sinus infection, based on the bacterial etiology for this
infection.

II. Antimicrobial Agents Most Often Used Against Upper Airway Infections in Children

A. Penicillins and β-Lactams

Penicillin, the first antibiotic to be discovered in 1928 by Alexander Fleming, and introduced in clinical practice in 1941 by Howard Florey, derives from the fungus *Penicillium notatum*. Penicillin, similarly to cephalosporin, is a β-lactam antibiotic because it has a β-lactam ring. Even though its mechanism of action has not been yet been fully determined, the bactericidal activity of penicillin includes the inhibition of cell wall synthesis and the activation of bacterial autolytic endogenous system. Penicillin is active against the cell wall, which contains peptideglycan. During the process of bacterial replication, penicillin inhibits the enzymes that bind to the peptide chains, preventing the development of the normal structure of peptideglycan. These enzymes (transpeptidase, carboxypeptidase, endopeptidase) are located under the cell wall and are called penicillin-binding proteins (PBPs). Bacteria, differ in the composition, types and concentration of PBPs and, consequently, in cell wall permeability to antibiotics. Therefore, there are different bacterial susceptibilities to penicillins. Penicillins are relatively safe agents and are the most frequently employed antibiotics for the treatment of upper airway infections in children.

Preparations and Characteristics of Penicillin G

- Crystalline penicillin G (aqueous)—parenteral use, preferably IV, although it may also be administered intramuscularly (IM). It is clinically used when fast effect or high drug serum concentrations are desired. It can be used in severe infections, such as meningitis, pneumonia and endocarditis, caused by susceptible bacteria. Pediatric doses range from 100,000 to 400,000 U/kg per day (the latter used for nervous system infections).
- Procaine penicillin (short half-life)—IM. It is more allergenic than the aqueous form and its clinical use should be limited to mild to moderate infections caused by penicillin-sensitive bacteria that do not tolerate oral formulations. The recommended doses in children range from 25,000 to 50,000 U/kg per day, administered once or twice a day.
- Benzathine penicillin (G benzathine penicillin)—Benzathine penicillin is awailable only IM and the recommended dose for children <25 kg is 50,000 U/kg and 1,200,000 U for children >25 kg, in a single dose. Appropriate serum levels should be maintained for a prolonged period of time (15–20 days). It is used also for the prophylaxis of rheumatic fever, prevention of infections caused by Group A, β-hemolytic *Streptococcus pyogenes* (GAS).
- Penicillin V (phenoxymethylpenicillin)—oral and parenteral preparations. Serum levels are maintained for about 4 h and it is indicated

for mild pharyngotonsil, respiratory tract or soft tissues infections caused by susceptible bacteria. The recommended dose is 25,000–50,000 U/kg per day, divided into three or four applications, or 125 mg dose for children <5 years and 250 mg dose BID (PO) for older children for prophylaxis of streptococcal infections in infantile rheumatic disease.

Action Spectrum of Penicillins

Penicillins are effective in treatment of infections caused by Group A *Streptococcus pyogenes* (GAS) and Group B *Streptococcus—Streptococcus agalactiae*. *S. pneumoniae* is sensitive to penicillin, except for strains with altered PBPs. *Staphylococcus* spp. are generally resistant to penicillin, as are Enterobacteriacae and *P. aeruginosa*.

The most common mechanism through which most bacteria have acquired resistance to penicillins is the production of the enzyme β-lactamase (an enzyme that destroys the β-lactam ring of the penicillin molecule and its by-products). Resistance caused by PBP modification is used by *S. pneumoniae*. Most *Moraxella catarrhalis* strains, as well as about half of the isolates of type b and about 20% of nontypable *H. influenzae* strains produce β-lactamase. About half of pigmented *Prevotella* and *Porphyromonas, Prevotella bivia, Prevotella disiens*, and *Fusobacterium nucleatum* that are the predominant anaerobic bacteria recovered in chronic respiratory infections produce primarily penicillinases.

β-lactamase-producing bacteria (BLPB) may have an important clinical role in infections. These organisms can have a direct pathogenic role in causing the infection as well as an indirect effect through their ability to produce the enzyme β-lactamase. BLPB may not only survive penicillin therapy but also may protect other penicillin-susceptible bacteria from penicillin by releasing the free enzyme into their environment.

S. pneumoniae resistance to β-lactam agents is a result of the modification of PBPs, leading to reduction of affinity between such enzymes and the antibiotics. Currently, pneumococci resistance is reported in all continents at rates of 40–50% in countries such as Spain, South Korea, Vietnam, France, Romania, Japan, South Africa, and the USA. Data analyzed from samples collected from different Brazilian states have contributed to include the country among those that have penicillin-resistance percentages (mostly intermediately resistance) in the range of 10–25%. About half of the penicillin-resistant strains are currently intermediately resistant (MIC of 0.1–1.0 mg/mL) and the rest are highly resistant (MIC > 2.0 mg/mL). However, doubling the dose of penicillins enables to still utilize these agent in the therapy of most respiratory infections.

A larger problem is multidrug-resistant pneumococci. Penicillin-resistant strains can also show resistance to other antimicrobial agents—including oral third-generation cephalosporins, trimethoprim–sulfamethoxazole (cotrimoxazole) and macrolides—but they are susceptible to vancomycin and the newer quinolones (i.e., levafloxacin, gatifloxacin, moxifloxacin). Intermediately resistant *S. pneumoniae* are still susceptible *in vitro* to high concentrations of penicillin or amoxicillin. Clindamycin and the oral second-generation cephalosporins, especially cefuroxime–axetil and cefprozil, are also effective *in vitro* against >95% of intermediately penicillin-resistant strains.

One disadvantage of the penicillins is the production of an allergic type phenomenon or hypersensitivity (including anaphylaxis and serum disease). Hypersensitivity is present in ~5% of the patients and cutaneous exanthema or rash is the most common manifestation. Anaphylactic manifestations are less frequent, present in 0.004–0.015% of patients receiving penicillin. Symptoms of anaphylaxis (hypotension or shock, urticaria, laryngeal edema, and bronchospasm) are generally manifested within 10–20 min after the administration of penicillin and require emergency treatment measures; because of this, it is recommended that patients who are injected with penicillin be maintained under observation for at least 30 min. Cutaneous patch tests are unreliable because a negative result does not rule out the possibility of a allergic reaction. There may be allergic cross-reaction with different penicillins (this is the reason why a patient allergic to one specific penicillin should be considered allergic to all of them) and with cephalosporins, there is cross-reaction in 10% of the cases.

Another disadvantage of the penicillins is their inactivation by penicillinase, an enzyme produced by most *Staph. aureus*, as well as other Gram-negative aerobic and anaerobic bacteria (see preceding text). Another important mechanism of resistance of *S. sureus* is to methicillin which is produced through PBP chromosomic alterations, reducing affinity to penicillins. In recent years, there has been a significant increase in the rate of infections by methicillin-resistance *S. aureus* strains, especially in hospital setting.

B. Aminopenicillins

Aminopenicillins are semisynthetic β-lactam antimicrobials formed by the addition of an amino group to benzathine penicillin. They are effective against *Streptococcus* sp. *S. pneumoniae*, *H. influenzae*, and β-lactamase nonproducing *M. catarrhalis*, some strains of *Escherichia coli* and a limited number of *Salmonella* sp. and *Shigella* sp. species. They are not effective against most *Staphylococcus* infections.

Similarly to penicillin G, the primary mechanism of bacterial resistance to aminopenicillin is through the production of β-lactamase. However, penicillin G or methicillin-resistance bacteria due to PBPs modifications, such as *S. pneumoniae* and *S. aureus*, respectively, present resistance to aminopenicillins as well.

Hydrochloridric acid inactivates ampicillin and its administration should take place two hours before or after the meals. Amoxicillin is not affected by the gastric juice and it may be administered with food. In ~7% of the cases, drug use is followed by cutaneous exanthema.

Amoxicillin is the preferred antibiotic for the treatment of mild to moderate acute upper and lower respiratory infections, such as otitis, sinusitis, bronchitis and pneumonia; the prevalence of *H. influenzae*, *M. catarrhalis*, and *S. pneumoniae* resistance should be considered in regions where it is going to be administered. The recommended mean dose is 40–50 mg/kg per day, divided into three administrations. In case of high prevalence of penicillin-resistant pneumococci, the dose may be doubled to 90 mg/kg per day.

- Ampicillin—oral and parenteral presentation.
- Amoxicillin—oral presentation.

C. Potentiated Penicillins

The combination of amoxicillin with clavulanic acid (as potassium clavulanate) for oral use was the first combination of penicillin and a β-lactamase inhibitor introduced for clinical use, in 1984. Pharmacokinetics of both drugs is similar. Amoxicillin–clavulanate is a broad-spectrum agent against aerobic Gram-positive bacteria such as methicillin-sensitive *S. aureus, S. epidermidis, S. pneumoniae*, *S. pyogenes*, and *S. viridans*. This combination is also effective against anaerobic bacteria including β-lactamase producing bacteria, which are important in chronic head and neck infections (*Prevotella*, *Porphyromonas*, and *Fusobacteria*). It has no activity against *P. aeruginosa*. It is especially recommended for the treatment of respiratory tract infections in which it is suspected or confirmed that β-lactamase-producing bacteria are the etiological agents. The use of this combination is recommended in areas where the prevalence of β-lactamase-producing *H. influenzae* strains is $\geq 30\%$ and in infections where *M. catarrhalis* (most of them β-lactamase-producers) is a predominant pathogen, especially in cases of otitis media, sinusitis, and other respiratory tract diseases.

Its main side effect is diarrhea which can be reduced when it is taken with food. The mean recommended dose varies from 25 to 45 mg/kg per day, administered twice to three times, depending on the formulation. For the recently approved 7:1 formulation (amoxicillin–clavulanate), 45 mg/kg per day in two doses is recommended. In instances where *S. pneumoniae* resistant to penicillin need to be covered, administration of an equal amount of amoxicillin for a total of 90 mg/kg per day is recommended. A new formulation that has a 14:1 formulation (amoxicillin: clavulanate), is available in some countries.

- Amoxicillin–clavulanate—the oral administration is more commonly used, but can also be administrated parenteral.

D. Broad-Spectrum Penicillins (Anti-Pseudomonas)

Carboxypenicillins (carbenicillin, ticarcillin, and ticarcillin/clavulanate) are semi-synthetic penicillins derived from ampicillin, whose carboxyl group is replaced by a side chain amine group. They are penicillins with higher activity against Gram-negative bacteria, such as *P. aeruginosa*. Coadministration with an aminoglycoside, may be associated with a synergetic effect (however, they should not be administered at the same time, because carboxypenicillin may inactivate aminoglycosides). Another benefit of the joint administration with an aminoglycoside is the prevention of resistance, because the administration of carboxypenicillin alone may lead to resistance, especially in the case of *P. aeruginosa*.

Both agents may be administered parenterally (preferably IV), they have short half-life ($\sim$1 h) and the recommended dose varies according to age and severity of the infection: carbenicillin—from 200 to 600 mg/kg per day, ticarcillin varies from 100 to 300 mg/kg per day.

E.   Cephalosporins

The first studies on cephalosporin date back from 1948, when fungus *Cephalosporium acremonium* was isolated in the sea close to a sewage tube on the coast of Sardinia, Italy. The currently available cephalosporins are semisynthetic compounds derived from one of the three isolated antibiotics of the culture broth of this fungus, cephalosporin C. As all other β-lactam antibiotics, cephalosporins inhibit cell wall synthesis and are considered to be bactericidal. The main inhibition mechanism takes place at the level of the reaction of transpeptidase, during the final phase of peptideglycan biosynthesis. Additional targets, for both penicillins and cephalosporins, are the PBPs. The mechanism of action varies in relation to the specificity of the affected PBP and its affinity to the various β-lactam antibiotics.

The cephalosporins vary according to their molecular configuration, providing a varied spectrum of activity. Some can be used as an alternative to penicillin to treat pneumococcal or streptococcal infections. Similarly, cephalosporins are an alternative for patients who present skin reactions to penicillin, but 10% of the patients have cross-hypersensitivity. Diarrhea is the main side effect.

The mechanisms of bacterial resistance to cephalosporins are:

- intrinsic structural differences in PBPs, which are the target of such drugs;
- development of PBPs with less affinity to antimicrobial agents;
- enzymatic destruction of the β-lactam ring by β-lactamase enzymes. This is the main bacterial defense mechanism against the cephalosporins. Both Gram-positive and Gram-negative bacteria are capable of producing enzymes at different degrees. Similarly, all cephalosporins present varied susceptibility to different β-lactamase.

Cephalosporins form a group of broad-spectrum antibiotics. Because of their low incidence of side effects, these agent may be overused and abused. Their administration should be made with care because they are costly and generally there are other similarly effective narrower-spectrum drugs, whose use reduces the risk of developing bacterial resistance.

Cephalosporins are classified by generations. This classification is based on the chronology of their introduction and their antibacterial activity.

First-Generation Cephalosporins

They are characterized by the activity against Gram-positive cocci, including penicillin-resistant *S. aureus*. This antibacterial activity is the reason for their frequent prophylactic and therapeutic used in otorhinolaryngological and head and neck surgeries to prevent and treat postoperative infections. They have no action against Gram-negative aerobic bacteria including *P. aeruginosa* and *H. influenzae*.

- Cephalexin—oral administration
- Cephalothin, cefazolin—parenteral administration
- Cefadroxil—oral administration.

Second-Generation Cephalosporins

These agents possess a broad spectrum of efficacy against infections caused by Gram-negative organisms, including β-lactamase-producing *H. influenzae* (important agent in the etiology of otitis media, sinusitis, epiglottitis, etc.). They are also active against *S. pneumoniae* and *S. pyogenes.*

All second-generation cephalosporins are active against *S. aureus* and *S. pyogenes* and also possess good activity against *E. coli, Klebsiella, Proteus, H. influenzae*, and *M. catarrhalis*. They are inefficient against *P. aeruginosa*. Some (cefuroxime–axetil, cefprozil) are also active against *S. pneumoniae* that is intermediately resistant to penicillin.

In general, second-generation cephalosporins are active in infections caused by *S. pneumoniae, H. influenzae*, and *M. catarrhalis.*

- Cefaclor* and cefuroxime–axetil—oral administration
- Cefoxitin—IM and IV administration
- Cefprozil—oral administration

Third-Generation Cephalosporins

They have a broad spectrum of activity against aerobic Gram-negative bacilli. Some third-generation cephalosporins, such as ceftazidime possess good activity against *P. aeruginosa*. They are very active in infections caused by *H. influenzae* and *M. catarrhalis* (including β-lactamase-producing strains). The oral ones are

---

*Bacterial resistance to cefaclor has increased and it is currently considered a cephalosporin between the first- and second-generation.

less efficient against pneumococcal infections than second-generation cephalosporins. However, ceftriaxone that is give parenterally is effective against penicillin resistant *S. pneumoniae*.

- Ceftazidime, ceftriaxone, cefotaxime, cefodizime (not yet approved for pediatric use) and cefoperazone—IM or IV administration
- Cefetamet–pivoxil, cefixime, and cefdinir, cefpodoxime–proxetil— oral administration

Fourth-Generation Cephalosporins

They have a broader spectrum of activity when compared to third-generation drugs. In addition, they have more stability against β-lactamase-mediated hydrolysis transmitted by plasmid or chromosome. They also present broad-spectrum against Gram-negative microorganisms, *P. aeruginosa*, most entero-cocci and *Serratia* sp. Cefepime is used for the treatment of pediatric patients with community or hospital-acquired infections.

- Cefepime—parenteral (IV) administration
- Cefpirome—parenteral (IV) administration. It has not been approved for pediatric use yet.

F. Other β-Lactam Agents: The Carbapenems (e.g., Imipenem, Meropenem)

These antimicrobials are similar to penicillins and cephalosporins as they have a β-lactam ring and are therefore classified as β-lactam antibiotics. They are often used in nosocomial infections as they are very active against infections produced by methicillin-sensitive *Staph. aureus*, but methicillin-resistant *Staph. aureus* have variable sensitivity against this class of antimicrobials. They are also useful in nosocomial infections caused by aerobic, anaerobic and especially Gram-negative microorganisms. As the antibacterial spectrum of activity of these drugs includes most pathogenic bacteria, they are appropriate for the treatment of severe hospital-acquired infections, especially when a mixed aerobic and anaerobic flora is responsible for the infection.

- Imipenem–cilastatin—parenteral administration.
- Meropenem—parenteral administration.

G. Sulfonamides

The drugs belonging to this group are generally bacteriostatic, but have an additional effect when given with another bacteriostatic agent and manifest a synergistic effect when coadministered with a bactericidal agent.

They have broad-spectrum activity against Gram-positive and Gram-negative organisms, including respiratory pathogens such as *S. pneumoniae*, *H. influenzae*, and *M. catarrhalis*.

The combination of trimethoprim–sulfamethoxazole (TMP/SMX) that has been marketed since 1968 is widely used and has become one of the most popular antimicrobial agents of the world due to it low cost, easy compliance (oral administration every 12 h) and pleasant taste. TMP/SMX is efficient against penicillin-resistant *H. influenzae* and *M. catarrhalis*. Its wide use, however, can lead to bacterial resistance, which has been increasingly reported in the literature by growing number of strains of *S. pneumoniae* and *H. influenzae* (1). TMP/SMX is not active against *S. pyogenes*.

These drugs can cause hypersensitivity reactions that include different skin reactions, such as morbilliform exanthema, and the risk of blood dyscrasia after long-term use.

● TMP/SMX—oral and parenteral administration.

H. Macrolides

Although there are similarities in their chemical structure, antibacterial spectrum, mechanism of action and resistance, the antibiotics of this group present different pharmacokinetic properties. This group comprises erythromycin, clarithromycin, and azithromycin. Macrolides are bacteriostatic agents that inhibit bacterial protein synthesis, but depending on the concentration or nature of the bacteria involved, they can also be bactericidal.

They are an alternative for patients allergic to penicillin and its derivatives. Macrolides have the same spectrum of β-lactam agents and are efficient against infections caused by *M. catarrhalis*, *Mycoplasma pneumoniae*, *Chlamydia* sp., *Legionella* sp., and *S. pneumoniae*.

Erythromycin is inactive against *H. influenzae* and some *S. pyogenes*. Resistance of GAS to erythromycin and other macrolides occurs in countries where these agents were overused (e.g., Japan, Finland, Spain, Taiwan, and Turkey) (2). Cross-resistance of *S. pneumoniae* is common among all macrolides. Azithromycin has improved efficacy against Gram-negative organisms (*H. influenzae* and *M. catarrhalis*), while clarithromycin is more efficient than erythromycin against Gram-positive organisms. Recent studies show, however, increased resistance of *S. pneumoniae* to all macrolides, and survival of azithromycin-susceptible *H. influenzae* in the middle ear and sinuses (2). These agents are indicated however in atypical primary pneumonia, in which young adults have prolonged productive cough course and other infections caused by *M. pneumoniae*.

Erythromycin is presented as stearate, estolate and ethylsuccinate. The estolate form can cause hepatotoxicity. In 10–15% of the cases, erythromycin can cause major gastrointestinal alterations and with the exception of stearate, should be given with the meals.

Clarithromycin is better absorbed with food and azithromycin is better absorbed 1–2 h before or after meals.

- Clarithromycin—oral administration
- Azithromycin—oral and parenteral (IV) administration

I. Chloramphenicol

Primarily bacteriostatic, this antimicrobial agent may have a bactericide action in some situations and with certain bacterial strains.

Chloramphenicol is a broad-spectrum antibiotic, very efficient in infections caused by *Streptococcus* sp., with excellent activity against *H. influenzae*, even those β-lactamase-producing microorganisms. Chloramphenicol is one of the antimicrobial agents most active against all anaerobic bacteria.

Originally isolated from *Streptomyces venezuelae*, chloramphenicol was commercially launched in 1949. It is widely used in penicillin-resistant infections because of its low cost. We should keep in mind, though, that the risk of fatal aplastic anemia is 13 times higher than with other antibiotics.

Chloramphenicol is extremely valuable in treating epiglottitis and meningitis caused by *H. influenzae* (it has good penetration through the brain–blood barrier).

The drug's toxicity must be remembered. The risk of fatal aplastic anemia with chloramphenicol is estimated to be approximately one per 25,000–40,000 patients treated. This serious complication is unrelated to the reversible, dosage-dependent leukopenic side effect. Other side effects are the production of the potentially fatal "gray baby syndrome" when given to neonates hemolytic anemia in patients with GGPD deficiency, and optic neuritis in individuals who take the drug for a prolonged time.

- Chloramphenicol—oral and parenteral administration.

J. Clindamycin

It is considered a bacteriostatic antibiotic, but has bactericide activity against streptococci and staphylococci strains and anaerobes which are important in chronic infections. It is active against GAS and *S. pneumoniae* and 90% of pneumococci with intermediate resistance are sensitive to clindamycin. There is a new potential use for clindamycin as a result of the increasing resistance of *S. pneumoniae* to penicillin in respiratory infections (3–5). It is one of the most active antimicrobial agents against anaerobes, such as the *Bacteroides fragilis* group and other anaerobic Gram-negative bacilli including those that produce β-lactamase, which are important in chronic head and neck infections (*Prevotella*, *Porphyromonas*, and *Fusobacteria*).

Its major role in otorhinolaryngological infections is in the treatment of mixed infections caused by microbial aerobic and anaerobic polyflora. Many of these polymicrobial infections are chronic and include chronic sinusitis (6). However, it causes high rates of diarrhea due to *Clostridium difficile* infection and it is not active against Gram-negative aerobic bacteria. The side effect of most concern with clindamycin is colitis. It should be noted that colitis has been associated with a number of other antimicrobial agents, such as ampicillin and many cephalosporins, and has been described in seriously ill patients in the absence of previous antimicrobial therapy.

- Clindamycin—oral and parenteral administration.

K. Quinolones

The "older" quinolones (i.e., ciprofloxacin, ofloxacin) are effective against *H. influenzae* and *M. catarrhalis* and ciprofloxacin is effective against many *P. aeruginosa* strains, but has minimal activity against *S. pneumoniae*. The "newer" quinolones (e.g., levofloxacin, gatifloxacin, moxifloxacin, and gemifloxacin) have improved activity against *S. pneumoniae* (7).

The development of resistance against quinolones can be very rapid and can occur even during treatment.

Laboratory studies with animals treated with quinolones have shown cartilage changes and interference in growth. Although these abnormalities have not been observed in children, the drug must not be used in patients younger than 18 years of age.

- Ciprofloxacin—parenteral and oral administration, topical preparation (excellent for otorrhea caused by *P. aeruginosa* in chronic otitis media).
- Ofloxacin—parenteral and oral administration, topical preparation.

L. Rifampicin

It is a semisynthetic derivative of rifampin B, a macrocyclical antibiotic, produced by *Streptomyces mediterranei*. Rifampicin is bactericidal for all tuberculosis bacilli populations, both intra- and extracellularly. It has bactericidal effect against many mycobacteria and can be an alternative agent for some resistant respiratory organisms. However, because of the reappearance of tuberculosis and the report of resistant strains, it should be reserved to treat this disease.

- Rifampicin—oral and parenteral administration.

M. Metronidazole

It is a bactericidal agent effective only against anaerobic bacteria especially Gram-negative bacilli such as *B. fragilis* group and other anaerobic Gram-negative bacilli including those that produce β-lactamase. Occasional strains of anaerobic Gram-positive cocci and nonsporulating bacilli are highly resistant.

Microaerophilic steptococci, *Propionibacterium acnes*, and *Actinomyces* species are almost uniformly resistant. Metronidazole is useful in the treatment of deep abscesses located in the cervical region, chronic sinusitis, infected cholesteatoma, and most anaerobic, orofacial and odontogenic infections. It is indicated for tonsillar or pharyngeal ulcers in Vincent's angina. It needs to be administered in combination with a penicillins, a cephalosporins or a macrolide to treat mixed infections (6). This is because most of these infections are polymicrobial due to aerobic–anaerobic bacteria.

Adverse reactions to metronidazole therapy are rare and include central nervous system toxicity symptoms of peripheral neuropathy, ataxia, vertigo, headaches, and convulsions. Gastrointestinal side effects include nausea, vomiting, metallic taste, anorexia, and diarrhea. Some animal studies have shown possible mitogenic activity associated with administration of large doses of this drug. However, no such evidence exists in humans.

- Metronidazole—oral or IV administration.

III. Antifungal Drugs

A. Amphotericin

Amphotericin is the most efficient drug against fungal systemic infections. It is excellent against *Aspergillus* sp. and mucormycosis that can infect the nose, paranasal sinuses, becoming invasive as a result of aging, weakness, diabetes, HIV, neoplasia, or use of corticoids.

- Amphotericin B—IV or intrathecal administration in cranial infections.

B. Ketoconazole

Ketoconazole, itraconazole, and fluconazole are oral antifungal drugs, excellent for the treatment of oral candidiasis.

- Ketoconazole—oral administration during the meals
- Itraconazole—oral administration
- Fluconazole—oral and parenteral administration.

IV. Antiviral Drugs

They are efficient in infections caused by *Herpes simplex* (HSV), *Varicella-zoster* (VZV), Epstein–Barr (EBV), Cytomegalovirus (CMV), Respiratory Syncytial (RSV) viruses.

- Acyclovir—oral or topical use on the lesions. Recommended for HSV and VZV infections.

- Valacyclovir—oral use (adults). Recommended for HSV infections.
- Fancyclovir and pencyclovir—oral use (adults). For HSV, VZV, and EBV infections.
- Gancyclovir—IV use. For CMV infections.
- Cidofovir—IV use. For CMV infections.
- Ribavirin—aerosol use. For RSV infections.

In the following text, we present a list of the main antibiotics previously referred to in the text.

V. List of Antimicrobial Agents and Their Doses

(As mentioned in the text, with US and Brazil brand names)

- Penicillin V (Beepen, Pen V): 20–50 mg/kg per day (PO)
- Aqueous penicillin G (Crystalline, Cristalina): 100,000–400,000 U/kg per day (parenteral)
- Procaine penicillin G (Wycillin): 25,000–50,000 U/kg per day (parenteral)
- Penicillin benzathine (Bicillin, Benzetacil): 50,000 U/kg (single dose)
- Ampicillin (Binotal): 50–100 mg/kg per day (PO), 100–200 mg/kg per day (parenteral)
- Amoxicillin (Amoxil): 40–45 mg/kg per day (PO) or 60–90 mg/kg per day (PO)
- Amoxicillin–clavulanate (Augmentin, Clavulin): 20–40 mg/kg per day (PO) TID administration (250 mg), and 45 mg/kg BID administration (400 mg)
- Cephalexin (Keflex): 25–50 mg/kg per day (PO)
- Cephalothin (Keflin): 75–150 mg/kg per day (parenteral)
- Cefazolin (Ancef, Kefazol): 50–100 mg/kg per day (parenteral)
- Cefadroxil (Duricef, Cefamox): 30 mg/kg per day (PO)
- Cefaclor (Ceclor): 20–40 mg/kg per day (PO)
- Cefdinir (omnicef): 14 mg/kg per day (PO)
- Cefuroxime–axetil (Ceftin, Zinnat): 30 mg/kg per day (PO, parenteral)
- Cefoxitin (Mefoxin): 80–160 mg/kg per day (parenteral)
- Cefprozil (Cefzil): 15 mg/kg per day (PO)
- Ceftazidime (Fortaz): 100–200 mg/kg per day (parenteral)
- Ceftriaxone (Rocephin, Rocefin): 50–75 mg/kg per day (parenteral)
- Cefotaxime (Claforan): 50–100 mg/kg per day (parenteral)
- Cefoperazone (Cefobid, Tricef): 100–150 mg/kg per day (parenteral)
- Cefixime (Suprax, Plenax): 8 mg/kg per day (PO)
- Cefpodoxime–proxetil (Vantin, Orelox): 10 mg/kg per day (PO)
- Cefpirome (Cefrom): 1 g (IV)
- Cefepime (Maxipeme, Maxcef): 50 mg/kg per day (IV)

- Imipenem (Primaxin, Tienam): 15 mg/kg QID (parenteral)
- Trimethoprim–sulfamethoxazole (Bactrim): 40/8 mg/kg per day or 5 mL/5 kg (PO)
- Erythromycin (E-mycin, Ilosone, Pantomicina): 30–50 mg/kg per day (PO), 20–50 mg/kg per day (parenteral)
- Clarithromycin (Biaxin, Klaricid): 15 mg/kg per day (PO)
- Azithromycin (Zithromax, Zitromax): 10 mg/kg per day on the first day and then 5 mg/kg per day (single daily dose) (PO)
- Chloramphenicol (Chloromycetin, Quemicetina): 50 mg/kg per day (PO), 50–100 mg/kg per day (parenteral)
- Clindamycin (Cleocin, Dalacin): 20–30 mg/kg per day (PO, parenteral)
- Ciprofloxacin (Cipro): 20 mg/kg per day (PO)
- Rifampicin (Rifadin, Rifaldin): 10–20 mg/kg per day (oral, parenteral)
- Metronidazole (Flagyl): 15–30 mg/kg per day (PO), 30–50 mg/kg per day (parenteral)
- Ketoconazole (Nizoral): 3.3–6.6 mg/kg per day (single dose) (PO)
- Itraconazole (Sporanox): 3.3–6.6 mg/kg per day (PO)
- Fluconazole (Diflucan, Zoltec): 4.0–8.0 mg/kg per day (parenteral)
- Acyclovir (Zovirax): 250 mg/m^2 body surface (TID) (IV).

VI. Paranasal Sinus Infections in Pediatrics

A. Definition and Classification of Sinusitis

Bacterial sinusitis is an inflammation of the paranasal sinus mucosa caused by bacterial overgrowth in a closed cavity. This disorder is also called rhinosinusitis, because the nasal epithelium is continuous with the mucosa that lines the paranasal sinuses, as the disease can affect both sites. Viral or allergic rhinitis typically precedes sinusitis, and sinusitis without rhinitis is rare. Many factors may predispose an individual to sinusitis. Evidence shows that viral upper respiratory tract infections and pharyngeal colonization with GAS predispose children to acute bacterial sinusitis. It may be appropriate to select antibiotics that are also effective against GAS, because *S. pyogenes* may be the concurrent infection in 15–20% of the children.

Sinusitis is classified on the basis of duration of symptoms and anatomic locations. Acute sinusitis symptoms last as long as 4 weeks. Subacute sinusitis has mild to moderate symptoms that are present for 4–12 weeks. Chronic sinusitis persists for >12 weeks and often has a pathophysiology that differs from acute sinusitis. Recurrent sinusitis is defined as four or more episodes in one year, each episode lasting more than 7 days, with complete resolution between episodes.

B. Microbiology of Sinusitis

In a study involving 50 children with acute maxillary sinusitis, Wald et al. demonstrated that bacteriology of sinus secretion is similar to that found in adults. Predominant organisms include *S. pneumoniae* (30%), *M. catarrhalis* (20%), and noncapsulated *H. influenzae* (20%). Both *Haemophilus* and *Moraxella* can produce β-lactamase and, as a result, be ampicillin resistant. It has been calculated that at least one-third of *H. influenzae* isolates and the majority of *M. catarrhalis* isolates are β-lactamase-producing organisms. According to β-lactamase prevalence data, some 20% of the maxillary paranasal sinus microbial pathogens are resistant to amoxicillin. *Staph. aureus* is rarely the cause of acute sinusitis. Jousemies-Somer et al. isolated *S. aureus* in <1% of samples obtained from patients with acute maxillary sinusitis (8). Anaerobic bacteria can be recovered in 8–10% of acute sinusitis especially in maxillary sinusitis associated with dental infections of the upper molars.

Bacteriology is the same in subacute sinusitis (persistent respiratory symptoms, that is, nasal secretion or cough present between 4 and 12 weeks), with predominance of pneumococci, followed by *H. influenzae* and *M. catarrhalis*.

The predominant pathogens isolated from pediatric patients with chronic sinusitis are *S. pneumoniae*, *M. catarrhalis*, *H. influenzae*, and anaerobes. Anaerobes (especially anaerobic Gram-negative bacilli such as *Prevotella*, *Porphyromonas*, and *Fusobacteria*), play an important role in chronic sinusitis (respiratory symptoms persisting for >3 months) and in those that follow dental infections. However, Gram-positive cocci as *Staph. aureus* and α-hemolytic *Streptococcus* are also frequently isolated. *Staph. aureus* is commonly associated with anaerobes in chronic sinusitis and is isolated in 15–20% of the cultures from well-characterized patients.

C. Antimicrobial Treatment of Sinusitis

Acute Sinusitis

A number of antimicrobial agents have been studied in the therapy of acute sinusitis over the past 25 years, with the use of pre- and post-treatment aspirate cultures. Appreciation of the high incidence of sinusitis and its impact on quality of life should stimulate primary care physicians to properly recognize the subtle clinical presentation of acute bacterial sinusitis and provide appropriate aggressive treatment. In an acute noncomplicated bacterial sinusitis episode, if the child has not received any antibiotic recently (<1 month), amoxicillin is the treatment of choice for most bacterial sinusitis cases in children. In addition to being efficient in most cases, amoxicillin is also inexpensive and safe.

However, since sinusitis has a spontaneous recovery rate of 40% many cases resolve spontaneously. However, untreated bacterial sinusitis may not resolve and progress to develop complications. Antibiotic use should be limited to carefully selected patients. Antibiotics should be used in children whose signs and symptoms persist for 10–14 days or longer without improvement. To manage bacterial sinusitis is often a challenging endeavour in which selection of the most appropriate antimicrobial agents remains a key decision.

This has become more difficult in recent years as all the predominant bacterial pathogens have gradually developed resistance to the commonly used antibiotics.

As a result of increased resistance of *S. pneumoniae* to β-lactam antibiotics, erythromycin and TMP/SMX association in many geographical regions, therapeutic options include high dose of amoxicillin (80–90 mg/kg per day) or clindamycin. The increase in the usual dose from 40 to 60–90 mg/kg per day represents an attempt to exceed the MIC (*minimum inhibitory concentration*) of most penicillin-resistant pneumococci.

In many geographical areas, the resistance of *S. pneumoniae* to TMP/SMX is higher than that to penicillin. Resistance of *H. influenzae* to TMP/SMX has increased significantly in recent years. Second-line agents should be used when resistant pathogens are suspected.

Although amoxicillin is indicated against most acute sinusitis cases, it is necessary to choose another antimicrobial agent when the child does not respond to amoxicillin treatment after 72 h, used this antibiotic in the previous 30 days, and lives in a geographical area with high prevalence of both resistant pneumococci and β-lactamase-producing *H. influenzae*. In such cases, other therapeutic alternatives include amoxicillin-clavulanate, cefuroxime–axetil, cefprozil, and cefpodoxime–proxetil as examples of cephalosporins.

Clindamycin can be used for infections caused by *S. pneumoniae*, but it does not eradicate *H. influenzae* or *M. catarrhalis* and, consequently, it is inappropriate for empirical therapy for sinusitis. Clindamycin can however be combined with a third-generation cephlosporin that can provide coverage for *H. influenzae* and *M. catarrhalis*. Macrolides (clarithromycin and azithromycin) may be acceptable second-line agents, specially in patients who are allergic to penicillin and cefdinir. However, resistance of pneumococci to these agents that has increased lately limits their use.

Cephalosporins offer broad coverage in sinusitis treatment, but first-generation agents have poor *H. influenzae* coverage. Cefaclor, a second-generation agent, provides better coverage, but resistance in *H. influenzae*, *M. catarrhalis*, and *S. pneumoniae* is a constant problem. Cefadroxil has poor activity against *S. pneumoniae* and some Gram-negative bacteria. Several second- and third-generation cephalosporins have excellent activity against all major pathogens, including cefuroxime–axetil, cefprozil, cefdinir, and cefpodoxime–proxetil.

Patients with acute sinusitis may require hospitalization due to major systemic toxemia or difficulties in taking the oral antimicrobial agent. These patients can be treated with IV cefotaxime at 200 mg/kg per day dose (divided into four doses).

Physicians should investigate immunological defects in children who do not respond to treatment. The majority of the children who have severe sinusitis have inadequate humoral defenses and received prolonged courses of antibiotics (9).

Antimicrobial therapy is beneficial and effective in the prevention of septic complications. The antimicrobial therapy should be maintained for 10–14 days (considered an appropriate treatment interval) (5) or seven days beyond the resolution of symptoms, whichever is longer. Most patients have an adequate response within 48 h, with less cough, nasal secretion and fever, if initially present. Another antimicrobial agent should be selected for patients that do not show an improvement after 72 h. Another week of treatment (total 21 days) should be considered when improvement is slow and patients are not totally asymptomatic 14 days after the beginning of treatment. In such cases, complete eradication of bacterial colonization of the sinus mucosa should occur.

Factors within the sinus cavity that may enable organisms to survive antimicrobial therapy are inadequate penetration of antimicrobial agents, a high protein concentration (can bind antimicrobial agents), a high content of enzymes that inactivate antimicrobial agents (i.e., β-lactamase), decreased multiplication rate of organisms that interfere with the activity of bacteriostatic agents and reduction in pH and oxygen partial pressure, which reduces the efficacy of some antimicrobial agents (e.g., aminoglycosides and quinolones).

Overuse of antibiotics, inappropriate dosing, and the use of broad-spectrum antibiotics as first-line treatment have contributed to the growing incidence of drug-resistant bacterial strains. Resistance will continue to emerge and render our first-line agents less useful. Some penicillin-resistant strains display multidrug resistance to TMP/SMX, macrolides, and some cephalosporins.

In the empirical choice of antimicrobial therapy for sinuses, several balances between narrow- and wide-spectrum antimicrobial agents must be made. If the patient fails to show significant improvement or shows signs of deterioration despite treatment, it is important to obtain a culture through sinus puncture, as this may reveal the presence of resistant bacteria. Culture of nasal pus or of sinus exudate obtained by rinsing through the sinus ostium can give unreliable information because of contamination by the resident bacterial nasal flora. Further antimicrobial treatment is based, whenever possible, and the agents should be effective against any potential organisms that may cause the infection.

In addition to antibiotics, other therapies have been utilized in the management of sinusitis. These include topical and systemic decongestants, corticosteroids, anti-inflammatory agents, mucolytic agents, humidification, antihistamines, nasal lavage or saline nasal spray, spicy food, and hot dry air.

Brook et al. (10) have shown that the administration of some β-lactam antibiotics selects β-lactamase-producing organisms in the respiratory tract. These organisms can spread within the family, from one household member to the other. Prophylactic use of amoxicillin also selects penicillin-resistant microorganisms.

Most patients with sinusitis are treated on an outpatient basis that requires appropriate follow-up to assess compliance. Follow-up times vary widely according to patient's age, risk factors and history. Additional evaluations are necessary if symptoms persist or worsen, perhaps because of resistant bacteria or poor antimicrobial coverage. Children should be considered at greater risk for recurrence if they are below the age of 6 months, attend daycare centers, live with a smoker, or have history of multiple upper respiratory infections.

Chronic Sinusitis

Many of the anaerobic pathogens isolated from inflamed sinuses, especially the Gram-negative bacilli are resistant to penicillins (5). Some of the aerobic isolates (*Staph. aureus* and *H. influenzae*) are also β-lactamase producers, and recent retrospective studies illustrate the superiority of therapy effective against both aerobic and anaerobic β-lactamase producers in chronic sinusitis.

Antimicrobial agents used for chronic sinusitis therapy should be effective against aerobic and anaerobic β-lactamase producers; these include the combination of a penicillin (e.g., amoxicillin) and a β-lactamase inhibitor (e.g., clavulanic acid), clindamycin, chloramphenicol, the combination of metronidazole and a macrolide. All of these agents (or similar ones) are available in oral and parenteral forms. Other effective agents are available only in parenteral form (e.g., cefoxitin, cefotetan, and cefmetazole). If Gram-negative organisms, such as *P. aeruginosa*, may be involved, parenteral therapy with aminoglycosides, a fourth-generation cephalosporin (cefepime or ceftazidime) or oral or parenteral treatment with a fluoroquinolone (only in postpubertal patients) is added. Parenteral therapy with a carbapenem (e.g., imipenem) is more expensive, but provides coverage for most potential pathogens, both anaerobes and aerobes.

The length of therapy is at least 21 days, and may be extended up to 10 weeks. Fungal sinusitis can be treated with surgical debridement of the affected sinuses and antifungal therapy. In contrast to acute sinusitis, which is generally treated vigorously with antibiotics, many physicians believe that surgical drainage is the mainstay of therapy in chronic sinusitis. When the patient does not respond to medical therapy, the physician should consider surgical drainage. Impaired drainage may be a major contribution to the development of chronic sinusitis, and correction of the obstruction helps to alleviate the infection and prevent recurrence. The use of antimicrobial therapy alone without surgical drainage of collected pus may not result in clearance of the infection. The chronically inflamed sinus membranes with diminished vascularity may be a poor means of carrying an adequate antibiotic level to the infected tissue, even though the blood level may be therapeutic. Furthermore, the reduction in the pH and oxygen tension within the inflamed sinus may interfere further with the activity of the antimicrobial agents, which can result in bacterial survival despite a high antibiotic concentration.

In the past, it was often necessary to resort to surgical intervention to cure chronic sinusitis. However, with improvements in the medical care, surgery is avoided more often. Functional endoscopic sinus surgery (FESS) has become the main surgical technique used; other surgical procedures serve only as a back up and are used especially when sinusitis is complicated by orbital and/ or intracranial involvement. Although endoscopic surgery can provide up to 80–90% success in adults and children (11,12), a substantial number of patients suffer from complications that warrant medical therapy being used to its full extent before resorting to surgery.

The surgeon's goals are to prevent persistence, recurrence, progression, and complications of chronic sinusitis. This is achieved by complete removal of diseased tissue, preservation of normal tissue, production of drainage (or obliteration if this is not possible) and consideration of the cosmetic outcome. Radical procedures should only be carried out if a simple approach—such as sinus lavage and medical therapy fails, or the disease is extensive.

VII. Conclusion

Variables influencing antimicrobial resistance form a complex multifactorial system. Appropriate antibiotic selection and duration of use is important to achieve efficacy and prevent antibiotic resistance. The therapeutic result obtained in the treatment of infections is affected by components such as susceptibility of the microorganism involved, host defense mechanisms and toxicity factors (13). Eradication, however, only occurs when the antibiotic reaches the infection site at adequate concentrations for the necessary time. The physician should be familiar with the pharmacodynamic and pharmacokinetic principles of these drugs in order to choose the appropriate antibiotic and anticipate whether the objectives will be reached or not.

In view of the development of new antimicrobial agents and the increased efficacy of existing ones, infections are being treated with more and more success. The benefit of one agent over another, however, has become a matter of subtle differences.

We would like to conclude this chapter with a reminder: the prevalence of antibiotic resistance among bacteria responsible for severe pediatric infections is increasing. There are geographical variations in resistance levels. We, physicians, should make a major effort to prevent emerging resistance resulting from inappropriate use of antimicrobial agents.

References

1. Block SL, Harrison CJ, Hedrick J, Tyler R, Smith A, Hedrick R. Restricted use of antibiotic prophylaxis for recurrent acute otitis media in the era of penicillin non-susceptible. Streptococcus pneumoniae. Int J Pediatr Otorhinolaryngol 2001; 61:47–60.
2. Dicuonzo G, Fiscarelli E, Gherardi G, Lorino G, Battistoni F, Landi S, de Cesaris M, Petitti T, Beall B. Erythromycin-resistant pharyngeal isolates of Streptococcus pyogenes recovered in Italy. Antimicrob Agents Chemother 2002; 46:3987–3990.
3. de Lencastre H, Tomasz A. From ecological reservoir to disease: the nasopharynx, day-care centres and drug-resistant clones of *Streptococcus pneumoniae*. J Antimicrob Chemother 2002; 50(suppl C):75–82.
4. Gwaltney JM Jr. Acute community acquired bacterial sinusitis: to treat or not to treat. Can Respir J 1999; 6(suppl A):46A–50A.

5. Pichichero ME, Reiner SA, Brook I, Gooch WM 3rd, Yamauchi T, Jenkins SG, Sher L. Controversies in the medical management of persistent and recurrent acute otitis media. Recommendations of a clinical advisory committee. Ann Otol Rhinol Laryngol 2000; 183(suppl):1–12.
6. Brook I, Shah K. Bacteriology of adenoids and tonsils in children with recurrent adenotonsillitis. Ann Otol Rhinol Laryngol 2001; 110(9):844–848.
7. Brook I. Anaerobic bacteria in upper respiratory tract and other head and neck infections. Ann Otol Rhinol Laryngol 2002; 111(5 Pt 1):430–440.
8. Penttila M, Savolainen S, Kiukaanniemi H, Forsblom B, Jousimies-Somer H. Bacterial findings in acute maxillary sinusitis—European study. Acta Otolaryngol 1997; 529(suppl):165–168.
9. Dykewicz MS. Rhinitis and sinusitis. J Allergy Clin Immunol 2003; 111(suppl 2):520–529.
10. Brook I. Failure of penicillin to eradicate group A beta-hemolytic streptococci tonsillitis: causes and management. J Otolaryngol 2001; 30:324–329.
11. Hartley BE, Lund VJ. Endoscopic drainage of pediatric paranasal sinus mucoceles. Int J Pediatr Otorhinolaryngol 1999; 50:109–111.
12. Jiang RS, Hsu CY. Functional endoscopic sinus surgery in children and adults. Ann Otol Rhinol Laryngol 2000; 109(12 Pt 1):1113–1116.
13. Brook I. Antibiotic resistance of oral anaerobic bacteria and their effect on the management of upper respiratory tract and head and neck infections. Semin Respir Infect 2002; 17:195–203.

28

Cough/Bronchitis in Children—The Importance of Judicious Use of Antimicrobial Agents

SCOTT F. DOWELL

Centers for Disease Control and Prevention, Atlanta, Georgia, USA

FRANCISCO GIMÉNEZ SÁNCHEZ

Unidad de Investigación en Medicina Tropical y Salud Internacional, Instituto de Salud Carlos III, Madrid, Spain

I. Background and Definitions

Bronchitis is defined as inflammation of the bronchial respiratory mucosa. This condition often does not exist in children as an isolated clinical entity, but rather is associated with several other conditions of the upper and lower respiratory tracts. The clinical definition of bronchitis in children is not well established. Clinicians typically make the diagnosis for a child with cough of relatively gradual onset, beginning 3–4 days after the appearance of rhinitis, with or without fever or sputum production. In a survey conducted in Georgia, physicians reported up to 102 different combinations of necessary findings to diagnose acute bronchitis, including presence of rhinitis, cough, wheeze, bronchial sounds, and fever (1). Almost half of these physicians used a certain duration of cough or of productive cough as an essential criterion.

This condition is marked by cough, and is designated in the literature with several terms including bronchitis, tracheobronchitis, wheezy bronchitis, and asthmatic bronchitis, often excluding more specific diagnoses such as pneumonia, bronchiolitis, and asthma. The term bronchitis does not reflect the clinical usage, or specific etiology; therefore, we will use the term cough/bronchitis. The establishment of a consensus on diagnosis and treatment of bronchitis is complicated due to the lack of a standardized case definition, the large number of combinations of symptoms reported, the difficulty of obtaining appropriate specimens for viral and bacterial diagnosis testing, the high rate of spontaneous resolution, and the lack of placebo-controlled treatment trials among children. Despite the need for additional knowledge, the available information is sufficient to provide principles that can be used to limit unnecessary prescription of antimicrobial agents for treatment of this condition (2).

II. Pathophysiology

The pathology of cough illness/bronchitis is an acute inflammatory disease of the larger air passages, including the trachea and the large- and medium-sized bronchi. The nose and nasopharyngeal mucosa may be affected by upper respiratory infections and the bronchial tree may be involved. In acute bronchial infection, the clinical features result from damage of the ciliated epithelia of the lower trachea and the large- and medium-sized bronchi, with hyperemic and edematous mucous membranes and increased bronchial secretions leading to a failure to eliminate secretions efficiently. The duration of symptoms probably depends upon the specific initial infectious agent, host conditions and secondary infections. Mild bronchial asthma has been found to be more common in patients with a history of recurrent acute bronchitis, establishing a relationship between acute bronchitis and airway reactivity (3). Therefore, in cases of prolonged cough, bronchospasm associated with acute respiratory infections may play an important role. Children with recurrent bronchitis may develop a severe bronchial inflammation associated with an increased mucous protein content and a reduction in the mucociliary function (4).

Neither the character nor the culture results of surrogate specimens such as sputum or nasopharyngeal secretions are sufficiently predictive of a bacterial infection of the bronchi. Sputum—comprising epithelial cells, polymorphonuclear lymphocytes, and noncellular elements—is a nonspecific response to airway inflammation, produced in response to both viral and bacterial infections as well as to noninfectious processes. In a study in children, bacteria were isolated in 17% of sputum samples and leukocytes were found in 82% of virus-positive sputum specimens and in 85% of bacteria-positive specimens (5).

III. Microbiology and Diagnosis

Classically, cough/illness bronchitis has been divided into three phases: first, a prodromal period with fever and upper respiratory symptoms; second, a 4–6-day period with cough and tracheobronchial symptomatology; and finally, a recovery period with cough that may last 1 or 2 weeks. Chest radiographic results are normal, or unchanged from baseline.

The term bronchitis does not imply any specific cause, but studies demonstrate that cough illness is commonly caused by viral pathogens (6–10). Since obtaining secretions directly from the bronchi of children is an invasive technique and the disease is generally mild and limited, establishing the cause of cough illness/bronchitis is difficult. The presence of bacteria in a culture of nasopharyngeal secretions also should not be used as an indication that the cough may be caused by a bacterial pathogen. Nasopharyngeal cultures are a poor predictor of the true bacterial infection of the bronchial mucosa, and the mere presence of bacteria at the level of the bronchi may not reflect a proven infection (11–13).

Several studies have demonstrated that viral pathogens such as parainfluenza virus, influenza virus, adenovirus, and respiratory syncytial virus are usually the agents identified among children with cough illness/bronchitis (8,14). Cases of acute bronchitis are particularly common during influenza epidemics. *Mycoplasma pneumoniae* (8) and *Chlamydia pneumoniae* (15) have also been identified in a small proportion of cases of cough illness in older children (16–18). There are no specific signs of cough caused by *M. pneumoniae.* Laboratory confirmation of the diagnosis is usually made by acute- and convalescent-phase serologic testing, although newer genetic-based tests are now available (19). *C. pneumoniae* is a relatively common cause for mild upper and lower respiratory infection in school-aged children and may present with prolonged cough (15,20). Some evidence for an association with reactive airway disease has also been reported (21,22). Laboratory tests for confirmation of *C. pneumoniae* infection include culture, the polymerase chain reaction assay, and serology, but these are not widely available outside research settings (23,24). The possible role of *Streptococcus pneumoniae* and *Haemophilus infuenzae* in acute bronchitis is not clear since these bacteria may be carried in the upper respiratory tract without symptoms. *Bordetella pertussis* classically causes paroxysm of cough followed by a characteristic inspiratory whoop. Particularly among older children and adults, pertussis also can present with a prolonged cough and no whoop (25). A diagnosis of pertussis can be confirmed by culture of the organism or antigen detection from nasopharyngeal secretions in the acute phase or serology in later phases of the illness. Commonly, a history of exposure to a family member with characteristic symptoms or an ongoing outbreak may help in assigning the presumptive etiologic agent.

Those children with significantly prolonged cough (4–8 weeks) should be investigated for other causes, such as reactive airway disease, tuberculosis, foreign body aspiration, cystic fibrosis, sinusitis, immunodeficiency, gastroesophageal reflux, or tracheoesophageal fistula (2). If possible, empiric antimicrobial therapy should be avoided in the initial management of a prolonged cough.

Children with other underlying chronic pulmonary disease (not including asthma) may have acute exacerbations with episodes characterized by cough, increased secretions, rales, rhonchi, and fever. These patients have an increased likelihood of bacterial colonization, impaired pulmonary clearance mechanisms, and immune compromise. Cystic fibrosis patients may be colonized by *Pseudomonas aeruginosa, Staphylococcus aureus*, or *H. influenzae*, producing acute exacerbations (26). Likewise, children with other underlying severe chronic lung diseases such as bronchopulmonary dysplasia, lung hypoplasia, ciliary dyskinesia, or chronic aspiration may suffer bacterial infections producing cough illness.

IV. Antimicrobial Treatment

Antimicrobial agents do not shorten the duration of the viral upper respiratory illness nor decrease the incidence of bacterial complications (27–30). However, in practice, antibiotics are frequently prescribed for children with bronchitis. Antibiotic prescriptions for bronchitis represented 9% of total prescriptions in the National Ambulatory Medical Care Survey (NAMCS), which was conducted in the USA in 1992 and evaluated patients younger than 18 years (31). In addition, antibiotics are prescribed in 72–88% of diagnosed cases of acute bronchitis (32). In a study conducted in pediatricians in Atlanta, 85% of children diagnosed with bronchitis were treated with antibiotics (1). Many practitioners believe that viral lower respiratory infections may suffer a bacterial superinfection which might be averted by prophylactic use of antimicrobial agents. The presence of fever in conjunction with cough is used by some practitioners to diagnose bronchitis and prescribe antibiotics. However, fever does not indicate that a cough is related to a bacterial infection and is a common sign found in viral respiratory infections, especially in the first 2 days of illness, and resolving over the ensuing few days (10,33,34).

In adults, most studies conclude that there is no evidence to support the use of antibiotic treatment for acute bronchitis (35). Several trials showed no difference or minimal improvement in outcome between those who received placebo and those treated with erythromycin, doxycycline, trimethroprim/sulfamethoxasole, or tetracycline (36–39). There are no randomized, placebo-controlled antibiotic trials of children with cough illness/bronchitis strictly defined by sputum production. However, several pediatric studies have evaluated the use of antibiotics in common practice for bronchitis defined as cough illness; these studies showed no benefits from antibiotic use for the cough (40,41). In addition, a meta-analysis of several trials concluded that antibiotics do not prevent or decrease the severity of bacterial complications subsequent to viral respiratory tract infections (42).

The majority of prolonged cough illnesses are viral, allergic, or postinfectious and do not require antibiotic therapy. Reactive airway disease has been recognized as one of the most common causes of recurrent or prolonged cough among children (43). Children with this disease may have minimal or no appreciable wheezing on physical examination but may respond to bronchodilator therapy; the cough will resolve and airway reactivity improve without antibiotics (44). In experimental rhinovirus colds, the cough continues for 14 days after onset of symptoms in up to 20% of subjects and does not itself indicate a bacterial infection of the bronchi (45,46).

Other specific pathogens may benefit from antimicrobial treatment and should be considered in the differential diagnosis. In a case in which *M. pneumoniae* infection with prolonged cough or pneumonia has been documented, treatment with effective antibiotics can shorten the illness and the duration of cough and perhaps reduce the spread of infections in contacts. The most active agents against *M. pneumoniae* are macrolides and tetracyclines (47). Because of adverse effects on developing teeth and bones, tetracyclines are restricted to patients older than 8 years of age. Erythromycin may be used at 30–50 mg/kg per day divided into three doses. Macrolides—azithromycin (10 mg/kg per day) and clarithromycin (15 mg/kg per day) commonly have fewer adverse effects and may be administrated in one or two doses, respectively, but are more expensive. In *C. pneumoniae* infection, as with *M. pneumoniae*, tetracyclines and macrolides are active against the organism, while penicillins and cephalosporins are not (48). When infection by *B. pertussis* is diagnosed, treatment with erythromycin is indicated. If started early in the course of disease, erythromycin may decrease the duration of symptoms but later only diminishes transmission of the organism (49).

Children with underlying chronic pulmonary disease (not including asthma) occasionally may benefit from antimicrobial therapy for acute exacerbations. In such cases differences in epidemiology, natural history, and pathogenesis must be considered. Cystic fibrosis patients may receive antibiotics directed at *P. aeruginosa*, *S. aureus*, or *H. influenzae* during the acute exacerbations (26), as may children with underlying severe chronic lung diseases (e.g., bronchopulmonary dysplasia, lung hypoplasia, ciliary dyskinesia, chronic aspiration). General principles of judicious antimicrobial use are particularly appropriate for these children to decrease the adverse effects from multiple courses of antibiotics and resultant colonization with antibiotic-resistant organisms.

References

1. Watson RL, Dowell SF, Jayaraman M, Keyserling H, Kolczak M, Schwartz B. Antimicrobial use for pediatric upper respiratory infections: reported practice, actual practice and parent beliefs. Pediatrics 1999.
2. O'Brien K, Dowell SF, Schwartz B, Marcy M, Phillips WR, Gerber MA. Cough-illness/bronchitis—principles of judicious use of antimicrobial agents. Pediatrics 1998; 101(suppl):178–181.
3. Aherne W, Bird T, Court SDM et al. Pathological changes in virus infections of the lower respiratory tract in children. J Clin Pathol 1970; 23:7–18.

4. Gaillard D, Jouet JB, Egreteau L et al. Airway epithelial damage and inflammation in children with recurrent bronchitis. Am J Crit Care Med 1994; 150:810–817.

5. Horn MEC, Reed SE, Taylor P. Role of viruses and bacteria in acute wheezy bronchitis in childhood: a study of sputum. Arch Dis Child 1979; 54:587–592.

6. Jafri HS. Treatment of respiratory syncytial virus: antiviral therapies. Pediatr Infect Dis J 2003; 22:S89–S92; discussion S92–S93.

7. Greensill J, McNamara PS, Dove W, Flanagan B, Smyth RL, Hart CA. Human metapneumovirus in severe respiratory syncytial virus bronchiolitis. Emerg Infect Dis 2003; 9:372–375.

8. Chapman RS, Henderson FW, Clyde WA, Collier AM, Denny FW. The epidemiology of tracheobronchitis in pediatric practice. Am J Epidemiol 1981; 114:786–797.

9. Glezen WP, Denny FW. Epidemiology of acute lower respiratory disease in children. N Engl J Med 1973; 288:498–505.

10. Monto AS, Cavallaro JJ. The Tecumseh study of respiratory illness II. Patterns of ocurrence of infection with respiratory pathogens, 1965–1969. Am J Epidemiol 1971; 94:280–289.

11. Gehanno P, Lenoir G, Barry B, Bons J, Boucot I, Berche P. Evaluation of naso-pharyngeal cultures for bacteriologic assessment of acute otitis media in children. Pediatr Infect Dis J 1996; 15:329–332.

12. Todd JK. Bacteriology and clinical relevance of nasopharyngeal and oropharyngeal cultures. Pediatr Infect Dis J 1984; 3:159–163.

13. Wald E, Milmoe G, Bowen A, Ledesma-Medina J, Salamon N, Bluestone C. Acute maxillary sinusitis in children. N Engl J Med 1981; 304:749–754.

14. Van der Veen J. The role of adenoviruses in respiratory disease. Am Rev Respir Dis 1963; 88:167–180.

15. Falck G, Gnarpe G, Gnarpe H. Prevalence of *Chlamydia pneumoniae* in healthy children and in children with respiratory tract infections. Pediatr Infect Dis J 1997; 16:549–554.

16. Denny FW, Clyde WA, Glezen WP. *Mycoplasma pneumoniae* disease clinical spectrum, pathophysiology, epidemiology and control. J Infect Dis 1971; 123:74–92.

17. Foy JH. Infections caused by *Mycoplasma pneumoniae* and possible carrier state in different populations of patients. Clin Infect Dis 1996; 17(suppl):S37–S46.

18. Foy HM, Cooney MK, Maletzky AJ, Grayston JT. Incidence and etiology of pneumonia, croup and bronchiolitis in preschool children belonging to a prepaid medical care group over a four-year period. Am J Epidemiol 1973; 97:80–92.

19. Nohynek H, Eskola J, Kleemola M, Jalonen E, Saiddu P, Leinonen M. Bacterial antibody assays in the diagnosis of acute lower respiratory tract infection in children. Pediatr Infect Dis J 1996; 14:478–484.

20. Normann E, Gnarpe J, Gnarpe H, Wettergren B. *Chlamydia pneumoniae* in children with acute respiratory tract infections. Acta Paediatr 1998; 87:23–27.

21. Emre U, Roblin PM, Gelling M et al. The asssociation of *Chlamydia pneumoniae* infection and reactive airway disease in children. Arch Pediatr Adolesc Med 1994; 148:727–732.

22. Emre U, Sokolovskaya N, Roblin PM, Schachter J, Hammerschlag M. Detection of anti-*Chlamydia pneumoniae* IgE in children with reactive airway disease. J Infect Dis 1995; 172:265–267.

23. Jantos CA, Roggendorf R, Wupperman FN, Hegemann JH. Rapid detection of *Chlamydia pneumoniae* by PCR-enzyme immunoassay. J Clin Microbiol 1998; 36:1890–1894.

24. Kutlin A, Roblin PM, Hammerschlag MR. Antibody response to *Chlamydia pneumoniae* infection in children with respiratory illness. J Infect Dis 1998; 177:720–724.

25. Mink CM, Cherry JD, Christenson P et al. A search for *Bordetella pertussis* infection in university students. Clin Infect Dis 1992; 14:464–471.

26. Moss RB. Cystic fibrosis: pathogenesis, pulmonary infection, and treatment. Clin Infect Dis J 1995; 21:839–851.

27. Steinman MA, Gonzales R, Linder JA, Landefeld CS. Changing use of antibiotics in community-based outpatient practice, 1991–1999. Ann Intern Med 2003; 138:525–533.

28. Hickman DE, Stebbins MR, Hanak JR, Guglielmo BJ. Pharmacy-based intervention to reduce antibiotic use for acute bronchitis. Ann Pharmacother 2003; 37:187–191.

29. Wilson SD, Dahl BB, Wells RD. An evidence-based clinical pathway for bronchiolitis safely reduces antibiotic overuse. Am J Med Qual 2002; 17:195–199.

30. McCaig LF, Besser RE, Hughes JM. Trends in antimicrobial prescribing rates for children and adolescents. J Am Med Assoc 2002; 287:3096–3102.

31. Nyquist AC, Gonzales R, Steiner JF, Sande MA. Antibiotic prescribing for children with colds, upper respiratory tract infections, and bronchitis. J Am Med Assoc 1998; 279:875–877.

32. Vinson DC, Lutz LJ. The effect of parental expectations on treatment of children with cough: a report from ASPN. J Fam Pract 1993; 37:23–27.

33. Cate TR, Couch RB, Fleet WF, Griffith WR, Gerone PJ, Knight V. Production of tracheobronchitis in volunteers with rhinovirus in a small-particle aerosol. Am J Epidemiol 1971; 94:269–279.

34. Hall WJ, Hall CB, Speers DM. Respiratory syncytial virus infection in adults. Ann Intern Med 1978; 88:203–205.

35. Orr PH, Scherer K, Macdonald A, Moffat MEK. Randomized placebo-controlled trials of antibiotics for acute bronchitis: a critical review of the literature. J Fam Pract 1993; 36:507–512.

36. Brickield FX, Carter WH, Johnson RE. Erythromycin in the treatment of acute bronchitis in a community practice. J Fam Pract 1986; 23:119–122.

37. Howie JGR, Clark GA. Double-blind trial of early dimethylchlortetracycline in minor respiratory illness in general practice. Lancet 1970; 2:1099–1102.

38. Stott NCH, West RR. Randomised controlled trial of antibiotics in patients with cough and purulent sputum. Br Med J 1976; 2:556–559.

39. Williamson HA. A randomised, controlled trial of doxycycline in the treatment of acute bronchitis. J Fam Pract 1984; 19:481–486.

40. Taylor B, Abbott GD, Mckerr M, Fergusson DM. Amoxycillin and cotrimoxazole in presumed viral respiratory infections of childhood: placebo-controlled trial. Br Med J 1977; 2:552–554.

41. Townsend EH. Chemoprophylaxis during respiratory infections in a private pediatric practice. Am J Dis Child 1960; 99:566–573.

42. Gadomski AM. Potential interventions for preventing pneumonia among young children: lack of effect of antibiotic treatment for upper respiratory infections. Pediatr Infect Dis J 1993; 12:115–120.

43. Cloutier MM, Loughlin GM. Chronic cough in children: a manifestation of airway hyperreactivity. Pediatrics 1981; 67:6–12.
44. Konig P. Hidden asthma in childhood. Am J Dis Child 1981; 135:1053–1055.
45. Gwaltney JM, Hendley JO, Simon G. Rhinovirus infections in an industrial population. Characteristics of illness and antibody response. J Am Med Assoc 1967; 202:494–500.
46. Gwaltney JM, Hendley JO, Simon G, Jordan WS. Rhinovirus infections in an industrial population. J Am Med Assoc 1967; 202:158–164.
47. Broughton RA. Infections due to *Mycoplasma pneumoniae* in childhood. Pediatr Infect Dis J 1986; 5:71–85.
48. Grayston JT. *Chlamydia pneumoniae* (TWAR) infections in children. Pediatr Infect Dis J 1994; 13:675–685.
49. American Academy of Pediatrics. Pertussis. In: Peter G, ed. Red Book. Report of the Committee on Infectious Diseases. 24th ed. Elk Grove Village, see: American Academy of Pediatrics, 1997:394–397.

29

Management of Chronic Rhinosinusitis in Children

HARVEY COATES

Princess Margaret Hospital for Children,
Perth, Australia

I. Introduction

Chronic sinusitis is persistent disease that cannot be alleviated by medical therapy alone and involves radiographic evidence of mucosal hyperplasia.

In children, it is defined as 12 weeks of persistent symptoms and signs or six episodes per year of recurrent acute sinusitis, each lasting at least 10 days, in association with persistent changes on computed tomography (CT), 4 weeks after medical therapy without intervening acute infection. The Consensus Meeting on Management of Rhinosinusitis in Children held in Brussels (September 1996) believed, however, that CT scanning in all children with suspected chronic rhinosinusitis is not feasible and omits that part of the definition. The true incidence of chronic sinusitis in childhood is not known, and there are controversies about its nature and where rhinitis ends and sinusitis begins. Acknowledging this, the Consensus Panel prefers to use the term rhinosinusitis to define a continuum of disease.

The burden of disease in children must be critically assessed. Many children with a mucopurulent rhinosinusitis will resolve their disease spontaneously over time with little morbidity. The judgment lies in determining which children require medical treatment and those few children who require progression to surgical intervention. Even the staging of surgery, the type of procedure, and allowance for different age groups within the pediatric spectrum is controversial.

However, in spite of these controversies, the last two decades have seen dramatic advances in our understanding of the etiology, pathogenesis, diagnosis, and management of chronic pediatric sinusitis. In particular, the widening usage of CT scanning and endoscopy has contributed much to our knowledge of the disease process and its management. It is our duty to impart this new knowledge to our pediatric and family practitioners to facilitate the treatment of this common condition in children and to allow early and appropriate referral of those children who require specialist care.

II. Etiologic Factors

Some authorities feel that the incidence of chronic pediatric rhinosinusitis is on the increase, from causes as diverse as the increase in urban environmental pollution, to the dramatic rise in daycare use and associated upper respiratory tract infections (URTI). The etiological factors can be broadly divided into inflammatory, anatomical, systemic, and miscellaneous factors (see Table 29.1). In the pediatric age group, viral upper respiratory infections play the major role in the causation of acute, recurrent acute, and chronic sinusitis. Attendance at a daycare unit may lead to a threefold increase in the incidence of URTI. If, in addition, the child has an allergic predisposition, then this will be aggravated by the development of an URTI. Allergic inflammatory disease is seen in up to 40% of the pediatric population, manifesting as either asthma, eczema, or hayfever with the associated otorhinolaryngological complications being otitis media with effusion, sinusitis, or adenotonsillar hypertrophy.

Gastroesophageal reflux has been suggested as a significant contributing factor to chronic sinusitis in young children. If the clinician suspects reflux as

Table 29.1 Etiological Factors for Chronic Sinusitis in Children

Inflammatory	Anatomical	Systemic	Miscellaneous
Upper respiratory tract infection	Ostiomeatal complex obstruction	Cystic fibrosis	Swimming
Allergy	Nasal septal deformity	Immotile cilia syndrome	Diving
Gastroesophageal reflux	Turbinate hypertrophy	Kartagener's syndrome	Flying
	Nasal polyps	Immunodeficiency syndrome	
	Adenoid hypertrophy		
	Foreign bodies		
	Cleft palate		
	Choanal atresia		

a causal factor in a young child with sinusitis, especially in the presence of continued erythema of the pharynx and the absence of obvious infection, then either empirical management with elevation of the head of the bed, antacids, or specific H2 antagonists, or referral to a gastroenterologist may be appropriate.

The essential abnormality in the development of chronic maxillary sinusitis in children and in adults is tissue changes occurring secondary to infection, allergy, or other factors in the region of the ostiomeatal complex, causing obstruction and secondary infections and change in the normal physiology of the sinus. The ostiomeatal complex is the keystone in sinus function and must be patent to ensure sinus clearance and normal sinus health. Blockage of the ostia creates hypoxic changes within the sinus causing the bacteriology to change from aerobic to anerobic. There is a retention of secretions which results in inflammatory changes and bacterial infection and this leads to thickening of the secretions. Damage to the delicate cilia epithelium of the mucous membrane occurs, causing mucosal thickening, which further aggravates the blocked ostium. Other anatomical abnormalities, such as a nasal septal deformity, turbinate hypertrophy, or the presence of polyps will cause disturbances of air through the nose and sinuses and may contribute to obstruction of the ostiomeatal complex.

Adenoid hypertrophy has been implicated as a causative factor in chronic sinusitis in children and this may be because it is a repository of bacteria. Certainly there is evidence that removal of the adenoids may cause spontaneous improvement in children with chronic sinusitis. Choanal atresia, cleft palate, and foreign bodies may also contribute to chronic sinusitis.

Systemically, cystic fibrosis is a major cause of chronic sinusitis and the main cause of nasal polyposis in children. The immotile cilia syndrome and Kartagener's syndrome contribute to chronic sinusitis by the immotile or absent cilia not providing normal or adequate drainage through the normal ostia.

Immunologic disorders, particularly those of antibody deficiencies are associated with chronic sinusitis. Gandhi et al. noted 29% of their 86 children with chronic sinusitis had a B-cell abnormality of either the immunoglobulin isotype IgG subclass, or were hyperresponsive to the pneumococcal polysaccharide vaccine. Sethi et al. noted 30% of their patients had an identifiable abnormality in their immune function or an abnormal immune mucosal response. Driscoll et al. noted a preponderance of lymphocytes of the helper phenotype in children with chronic sinusitis regardless of their associated medical conditions, suggesting a difference between children and adults. Shapiro et al., noted that in their children with recurrent or chronic sinusitis that 67% had recurrent otitis media associated with this, 35% had asthma, and 11% had pneumonia. They noted that 40% had elevated IgG or positive skin tests and that 5.6% had abnormal immune studies. Children with acquired immunodeficiency syndrome, such as with HIV infection, have a high incidence of chronic sinusitis.

In susceptible children, certain physical activities such as swimming, diving, or flying, particularly with an URTI, may precipitate sinus disease.

III. Symptoms and Signs

Wald suggested a triad of presenting symptoms that included nasal discharge with congestion or obstruction, daytime cough often becoming worse at night or early morning, and malodorous breath. She noted that headaches were not a common complaint, whereas Parsons and Phillips noted that 90% of their children exhibited this symptom, particularly those children who were older than 5 years of age. They felt that chronic sinusitis in children can be described as having seven major presenting symptoms (see Table 29.2).

These symptoms must be differentiated from allergic symptoms and are presented in Table 29.3.

Parsons and Phillips noted that the greatest complaint was chronic nasal obstruction followed by prolonged purulent nasal discharge and postnasal drip. In addition, chronic cough and halitosis and headache were noted in over two-thirds of all the children in his retrospective study. Interestingly, almost

Table 29.2 Major Presenting Symptoms of Chronic Sinusitis in Children (After Parsons and Phillips)

1. Persistent purulent nasal discharge
2. Chronic nasal obstruction
3. Postnasal drainage
4. Cough, normally worse at bed time or upon arising
5. Malodorous breath
6. Headaches, dental pain, or head pains
7. Behavioral problems

Table 29.3 Typical Allergic Nasal
Symptoms in Children

1. Nasal obstruction
2. Nasal congestion
3. Itchy runny nose
4. Paroxysmal sneezing
5. Itching of nose, ears, and eyes
6. Thin watery discharge
7. Other allergic symptoms and signs

two-thirds of the parents reported that their children exhibited unpleasant beha-vioral changes when they had exacerbation of their sinus symptoms, including irritability, hostile behavior, head banging, or crying while holding their head.

Examination of the ears may often reveal an associated otitis media with effusion (1,2). Examination of the nose, although not revealing the status of the sinuses, may show boggy erythematous nasal mucosa, the presence of puru-lent discharge, or on occasion a foreign body. There may be facial tenderness particularly over the antra or edema and halitosis may be present. Examination of the nose in younger children with an otoscope facilitates their cooperation and older children may cooperate with flexible or rigid endoscopy. Transillumi-nation in children is not of great value.

Topical vasoconstrictors such as Neosynephrine 0.5% with 5% lidocaine, allow sufficient anesthesia and decongestion to examine the nose in older children. Septal deformities should be noted and polyps, when present, are highly suggestive of cystic fibrosis.

The general examination, apart from noticing the presence of cough, hypo-nasal speech, edema, and discoloration of the periorbital region, may show signs of adenotonsillar hypertrophy. In addition there may be the classical facial fea-tures of the atopic child, with Dennie's line, transverse nasal crease, periorbital "allergic shiners," and circum-nasal and oral pallor (Fig. 29.1).

Chronic sinusitis may present with complications as the initial symptoms. The most common of these are orbital complications, including periorbital edema, proptosis, progressing to ophthalmoplegia. Intracranial complications may occur including meningitis, epidural abscess, subdural abscess, intracerebral abscess, and cavernous sinus thrombosis.

IV. Radiology and Imaging

The role of standard radiographic views including an antero-posterior, a lateral, and an occipito-mental view is controversial. The Water's view, or occipto-mental view, may detect disease in the maxillary sinuses in children over the age of 1 year, but as an air fluid level is an uncommon radiological finding in

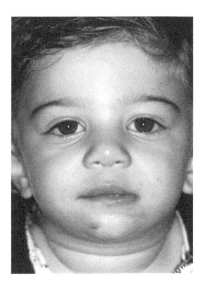

Figure 29.1   Clinical photograph of a child with the allergic facies, and classical Dennie's lines.

children under the age of 5 years there may be some difficulty differentiating the presence of fluid or mucosal swelling. The plain films provide rapid and noninvasive evaluation of the lower third of the nasal cavity in the maxillary, frontal, sphenoid, and posterior ethmoid sinuses, but are inadequate for evaluation of the anterior ethmoid air cells, the upper two-thirds of the nasal cavity and the middle meatus and frontal recess air passages (3). The lateral X-ray is useful for examination of the sphenoid and ethmoid sinuses and also gives an indication of the size of the adenoid mass. The Caldwell view, which I do not use routinely in children under the age of 7 years, will demonstrate the frontal sinuses and anterior ethmoid sinuses.

As plain sinus X-rays may miss significant disease in the maxillary and ethmoid sinuses, and do not delineate the ostiomeatal complex, there is a strong tendency in many centers for CT scanning of the sinuses to be performed. In our center, limited 5 mm cuts in the coronal plane are performed. These are usually adequate to delineate the sinus disease (see Fig. 29.2), and are equivalent in cost to the plain sinus film series. If surgery is contemplated, then a full set of coronal CT views should be obtained and axial views are necessary if there are orbital complications. Coronal sections may be technically difficult to obtain in children less than 4 years of age, as the position may precipitate airway obstruction in the younger sleeping child.

MRI may be used in the diagnosis of sinus disease, but has a number of limitations including cost, the need for sedation or a general anesthetic in young children, and lack of ability to display the bony landmarks. MRI may

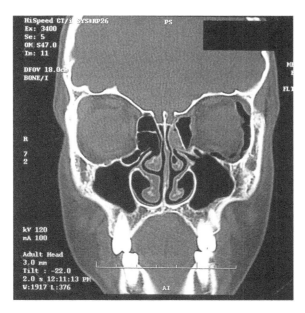

Figure 29.2 CT scan demonstrating a patent ostio-meatal complex on the right, and obstruction on the left, with ethmoiditis.

be considered in the case of suspected tumor or fungal infection of the sinuses (4). In the author's practice plain films are used to help in the diagnosis of chronic sinusitis and establish other associated factors, for example, adenoid hypertrophy. If, after maximal medical therapy there is a lack of clinical improvement, then a modified CT scan in the coronal plane will be ordered. In many cases this will be adequate for surgical management, but on occasion full CT scanning in both the coronal and axial planes will be necessary, particularly where there are complications such as periorbital abscess.

V. Microbiology

Microbiologic assessment is not routinely performed in children with uncomplicated chronic rhinosinusitis. Table 29.4 details the principal indications for sinus puncture.

The Consensus Group in Brussels could not agree whether middle meatal cultures could substitute for sinus punctures. Culture specimens obtained from the middle meatus or from the ethmoid bulla have a higher incidence of positive results than those obtained from the maxillary antrum. Organisms that have been found in chronic sinusitis are delineated in Table 29.5.

Brook (5) noted that anerobic Gram-positive cocci such as staphylococci and streptococci as well as anerobes were most commonly found during culture at the

Table 29.4 Principal Indications of Sinus
Puncture in Children

---

1. A severe illness or toxic condition in a child
2. Acute illness in a child that does not improve
   with medical therapy in 48–72 h
3. An immunocompromised host
4. The presence of suppurative (intraorbital or
   intracranial) complications, excepting orbital
   cellulitis

---

time of sinus surgery. However, Muntz and Lusk noted that the tissue culture bacteriology from the ethmoid bullae of children undergoing functional endoscopic sinus surgery (FESS) had the principal organisms isolated being alpha hemolytic *Streptococcus* (23%), *Staphylococcus aureus* (19%), *Moraxella catarrhalis* (7%), *Haemophilus influenzae* (7%), with anerobic organisms isolated in only 7% of cases. They concluded that the course of chronic sinusitis was more that of obstruction and mucostasis with overgrowth of colonizing bacteria, rather than a primarily infectious process. Fungal sinusitis is uncommon (6).

VI. Additional Investigations

A. Allergy Testing

As there is a strong association between the presence of perennial allergic rhinitis, seasonal allergic rhinitis, and chronic sinusitis, allergy testing is performed in those children where there is a high suspicion of allergic disease. This is based on clinical grounds and often there will be a family history of atopy and a personal history of either asthma, eczema, or hayfever. In addition, there may be clinical symptoms of allergic rhinitis as previously mentioned and the clinical features of allergic rhinitis including Dennie's line, transverse nasal crease, and allergic shiners.

Table 29.5 Typical Microorganisms Found in Chronic
Sinusitis

Microorganisms

Streptococcus pneumoniae
Haemophilus influenzae
Moraxella catarrhalis
Staphylococcus aureus
Anerobes

In children over the age of 3 years, skin prick testing is performed, particularly investigating for dust mite, pollen, grasses, moulds, and animal hair to which the child may be exposed. The radioallergosorbent test (RAST) is an alternative means of determining measurement of allergen/specific IgE, but these tests are more costly and somewhat less sensitive than skin testing. They may be useful in younger children, and are helpful for titration of the antigen dosage in sublingual desensitization. Food allergies may be detected by a process of avoidance and provocation testing, and this applies particularly to dairy products, wheat, yeast, eggs, citrus fruit, and soy allergies which are the most common food allergies noted.

If there is a concern regarding systemic underlying causes of rhinosinusitis, then full blood count and immunoglobulin testing (including the subclasses) may be arranged. In addition, antipneumococcal (antibody) testing may be performed to help determine the immune status of the child.

VII. Medical Management

Chronic sinusitis in young children tends to spontaneously resolve. Therefore, there should be a treatment regimen which commences with relatively simple avoidance and therapeutic measures, and progressing to maximal medical therapy, and then to a graduated surgical approach (7,8). The ultimate objective of treatment is to rapidly sterilize sinus secretions and re-establish normal sinus drainage, and this objective may be achieved by medical and surgical therapy. A stepped protocol of therapy options for pediatric chronic sinusitis may be used (see Table 29.6).

Table 29.6 Stepped Protocol for Treatment Options for Pediatric Chronic Sinusitis

Less intensive . . . . More intensive
Reduced daycare attendance
Dust mite control
Trial of dairy free diet
Daily nasal saline lavage
Nasal sodium cromolyn (children under 4)
2 Weeks broad spectrum antibiotics (with repeat if necessary)
Topical nasal steroids
Age-appropriate allergy testing and sublingual immunotherapy
Antibiotic prophylaxis
Adenoidectomy (where appropriate)
Antral lavage or mini natural ostium antrostomy
Endoscopic ethmoidectomy and antrostomy
Intravenous gamma-globulin for documented immunodeficiency

Source: Adapted from Manning, with permission.

The author believes that the increase in chronic sinusitis together with middle ear disease is related to the increase in use of daycare facilities in the 1980s and 1990s, as well as the increasing incidence of allergic disease and air pollution. Therefore, change from full daycare to part-time daycare, or home-based daycare may reduce exposure to URTIs. The author finds that empirical measures to reduce dust mite exposure in the home, together with a 2-week trial of a dairy-free diet in young children is very valuable in reducing allergic rhinosinusitis symptoms in a significant number of children. In children under the age of 4, nasal sodium cromolyn may be used three to four times a day, possibly alternating with nasal saline lavage, although there are practical problems with this degree of intensive therapy if the parent works.

Antibiotic therapy is initially for 2 weeks. If there is no improvement with this regimen, then the antibiotic may be changed to one such as amoxicillin/clavulanate for a further 2 weeks, and maximal medical therapy dictates a third 2-week course if the child does not demonstrate improvement.

If the antibiotic is changed, the author does not obtain sinus secretions as this may be traumatic to the child. The author tends to use amoxicillin or cefaclor in the first instance, although it is noted in the Consensus Panel in Brussels that the following antibiotics are not recommended as first choice for the treatment of rhinosinusitis:

- combination of sulfamethoxazole and trimethoprim
- clarithromycin
- cefixime
- ceftibuten
- doxycycline monohydrate
- cefaclor.

These agents have known serious side effects or are not effective against antimicrobial resistant bacterial pathogens, or both.

If the child does not respond in the first 2 weeks to amoxicillin or cefaclor, then amoxicillin/clavulanate is substituted for the next 2-week course. On occasion, if there is no improvement with oral antimicrobial antibiotic therapy, consideration of admission to hospital and intravenous antibiotic therapy may be necessary.

As 40% of children in the author's practice have an atopic background, maximal medical therapy includes a 1-month trial of a nasal steroid spray, which may in the first 5 days be preceded by a decongestant spray to facilitate absorption of the steroid spray. The author does not use antihistamine/decongestants, as these may cause drying up and stasis of secretions in chronic sinusitis. In addition, they will interfere with subsequent allergy testing (particularly the long acting antihistamines).

VIII. Surgical Management

Surgical management of chronic sinusitis in children follows failed maximal medical therapy with antibiotics, nasal irrigations of saline and nasal steroids (9). The Consensus Panel from Brussels felt that indications for sinus surgery should be divided into absolute and possible indications (see Table 29.7).

Prior to the development of functional endoscopic sinus surgery (FESS), chronic rhinosinusitis in young children was often managed with an adenoidectomy and sinus washout, or inferior meatus antrostomy. Takahashi et al. and Rosenfeld have reported on the efficacy of adenoidectomy in cases of chronic sinusitis in children. Van den Berg and Heatley studied 48 children aged between 1 and 12 years with a 5-month to 2-year followup. They noted resolution of symptoms in 58%, some improvement in 21%, and minimal to no improvement in 9% of cases. Of the 48 children, only 3 (6%) required endoscopic sinus surgery. Antral sinus and maxillary sinus lavage usually has only a transient effect, and a number of papers have shown that inferior meatus antrostomy has a high rate of closure and little therapeutic efficacy.

The author, however, believes that in selected children, particularly those under the age of 5, an adenoidectomy where indicated (see Fig. 29.3), together with a natural inferior ostium antrostomy will allow both drainage and ventilation of the sinuses, albeit for only 6 months or so. These procedures are relatively safe in young children compared with the possible risks of surgery in the middle meatal region in the hands of the average otorhinolaryngologist. The nasal antral window through the inferior meatus has a potential for injury to the developing teeth.

Table 29.7 Indications for Sinus Surgery

Absolute
Complete nasal obstruction in cystic fibrosis due to massive polyposis
Antrochoanal polyp
Intracranial complications
Mucoceles and mucopyoceles
Orbital abscess
Traumatic injury in the optic canal (decompression)
Dacryocystorhinitis due to sinusitis and resistant to appropriate medical treatment
Fungal sinusitis
Some meningoencephaloceles
Some neoplasms
Possible
Chronic rhinosinusitis persisting despite optimal medical therapy

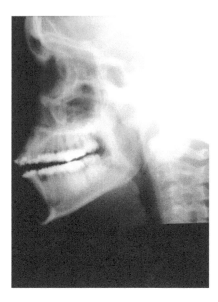

Figure 29.3 Plain lateral X-ray demonstrating the combination of moderate adenoid hypertrophy together with significant posterior tip of the inferior turbinate hypertrophy.

The Caldwell–Luc approach is rarely indicated in children because of potential for permanent sinus hypoplasia with facial and dental abnormalities.

When in the last decade endoscopic sinus surgery was pioneered, the advocates of this procedure extolled the virtues of middle meatus surgery being more physiologic than previous surgery. There was improved visualization of the anatomy with endoscopic techniques in conjunction with the CT scan findings. As described by Lazar, FESS is a functional rather than an exenterative or ablative procedure. The ostiomeatal complex is a key to this surgery, and abnormal mucosal tissue or bony tissues can be removed, whilst leaving the normal mucosa in place. Success rates reported in with FESS ranged from 80% to 93%. Up to this time, there are no prospective controlled studies which show the effectiveness of functional endoscopic sinus surgery. Endoscopic sinus surgery has been shown in young animal models to impair facial growth (10).

There is thus a controversy amongst those that are more conservative, and those who advocate middle meatus surgery. When it is indicated, endoscopic sinus surgery should be more conservative in children than in adults, and is primarily a natural middle ostium nasal antral window. Generally, endoscopic sinus surgery should be reserved for older children rather than those under the age of 5 years. A symposium discussing the controversies over the treatment of chronic rhinosinusitis in children concluded that there was significantly less need for surgery for sinonasal conditions in children when compared with adults. It was noted by Stammberger, in the paper by Lund et al., that <2% of his many thousands of surgical cases had been children.

Research has also acknowledged that factors other than anatomic abnormalities and ostiomeatal complex obstruction affect the outcomes of FESS in children with chronic sinusitis (see Table 29.8).

IX. Complications of Functional Endoscopic Sinus Surgery

The most frequently noted complication following endoscopic sinus surgery is the formation of adhesions between the middle turbinate and the lateral nasal wall which may cause ethmoid obstruction. Other general complications may include damage to the nasolacrimal duct, bleeding from the sphenopalatine and anterior ethmoid arteries, as well as orbital injuries and cerebrospinal fluid leak.

Management of significant adhesions postoperatively may include a further surgical procedure to remove the adhesions and crusting. Nasal packing may aggravate this condition, and in particular paraffin-soaked nasal gauze is contra indicated. If a child has significant nasal polyps then preoperative systemic steroids may reduce peroperative bleeding and postoperative inflammatory reactions. Generally, prolapse of orbital fat following surgery is not a major problem, unless there is entrapment of the medial rectus muscle or hemorrhage intraorbitally. The uncommon complication of intraorbital bleeding is managed by removal of packing and consideration of an external ethmoidectomy for ligation of the anterior ethmoid arteries and partial orbital decompression. Occasionally, a lateral canthotomy is required if there are signs of increased orbital pressure noted by the ophthalmologist.

Cerebrospinal fluid leak is managed by either a free graft if it is noted in the course of the procedure with postoperative packing for 5–6 days, or abdominal fat, muscle, and temporalis fascia in larger defects.

X. Surgical Management of Complications of Sinusitis

A. Periorbital Abscess

Periorbital abscess is a complication of acute and chronic sinusitis which presents with periorbital cellulitis (see Fig. 29.4), some orbital signs such as proptosis and gaze restriction, and is often initially managed with intravenous antibiotics, and a CT scan (see Fig. 29.5) performed if there is no improvement in 24–48 h or if

Table 29.8 Factors Affecting the Outcome of FESS in Children

1. The extent of the disease
2. Daycare attendance
3. Significant exposure to a smoke-filled environment
4. Postoperative nasal endoscopy findings
5. The presence of systemic disease

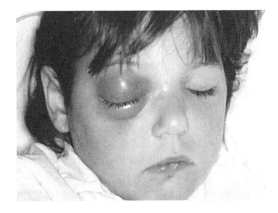

Figure 29.4 Clinical photograph of a child with periorbital cellulitis.

there are signs of increasing orbital complications. An external ethmoidectomy approach has been used in the past and continues to be a relatively safe and effective means of drainage of the periorbital abscess, but endoscopic techniques can be used when there is a sub periostial abscess present.

B.   Intracranial Suppurative Complications

Intracranial suppurative complications, particularly in the region of the frontal sinus and frontal lobe, may occur, and these are often treated with long-term antibiotics parenterally and/or surgical drainage for refractory disease.

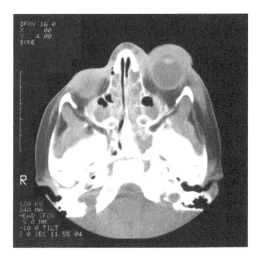

Figure 29.5   CT scan of patient with left proptosis, periorbital cellulitis, and bilateral ethmoiditis.

C. Nasal Polyposis

As true nasal polyps are uncommon in children, the differential diagnosis of a polyp or cyst in the nasal cavity should be carefully reviewed (see Fig. 29.6). The majority of nasal polyps in children are associated with cystic fibrosis, but antrochoanal polyps, tumors, and foreign bodies may be associated with a polypoid appearance. An adolescent may present with a nasopharyngeal angiofibroma, and in younger children, rhabdomyosarcomas may also present as a unilateral nasal mass.

Nasal polyps may cause significant airway obstruction as well as recurrent sinusitis and removal usually gives significant relief, although there is a high incidence of recurrence, particularly in children with cystic fibrosis. New techniques using mechanical debriders can remove polyps easily with little hemorrhage, and thus enable easier visualization of the anatomy.

XI. Post-operative Management

In the immediate postoperative period, the child may require saline nasal irrigations, systemic antibiotics, and inhaled nasal steroid spray. It is crucial that, at this time, the parents of the child are counseled that surgery is not a cure for allergy in those children with an obvious atopic background. If the child has not been investigated for allergies, or had topical or systemic therapy for allergic rhinitis then this should be instituted. It should be emphasised to the parents that chronic sinusitis will usually resolve over time in children and that the mucosal

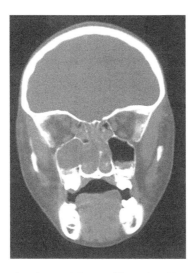

Figure 29.6 CT scan showing a right maxillary sinusitis with some polyposis, and ethmoiditis with displacement of the septum to the left.

changes are not usually irreversible particularly if ongoing and supportive medical treatment is carried out.

XII. Summary

Chronic sinusitis in children appears to be increasing in children with increasing utilization of daycare centers, environmental pollution, and allergies. The majority of children with chronic sinusitis have a disease process which spontaneously improves over time, but there are a small group of children who will require medical intervention. Those children who have anatomical factors leading to intractable sinus disease which does not settle with maximal medical therapy may require surgical management. This can be a progressive surgical approach commencing with an adenoidectomy, and an inferior ostium nasal antral window, and progress to functional endoscopic sinus surgery. It is important to manage coexisting disease such as allergic rhinitis and immunodeficiencies.

Acknowledgment

My profound thanks to Ms Kim Gifkins for her untiring efforts to assist and help edit the manuscript.

References

1. Cunningham JM, Chiu EJ, Landgraf JM, Gliklich RE. The health impact of chronic recurrent rhinosinusitis in children. Arch Otolaryngol Head Neck Surg 2000; 126(11):1363–1368.
2. Kay DJ, Rosenfeld RM. Quality of life for children with persistent sinonasal symptoms. Otolaryngol Head Neck Surg 2003; 128(1):17–26.
3. Sivasli E, Sirikci A, Bayazyt YA, Gumusburun E, Erbagci H, Bayram M, Kanlykama M. Anatomic variations of the paranasal sinus area in pediatric patients with chronic sinusitis. Surg Radiol Anat 2002; 24(6):399–404.
4. Younis RT, Anand VK, Davidson B. The role of computerised tomography and magnetic resonance imaging in patients with sinusitis with complications. Laryngoscope 2002; 112(2):224–229.
5. Brook I. Sinusitis—overcoming bacterial resistance. Int J Pediatr Otorhinolaryngol 2001; 58(1):27–36.
6. McClay JE, Marple B, Kapadia L, Biavati MJ, Nussenbaum B, Newcomer M, Manning S, Booth T, Schwade N. Clinical presentation of allergic fungal sinusitis in children. Laryngoscope 2002; 112(3):565–569.
7. Don DM, Yellon RF, Casselbrant ML, Bluestone CD. Efficacy of a stepwise protocol that includes intravenous antibiotic therapy for the management of chronic sinusitis in children and adolescents. Arch Otolaryngol Head Neck Surg 2001; 127(9):1093–1098.

8. Picichero ME. Short course antibiotic therapy for respiratory infection: a review of the evidence. Pediatr Inf Dis J 2000; 19(9):929–937.
9. Manning S. Surgical intervention for sinusitis in children. Curr Allergy Asthma Rep 2001; 1(3):289–296.
10. Bothwell MR, Piccirillo JF, Lusk RP, Ridenour BD. Long-term outcome of facial growth after functional endoscopic sinus surgery. Otolaryngol Head Neck Surg 2002; 126(6):628–634.

30

Rhinitis and Rhinosinusitis Treatment with Corticosteroids in Children

ISAAC SHUBICH

Miami Children's Hospital,
Miami, Florida, USA

JAVIER DIBILDOX

Autonomous University of San Luis Potosí,
San Luis Potosí, Mexico

Rhinitis belongs to a heterogeneous group of nasal disorders manifested by one or more of the following symptoms: sneezing, rhinorrhea, nasal itching, and nasal congestion (1). The inflammation of the nasal mucosa and intranasal structures are caused frequently by allergic and nonallergic rhinitis. In a significant proportion of the population, allergic rhinitis is the most frequent cause of chronic rhinitis (1–3). Nonallergic rhinitis occurs in 30–50% of patients with rhinitis (1). Patients with allergic and nonallergic rhinitis share common symptoms such as nasal congestion, rhinorrhea, sneezing, and postnasal drip (1,2,4).

The incidence of allergy has increased markedly during the last 40 years, and allergies affect about 10% of children and up to 20% of adolescents and adults (5). Allergic rhinitis is defined as an inflammation of the mucosal lining of the nose manifested by early and late phase responses. Each type of response is characterized by sneezing, congestion and rhinorrhea, but nasal congestion predominates in the late phase response (2). The clinical manifestations of allergic rhinitis may also include a variety of signs and symptoms such as nasal obstruction, pruritus of eyes, ears or palate, red or watery eyes, chronic pharyngitis, hoarseness, chronic cough, postnasal drip, eustachian tube dysfunction, sleep disorders, asthma, and recurrent infections of ear, nose, and sinuses (2). In children a persistent nasal congestion may be the only complaint.

The inflammation of the nasal mucosa in patients with allergic rhinitis is characterized by infiltration of T-lymphocytes in the submucosa and the epithelium, as a reaction from an increase in the recruitment of inflammatory cells and a prolonged survival of these cells in the nasal mucosa (1,2). Other conditions associated with allergic rhinitis are asthma, rhinosinusitis, conjuntivitis, otitis media, nasal polyposis, lower respiratory tract infection, and dental occlusion (2). Lack of appropriate treatment can aggravate these comorbid conditions (6).

Nonallergic, noninfectious rhinitis usually develops in middle-aged patients, and is rare in children (2,6). Nonallergic rhinitis, demostrated by negative allergen skin testing, is not mediated by the immunoglobulin E (IgE) and consists of diverse conditions including infectious rhinitis, nonallergic rhinitis with eosinophilia syndrome (NARES), occupational rhinitis, hormonal rhinitis, drug-induced rhinitis, gustatory rhinitis, and idiopathic (vasomotor) rhinitis (1,2,4). The most common cause of nonallergic rhinitis in children is infectious rhinitis.

Nonallergic rhinitis is manifested by sporadic or persistent symptoms such as nasal obstruction, rhinorrhea, postnasal drip, sneezing, and nasal itching (1,4). The pathophysiology of nonallergic, noninfectious rhinitis is less well known (1,6). In contrast to allergic rhinitis, nonallergic, noninfectious rhinitis usually develops in midde-aged persons (1,6). Another group of patients with nonallergic rhinitis present eosinophilic inflammation similar to the inflammation seen in patients with allergic rhinitis (1,6).

Rhinosinusitis is defined as the inflammation of the respiratory mucosa of one or more paranasal sinuses, usually secondary to infections. The incidence of rhinosinusitis in children tends to increase with age, and in children who experience frequent upper respiratory tract infections and allergic rhinitis (3). Rhinosinusitis without rhinitis is rare, and is manifested by nasal congestion, purulent rhinorrhea, postnasal drip, facial and dental pain, headaches, anosmia, hyposmia, halitosis, and cough. Rhinosinusitis and allergic rhinitis share the pathologic features of edema of the nasal mucsa, mucociliary dysfunction, and increase of mucus production, thus increasing the risk of developing acute and chronic rhinosinusitis (2).

Acute rhinosinusitis is more often associated with a bacterial or viral infection. Noninfectious inflammation with mucosal hyperplasia and predominance of eosinophils and mixed mononuclear cells is related to chronic rhinosinusitis (1). The incidence of chronic rhinosinusitis is higher in allergic children. In one study, 70% of the children with allergic and chronic rhinosinusitis were found to have abnormal sinus X-rays (2).

Nasal polyps are chronic inflammatory formations that originate from the mucosal lining of the paranasal sinuses and frequently coexist with asthma, rhinitis, and rhinosinusitis. The prevalence of nasal polyps in allergic patients is low and usually under 5.0% (1,2). The polyps associated with asthma, chronic rhinosinusitis, and aspirin sensitivity show an eosinophilic infiltrate (1). Nasal polyps are infrequent in children younger than 10 years old, except in the presence of cystic fibrosis. In cystic fibrosis, the polyps show a neutrophil infiltrate and the incidence of polyps varies from 6% to 48% (1,2). Nasal polyps can also occur in children with primary ciliary dyskinesia.

I. Treatment

The goal of treatment in children with rhinitis is to obtain the best results with the least risk. The patients should be carefully evaluated to determine the best form of therapy for each patient. Treatment should be selected according to the patient's clinical manifestations and type of rhinitis, and in severe cases several medications may be required (1).

Intranasal corticosteroids are the most effective anti-inflammatory medication for the treatment of allergic rhinitis (1,2,6,7). Currently, they are indicated in the treatment and prophylaxis of seasonal and perennial allergic rhinitis (1–3,8). Other therapeutic uses for corticosteroids include nonallergic rhinitis, chronic rhinosinusitis, and nasal polyposis (1,2,4).

Steroids with a high topical potency and low systemic bioavailability were introduced for the treatment of perennial rhinitis in 1974 and found to be as effective as corticosteroids administered systemically (7). The newer steroids require less frequent dosing, have a higher safety profile and generally do not cause systemic adverse events when used at recommended doses. These preparations include beclomethasone dipropionate, flunisolide, triamcinolone acetonide, budesonide, fluticasone propionate, and mometasone furoate.

Most intranasal corticosteroids are recommended for use in children older than 6 years. Fluticasone has been approved for use in children age 4 and older, and mometasone furoate was approved for the treatment of symptoms of allergic rhinitis for adults and children age 3 and older. Since July 2002, the US Food and Drug Administration (FDA) has approved the expansion of the indication of mometasone furoate for the treatment of seasonal and perennial nasal allergy symptoms to include children 2 years of age and older.

Although the mode of action is complex, intranasal corticosteroids are the most potent medications currently available for the treatment of allergic and nonallergic rhinitis (1,2,7). The corticosteroid binds to the glucocorticoid receptor in the cytoplasm of the target cells, moves to the nuclear compartment and increases or inhibits gene transcription through processes known as transactivation and transrepression, respectively (2,7). Corticosteroids act, in large part, through their ability to upregulate or downregulate gene transcription within various cells. The rationale for using intranasal corticosteroids in the treatment of rhinitis is that high concentrations can be achieved at the receptor sites in the nasal mucosa, with a minimal risk of systemic adverse events (2,3).

The onset of action of the newer, more potent corticosteroids is as short as 24 h, and improvement can occur in just a few hours with fluticasone and mometasone (6,7). Maximum relief of symptoms may take as long as 3 weeks of therapy and are most effective when used regularly.

The ideal treatment for allergic rhinitis is avoidance of the offending antigens. However, because this is often difficult or impossible, pharmacotherapy for symptomatic relief may be indicated. Antihistamines, decongestants, mast cell stabilizers, and anticholinergic drugs may provide effective relief from one or more symptoms of allergic rhinitis, but do not have a significant effect upon the underlying late inflammatory response. The symptoms of allergic rhinitis are attributed to the accumulation and activation of infiltrating cells, which release mediators and cytokines resulting in allergic inflammation. Intranasal steroids deposited in the receptor sites in the nasal mucosa can suppress many stages of the allergic inflammation (2,7), and significantly affect the production and/or activity of proinflammatory mediators such as cytokines, adhesion molecules, mast cells, and eosinophils (2,7).

Intranasal steroids are frequently used for several weeks in the treatment of rhinitis exacerbations, prolonged pollen season and in severe, chronic, perennial rhinitis. Corticosteroids relieve most effectively nasal congestion, rhinorrhea, itching, and sneezing in patients with allergic rhinitis (2,3). Treatment of allergic rhinitis with intranasal corticosteroids is superior to treatment with both antihistamines and cromones (2,6,9), and corticosteroids are better tolerated than decongestants, but do not seem to be effective in reducing ocular symptoms (6).

Other benefits including improvement in quality of life, improvement of sleep disturbances, and reduction of adenoid enlargement associated with airway obstruction in children have been reported with the use of intranasal corticosteroids.

Systemic steroids are rarely needed for the treatment of allergic rhinitis in children, although, in patients with severe symptoms refractory to other therapy, a short course of oral, short-acting steroids such as prednisone may be helpful.

In children 3–11 years of age with seasonal allergic rhinitis, 100 mg of mometasone furoate aqueous nasal spray once daily provides greater symptomatic relief than placebo and relief similar to that of 84 mg of beclomethasone dipropionate administered twice daily (8).

Nonallergic, noninfectious rhinitis with a poorly defined etiology and pathophysiology are generally difficult to treat, with the exception of aspirin-induced rhinitis, nasal polyposis, and other rhinitic forms, which respond to corticosteroids (1). The mechanism by which corticosteroids work in patients with nonallergic rhinitis is not known, but may be attributed to their vasoconstrictive properties (6). The newer corticosteroid preparations tend to be more potent vasoconstrictors so they may be more effective for the treatment of nonallergic rhinitis (6).

Intranasal corticosteroids are effective in the treatment of patients with NARES, and may be useful in some patients with idiopathic (vasomotor) rhinitis (1). Intranasal corticosteroids may facilitate the withdrawal of the topical decongestants in patients with rhinitis medicamentosa caused by prolonged use of topical nasal decongestants. The management of bacterial rhinosinusitis usually requires antibiotics, but the treatment of underlying allergic rhinitis is useful in ameliorating the signs and symptoms of rhinosinusitis (3).

Patients with eosinophilic nonallergic rhinitis typically respond well to intranasal corticosteroids, although patients with more severe disease with nasal polyps and rhinosinusitis may require systemic corticosteroids (1,6). Intranasal corticosteroids are effective in reducing the size and in preventing continued growth of nasal polyps, including those associated with cystic fibrosis. They are also helpful in reducing polyp size and in controlling polyp formation following polypectomy (1,2,4).

II. Adverse Events

The intranasal corticosteroids are generally well tolerated and safe when used appropriately. There is a genuine concern, however, among physicians and parents about the use of topical steroids in children due to the potential systemic and local adverse events caused by the corticosteroids and because children may require treatment with long-term use of intranasal topical steroids, thus causing systemic and local adverse events, such as growth retardation in children and adolescents, hypothalamic–pituitary–adrenal axis suppression, and damage to the septum and nasal mucosa that may result from a cumulative effect of the medication (2,3,8,9).

The systemic effects of intranasal corticosteroids depend on the systemic bioavailability of the drug through direct intranasal and gastrointestinal absorption. The oral bioavailability has been well established for most of the corticosteroids, and is important because approximately 80% of the intranasal dose is swallowed (6). The oral bioavilability of triamcinolone acetonide is reported to be 23%, 20% for flunisolide, 11% for budesonide, and less than 0.1% for fluticasone propionate and mometasone furoate (6). The total bioavailability is determined by the oral and intranasal absorption of corticosteroids. The total bioavailability of mometasone furoate is reported at 0.1%; for fluticasone propionate it is 0.5 to <2%, for budesonide it is 20% and for flunisolide it is 40–50% (6). Budesonide is well absorbed through the nasal mucosa directly into the systemic circulation.

The absorption from the nasal mucosa of fluticasone propionate and mometasone furoate is very low (7). The clinical efficacy of intranasal corticosteroids with very low systemic bioavailability such as mometasone furoate, fluticasone propionate, and budesonide may indicate that the therapeutic effect is achieved through local actions in the nasal mucosa (7).

Beclomethasone dipropionate aqueous nasal spray 168 mg BID was compared with placebo in a double-blind randomized trial for 12 months in 100 children 6–9 years of age with perennial allergic rhinitis. The study resulted in a significant suppression of growth in children compared to placebo (10). In a similar study, mometasone furoate 100 mg/day was compared to placebo in a double-blind, randomized trial for 12 months. Height was measured six times by stadiometry and hypothalamic–pituitary–adrenal axis function was assessed by cosyntropin stimulation testing. The rate of growth was similar for both groups throughout the study, and no adverse events on the hypothalamic–pituitary–adrenal axis were found (5).

In one study to assess the long-term safety of 100 µg of mometasone furoate and 168 mg of beclomethasone dipropionate BID in children 6–11 years of age, no significant changes from baseline intraocular pressure or posterior subcapsular cataracts were detected after 12 months of treatment for either treatment group, nor was there evidence of hypothalamic–pituitary–adrenal axis supression in the patients tested with cosyntropin stimulation at weeks 26 and 52 (8).

The lower bioavailability of mometasone furoate and fluticasone propionate among the presently available topical nasal steroids, may be clinically significant in children requiring long-term use of intranasal topical steroids, particularly in those cases of simultaneous use of topical or inhaled steroids in the treatment of asthma, perennial allergic rhinitis and eczema, due to potential adverse events such as hypothalamic–pituitary–adrenal axis supression, osteoporosis, and growth retardation.

Local adverse events may occur during prolonged topical nasal steroids use, because of the inflammation of the nasal mucosa caused by nonallergic and allergic disease; the spray could increase the risk of mucosal irritation, dryness, crusting, bleeding, and septal perforations. Mild epistaxis is probably the most bothersome side effect (6). Rare occurrences of nasal septal perforation in adults and children have been reported. Other infrequent complaints include unpleasant smell or taste, stinging, and burning (6). All patients using a nasal topical steroid must be cautioned to consult their physician in cases of persistent nasal irritation, crusting, or epistaxis.

Comparative biopsies of the nasal mucosa before and after one year treatment with mometasone furoate aqueous nasal spray in adults showed in the posttreatment biopsies improvement in the appearance of the epithelium and reduction of the inflammatory cell infiltrate, particularly eosinophils and mast cells with no signs of nasal mucosa atrophy (2,8).

There have also been case reports of glaucoma associated with intranasal corticosteroid use, but large epidemiologic studies have not shown any association with glaucoma or cataracts and these drugs (2,6).

Even though the long-term use of these medications in children has been shown to be safe (2,5,8), the nasal corticosteroid should be titrated to the lowest dose at which effective control of rhinitis is maintained.

III. Conclusion

Intranasal corticosteroids are safe and highly effective drugs for treating children with seasonal and perennial allergic rhinitis, nonallergic rhinitis, chronic sinusitis, and nasal polyposis. The nasal corticosteroid should be titrated to the lowest dose at which effective control of rhinitis is maintained. All inhaled corticosteroids have the potential to cause systemic side-effects. It is recommended that the height of children receiving prolonged treatment with nasal corticosteroids is regularly monitored, and examination of the intranasal structures should be done in each visit to the attending physician. Also, the parents and patients must be cautioned to consult their physician in cases of persistent nasal irritation, crusting, or epistaxis.

References

1. Dykewicz MS. Rhinitis and sinusitis. J Allergy Clin Immunol 2003; 111:S520–S529.
2. Bousquet J, van Cauwenberge P, Khaltaev N. Allergic rhinitis and its impact on Asthma: ARIA workshop report. J Allergy Clin Immunol 2001; 108:S147–S334.
3. Fireman P. Therapeutic approaches to allergic rhinitis: treating the child. J Allergy Clin Immunol 2000; 105:S616–S621.
4. Settipane RA, Lieberman P. Update on nonallergic rhinitis. Ann Allergy Asthma Immunol 2001; 86:494–507.
5. Schenkel EJ, Skoner DP, Bronsky EA, Miller SD, Pearlman DS, Rooklin A, Rosen JP, Ruff ME, Vandewalker ML, Wanderer A, Damaraju CV, Nolop KB, Messarina-Wicki B. Abscence of growth retardation in children with perennial allergic rhinitis after one year of treatment with mometasone furoate aqueous nasal spray. Pediatrics 2000; 105:E22.
6. Williams PV. Treatment of rhinitis. Corticosteroids and cromolyn sodium. Immunol Allergy Clin North Am 2000; 20(2):369–381.
7. Mygind N, Nielsen LP, Hoffmann HJ, Shukla A, Blumberga G, Dahl R, Jacobi H. Mode of action of intranasal corticosteroids. J Allergy Clin Immunol 2001; 108:S16–S25.
8. Dibildox J. Safety and efficacy of mometasone furoate aqueous nasal spray in children with allergic rhinitis: results of recent clinical trials. J Allergy Clin Immunol 2001; 108:S54–S58.
9. Scadding GK. Corticosteroids in the treatment of pediatric allergic rhinitis. J Allergy Clin Immunol 2001; 108:S59–S64.
10. Skoner DP, Rachelefsky GS. Meltzer EO, Chervinsky P, Morris R, Seltzer J et al. Detection of growth suppression in children during treatment with intranasal beclomethasone dipropionate. Pediatrics 2000; 105:E23.

31

Obstructive Sleep Apnea and Snoring in Children

ELLEN DEUTSCH* and **JAMES S. REILLY***

Jefferson Medical College,
Philadelphia, Pennsylvania, USA

I. Introduction

Snoring is so common among both children and adults that many parents consider it normal. However, snoring is a symptom of turbulent airflow, resulting from varying degrees of upper airway obstruction. The clinical significance of snoring varies widely, ranging from being merely a benign nuisance to being a marker of a disease process with life-threatening complications. When snoring is persistent and a child's parents are concerned, or if the physician suspects clinically significant airway obstruction, a thorough evaluation should be completed.

Some snoring is considered to be "primary snoring," that is, habitual snoring without associated hypoxemia, hypercapnia, sleep disruption, or daytime

*Nemours Childrens Clinics, Alfred I duPont Hospital for Children, Wilmington, Delaware, USA.

symptoms (1). In contrast, snoring may be a symptom of severe chronic hypoventilation, which can result in life-threatening conditions such as cor pulmonale, cardiomegaly, right ventricular hypertrophy, pulmonary hypertension, congestive heart failure, permanent neurologic damage, or even death (1–8). Conditions causing snoring may also result in failure to thrive because of the increased energy expenditure caused by the increased effort of breathing during sleep (1,9,10).

For most children with obstructive sleep disorders, the manifestations are not life-threatening, but still may adversely affect the child's quality of life, behavior, and cognitive capabilities. Obstructive sleep disorders with concomitant chronic sleep deprivation can contribute to inattention, daytime hypersomnolence, deficits in learning, memory, and vocabulary, attention deficit hyperactivity disorders, irritability, hyperactivity, aggressive behavior, discipline problems, and neurobehavioral disturbances (11–15).

In addition, obstructive sleep disorders due to adenotonsillar hypertrophy can contribute to enuresis, short stature, dysphagia, speech disorders and distortions including hyponasality, chronic rhinorrhea, malocclusion, and chronic otitis media with effusion (16–23). Snoring may also cause sleep deprivation and emotional stress for parents, who stay awake at night to cope with their child's sleep disorder (11,16,24).

The challenge to physicians caring for children is to sort out those children who merely snore from those who have clinically significant upper airway obstruction, and to determine appropriate management based on the source and the severity of the problem.

II. Definitions

Obstructive sleep apnea (OSA) is the term reserved for the most serious manifestation of this spectrum of disease. OSA occurs when there is lack of nasal and oral airflow in a sleeping child despite respiratory effort. In children, OSA most commonly results from relative enlargement of the tonsils or adenoids. This can be contrasted with central apnea, occurring more commonly in infants, where there is lack of airflow due to lack of respiratory effort. Although the definition of OSA is simple, the precise criteria are not well established. Various authorities define OSA as cessation of oral-nasal airflow lasting 8, 10, or 15 s, or even just 6 s in younger children with more rapid respiratory rates (25,26). Others monitor the average breath duration, considering obstruction in respiration lasting longer than 2 or $2\frac{1}{2}$ breaths important (1,27). The most inclusive criteria, put forth by Marcus et al. (28) is that an interruption of air movement of any duration, despite continued respiratory effort, is abnormal and interferes with quality sleep.

Airway obstruction without frank apnea also occurs in children. Obstructive sleep hypopnea, or partial airway obstruction without frank apnea, is probably more common in children than true OSA, but may be just as clinically and physiologically significant (29,30). Hypopnea is even more difficult to define and measure objectively than apnea. Hypopnea is generally defined as a decrease in the measured amplitude of oral-nasal airflow of at least 50%, despite maintenance of respiratory effort (27). Children with hypopnea do not have complete cessation of airflow, but do have chronically increased work of breathing because of partial or intermittent airway obstruction.

Both apnea and hypopnea may have similar consequences. The term "obstructive sleep apnea syndrome" (OSAS) is sometimes used to denote the range of manifestations of airway obstruction.

III. Etiologies

The most common curable cause of OSA in children is relative enlargement of the tonsils or adenoids. The size of the tonsils should be assessed relative to the space within the pharynx which contains them (31). Hyperplasia of adenoidal and tonsillar tissue seems to peak at about age 4 years, with a range of age 2–10 years (18,32). This proliferation of lymphoid cells occurs more frequently in the presence of infections, which are also more common within this age group.

The airway obstruction which occurs in OSA is frequently dynamic; therefore, the manifestations may change with body position and during sleep. Obstruction is usually most pronounced when the child is recumbent and sleeping, when the tonsils can prolapse and the surrounding tissues of the pharynx are most compliant (31).

Acute tonsillar enlargement may occur during acute tonsillitis, particularly during viral infections such as infectious mononucleosis caused by Epstein Barr virus. Some improvement in the symptoms of acute enlargement may be obtained with steroids or antibiotics.

OSA probably results from a complex interaction involving both the size of the tonsils and adenoids, and other anatomic, mucosal, and neuromuscular factors which may affect pharyngeal collapsibility. Conditions which may cause or contribute to upper airway obstruction include obesity, craniofacial abnormalities such as micrognathia, midface hypoplasia, macroglossia, choanal atresia or stenosis, nasal foreign body, nasal or antrochoanal polyps, deviated nasal septum, velopharyngeal flap, cleft palate repair, mucopolysaccharidoses, neuromuscular abnormalities including cerebral palsy and hypothyroidism, mucosal abnormalities such as inhalent allergies and allergic rhinitis, and upper respiratory tract infections (11,18,20,25,33–36).

IV. Clinical Evaluation

As clinicians, we work to sharpen our skills in an effort to make an accurate determination of the significance of a child's snoring by carefully evaluating the child's history and physical examination. The literature both supports and refutes the reliability of clinical evaluation in determining the severity of airway obstruction.

Some investigators assert that clinicians are, indeed, able to diagnosis OSA based on parental history and physical examination. Brouillette et al. found that "in a general office practice, a history of frequent snoring and difficulty breathing during sleep or of obstructive apnea observed by the parents strongly suggests that the child has OSA." They devised a mathematical "OSA score," based on parental assessment of difficulty in breathing, apnea, and snoring during sleep, and compared the prediction of OSA with formal polysomnograms. In the absence of confounding factors, such as neurologic disease, high and low scores were predictive of the presence or absence of OSA, respectively, and scores in the middle required further investigation (12). Other authors have confirmed their findings (37).

Other authors refute the assertion that either parents or physicians can accurately predict the presence or severity of upper airway obstruction during sleep, particularly when trying to distinguish between primary snoring and OSA (1,25,38). Several explanations are possible. Parental perceptions of snoring and thresholds for concern are quite variable (1). Some consider snoring to be normal because it is the baseline state of the child or of another family member; some incorrectly ascribe the airway symptoms to constant colds, allergy, or asthma. Demonstrating the sounds of obstruction, snoring, snorting, gasping, or catching up after an obstructive pause in breathing helps parents recognize these manifestations in their children.

In addition, the perceptions and thresholds of physicians are variable, as are their opportunities for observation. The circumstances of typical examinations by physicians involve factors which may contribute to underestimating the severity of an upper airway problem in a child. First, physicians most often examine children while the children are awake, frequently in an office setting. Under these circumstances, the child may not manifest the severity of symptoms which occur during sleep. Second, as examinations are often intermittent, physicians may not appreciate the chronicity of the child's symptoms. The frequency and chronicity of nasal obstruction and rhinorrhea are factors which should be considered in making treatment decisions.

V. Laboratory Evaluation

Additional data may aid in assessing the etiology and severity of airway obstruction.

Lateral neck radiographs are frequently used to evaluate the relative size of the adenoids, and have been shown to demonstrate reasonable correlation with intraoperative findings (39). They are relatively easily available, and are usually well tolerated by children. However, they are limited by being static studies. In selected, complex children, sleep videofluoroscopy may reveal dynamic airway collapse not observed on static radiographs (18,29,40).

Fiberoptic nasopharyngoscopy employs a fiberoptic telescope passed through the nose to view the adenoids in the choanae, and may provide a dynamic view of the adenoids in the nasopharynx. With the newer, thinner naso-pharyngoscopes, this study is well tolerated by many children. However, this examination is stressful for some children, and is difficult to accomplish in an uncooperative child.

Tape recordings of snoring are occasionally advocated, but there is limited documentation of their validity (27). Typically, 2–10 min of the tapes are subjec-tively evaluated for episodes of obstruction and quality of snoring. Sampling error is possible.

Sonography consists of computer analysis of recorded sleep sounds. Although it has been validated, it is not commonly used (37,41).

"Sleep studies," pneumograms, and polysomnograms are the most defini-tive methods for documenting OSA. At a minimum, the following four parameters must be included: (1) nasal or oral airflow, usually measured by thermistor; (2) chest wall motion, usually measured by plethysmography; (3) oxygen saturation (SaO_2), usually measured by pulse oximetry; and (4) heart rate. Episodes of partial or total lack of airflow, oxygen desaturation, and bradycardia are assessed. Precise criteria are not standardized. More sophisticated polysomnograms may include end-tidal CO_2, electroencephalogram, electro-oculograms, and electromyograms for assessment of sleep stage and arousals, infrared video observation, and esopha-geal pressure measurements. An esophageal pH probe may be included to evaluate gastroesophageal reflux (15,26,28,42).

Overnight studies are expensive, so shorter "nap" studies are sometimes obtained. In the study by Marcus et al., nap polysomnograms which were positive for sleep-disordered breathing were confirmed by overnight polysomnography. However, some children had negative nap studies with positive overnight studies, indicating that nap polysomnography underestimated abnormalities detected by overnight polysomnography (28).

Although nocturnal polysomnography has been considered the gold refer-ence standard of diagnosis of OSAS in adults, a negative polysomnogram by con-ventional criteria may not fully exclude an obstructive sleep disorder in children (27,43). Most children with serious sleep-related upper airway obstruction have chronically increased upper airway resistance during sleep but do not have repeti-tive complete obstructive apneas (43). The manifestations of partial upper airway obstruction lie in a continuum between primary snoring and OSAS (1). Several authors assert the concept of an upper airway resistance syndrome (UARS). Chil-dren with UARS have snoring with increased upper airway resistance during sleep and exhibit the same symptoms as OSAS, such as restlessness, behavioral problems, poor school performance, and excessive daytime somnolence, but do not have classically defined apneas or hypopneas or significant drops in blood oxygen levels. Rather they have continuous partial obstructive hypoventilation characterized by increased respiratory effort followed by arousal, cyclic decreases in SaO_2, hypercarbia, labored paradoxical respiratory efforts, sleep fragmentation, and snoring (1,29,42,43). For children who are affected, the increased airway resistance may be compensated for by increased respiratory effort during non-rapid eye movement sleep, which allows for the maintenance of appropriate minute ventilation (42).

VI. Management

Adenotonsillectomy is a well-established and effective treatment for children who have OSAS or UARS due to enlargement of the tonsils or adenoids. Most of the complications of OSAS improve or resolve after tonsillectomy or adenoidectomy (2–5,7,9,11,13,19,23,29,44–46). The procedure is usually performed under general anesthesia, often on an outpatient basis. Children usually experience throat pain for 3–7 days after surgery, adolescents often have discomfort for up to 2 weeks. Throat pain, time to recovery, and risk of postoperative hemorrhage is greater after tonsillectomy than after adenoidectomy alone.

Although there is a traditional reluctance to perform adenotonsillectomy in children under 3 years of age, the decision to perform tonsillectomy should be made without regard to the age of the patient, provided that the surgery is carried out for appropriate indications and is performed in an appropriate institution (47). In the group of 22 children reported by Brouillette et al. (29) 21 patients were <3 years old when their breathing difficulties began, and delays in referrals averaged 23 ± 15 months.

Other surgical options include tracheotomy and uvulopalatopharyngoplasty (UPPP). Tracheotomy is curative, but is usually reserved for children with additional neuromuscular or anatomic abnormalities. Maintaining a child with a tracheotomy entails significant medical, economic, and social morbidity, so it should be avoided if other options can be effective. UPPP is performed more often in adults than in children, and is generally more effective for snoring than for apnea (11). Mandibular advancement and hyoid resuspension (11) and advancement of the base of the tongue are not commonly performed.

The most common medical management of OSA is to supplement inspiratory nasal airflow with continuous positive airway pressure (CPAP) or bilevel positive airway pressure (BiPAP). The airflow may act as a pneumatic splint (48). CPAP may be useful for patients with OSAS without adenotonsillar hypertrophy, patients with an inadequate response to adenotonsillectomy, or patients who would prefer to avoid surgery (11). For some patients, such as those with craniofacial abnormalities, proper mask fit for BiPAP cannot be accomplished. An external nasal dilator has been shown to reduce the frequency of obstructive respiratory events in infants (49).

Respiratory stimulants have limited success in adults and are rarely indicated in children (11). Oxygen supplementation alone is usually inadequate (11). Weight loss is important for obese children, but is difficult and slow to accomplish.

VII. Summary

Snoring is a common condition in both children and adults. Its significance varies from being a benign nuisance to being a marker of a life-threatening disease process. For most children with obstructive sleep disorders, the manifestations are not life-threatening, but still may adversely affect the child's quality of life, behavior, and cognitive capabilities. Chronic increased airway resistance, with partial or intermittent airway obstruction, is probably more common in children than frank apnea. The obstruction is usually most pronounced when the child is recumbent and sleeping.

The most common curable cause of obstructive sleep disorders in children is relative enlargement of the tonsils or adenoids. Adenotonsillectomy is a well-established and effective treatment for these children. In some children, additional anatomic, mucosal, and neuromuscular conditions may contribute to fixed anatomical obstruction or dynamic pharyngeal collapsibility.

Clinical evaluation is an important part of assessing the severity of airway obstruction; however, the literature both supports and refutes the accuracy of clinical examination. Additional diagnostic data may be obtained from lateral neck radiographs, fiberoptic nasopharyngoscopy, and "sleep studies," in selected patients. A negative polysomnogram by conventional criteria may not identify children with serious sleep-related upper airway obstruction who have chronically increased upper airway resistance during sleep but do not have repetitive complete obstruction.

It is hoped that understanding the symptoms and the dynamic nature of the process of upper airway obstruction during sleep will help clinicians to continue to sharpen their diagnostic skills.

References

1. Carroll JL, McColley SA, Marcus CL et al. Inability of clinical history to distinguish primary snoring from obstructive sleep apnea syndrome in children. Chest 1995; 108:610.
2. Levy AM, Tabakin BS, Hanson JS et al. Hypertrophied adenoids causing pulmonary hypertension and severe congestive heart failure. N Engl J Med 1967; 277:506.
3. Lind MG, Lundell BPW. Tonsillar hyperplasia in children. A cause of obstructive sleep apneas, CO_2 retention, and retarded growth. Arch Otolaryngol 1982; 108:650.
4. Macartney FJ, Panday J, Scott O. Cor pulmonale as a result of chronic naso-pharyngeal obstruction due to hypertrophied tonsils and adenoids. Arch Dis Child 1969; 44:585.
5. Noonan J. Reversible cor pulmonale due to hypertrophied tonsils and adenoids. Studies in two cases (abstract). Circulation 1965; 32:164.
6. Sie KCY, Perkins JA, Clarke WR. Acute right heart failure due to adenotonsillar hypertrophy. Int J Pediatr Otorhinolaryngol 1997; 41:53.

7. Sofer S, Weinhouse E, Tal A et al. Cor pulmonale due to adenoidal or tonsillar hypertrophy or both in children. Chest 1988; 93:119.

8. Wilkinson AR, McCormick MS, Freeland AP et al. Electrocardiographic signs of pulmonary hypertension in children who snore. Br Med J 1981; 282:1579.

9. Everett AD, Koch WC, Saulsbury FT. Failure to thrive due to obstructive sleep apnea. Clin Pediatr 1987; 26:90.

10. Marcus CL, Carroll JL, Koerner CB et al. Determinants of growth in children with the obstructive sleep apnea syndrome. J Pediatr 1994; 125:556.

11. Brooks LJ. Sleep-disordered breathing in children. Respir Care 1998; 43:394.

12. Brouillette RT, Hanson D, David et al. A diagnostic approach to suspected obstructive sleep apnea in children. J Pediatr 1984; 105:10.

13. Chervin RD, Dillon JE, Bassetti C et al. Symptoms of sleep disorders, inattention, and hyperactivity in children. Sleep 1997; 20:1185–1192.

14. Mangat D, Orr WC, Smith RO. Sleep apnea, hypersomnolence, and upper airway obstruction secondary to adenotonsillar enlargement. Arch Otolaryngol 1977; 103:383.

15. Rhodes SK, Shimoda KC, Waid LR et al. Neurocognitive deficits in morbidly obese children with obstructive sleep apnea. J Pediatr 1995; 127:741.

16. Ahlqvist-Rastad J, Hultcrantz E, Svanholm H. Children with tonsillar obstruction. Indications for and efficacy of tonsillectomy. Acta Paediatr Scand 1988; 77:831.

17. Bate TWP, Price DA, Holme CA et al. Short stature caused by obstructive sleep apnoea during sleep. Arch Dis Child 1984; 59(1):78.

18. Brodsky L. Modern assessment of tonsils and adenoids. Pediatr Clin North Am 1989; 36:1551.

19. Hultcrantz E, Larson M, Hellquist R et al. The influence of tonsillar obstruction and tonsillectomy on facial growth and dental arch morphology. Int J Pediatr Otorhinolaryngol 1991; 22:125.

20. Hunt CE, Brouillette RT. Disorders of breathing during sleep. In: Chernick V, Kendig EL, eds. Kendig's Disorders of the Respiratory Tract in Children. WB Saunders Company, 1990:1004–1015.

21. Maw AR. Chronic otitis media with effusion (glue ear) and adenotonsillectomy. Prospective randomised controlled study. Br Med J 1983; 287:1586.

22. American Academy of Pediatrics. Tonsils and Adenoids: Guidelines for Parents. American Academy of Pediatrics, 1994.

23. Weider DJ, Sateia MJ, West RP. Nocturnal enuresis in children with upper airway obstruction. Otolaryngol Head Neck Surg 1991; 105:427.

24. Deutsch ES, Isaacson GC. Tonsils and adenoids: an update. Pediatr Rev 1995; 16:17.

25. Brooks LJ, Stephens BM, Bacevice AM. Adenoid size is related to severity but not the number of episodes of obstructive apnea in children. J Pediatr 1998; 132:682.

26. Frank Y, Kravath RE, Pollak CP et al. Obstructive sleep apnea and its therapy. Clinical and polysomnographic manifestations. Pediatrics 1983; 71:737.

27. Goldstein NA, Sculerati N, Walsleben JA et al. Clinical diagnosis of pediatric obstructive sleep apnea validated by polymnography. Otolaryngol Head Neck Surg 1994; 111:611.

28. Marcus CL, Keens TG, Bautista DB et al. Obstructive sleep apnea in children with Down syndrome. Pediatrics 1991; 88:132.

29. Brouillette RT, Fernbach SK, Hunt CE. Obstructive sleep apnea in infants and children. J Pediatr 1982; 100:31.

30. Mauer KW, Staats BA, Olsen KD. Upper airway obstruction and disordered nocturnal breathing in children. Mayo Clin Proc 1983; 58:349.
31. Bluestone CD. Current indications for tonsillectomy and adenoidectomy. Ann Otol Rhinol Laryngol 1992; 101:58.
32. Bicknell PG. Role of adenotonsillectomy in the management of pediatric ear, nose and throat infections. Pediatr Infect Dis J 1994; 13:S75.
33. Marcus CL, Keens TG, Davidson Ward SL. Comparison of nap and overnight polysomnography in children. Pediatr Pulmonol 1992; 13:16.
34. McColley SA, Carroll JL, Curtis S et al. High prevalence of allergic sensitization in children with habitual snoring and obstructive sleep apnea. Chest 1997; 111:170.
35. Potsic WP. Obstructive sleep apnea. Pediatr Clin North Am 1989; 36:1435.
36. Rodgers GK, Chan KH, Dahl RE. Antral choanal polyp presenting as obstructive sleep apnea syndrome. Arch Otolaryngol Head Neck Surg 1991; 117:914.
37. Bobin S, Attal P, Trang H et al. Childhood obstructive sleep apnea: diagnostic methods. Pediatr Pulmonol 1997; (suppl 16):289.
38. Suen JS, Arnold JE, Brooks LJ. Adenotonsillectomy for treatment of obstructive sleep apnea in children. Arch Otolaryngol Head Neck Surg 1995; 121:525.
39. Cohen LM, Koltai PJ, Scott JR. Lateral cervical radiographs and adenoid size: do they correlate? ENT J 1992; 71:638.
40. Felman AH, Loughlin GM, Leftridge CA et al. Upper airway obstruction during sleep in children. AJR AM J Roentgend 1979; 133:213.
41. Potsic WP. Comparison of polysomnography and sonography for assessing regularity of respiration during sleep in adenotonsillar hypertrophy. Laryngoscope 1987; 97:1430.
42. Guilleminault C, Pelayo R, Leger D et al. Recognition of sleep-disordered breathing in children. Pediatrics 1996; 98:871.
43. Rosen CL, D'Andrea L, Haddad GG. Adult criteria for obstructive sleep apnea do not identify children with serious obstruction. Am Rev Respir Dis 1992; 146:1231.
44. Guilleminault C, Winkle R, Korobkin R et al. Children and nocturnal snoring. Evaluation of the effects of sleep related respiratory resistive load and daytime functioning. Eur J Pediatr 1982; 139:165.
45. Potsic WP, Pasquariello PS, Baranak CC et al. Relief of upper airway obstruction by adenotonsillectomy. Otolaryngol Head Neck Surg 1986; 94:476.
46. Williams III EF, Woo P, Miller R et al. The effects of adenotonsillectomy on growth in young children. Otolaryngol Head Neck Surg 1991; 104:509.
47. Berkowitz RG, Zalzal GH. Tonsillectomy in children under 3 years of age. Arch Otolaryngol Head Neck Surg 1990; 116:685.
48. Strohl KP, Redline S. Nasal CPAP therapy, upper airway muscle activation, and obstructive sleep apnea. Am Rev Respir Dis 1986; 134:555.
49. Scharf MB, Berkowitz DV, McDannold MD et al. Effects of an external nasal dilator on sleep and breathing patterns in newborn infants with and without congestion. J Pediatr 1996; 129:804.

D. Surgery

32

Choanal Atresia

FRANS GORDTS and PETER A. R. CLEMENT

Free University of Brussels
Brussels, Belgium

I. Introduction

The abundant literature dealing with choanal atresia contrasts with the rather low incidence of this pathology. Since the first description by Johann Roederer in 1755 and the first documented operation by Emmerett in 1854, more than 350 papers have been published dealing with the various aspects of this entity (1).

Nevertheless, congenital choanal atresia remains a challenging clinical problem. Neonates are predominantly obligate nasal breathers and bilateral choanal atresia therefore requires prompt diagnosis and appropriate intervention in order to avoid severe hypoxia.

II. Nasal vs. Oral Breathing

The infant larynx is situated considerably higher in the neck than in adults. The superior border of the larynx is located as high as the first cervical vertebra. This superior location helps to explain obligate nasal breathing. On inspiration, the cartilaginous tip of the epiglottis touches the posterior edge of the soft palate forming a veloepiglottic sphincter favoring nasal and impeding oral breathing. On swallowing, the airway is protected as the epiglottis falls back (2).

In theory, this obligate nasal breathing lasts for the first 9 months of life (3), while mouth breathing, a learned response by neonates, starts developing progressively 4–6 weeks after birth (4).

However, this axiomatic theory of "obligatory" nose breathing is challenged by the survival of infants born with bilateral choanal atresia or pyriform aperture stenosis. An amazing example of a child who reached the age of 4 years before the diagnosis of bilateral choanal atresia was established has previously been documented (5).

The most important anatomical parameter that facilitates the switch from nasal to oral ventilation in human infants is a cervical extension, creating a lordosis of the neck that results in an opening of the veloglossal and veloepiglottic sphincters (6).

Therefore, oral respiration evident prior to 2 months of age should give rise to the suspicion of bilateral nasal obstruction (7). Moreover, children born with bilateral atresia can be trained to breathe through the mouth with the aid of indwelling oral appliances discussed hereafter (8). However, it is well established that infants with unrepaired bilateral choanal atresia may suddenly die due to an inadequate oral airway (8). In the long term, persistent mouth breathing is supposed to create another—obviously less urgent—problem: facial maldevelopment might result in the long-face or adenoid facies syndrome. Some reports suggest, however, that children with choanal atresia do not exhibit long-face syndrome (9) and that the growth of their sinuses is independent of nasal ventilation (10).

III. Epidemiology and Associated Anomalies

The epidemiology of choanal atresia is not always clear. Fortunately, it is a relatively rare malformation having an incidence of between 1 in 5000 and 1 in 8000 live births (8). Recent data (11) based on more than 5 million births suggest an even lower average rate of 0.82 per 10,000 births. Depending on the source consulted, there is a twice as high (8) to nonexisting (11) female-to-male preponderance. No statistically significant difference between races is observed, even though white infants have a higher rate than those of other races (11).

Choanal atresia is very often associated with other congenital anomalies. In a series with 50 children, up to 72% presented such associated pathologies. Thirty per cent of these patients had the CHARGE association (see later), 26% had other multiple major anomalies, and 16% had a single anomaly (12).

In another study that included 444 infants with choanal atresia, chromosome anomalies were found in 6% of the children, and 5% had monogenic syndromes or conditions (11). Associated malformations were present in 47% of the infants without chromosome anomalies (11).

The mnemonic "CHARGE" was suggested (13) for the first time in 1981 to describe associated anomalies in patients with either choanal atresia or ocular coloboma: C—coloboma, H—heart disease, A—atresia choanae, R—retarded growth and retarded development and/or CNS anomalies, G—genital hypoplasia, and E—ear anomalies and/or deafness. Later reports recommend limiting the use of the CHARGE acronym to cases where malformations are present in at least four of the six categories (14). A recent paper (11) warns that only a small proportion of infants with choanal atresia and other elements of the CHARGE complex truly represent this entity. These authors state that the term CHARGE association is overused in clinical practice. They restrict the use of the acrocrym to infants with choanal atresia and/or coloboma combined with at least three cardinal malformations (heart, ear, and genital), while growth retardation should not be used in the definition.

Other associated congenital malformations are numerous and can affect nearly every part of the child's body. Table 32.1 lists some of the possible defects. Only a few papers provide either clear and concise tables (15) with figures derived from literature surveys or personal series (12,13).

IV. Classification and Anatomy

Choanal "atresia" consists of complete congenital blockage between the nasal cavity and the nasopharynx while choanal "stenosis" refers to an incomplete blockage. About 65% to 75% of choanal atresias are unilateral (8) and, according to at least one study (12) with a predominance on the right side (66%). A more recent paper (11) has not shown an obvious predilection for either the right or the left side. Traditionally, choanal atresia has been described as 90% bony and 10% membranous, but a recent review (16) failed to demonstrate purely membranous atresias: on computed tomography scans (CT), 71% of the atresias were mixed bony–membranous and 29% pure bony. Therefore, a new classification with the inclusion of bony, mixed, and membranous atresias is suggested (16).

The "anatomy" of a typical choanal atresia reveals narrowing of the posterior nasal cavity due to a medial displacement of the pterygoid plate and thickening of the (posterior) vomer together with the actual (bony more

Table 32.1 Anomalies Associated with Choanal Atresia

Skull
  Microcephaly
  Craniosynostosis
CNS
  Micro-, hydrocephalus
  Meningo-(encephalo)cele
  Facial palsy
Ophtalmologic
  Microphtalmia
  Coloboma
  Hypoplastic orbit
  Ptosis
Otic
  Pinna anomalies
  Meatal atresia
  Ossicular and cochleovestibular anomalies
Nasal
  Absent septum
  Nasolacrimal defects
Oropharyngeal
  Macroglossia
  Cleft palate
Larynx
  Web
  Subglottic stenosis
Cardiac
  Patent ductus arteriosus
  Fallot's tetralogy
  Wolf–Parkinson–White syndrome
Gastrointestinal
  Tracheo-oesophageal fistula
  Pyloric stenosis
  Imperforate anus
Genitourinary
  Genital defects in males
  Upper urinary tract anomalies
Skeletal
  Polydactyly
  Anomalous ribs
  Short neck
  Congenital dislocation of the hip
Syndromes
  Acrocephalosyndactyly (Apert's syndrome)
  Mandibulofacial dysostotis (Treacher Collins syndrome)
  Craniofacial dystosis (Crouzon's syndrome)

frequently than membranous) obstruction (17) and elevation of the posterior nasal floor. Choanal orifices normally measure (from the lateral wall of the nasal caviy to the vomer) greater than 0.67 cm at birth and 0.70 cm under 2 years, while the vomer width does not exceed 0.23 cm in children less than 8 years of age (18). Normal choanae enlarge at a rate of 0.208 mm/year (19).

V. Signs and Symptoms

Symptomatology is obviously quite different depending on whether the choanal atresia is uni- or bilateral. Unilateral atresia may go unrecognized until adulthood and even then the pathology can mimic septal deviation (the septum does usually deviate to the affected side) unless posterior rhinoscopy or endonasal endoscopy reveals atresia. However, persistent unilateral rhinorrhea in children should arouse suspicion of either a corpus alienum or a unilateral atresia. Moreover, when occlusion of the normal side by acquired disease produces symptoms, the diagnosis may be sought at an earlier age. In one series (12), diagnosis of unilateral atresia was made on average at 18 months.

Bilateral atresia in newborns presents as acute respiratory distress. The severity and duration of the unattended distress may vary according to the adaptability of the neonate in acquiring oral respiration, which again is related to the degree of neurologic development and maturity (20). Typically, bilateral choanal atresia causes "cyclic" cyanosis relieved by crying (unlike cyanosis of laryngeal origin, which is usually aggravated by crying). The cycle starts with vigorous efforts by the infants to breathe. The whole length of a neonate's tongue is in apposition to the hard and soft palates, creating a vacuum. The greater the effort to breathe, the more tightly the mouth appears to close, the chest retracts, and cyanosis develops. When crying ensues, the cycle is broken.

VI. Diagnosis

For children born in a hospital, a catheter is usually passed through each nostril into the nasopharynx as part of the standard newborn examination.

If any probe with a diameter of 2–3 mm can be inserted more than 44 mm from the ostium externum of the nose, the pharyngeal wall is reached, demonstrating a free passage (21). When the catheter fails to pass into the oropharynx, choanal atresia is probable. However, misdirection or coiling of a flexible catheter can lead to an erroneous diagnosis of choanal atresia. Furthermore, this traditional clinical test provides little information about the nature, position, or thickness of the atretic plate. Therefore, high-resolution computed tomography (CT) not only confirms the diagnosis, but also gives anatomic information that ultimately can influence the choice of surgical repair. The advantages of CT in the radiographic evaluation of choanal atresia are numerous (22): contrast medium is unnecessary, thus avoiding the risk of aspiration. High-resolution

CT provides accurate vizualization of the narrowing of the pterygoid plates at the choanae. The thickness and shape of the vomer deformity is well visualized and CT clearly demonstrates whether the atresia is bony or membranous. The thickness of the atretic plate and depth from the nasal sill can be accurately measured. In addition, CT visualizes whether the nasopharynx is patent. CT is, however, not immune from pitfalls: among 22 patients that underwent preoperative axial CT, seven scans were misleading regarding the type of atresia (12). In one case the CT scan was consistent with a meningoencephalocoele, but at operation the only abnormality was a unilateral bony choanal atresia (12). In another case with bilateral bony choanal atresia in a child, CT showed mucoid nasal secretions (with an attenuation resembling brain parenchyma) adjacent to a radiolucent cribiform plate. The preoperative diagnosis of nasopharyngeal encephalocele resulted in surgical exploration where the not yet ossified cribiform plate was found to be intact (23).

Therefore, a proper CT should be obtained according to the following guidelines:

> Thin-cut axial scans should parallel the posterior hard palate at the level of the pterygoid plates (18) or the infraorbitomeatal line (5).
>
> In order not to confound ordinary snot with brain tissue (12,23) it is of the utmost importance to have the nose properly suctioned prior to the examination (Fig. 32.1).
>
> Furthermore, the accuracy of CT is optimized by application and subsequent aspiration of an age-appropriate topical decongestant to the nasal cavity prior to the actual (12,18) scanning.

(Para)sagittal reconstruction not only defines the vertical height and thickness of the atretic plate (22) but also helps to avoid an inadvertent passage ("false route") into the clivus by vizualization of the slope of the palate.

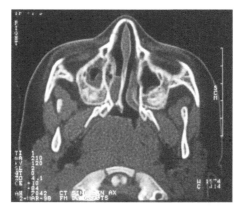

Figure 32.1 Accumulation of nasal secretions anterior to the atresia hampers an accurate interpretation of the choanal anatomy.

When available, three-dimensional reconstruction allows identification of associated craniofacial anomalies, and is useful in computer-assisted surgery (22). Frequently, a combination of these associated anomalies constitute the CHARGE complex. In suspected CHARGE cases, CT or MRI scanning of the temporal bone is very helpful to the ENT surgeon to visualize abnormalities of the inner ear (aplasia of the semicircular canals, dysplastic cochlea, etc.) or middle ear (absence of oval window, stapedius muscle, abnormalities of incus and stapes, etc.) (24,25).

In the differential diagnosis of choanal atresia, both common and very rare pathologies have to be considered: adenoid hypertrophy, nasal mucosal congestion (12), hypertrophy of the inferior turbinate (22), choanal stenosis (12), congenital syphilis (7), congenital nasal pyriform aperture stenosis, congenital nasolacrimal duct cysts (26). Some authors (7) group these pathologies together and term them as nasal obstruction without choanal atresia (NOWCA). Finally, other masses or abnormalities within the nose such as gliomas, dermoids or encephaloceles have to be excluded (27).

VII. Management

Unilateral choanal atresia is seldom urgent. Surgery can be delayed for at least 1 year. Meanwhile, the operative site can be expected to enlarge to approximately twice the size of that of a newborn (8). Definite therapy can be carried out at any time during childhood, usually before the patient starts school, to stop rhinorrhea (4). The best results are obtained in children of 3 years or older (28).

Even bilateral choanal atresia is not a surgical emergency (29). There should nevertheless be immediate concern for the airway: the infant can be stimulated to cry and a finger can be inserted into the mouth until an airway is established (8). Tracheotomy is rarely necessary, if no other anomalies exist. However, in the presence of Crouzon's or Apert's disease and Treacher Collins syndrome, the likelihood of a tracheotomy becomes much higher (30). Endotracheal intubation usually is unnecessary unless the infant requires mechanical ventilation (8). A plastic anesthesia oropharyngeal airway (for instance a Güdel-canula), like the insertion of a finger into the mouth, pushes the tongue downward and prevents thereby apposition with the soft palate (31). However, the infant cannot feed through this. A McGovern nipple (32) serves the same purpose and can be used for gavage feeding. A McGovern nipple is an ordinary, large nipple with the end cut off (or a nipple with two additional lateral holes). This nipple allows an infant to mouth breathe between swallows while feeding. It is secured either with large tapes to the face (12) or with the ribbons of a surgeon's mask tied around the suboccipital area (8). With this method, definitive management is delayed to allow time for a complete workup to rule out other anomalies (8). Some authors (29) use the rule of 10 to optimize the timing of surgical repair (10 lb, 10 g of haemoglobin, 10 weeks of age) and prefer to wait until the infant has acquired mouth breathing; this adds an additional safety factor in case stent obstruction occurs during the postoperative period. Other surgeons (33) choose to operate as soon as possible because (1) the atretic plate offers little resistance in the neonate, (2) nasal breathing allows normal facial resistance in the neonate, (3) a nasal stent is well tolerated in the neonate, and (4) total hospital time is shortened.

Various means of surgical correction have been proposed in the past. The number of procedures available is evidence that no one type of repair provides for every case complete success without complications. No single controlled series has statistically established the superiority of one technique over another (34).

Although many methods are described, the key points are removal and shortening of the posterior bony septum and removal of the superolateral nasal wall and lateral pterygoid plate (8). Preservation of mucosal flaps for relining the lumen is claimed to be important too, but some authors (16) do not try to create these flaps as they are very difficult to retain during a drill-out procedure and probably do not survive during stenting.

Two very effective surgical techniques have little or no indication in infants and younger children due to their potential for damaging the developing facio-maxillary skeleton (35): the transantral and transseptal approaches. The former is helpful in opening the posterior choana into a common cavity with a maxillary sinus to prevent restenosis in cases of recurrent stenosis. The latter has been advocated in older patients with unilateral atresia (36,37) while, however, the sublabial variant is claimed to be suitable for infants (38).

Today the transpalatal and transnasal approaches are undoubtedly the two most common procedures to correct choanal atresia. In the past, the transnasal approach has been stigmatized by the risk of complications with a blind technique (34) while the transpalatal approach has been touted for its greater visibility. The better visualization and hence ease of surgical exposure together with short-term stenting and good postoperative results make the transpalatal approach still a popular technique. However, risk of injury to the greater palatine neurovascular bundle, greater blood loss, longer operative time, problems with postoperative oral intake, and risk of palatal fistulization have all to be taken into account (39). Most of all, destruction of the posterior two-thirds of the median palatal suture has been shown to reduce the transversal maxillary growth (40). A cross-bite frequency has been observed in up to 52% of 51 patients operated by the transpalatal approach (41). Since the essential spurt in growth of the hard palate is within the 5 first years of life (42), transpalatal surgery should be reserved for the elective management of unilateral choanal atresia, which permits postponement of surgery. The transpalatal approach is also suitable for third-time surgery or other revision surgery (8). For all these reasons, the last decades have witnessed a gradual shift of interest in favor of the transnasal approach. Once described as a blind technique prone to very serious compli-cations (see later), the endoscopic endonasal approach has evolved into a simple, safe, and reliable procedure that can be employed in the management of bilateral choanal atresia even in the newborn (43). The introduction of the operating microscope, otologic microdrill, endoscopes, microinstruments, and back-biting forceps all have significantly contributed to this positive development. According to Morgan and Bailey (12) and Reddy et al. (43), Dehaen and Clement (21) were probably one of the first to combine a 110° endoscope to inspect the nasopharynx while the atresia is being visualized transnasally with the operating microscope. By means of a microneedle on a curved shaft, the atretic plate is perforated and enlarged with an otologic microdrill. The thinnest portion of the atresia is generally at the junction of the plate, hard palate, and vomer (21,27). A more recent milestone in the transnasal treatment of choanal atresia is the use of endoscopes. Stankiewicz (44) is credited with the application of endoscopic technology, which has greatly improved visualization for this procedure. The ideal patient for a transnasal approach has thin or membranous (very rare!) choanal atresia with good access through both nasal airways (45). This transnasal approach, seemingly the most logical way for choanal atresia correction, has some general shortcomings of endoscopy: no binocular vision, fogging of light, one hand not free for surgery (43). Furthermore, the space available for manipulation of instruments in the nasal cavities is small, especially in cases of bilateral choanal atresia in the newborn (43). Craniofacial anomalies, severe turbinate hypertrophy, and deviations of the septum are poor candidates for endoscopic repair. Also, if the atretic plate is very thick (by CT) it is advisable to use the transpalatal route (43).

For the near future microdebrider/suction drill technology (34) for rapid removal of bony tissue and new laser innovations like the holmium:yttrium–aluminium–garnet (Ho:YAG) laser (46), capable of bone ablation, may be advantageous in the transnasal repair of choanal atresia.

VIII. Stenting and Postoperative Care

Postoperative stenting is the subject of differences of opinion. Stents can serve as a nidus for infections, and there is a question as to whether this foreign body may contribute to choanal restenosis, much as an endotracheal tube may cause subglottic stenosis (16). Some authors do not use stents after transnasal CO_2-laser vaporization or after combined transseptal/transnasal procedures in older children and adults ("Endonasal Surgery of Choanal Atresia," H. Rudert, personal communication, E.R.S. and I.S.I.A.N. Meeting, July 28–Aug 1, 1998, Vienna, Austria). In cases of revision surgery with the microdebrider/suction drill, stenting is sometimes omitted in adult patients (34). However, in spite of a great variability in the materials used, the relative size or method of placing/securing the stent, many authors advise postoperative stenting. The duration of stenting is individualized, but the stent should be left in place until the operated choana is mucosalized, which takes about 4–6 weeks (16).

After surgery, the infants should be maintained for several days in the neonatal intensive care unit. Patients may be discharged (on an apnea monitor) when there is no further respiratory distress and when the parents are able to suction and care for the stents. Most studies advise broad-spectrum antibiotics for the entire time of stenting. Since prolonged use of antibiotics may occasionally cause the growth of resistant strains of microorganisms, some authors limit the use of antibiotics to episodes of purulent rhinitis (27). When adequate local care (frequent aspiration and cleaning) is available, antibiotic therapy is not necessary. The use of antireflux drugs (47) or topical corticosteroids after removal of the stents (12,27,45) is optional. Following stent removal, probably under general anesthesia, which allows for removal of any granulation tissue, the child is frequently checked for airway problems.

IX. Complications

Some complications are probably historical and related to the blind, transnasal puncture, a procedure no longer performed: creation of a "false route" to the anterior fossa or slipping of an instrument with serious lesions between atlas and occipital bone, CFS leaks, midbrain trauma, Gradenigo syndrome (4). Palatal fistulization or occurrence of a submucosal tunnel are two of the other possible intraoperative complications (12). Postoperative complications are often related to the stenting: airway obstruction and respiratory distress due to plugging of nasal stents, inadvertent dislocation of the stents, pressure necrosis with alar or columellar ulceration, and septal erosion.

X. Results

As for the nearly impossible task of comparing the results of such diverse surgical options in such a rare pathology, the interested reader is referred to the publications of Pirsig (42), Morgan and Bailey (12), and Vickery and Gross (34) or to the most recent and largest reported study of choanal atresia to date ("Management and Outcome of Choanal Atresia Correction," N.R. Friedman et al., personal communication, 7th International Congress of Pediatric Otorhinolaryngology, Jun 7–10, 1998, Helsinki, Finland).

XI. Personal Series

Between 1979 and 1999, seven cases of choanal atresia were diagnosed and treated at our institution (Table 32.2). In contrast with data from some reports (11), the majority of our patients were female. Otherwise in accordance with the literature, atresias were more often uni- than bilateral (17), with the right

Table 32.2 Summary of Clinical Records of Choanal Atresia Patients

No.	Sex	Type atresia	Associated anomalies	Age at surgery elsewhere	Age at surgery	Type of surgery	Revision surgery		Length follow-up	Outcome
							Age	Type		
1	F	B	Polydactylia Daughter of No. 2		9 weeks	TND	3 years	TND	7.5 years	OK
2	F	R	Mother of No. 1	4 years	29 years	TS	7 years	TS	4 years	OK
3	F	L			11 years	TS			17 months	OK
4	M	B	CHARGE complex	4 days	10 months	TND	5 years	TND	6 years	OK
5	F	B	Treacher Collins syndrome		3 weeks	TND	1 year	Elsewhere	9 years	OK
6	F	R			2.5 years	TND	Awaits	Revision surgery	13 months	Obliteration
7	M	L	Down syndrome							

Note: F, female; M, male; B, bilateral; R, unilateral right; L, unilateral left; TND, transnasal drill-out; TS, transseptal.

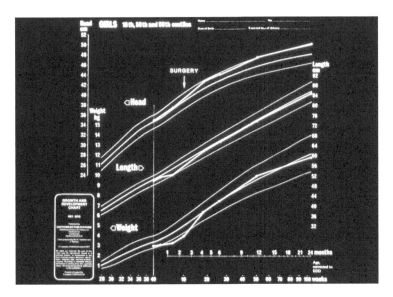

Figure 32.2 Growth chart: growth improvement after surgery is evident.

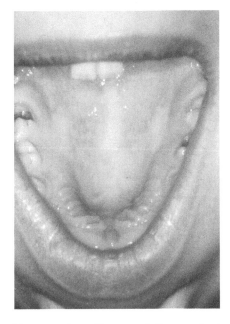

Figure 32.3 Normal transversal maxillary growth 7 years after transnasal correction of bilateral choanal atresia.

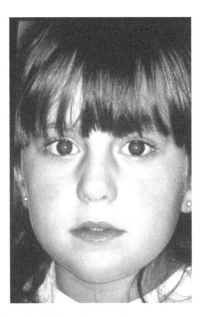

Figure 32.4 Harmonious facial development 7 years postoperatively.

side being as frequently affected as the left side (11) and without a single purely membranous atresia (16).

Only in two out of our seven patients did choanal atresia present as a solitary finding. Of particular interest is the first case with bilateral choanal atresia in

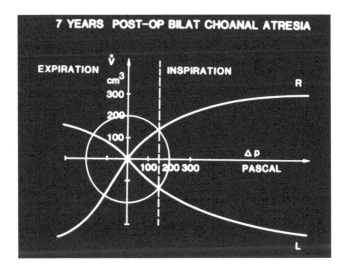

Figure 32.5 Active anterior rhinomanometry.

whom a peculiar hereditary trend was noted. As an associated anomaly, this girl presented with polydactylia, a feature also noted in her paternal grandmother. Furthermore, the girl's own mother (case 2) had a unilateral choanal atresia. At the age of 5 weeks, the daughter had learned to breathe by mouth but because of failure to thrive, due to extreme feeding difficulties and persisting signs of respiratory distress, it was decided to operate her at the age of 9 weeks. The growth improvement after surgery was evident (Fig. 32.2).

Both mother and daughter are representative of the long-term repercussion of choanal atresia and its management on facial and palatal growth. More than 7 years after transnasal correction of the bilateral atresia, the child's palate and face (Figs. 32.3 and 32.4) have harmonious proportions while the functional results (Fig. 32.5) are very satisfactory. In the mother, definitive correction of unilateral choanal atresia was only performed at the age of 29 years.

Nevertheless, and as reported before (9,10) no obvious facial maldevelopment was noted (Figs. 32.6 and 32.7).

In three children associated anomalies were more serious: CHARGE complex, Treacher Collins syndrome (Figs. 32.8 and 32.9), and Down syndrome. Down syndrome is not mentioned (12,13,15) as a common major congenital malformation associated with choanal atresia. However, in the presence of Down syndrome there exists a 100 times risk increase for choanal atresia (48).

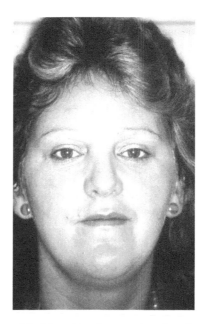

Figure 32.6   Absence of facial maldevelopment in spite of a very late correction of unilateral choanal atresia.

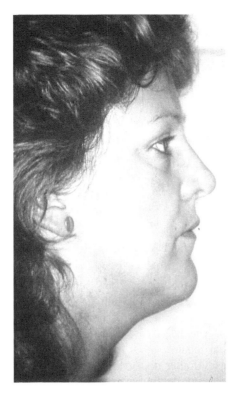

Figure 32.7 Absence of facial maldevelopment in spite of a very late correction of unilateral choanal atresia.

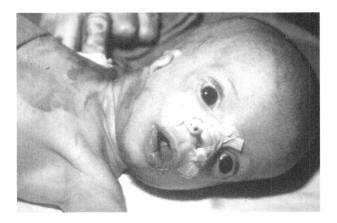

Figure 32.8 Postoperative stenting in a girl with Treacher–Collins syndrome.

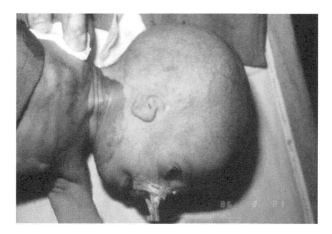

Figure 32.9   Postoperative stenting in a girl with Treacher–Collins syndrome.

The two oldest patients (cases 2 and 3) had a transseptal correction of their unilateral choanal atresia. The initial approach in all other children was by means of a transnasal microscopic/endoscopic drill-out procedure (Figs. 32.10–32.13). The latest case with unilateral atresia in a Down syndrome awaits surgical repair.

Only once (case 4) after revision surgery was postoperative stenting not applied. The postoperative stenting after transseptal surgery lasted for 1 week while stenting duration after the other procedures varied from 1 to 8 months.

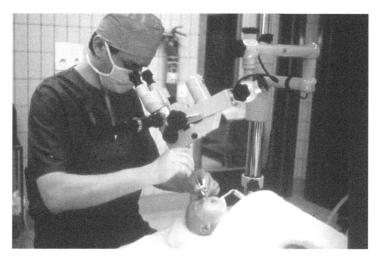

Figure 32.10   Position of the surgeon during the transnasal microscopic/endoscopic drill-out procedure.

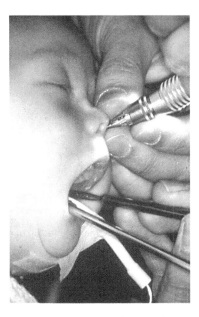

Figure 32.11 Simultaneous endoscopic visualization of the nasopharyngeal side of the atresia while retracting the soft palate with a columella nasi retractor.

Two patients had been operated on elsewhere before they underwent revision surgery at our institution. Two children with bilateral choanal atresia and operated either in our own or another institution at a very young age needed two subsequent revision procedures. After stent removal, case 6 was lost for follow-up

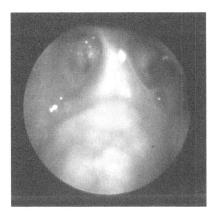

Figure 32.12 Nasopharyngeal view during surgery of bilateral choanal atresia.

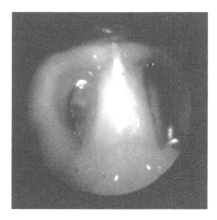

Figure 32.13   Same view as in Fig. 32.12 but with the tip of the suction visible through the choana.

during one entire year, after which the child reappeared with an obliterated choana. In all other children, the final outcome was favorable and without important complications.

Acknowledgment

The authors would like to express their gratitude to Prof. Dr. Paul Wylock and Dr. Greta Mullie, Department of Plastic and Reconstructive Surgery, for providing Figs. 32.8 and 32.9.

References

1.   Deutsch E, Kaufman M, Eilon A. Transnasal endoscopic management of choanal atresia. Int J Pediatr Otorhinolaryngol 1997; 40:19–26.
2.   Strauss M, Widome MD, Roland PS. Nasopharyngeal hemangioma causing airway obstruction in infancy. Laryngoscope 1981; 91:1365–1368.
3.   Cotton RT, Reilly JS. Congenital malformations of the larynx. In: Bluestone CD, Stool SE, Kenna ME, eds. Pediatric Otolaryngology. 3rd ed. Philadelphia, PA: WB Saunders, 1996:1299–1306.
4.   Hengerer AS, Yanofsky SD. Congenital malformations of the nose and paranasal sinuses. In: Bluestone CD, Stool SE, Kenna ME, eds. Pediatric Otolaryngology. 3rd ed. Philadelphia, PA: WB Saunders, 1996:831–842.
5.   Crockett DM, Healy GB, McGill TJ, Friedman EM. Computed tomography in the evaluation of choanal atresia in infants and children. Laryngoscope 1987; 97:174–183.
6.   Shatz A, Arensburg B, Hiss J, Ostfeld E. Cervical posture and nasal breathing in infancy. Acta Anat Basel 1994; 149:141–145.

7. Derkay CS, Grundfast KM. Airway compromise from nasal obstruction in neonates and infants. Int J Pediatr Otorhinolaryngol 1990; 19:241–249.

8. Brown K, Brown OE. Congenital malformations of the nose. In: Cummings CW, ed. Pediatric Otolaryngology Head and Neck Surgery. 3rd ed. St. Louis, MO: Mosby, 1998:92–103.

9. Nicklaus PJ, Kelley PE. Nasal obstruction and craniofacial growth. Curr Opin Otolaryngol Head Neck Surg 1996; 4:424–428.

10. Klossek JM, Ferrie JC, Fourcroy PJ, Desmons C, Basso-Brusa F, Fontanel JP. Unilateral choanal atresia and paranasal sinus growth. Ann Otolaryngol Chir Cervicofac 1996; 113:392–396.

11. Harris J, Robert E, Kallen B. Epidemiology of choanal atresia with special reference to the CHARGE association. Pediatrics 1997; 99:363–367.

12. Morgan DW, Bailey CM. Current management of choanal atresia. Int J Pediatr Otolaryngol 1990; 19:1–13.

13. Pagon RA, Graham JM, Zonana J, Yong SL. Colomba, congenital heart disease, and choanal atresia with multiple anomalies: CHARGE association. J Pediatrics 1981; 99:223–227.

14. Dobrowski JM, Grundfast KM, Rosenbaum KN, Zajtchuk JT. Otorhinolaryngic manifestations of CHARGE association. Otolaryngol Head Neck Surg 1985; 93:798–803.

15. Bergstrom LV, Owens O. Posterior choanal atresia: a syndromal disorder. Laryngoscope 1984; 94:1273–1276.

16. Brown OE, Pownell P, Manning SC. Choanal atresia: a new anatomic classification and clinical managament applications. Laryngoscope 1996; 106:97–101.

17. Brown OE, Burns DK, Smith TH, Rutledge JC. Bilateral posterior choanal atresia: a morphologic and histologic study, and computed tomographic correlation. Int J Pediatr Otorhinolaryngol 1987; 13:125–142.

18. Slovis TL, Renfro B, Watts FB, Kuhns LR, Belenky W, Spoylar J. Choanal atresia: precise CT evaluation. Radiology 1985; 155:345–348.

19. Sweeney KD, Deskin RW, Hokanson JA, Thompson CP, Yoo JK. Establishment of normal values of nasal choanal size in children: comparison of nasal choanal in children with and without symptoms of nasal obstruction. Int J Pediatr Otorhinolaryngol 1997; 39:51–57.

20. Belenky WM, Madgy DN. Nasal obstruction and rhinorrhea. In: Bluestone CD, Stool SE, Kenna ME, eds. Pediatric Otolaryngology. 3rd ed. Philadelphia, PA: WB Saunders, 1996:765–779.

21. Dehaen F, Clement PAR. Endonasal surgical treatment of bilateral choanal atresia under optic control in the infant. J Otolaryngol 1985; 14:95–98.

22. Brown OE, Smith T, Armstrong E, Grundfast K. The evaluation of choanal atresia by computed tomography. Int J Pediatr Otorhinolaryngol 1986; 12:85–98.

23. Black CM, Dungan D, Fram E, Bird CR, Rekate HL, Beals SP, Raines JM. Potential pitfalls in the work-up and diagnosis of choanal atresia. Am J Neuroradiol 1998; 19:326–329.

24. Admiraal RJ, Joosten FB, Huygen PL. Temporal bone CT findings in the CHARGE association. Int J Pediatr Otorhinolaryngol 1998; 45:151–162.

25. Dhooge I, Lemmerling M, Lagache M, Standaert L, Govaert P, Mortier G. Otological manifestations of CHARGE association. Ann Otol Rhinol Laryngol 1998; 107:935–941.

26. Calcaterra VE, Annino DJ, Carter BL, Woog JJ. Congenital nasolacrimal duct cysts with nasal obstruction. Otolaryngol Head Neck Surg 1995; 113:481–484.

27. Richardson MA, Osguthorpe JD. Surgical management of choanal atresia. Laryngoscope 1988; 98:915–918.
28. Lazar RH, Younis RT. Transnasal repair of choanal atresia using telescopes. Arch Otolaryngol Head Neck Surg 1995; 121:517–520.
29. Maniglia AJ, Goodwin WJ. Congenital choanal atresia. Otolaryngol Clin North Am 1981; 14:167–173.
30. Sculerati N, Gottlieb MD, Zimbler MS, Chibbaro PD, McCarthy JG. Airway management in children with major craniofacial anomalies. Laryngoscope 1998; 108:1806–1812.
31. Legler U. Misbildungen der Nase. In: Berendes J, Link R, Zöllner F, eds. Hals-Nasen-Ohren-Heilkunde in Praxis und Klinik, Band 1, Obere und untere Luftwege I. 2nd ed. Stuttgart: Georg Thieme, 1977:5.1–5.40.
32. McGovern FH. Bilateral congenital choanal atresia in the newborn: a method of medical management. Laryngoscope 1961; 71:480–483.
33. Lantz HJ, Birck HG. Surgical correction of choanal atresia in the neonate. Laryngoscope 1981; 91:1629–1634.
34. Vickery CL, Gross CW. Advanced drill technology in treatment of congenital choanal atresia. Otolaryngol Clin North Am 1997; 30:457–465.
35. Osguthorpe JD, Singleton GT, Adkins WY. The surgical approach to bilateral choanal atresia. Arch Otolaryngol 1982; 108:366–369.
36. Hall WJ, Watanabe T, Kenau PD, Baylin G. Trans-setpal reapir of unilateral choanal atresia. Arch Otolaryngol 1982; 108:659–661.
37. McIntosh WA. Transseptal approach to unilateral posterior choanal atresia. J Laryngol Otol 1986; 100:1133–1137.
38. Krespi YP, Husain S, Levine TM, Reede DL. Sublabial transseptal repair of choanal atresia or stenosis. Larynscope 1987; 97:1402–1406.
39. Owens H. Observations in treating twenty-five cases of choanal atresia by the transpalatine approach. Laryngoscope 1965; 75:84–104.
40. Freng A. Surgical treatment of congenital choanal atresia. Ann Otol 1978; 87:346–350.
41. Freng A. Growth in the width of the dental arches after partial extirpation of the midpalatal suture in man. Scand J Plast Reconstr Surg 1978; 12:267–272.
42. Pirsig W. Surgery of choanal atresia in infants and children: historical notes and updated review. Int J Pediatr Otorhinolaryngol 1986; 11:153–170.
43. Reddy TN, Dutt SN, Raza M. Emergency management of bilateral choanal atresia in the newborn by the endoscopic endonasal approach: a clinical record and review of literature. Int J Pediatr Otorhinolaryngol 1996; 38:21–30.
44. Stankiewicz JA. The endoscopic repair of choanal atresia. Otolaryngol Head Neck Surg 1990; 103:931–937.
45. Jacobs IN. Current surgical techniques. Choanal atresia repair. Curr Opin Otolaryngol Head Neck Surg 1996; 4:434–439.
46. Panwar SS, Martin FW. Trans-nasal endoscopic holium:YAG laser correction of choanal atresia. J Laryngol Otol 1996; 110:429–431.
47. Beste DJ, Conley SF, Brown CW. Gastroesophageal reflux complicating choanal atresia repair. Int J Pediatr Otolaryngol 1994; 29:51–58.
48. Kallen B, Mastroiacovo P, Robert E. Major congenital malformations in Down syndrome. Am J Med Genet 1996; 65:160–166.

33

Surgical Management of Chronic Rhinosinusitis in Children

PATRICK FROEHLICH

E. Herriot Hospital,
Lyon, France

I. Introduction

Functional endoscopic sinus surgery (FESS) has been developed for use in children since 1989, leading to new therapeutic solutions in rhinosinusitis management (1). Given this new surgical approach, a clear definition of the concept of rhinosinusitis in children seemed to be required, the most difficult being to determine the place of surgery in its management. After excessive enthusiasm for surgery in the early years, indications have shrunk to well-defined situations. There have also been technical improvements, which made a minimal invasive approach possible compared to the initial large surgical cavities.

In all cases, surgery seeks to relieve the obstruction of the nose and sinuses caused by anatomic variants and/or by inflammatory or fibrous mucosal tissue. Surgery can help to achieve normal physiologic conditions, but it will not cure abnormal or diseased inflammatory mucosa. Surgery can help in cases of obstructed nose, facial pain, or headache resulting from an obstructed sinus or infection secondary to mucus retention in sinus cavities.

II. Surgical Basis in Minimal Invasive Sinus Surgery in Children

The possibility of surgery is considered only after the treatment of other factors contributing to rhinosinusitis has been looked into (2). Preventive or curative therapy has to be applied first (Table 33.1). Once this has been done as thoroughly as possible, if certain symptoms are observed to persist, then surgery is to be considered (3).

Three elements guide the decision as to whether surgery could help and if so, which procedure is to be performed: observed symptoms, nasal fiberoptic examination, and CT-scan of the nose and sinus. Endoscopy of the nose in children is most easily performed with a pediatric flexible 1.8–2.2 mm nasal endoscope. CT-scan of the nose and sinus is not indicated at this stage. The new generations of spiral CT-scans allow rapid enough image acquisition for acceptance in children (4,5).

The radiation delivered in one scan is equivalent to 1 year of natural radiation. As the crystalline lens lies within the scan radiation field, excessive CT-scanning could increase the risk of cataract.

These three elements help decide whether the observed symptoms are consistent with obstruction of a diseased sinus as identified by endoscopy and radiology (6) (Table 33.2). If so, it can be reasonably predicted that the symptom secondary to obstruction will be relieved by surgery. In no way is surgery indicated to correct an abnormality discovered on endoscopy or CT-scan if no symptom can be associated thereto; nor is it ever indicated to cure a symptom not associated with an obstructive anatomical variant or hyperplastic mucosa or polyps.

Table 33.1 Step-by-step Management of Children with Chronic Rhinosinusitis

First stage	Environmental factors (smoke, pollution, other irritants)
	Adenoid hypertrophy
Second stage	Allergy
	Gastroesophageal reflux
Third stage	Drainage
	Local steroids
Fourth stage	Hypogammaglobulinemia
	Immunosuppression
Fifth stage	CT-scan and surgery

Table 33.2 Findings for Surgical Indication

Symptoms	Endoscopic finding	CT-scan
Nasal obstruction	Enlarged inferior turbinate	Sinus opacity
Headache, facial pain	Septal deviation	Anatomic variation
Cough	Mucosal edema	Concha bullosa
Postnasal discharge	Mucosal inflammation	Septal deviation
Purulent nasal discharge	Clear mucoid drainage	Paradoxical turbinates
Fetid breath	Purulent nasal discharge	Infraorbital cell
Behavior changes	Polyps	Hypoplastic maxillary sinus
		Pneumatized uncinate process

III. Chronic Rhinosinusitis: Surgical Management of the Obstructed Nose

Chronic bilateral nasal obstruction is above all due, apart from adenoid hypertrophy, to hyperplastic inferior turbinate mucosa. When the elimination of the identified causal factors and medical anti-inflammatory therapy (local steroids) fail to control symptoms or to prevent recurrence, then turbinectomy can provide a very effective solution. Sinus surgery is never indicated for the obstructed nose as such, even if sinus abnormalities can be identified on CT-scan, unless other symptoms are being caused by the diseased sinus.

Patients at this stage are usually aged over 8 years and most present with diffuse chronic airway mucosa inflammatory disease, especially involving asthma.

The surgical procedure consists in partial inferior turbinate resection under general anesthesia. Total resection is avoided, so as to limit the risk of postoperative crusting. The resection also avoids the latero-posterior part of the inferior turbinate in order to keep well away from the sphenopalatine artery. A nasal packing can be left in place at the end of surgery, to be removed under general anesthesia after 48 h: this is to control any possible bleeding.

Results are usually excellent, and prove enduring on long-term follow-up.

Alternatives such as electrocauterization may be more respectful of the anatomy but carry the risk of a merely temporary improvement. A solution along these lines may yet come from radio-frequency thermal mucosal ablation.

Other causes of nasal chronic obstruction also exist.

Septal deviation can entail unilateral but rarely bilateral obstruction. In children, septoplasty is only indicated in case of major obstruction with progressive lateral deviation of the nose. Minimal cartilage resection, avoiding growth centers is recommended in order to limit nasal growth defects, especially during puberty.

Cases of unilateral choanal atresia can have been unnoticed, being recognized only in children with persistent chronic unilateral nasal obstruction. Endoscopic correction can then be decided upon.

IV. Surgical Management of the Obstructed Sinus

Initially, wide sinus opening and resection as performed in adults was also pre-scribed for children. The wide opening concept then gradually came to be replaced by minimal invasive surgery specifically developed for children and applied to FESS (7). There were various reasons for this, including facial growth consider-ations, restoration of physiological sinus drainage, progress in surgical techniques and, above all, improved understanding of chronic childhood rhinosinusitis.

The major idea behind FESS is to ensure free physiological mucociliary sinus drainage. An anatomical key-point is that the ostiomeatal complex, where maxillary sinus, anterior ethmoid, and frontal sinus drainage take place and, within the ostiomeatal complex, the precise drainage opening, have been accurately described from an endoscopic approach. Surgery thus aims specifi-cally to free the obstructed opening by correcting an anatomical variant or resect-ing any interfering mucosal tissue or polyps.

After adequate medical management, FESS becomes indicated when a coherent pattern of observed symptoms, endoscopic obstruction, and radiological opacity of the implicated sinus emerges.

The symptoms most amenable to cure by surgery are facial pain and head-ache of sinus origin. Pain is at first suspected to be of sinus origin when its pro-jection is facing the implicated sinus. Frequent sinus infection complicating postnasal drainage can also be limited by associating surgical drainage to medical management. Other possibly sinus-linked symptoms, that is, cough, postnasal drainage, are likely to persist despite surgery. Surgery will not cure inflamed mucosa or affect symptoms secondary to such inflammation.

Surgery employs pediatric instrumentation and powered instrumentation (8) with microdebriders with adequate straight and curved pediatric blades. Thorough local anesthetic completing the general anesthesia helps limit preoperative bleeding so as to obtain excellent endoscopic visualization. Topical oxymetazoline along with adrenaline injection is one possible choice. A wide-angle $0°$ and $30°$ 4 mm, or if this is too large 2.8 mm, telescope can be used. As regards stents, the tendency is not to leave them in place at the end of the procedure. Postoperative care consists of salt water rinse. Over and above many points, a lot of variants have been described by different teams.

For minimal invasive surgery, instruments should keep a safe distance from such danger zones as orbit and dura. Enhanced safety and precision could, however, be obtained in the near future by means of surgical instrument tracking using preoperative navigation imaging systems that are being developed.

V. Conclusion

Minimal invasive surgery applied to FESS is a useful means of treatment of chronic rhinosinusitis in children. Cautious indications are based on clinical history and symptomatology, flexible endoscopy, and CT-scan. These indications are now well established and obstruction of the diseased nose and sinus can be efficiently relieved.

References

1. Gross CW, Lazar RH, Gurucharri MJ. Pediatric functional endonasal sinus surgery. Otolaryngol Clin North Am 1989; 22:733–738.
2. Burton MD, Pransky SM, Katz RM. Pediatric airway manifestations of gastroesophageal reflux. Ann Otol Rhinol Laryngol 1992; 101:742–749.
3. Clement PA, Bluestone CD, Gordts F, Lusk RP, Otten FW, Goossens H, Scadding GK, Takahashi H, van Buchen FL, Van Cauwenberge P, Wald ER. Management of rhinosinusitis in children. Consensus Meeting, Brussels, Belgium, Sept. 13, 1996. Arch Otolaryngol Head Neck Surg 1998; 124:31–34.
4. April MM, Zinreich SJ, Baroody FM, Naclerio RM. Coronal CT scan abnormalities in children with chronic sinusitis. Laryngoscope 1993; 103:985–990.
5. Milczuk HA, Dalley RW, Wessbacher FW, Richardson MA. Nasal and paranasal sinus anomalies in children with chronic sinusitis. Laryngoscope 1993; 103:247–252.
6. Lesserson JA, Kieserman SP, Finn DG. The radiographic incidence of chronic sinus disease in the pediatric population. Laryngoscope 1994; 104:159–166.
7. Settliff RC. Minimally invasive sinus surgery: the rationale and the technique. Otolaryngol Clin North Am 1996; 29:115–129.
8. Parsons DS. Rhinologic uses of powered instrumentation in children beyond sinus surgery. Otolaryngol Clin North Am 1996; 29:105–114.

34

The Minimally Invasive Approach in Pediatric Functional Endoscopic Sinus Surgery

DAVID S. PARSONS

Pediatric Otolaryngology and Sinus Care,
Greenville, South Carolina, USA

MARCELLA BOTHWELL

Washington University Hospital,
St. Louis, Missouri, USA

Rhinosinusitis is a very common disease in children (1). The average toddler raised in the home environment has six to eight upper respiratory infections (URIs) each year while the child in daycare may have up to 20–22 URIs each year. Sinusitis may be the result in 0.5% of these infectious processes (2). In older children, 3–4% of all otherwise healthy children will develop sinusitis each year. The majority of these episodes resolve without intervention or only require one course of antibiotics. Some children develop recurrent or chronic rhinosinusitis that responds poorly or transiently to intensive medical management. Functional endoscopic sinus (FES) surgery may be considered when extensive medical management has failed (3).

The authors briefly, review "maximal medical management." An extensive medical evaluation should always precede maximal medical therapy, and the therapy should be given for an extended period of time in hopes of resolving rhinosinusitis before considering FES surgery. The medical evaluation should include a screen for allergy, gastroesophageal reflux, immune compromise, ciliary dyskinesia, or cystic fibrosis. The history obtained from the parents should address risk factors for chronic rhinosinusitis including environmental irritants such as smoking history (second hand or primary) and daycare exposure to other ill children. A history of chronic nasal obstruction could suggest adenoid hypertrophy; the authors strongly believe that adenoidectomy should not be done with sinus surgery but should precede it as a separate procedure as most children show marked improvement in their sinus symptoms following adenoidectomy (4). Only after exhaustive and prolonged medical management directed at all positive findings has been attempted, should FES surgery be considered in children (5).

The "mini FES" is a successful minimally invasive surgical technique for children and adults with chronic or recurrent rhinosinusitis. The surgical principles of the technique are simple; however, mastery of the precise and delicate approach is required for optimal outcome. The steps of the procedure include: removal of lateral wall of obstructive concha bullae if necessary, creation of a "window" in the lower portion of the uncinate process to identify the natural ostia, removal of entire lower uncinate process, opening the bullae ethmoidalis in a manner that includes its natural ostia, and finally inspection of the internal mucosa.

The underlying concept of the minimally invasive approach to functional surgery is an improvement over previous surgical approaches. The ostiomeatal complex (OMC) is the frequent site of the mucus membrane disease process. This more conservative FES technique is not aimed at the extent of the sinus disease as defined by computed tomography (CT), but rather at restoring ventilation and function to the OMC (6). Aggressive dissection is generally not required or recommended. Restoring adequate ventilation and drainage to the OMC area usually allows recovery of other sites of sinus disease (7,8).

After deciding to pursue pediatric FES surgery, the child should be screened for hematological abnormalities and recent aspirin or ibuprofen ingestion. The most common etiology of FES complications is poor visibility caused by excessive bleeding. Using vasoconstrictive and hemostatic agents in the operative field minimizes surgical bleeding (9).

The surgery is started by injecting no more than 7 mg/kg of lidocaine with 1:100,000 epinephrine into the greater palatine foramen and the root of the middle turbinate, and then placing oxymetazoline soaked cottonoid under the middle turbinate.

A 135° probe (Medtronics-Xomed) is placed within the infundibulum to minimally displace the uncinate process anteriomedially making it easier to insert the backbiter blade (Fig. 34.1).

The uncinate process dissection is performed with a backbiter, rarely a sickle knife. The use of the sickle knife is discouraged in children, as the cut is made from the medial to the lateral toward the lacrimal drainage system and the orbit. The backbiter blade is active in a lateral to medial direction and thus substantially reduces the potential for injury [Figs. 34.2(a) and (b)].

A "window" is then created within the lower half of the uncinate process and redundant tissue is removed from its edges using the microdebrider [Fig. 34.3(a)]. The posterior exit of the infundibulum identifies the final common

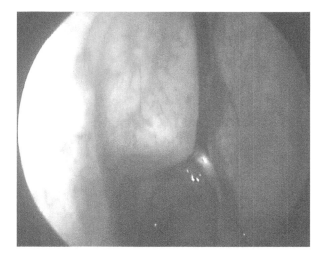

Figure 34.1 Use of 135° probe to manipulate uncinate.

pathway of the infundibulum, which is followed anteriorly. The natural ostium will be found with rare exception within 1–2 mm of the anterior uncinate as it inserts into the lateral nasal wall. The natural ostium is almost always in the most anterior and superior portion of the fontanelle. The technique produces little bleeding and an excellent "tried and true" method for identifying the natural ostium. It is critical that all the lower uncinate bone be removed to the limits of the anterior and inferior infundibulum. The anterior portion of the lower half of the uncinate process covers the natural ostium and prevents the surgeon from identifying this essential structure [Fig. 34.3(b)]. Failed FES surgeries are often due to incomplete removal of residual uncinate process that hides the natural ostium.

Three pearls of wisdom for identifying natural ostia are offered. First, natural ostia do not lie in the same plane as the lateral nasal wall. The anterior lip is more lateral than the posterior lip so the natural ostia lie in an oblique plane. Second, accessory ostia tend to be circular but the natural ostia are consistently oval in shape. Third, the natural ostia are almost always anterior and/or superior to the accessory ostia. Natural ostia should not be in the same plane as the lateral wall or perfectly circular and should be in the anterior–superior area of the fontanelle. If all these criteria are not met, one should consider that the hole identified is an accessory ostium and further evaluation should continue to find the natural ostium.

The most common cause of FES failure is a "missed ostium sequence" or failure to identify the natural ostium of the maxillary sinus. This is usually caused by failure to completely remove the lower uncinate process. The antrostomy

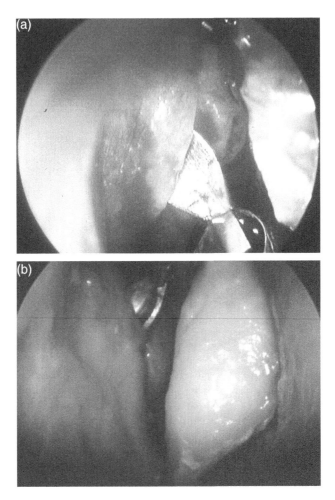

Figure 34.2   (a, b) Backbiting of the uncinate process.

created by the surgeon is therefore an accessory ostium. The mucociliary flow
pattern continues to beat mucus toward the small diseased natural ostium,
which is still intact and obstructed. The purulence escapes through the diseased
natural ostium and re-enters the maxillary sinus through the ineffective but larger
accessory ostium. This is known as the "recirculatory phenomenon" (Fig. 34.4).

The uncinate process is often the single cause of obstruction to the maxillary ostium. By simply removing the entire lower uncinate process, surgical
therapy is often successful. Enlargement of the natural ostium may or may not
be necessary.

If it is necessary to enlarge the maxillary ostium, then one should only
remove the posterior fontanelle. The anterior fontanelle is only 1–2 mm in

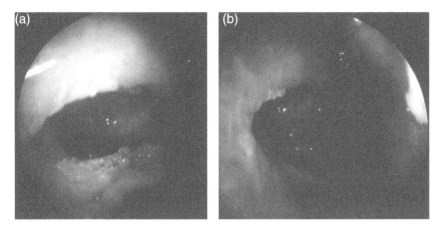

Figure 34.3   (a) Window in uncinate. (b) Removal of lower uncinate process from window.

length and protects the lacrimal duct system. The posterior fontanelle is significantly longer and often up to 20 mm in length. It is the site of most of the accessory ostia to the maxillary sinus. The cut is made from the natural ostium posteriorly staying as close to the roof of the maxillary sinus as possible. A precise incision can simply be made using the 0° Thru Cut instrument (Medtronics-Xomed). The incision should include any accessory ostia and the large lower flap is then sharply removed with the microdebrider. The anterior edge of the middle meatus antrostomy is always the anterior lip of the natural

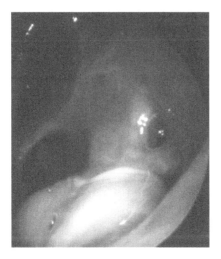

Figure 34.4   Recirculatory phenomenon.

ostium. Examination of the maxillary ostium should always be performed with a 30°, 45°, or 70° telescope after removal of the anterior uncinate process.

A 0° telescope is then used to identify the bulla ethmoidalis and its lower medial portion is removed. The natural ostium of the bulla is on its posterior side and is very large. The dissection of the lower medial bulla must continue until the natural ostium is part of the created opening. This creates a functional opening.

If the inspection of the anterior ethmoid is unremarkable, the surgery is concluded with the placement of a folded Merogel (Medtronic Xomed, Jacksonville FL) dressing. It is important to thoroughly moisten the stent by injecting saline to reconstitute the hyaluronic acid gelatin. If blood is used to "moisten" Merogel then the stent will not easily be absorbed.

Even if the mucus membrane is diseased, surgery can be terminated as ventilation and function is now restored. Exceptions to this include fungal sinusitis, mucopyocele in other sinus areas, and cystic fibrosis. This approach will work for most children with chronic or recurrent rhinosinusitis. There is less risk of surgical complications and bleeding when performing the "mini FES," however, prudent caution should always be considered. For those children whose symptoms persist after "mini FES," no bridges are burned. Revisions may be done with the initial steps of the FES already done and most importantly with all the landmarks preserved.

Children who have undergone this procedure have shown complete resolution or marked improvement in their rhinosinusitis symptoms. In data to be published, Lusk and Bothwell found an 81% "much improved and 15% somewhat improved" change in rhinosinusitis symptoms for a total of 96% improvement in a 10-year follow-up study after FES surgery. Furthermore, 81% of children and families were extremely satisfied and 13% moderately satisfied with their FES surgery for a total of 94% satisfaction at 10-year follow-up from surgery as compared to continued maximal medical management.

Theoretically, long-term risk of facial growth has been cautioned by Mair et al. (10) in animal models. In a newly published study by Bothwell et al. (11), no clinical or anthropomorphic difference was noted between children with chronic rhinosinusitis and FES surgery and children with chronic rhinosinusitis and no FES surgery. This paper suggests that if FES surgery is necessary after maximal medical management has failed, long-term risks of facial growth should not be a concern for parents.

References

1. Dingle JH. Illness in the Home: A Study of 25,000 Illnesses in a Group of Cleveland Families. Cleveland, OH: Press of Western Reserve University, 1964.
2. Wald ER. Diagnosis and management of sinusitis in children. Adv Pediatr Infect Dis 1996; 12:1–20.
3. Lusk RP, Muntz HR. Endoscopic sinus surgery in children with chronic sinusitis: a pilot study. Laryngoscope 1990; 100:654–658.

4.   Bolger WE, Parsons DS, Potempa L. Preoperative hemostatic assessment of the adenotonsillectomy patient. Otolaryngol Head Neck Surg 1990; 103:396–405.
5.   Parsons DS. Chronic sinusitis: a medical or surgical disease? Otolaryngol Clin North Am 1996; 29(1):1–9.
6.   Bolger WE, Butzin CA, Parsons DS. Paranasal sinus bony anatomic variations and mucosal abnormalities: CT analysis for endoscopic sinus surgery. Laryngoscope 1991; 101:56–64.
7.   Parsons DS, Pransky SM. Functional endoscopic sinus surgery in infants and young children. Instructional Courses AAO-HNS 1992; 5:159–164.
8.   Parsons DS, Wald E. Otitis media and sinusitis: similar diseases. Otolaryngol Clin North Am 1996; 29(1):11–25.
9.   Bolger WE, Kennedy DW. Complications in surgery of the paranasal sinuses. In: Eisele D, ed. Complications in Head and Neck Surgery. St Louis, MO: Mosby Yearbook, 1993:chap 50.
10. Mair EA, Bolger WE, Breisch EA. Sinus and facial growth after pediatric endoscopic sinus surgery. Arch Otolaryngol Head Neck Surg 1995; 121:547–522.
11. Bothwell MR, Lusk RP, Picirrillo JF, Ridenour BD. Long-term outcome of facial growth after functional endoscopic sinus surgery. Otolaryngol Head Neck Surg 2002; 126(6):628–634.

35

Surgical Treatment of Hypertrophy of the Inferior Turbinate

DESIDERIO PASSÀLI, VALERIO DAMIANI, LUISA BELLUSSI, and MARCO ANSELMI

University of Siena,
Siena, Italy

FRANCESCO MARIA PASSÀLI and GIULIO CESARE PASSÀLI

University of Genova,
Genova, Italy

Although it is not a life-threatening condition, nasal obstruction can interfere with the quality of life. After exclusion of septal deviations, the main structures contributing to this problem are the nasal turbinates, especially the inferior turbinates. Perennial allergic and nonallergic rhinitis are the most common non-infectious causes of mucosal swelling of the inferior turbinates reducing nasal air flow. Untreated, these conditions may result in permanent nasal obstruction secondary to dilation of the venous sinuses or fibrosis.

Surgical procedures on the enlarged inferior, and sometimes middle, turbinates are the only effective therapy in these cases. However, selection of the procedure of choice among the several available techniques appears to be based more on personal attitudes than on a critical assessment of the treatment outcomes. In fact since the first experiences in turbinal surgery performed by Hartman in the 1980s (1), the reported benefits from large number of surgical procedures suggests a lack of consensus about the most effective technique.

The principal procedures in current use are cauterization, cryosurgery, submucosal resection with or without outfracture, and resection of the turbinate.

Every procedure is performed, in our experience, following standardized steps:

1. *Electrocautery*: Inferior turbinate cauterization is done by applying a high frequency coagulation current via a round point electrode at constant power. The electrode is introduced as far as the posterior end of the nasal cavity. The coagulation is carried out on the medial surface from behind forward two to four times 10 s each time. At the end of the intervention Merocel packs is placed for three days to avoid the formation of synechiae between turbinate and septum (2).

2. *Cryotherapy*: The nasal probe of a standard cryogenic unit using nitrogen protoxide is applied along the free edge and then on the medial face at two overlapping levels for 2 min, at a temperature of $-80°C$. Merocel nasal packing is left in both sides for three days (3–5).

3. *Laser cautery*: Coagulation of the inferior turbinates is done using a carbon dioxide laser (Coherent MP20 laser) delivering 300 impulses per second at 10–15 W. The size of laser spot is the same as the point of the electrocautery needle. A 2.5 ms interval is left between consecutive applications to avoid excessive carbonization. Usually, packing is not necessary (6,7).

4. *Submucosal resection without lateral displacement*: Through a 3–4 mm incision on the head of inferior turbinate, the submucosal tissue is dissected from the medial surface and inferior edge from the bone by an elevator. Excess cavernous tissue is removed with Hartmann forceps with resection of the posterior end of the turbinate. Merocel packing is used (8–10).

5. *Submucosal resection with lateral displacement*: As the previous one, the submucosal resection begins with a 3–4 mm large incision performed on the head of the inferior turbinate (Fig. 35.1); the submucosal tissue is then dissected from the medial surface and inferior edge of the bone by an elevator (Fig. 35.2); through the tunnel in this way obtained, the excess cavernous tissue is then removed by Weil forceps, paying attention to the superior mucosal layer (Fig. 35.3). When there is a hypertrophy of the turbinal bone, it is possible to perform an outfracture and lateral displacement of the turbinate with a displacer (Fig. 35.4). The bleeding can make difficult to establish the entity of the tissue to be removed and the necessity of a lateral displacement.

To make this method more efficient, we use from 2 years a special straight dissector–aspirator with a 3 mm sharp extremity and with a very strong body.

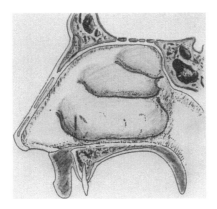

Figure 35.1 Incision on the head of the inferior turbinate.

This peculiarity permits the instrument to be introduced from the head of the inferior turbinate and then to perform the submucosal dissection. The contemporary aspiration made by the instrument with the endoscopic control, that we usually perform with a 25° optic, permits to carry out the surgical act following the real necessity case by case.

When necessary, by rotating the instrument, it is possible to obtain the lateral displacement of the whole bone. The time needed for this technique is moreover extremely shorter compared with the traditional surgical way.

6. *Turbinectomy*: After medial and upward fracture, the inferior turbinate is resected by angled scissors along the insertion close to the lateral nasal wall. Merocel nasal packing is used for three days to control bleeding (11–13).

Each procedure has recognized advantages and disadvantages.

We reviewed our experience with each of these procedures in patients with inferior turbinate hypertrophy unresponsive to medical therapy.

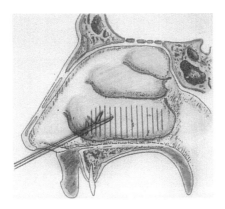

Figure 35.2 The submucosal tissue is dissected from the bone.

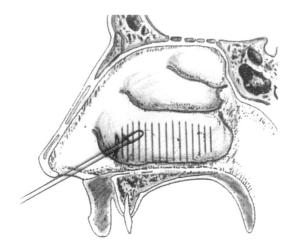

Figure 35.3   The excessive cavernous tissue is removed.

Four hundred and fifty-seven patients, 256 males and 201 females (age range 8–70 years, median age 38 years) with intractable nasal obstruction due to chronic allergic or vasomotor rhinitis and operated on at the ENT Clinic of the University of Siena were studied.

Patients with infectious rhinitis or marked septal deviation were excluded from the trial. Other exclusion criteria were: previous nasal surgery, nasal polyps or sinusitis contributing to the nasal obstruction, significant improvement after medical treatment with steroid nasal sprays or other major nasal diseases.

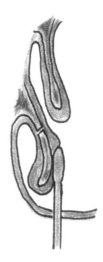

Figure 35.4   Displacement of the turbinate.

Each patient underwent the following diagnostic protocol:

A. Clinical history.
B. Clinical examination.
C. Skin tests by prick testing for Graminacee, Parietaria and Dermatophagoides to identify hypersensitive subjects.
D. Dosage of blood specific IgE by RAST.
E. Nasal decongestion test (NDT). NDT was carried out by (1) baseline recording of nasal resistance by anterior active rhinomanometry (Rynosystem Amplifon) according to the Committee report on the standardization of rhinomanometry (14); (2) insufflation of a local vasoconstrictor (tramazoline) into each nasal cavity; and (3) repeated recording of nasal resistance after ten minutes. If nasal resistance normalized or improved the test was considered positive. If the nasal resistance remained unchanged the test was judged to be abnormal (14). All the patients in the present study had abnormal NDT results.
F. Acoustic rhinometry performed by RHINOKLACK RK 1000 to assess the morphological and geometrical situation of the nasal cavity.
G. Measurement of nasal mucociliary transport time (MCTt) using charcoal powder placed on the inferior turbinate. Normal time to appearance of the charcoal indicator into the oropharynx was 13 ± 2 min (15). When the MCTt exceed 30 min we consider it blocked and interrupt the observation.
H. Measurement of nasal secretory IgA. Specimen were obtained by inserting two small cottonwool swabs into each nasal fossa, between the septum and the middle and inferior turbinates, under anterior rhinoscopy. Twenty minutes later the swabs were removed by a bayonet forceps and inserted into an insulin syringe to squeeze out the secretion into a test tube. Specimens were analyzed immediately or frozen for later analysis (16).
I. Questionnaire on symptoms that was collected every year during the controls. The patients graded the following symptoms: nasal obstruction during day and night, nasal discharge during day and night, sensation of ear fullness according to a 1–6 scale (Table 35.1).

Electrocautery was performed in 62 patients (first group); cryotherapy in 58 patients (second group); laser cautery in 54 patients (third group); submucosal resection without lateral displacement in 69 patients (fourth group); submucosal resection with lateral displacement in 94 patients (fifth group); turbinectomy in 45 patients (sixth group). Patients were assigned randomly to one of the six groups. Each of the 10 surgeons involved performed a balanced percentage of each type of operation, using the same technique. Residents were not involved. All the surgical procedures were carried out under local anesthesia.

In all cases nasal packing was used without a topical antibiotic. All the patients received a second generation cephalosporin for 6 days.

Table 35.1 Questionnaire on Symptoms Data Collected Every Year in Controls

1. Please express your evaluation on:						
—nasal obstruction during the day:	1	2	3	4	5	6
—nasal obstruction during the night:	1	2	3	4	5	6
2. Please express your evaluation on:						
—nasal discharge during the day:	1	2	3	4	5	6
—nasal discharge during the night:	1	2	3	4	5	6
3. Please express your evaluation on sensation of ear fullness:						
	0	1	2	3	4	5	6

Note: Symptoms must be graded according to a 1–6 scale where 1 is the absence of symptom and 6 is maximum severity of symptom.

Of the 457 patients initially entered into the trial 382 were available for follow-up. The follow-up was of 4 years in 100 patients, of 3 years in 91 patients, of 2 years in 107 patients, and of 1 year in 84 patients.

Forty percent (182) of the patients admitted to the study proved to be allergic. Nasal hyperactivity was triggered by Dermatophagoides in 30% (54) of cases, by grass pollen in 10% (18) of cases, and by both allergens in 60% (110).

Results were assessed by measuring of (1) patency as indicated by nasal resistance and acoustic rhinometry, (2) mucociliary transport time, (3) secretory IgA, (4) symptom score, and (5) complications.

I. Patency

Nasal resistance values are presented in Table 35.2. Although the average resistance values were improved in all groups from the preoperative level, the duration of improvement varied by treatment group. The least improvement occurred in the electrocautery group and these values worsened yearly again to become abnormal by the third postoperative year. Normal nasal patency was restored in the other groups and remained normal for the remainder of the study period. The greatest improvement was seen in the turbinectomy group.

Table 35.3 shows the morphological status of the nasal cavities as documented by acoustic rhinometric measurements. All groups had an increased volume during the first year with a decrease in the electrocautery, laser, and cryotherapy groups in the following years. It is well known that acoustic rhinometry measures the volume of nasal cavity. So the acoustic rhinometry will register an increase of the volume of nasal cavity after surgery as the size of the turbinates is decreased. Unfortunately, so far rhinometry is not standardized and the normal values are not established. However, we believe that the absolute values are not very important but it is very interesting to evaluate their trend during the follow-up years.

Table 35.2 Nasal Resistance Values Measured by Rhinomanometry

Follow-up (years)	Group 1 ($Pa/cm^3/s$)	Group 2 ($Pa/cm^3/s$)	Group 3 ($Pa/cm^3/s$)	Group 4 ($Pa/cm^3/s$)	Group 5 ($Pa/cm^3/s$)	Group 6 ($Pa/cm^3/s$)
First (100 subjects)	0.80 ± 0.13 (15 subjects)	0.6 ± 0.11 (16 subjects)	0.5 ± 0.09 (14 subjects)	0.45 ± 0.09 (20 subjects)	0.45 ± 0.09 (24 subjects)	0.3 ± 0.09 (11 subjects)
Second (191 subjects)	0.85 ± 0.14 (29 subjects)	0.6 ± 0.12 (30 subjects)	0.55 ± 0.10 (27 subjects)	0.45 ± 0.09 (39 subjects)	0.45 ± 0.09 (49 subjects)	0.3 ± 0.09 (21 subjects)
Third (298 subjects)	1.2 ± 0.33 (47 subjects)	0.9 ± 0.26 (45 subjects)	0.5 ± 0.10 (43 subjects)	0.5 ± 0.11 (53 subjects)	0.45 ± 0.10 (75 subjects)	0.45 ± 0.10 (35 subjects)
Fourth (382 subjects)	1.5 ± 0.41 (62 subjects)	1.0 ± 0.29 (58 subjects)	0.6 ± 0.14 (54 subjects)	0.5 ± 0.12 (69 subjects)	0.45 ± 0.12 (94 subjects)	0.45 ± 0.09 (45 subjects)

Note: Before surgery, mean value of resistance was $1.2 \, Pa/cm^3$ per second. Group 1 = electrocautery; Group 2 = cryotherapy; Group 3 = laser; Group 4 = submucosal resection; Group 5 = submucosal resection with displacement; Group 6 = turbinectomy.

Passàli et al.

Table 35.3 Nasal Volumes Measured by Acoustic Rhinometry

Follow-up (years)	Group 1 (cm³)	Group 2 (cm³)	Group 3 (cm³)	Group 4 (cm³)	Group 5 (cm³)	Group 6 (cm³)
First	8.5 ± 1.35	9.3 ± 1.31	10.4 ± 2.52	12.4 ± 2.96	11.5 ± 2.34	12.5 ± 1.95
(100 subjects)	(15 subjects)	(16 subjects)	(14 subjects)	(20 subjects)	(24 subjects)	(11 subjects)
Second	7.3 ± 1.28	7.6 ± 1.14	9.5 ± 2.37	10.2 ± 2.05	10.2 ± 2.15	11.8 ± 2.15
(191 subjects)	(28 subjects)	(30 subjects)	(27 subjects)	(39 subjects)	(45 subjects)	(21 subjects)
Third	5.5 ± 1.12	5.7 ± 1.03	8.1 ± 2.12	11.3 ± 2.14	11.1 ± 2.47	11.7 ± 2.03
(298 subjects)	(47 subjects)	(45 subjects)	(43 subjects)	(53 subjects)	(75 subjects)	(35 subjects)
Fourth	4.5 ± 1.13	4.9 ± 0.98	7.4 ± 1.93	11.4 ± 2.41	11.7 ± 2.39	11.8 ± 2.01
(382 subjects)	(62 subjects)	(58 subjects)	(54 subjects)	(69 subjects)	(94 subjects)	(45 subjects)

Note: Mean value before surgery was 4.8 cm³. Group 1 = electrocautery; Group 2 = cryotherapy; Group 3 = laser; Group 4 = submucosal resection; Group 5 = submucosal resection with displacement; Group 6 = turbinectomy.

II. Mucociliary Transport Time

The mucociliary clearance test results are shown in Table 35.4. The average mucociliary transport times remained abnormal except in the two groups undergoing submucosal resection.

III. Secretory IgA

A similar trend occurred with secretory IgA production (Table 35.5). Normal average values (80–100 mg/100 mL) were reached only in patients receiving submucosal resection and the combination with lateral displacement assured the best results.

IV. Symptom Severity Score

The trend of the symptom score in each group is recorded in Table 35.6 and shows the best results in patients treated by submucosal resection. Symptoms worsened in groups 1 and 2 in parallel to the decrease in nasal patency.

V. Complications

Surgical complications are presented in Fig. 35.5 and Table 35.7. The patients in groups 1–3 had the greatest problem with chronic crusting, due to the nasal physiology impairment, and synechiae formation. Bleeding was only noted in groups 4–6, reaching clinically troublesome levels only in group 6, with true hemorrhages in 25 patients in the total turbinectomy group.

Bleeding was absent in electrocautery, cryotherapy and laser groups.

Atrophy was absent in both submucosal resection groups.

VI. Composite Analysis

To compare the effectiveness of the procedures, analysis of variance was performed. The ANOVA was done year by year. Using rhinomanometric results, a statistically significant difference ($p = 0.05$) was found in favor of submucosal resection with lateral displacement (group 5) in comparison with groups 1–3.

A statistically significant difference between group 5 and groups 1, 2, 3, and 6 was noted using as the dependent variable (a) acoustic rhinometry results ($p = 0.01$), or (b) mucociliary transport time, or (c) the symptomatolgical scores ($p = 0.01$).

Cauterization, cryotherapy, and laser cautery are associated with only short-term benefit on airway patency and with troublesome complications of crusting. The decreased bleeding, lack of postoperative pain, and faster healing

Table 35.4 Mucociliary Transport Time

Follow-up (years)	Group 1 (cm^3)	Group 2 (cm^3)	Group 3 (cm^3)	Group 4 (cm^3)	Group 5 (cm^3)	Group 6 (cm^3)
First	26 ± 1.64	25 ± 1.92	27 ± 1.78	20 ± 2.45	21 ± 2.15	29 ± 0.92
(100 subjects)	(15 subjects)	(16 subjects)	(14 subjects)	(20 subjects)	(24 subjects)	(11 subjects)
Second	25 ± 1.57	26 ± 2.15	27 ± 1.67	20 ± 2.36	18 ± 1.83	28 ± 0.73
(191 subjects)	(28 subjects)	(30 subjects)	(27 subjects)	(39 subjects)	(45 subjects)	(21 subjects)
Third	26 ± 1.149	26 ± 2.05	26 ± 1.83	18 ± 2.15	15 ± 1.75	29 ± 0.85
(298 subjects)	(47 subjects)	(45 subjects)	(43 subjects)	(53 subjects)	(75 subjects)	(35 subjects)
Fourth	25 ± 1.93	25 ± 1.93	27 ± 1.90	20 ± 2.41	15 ± 1.68	29 ± 0.95
(382 subjects)	(62 subjects)	(58 subjects)	(54 subjects)	(69 subjects)	(94 subjects)	(45 subjects)

Note: Data are in minutes (mean ± SD). Normal value (for charcoal powder) is 13 ± 2. Group 1 = electrocautery; Group 2 = cryotherapy; Group 3 = laser; Group 4 = submucosal resection; Group 5 = submucosal resection with displacement; Group 6 = turbinectomy.

Table 35.5 SIgA Concentration in Nasal Secretions

Follow-up (years)	Group 1 (mg/100 mL)	Group 2 (mg/100 mL)	Group 3 (mg/100 mL)	Group 4 (mg/100 mL)	Group 5 (mg/100 mL)	Group 6 (mg/100 mL)
First (100 subjects)	10 ± 2.5 (15 subjects)	08 ± 2.2 (16 subjects)	10 ± 2.4 (14 subjects)	40 ± 8.3 (20 subjects)	38 ± 8.1 (24 subjects)	20 ± 5.3 (11 subjects)
Second (191 subjects)	10 ± 2.6 (29 subjects)	12 ± 2.8 (30 subjects)	11 ± 2.2 (27 subjects)	35 ± 7.8 (39 subjects)	40 ± 8.6 (49 subjects)	15 ± 4.6 (21 subjects)
Third (298 subjects)	12 ± 2.9 (47 subjects)	10 ± 2.7 (45 subjects)	15 ± 2.9 (43 subjects)	40 ± 8.4 (53 subjects)	52 ± 9.5 (75 subjects)	18 ± 4.8 (35 subjects)
Fourth (382 subjects)	18 ± 3.1 (62 subjects)	15 ± 2.8 (58 subjects)	10 ± 2.5 (54 subjects)	53 ± 9.2 (69 subjects)	70 ± 12.8 (94 subjects)	20 ± 5.5 (45 subjects)

Note: Normal value = 80–100 mg/100 mL. Group 1 = electrocautery; Group 2 = cryotherapy; Group 3 = laser; Group 4 = submucosal resection; Group 5 = submucosal resection with displacement; Group 6 = turbinectomy.

Table 35.6 Total Symptom Score

Follow-up (years)	Group 1 (mg/100 mL)	Group 2 (mg/100 mL)	Group 3 (mg/100 mL)	Group 4 (mg/100 mL)	Group 5 (mg/100 mL)	Group 6 (mg/100 mL)
First (100 subjects)	20 ± 2.25 (15 subjects)	21 ± 3.11 (16 subjects)	21 ± 2.45 (14 subjects)	10 ± 1.59 (20 subjects)	10 ± 1.43 (24 subjects)	21 ± 2.43 (11 subjects)
Second (191 subjects)	22 ± 2.78 (29 subjects)	22 ± 3.34 (30 subjects)	24 ± 3.10 (27 subjects)	12 ± 1.79 (39 subjects)	10 ± 1.67 (49 subjects)	20 ± 2.35 (21 subjects)
Third (298 subjects)	26 ± 3.76 (47 subjects)	27 ± 3.85 (45 subjects)	18 ± 2.11 (43 subjects)	12 ± 1.81 (53 subjects)	10 ± 1.85 (75 subjects)	22 ± 2.72 (35 subjects)
Fourth (382 subjects)	26 ± 3.82 (62 subjects)	25 ± 3.78 (58 subjects)	20 ± 2.23 (54 subjects)	12 ± 1.89 (69 subjects)	10 ± 1.72 (94 subjects)	20 ± 2.11 (45 subjects)

Note: Questionnaire on symptoms was collected every year at the control visit. Patients graded the following symptoms: nasal obstruction during day and night, nasal discharge during day and night, sensation of ear fullness according to 1–6 scale. Group 1 = electrocautery; Group 2 = cryotherapy; Group 3 = laser; Group 4 = submucosal resection; Group 5 = submucosal resection with displacement; Group 6 = turbinectomy.

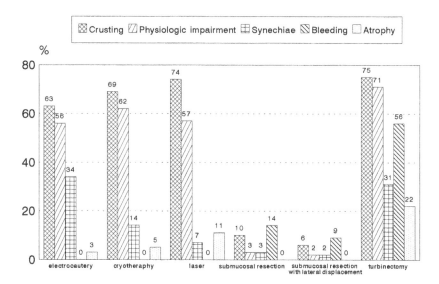

Figure 35.5 Surgical complications: percentage of patients having complications. Bleeding was absent in electrogroup 1, group 2, and group 3. Atrophy was absent in groups 4 and 5.

after laser cauterization do not justify the disadvantages such as the expensive instrumentation and risk of synechiae formation. Thus, the laser offers no advantage over simpler surgical instruments.

Submucosal resection of the vascular tissue within the turbinate had the least complications (bleeding, crusting) and the greatest improvement in mucociliary clearance and local SIgA production. The longer hospital stay is counterbalanced by the absence of bleeding and the minimal crusting. This conservative technique gives good results in the majority of the cases and is well tolerated. In our country we have to consider also this parameter (i.e., hospital stay) because, differently from other country, we hospitalized patients that have to be submitted to turbinate surgery.

The 94 patients who underwent submucosal resection (groups 4 and 5) obtained the best results. Adding lateral displacement (group 5) to the procedure incurred no additional risk and resulted in marginally better results. In fact the long lasting increase of nasal patency which come back to normal values was accompanied by the normalization of mucociliary transport time and local SIgA production. Therefore, we recommend the additional step of turbinate outfracture when performing submucosal resection of the turbinate tissue.

Outfracture of the inferior turbinate (without submucosal resection) does not significantly affect the nasal airway even when combined with amputating the posterior end of the turbinate. In fact, anterior rhinomanometry showed

Table 35.7 Complications

Complications	Group 1 (62 subjects)	Group 2 (58 subjects)	Group 3 (54 subjects)	Group 4 (69 subjects)	Group 5 (94 subjects)	Group 6 (45 subjects)
Crusting	39 subjects	40 subjects	40 subjects	7 subjects	6 subjects	34 subjects
Nasal physical impairment	35 subjects	36 subjects	31 subjects	2 subjects	2 subjects	32 subjects
Synechiae	21 subjects	8 subjects	4 subjects	2 subjects	2 subjects	14 subjects
Bleeding	0 subjects	0 subjects	0 subjects	10 subjects	8 subjects	25 subjects
Atrophic sequences	2 subjects	3 subjects	6 subjects	0 subjects	0 subjects	10 subjects

Group 1 = electrocautery; Group 2 = cryotherapy; Group 3 = laser; Group 4 = submucosal resection; Group 5 = submucosal resection with displacement; Group 6 = turbinectomy.

that any eventual improvement is not predictable in any specific patient and it is short lived. Therefore, outfracture whose advantages are the absence of risk of postoperative nasal adhesions and minimal possibility of developing atrophic rhinitis produces modest increase in nasal patency (17) or is unable to correct the nasal obstruction.

In contrast lateral displacement of inferior turbinate improves the results obtained with submucosal resection because hypertrophy reduction and lateralization are both obtained. Although a statistically significant difference was not observed in the present study comparing with submucosal resection with and without lateral displacement, the additional surgical step appears to improve outcome without any additional risk.

Turbinectomy had the greatest effect on nasal obstruction, but its adverse effect on the other nasal functions as showed by poor results of MCTt and SIgA dosage, and secondary hemorrhage limits the usefulness of this technique. Increased airflow and the macroturbulence produced by the modified nasal anatomy are responsible for excessive drying of nasal secretion and crusting.

Epiphora due to the damage of the opening of the nasolacrimal duct is uncommon except for the case of unusual duct opening up 10 mm below the attachment of the inferior turbinate. Dawes (18) and Cook et al. (19) noted a significant risk of primary hemorrhage following turbinectomy (8.9–10% of patients). Salam and Wengraf (20) noted the increase of nasal airflow corresponded to the decrease in the humidifying activity of the nasal mucosa.

Although atrophic rhinitis is a rare complication of total inferior turbinectomy, more frequent in patients with poor hygiene and nutrition, many authors recommended removal of the portion of the turbinate necessary to treat the airway obstruction, avoiding radical resection of the inferior turbinate.

Each procedure for surgical management of chronic nasal obstruction has been noted to have distinct advantages and drawbacks, leading to the general teaching that no one operation is "right" for every case and that surgery should be individualized. However, the results of this study permit us to draw specific conclusions. It is clear that the more conservative techniques must be preferred because they provide effective control of the vasomotor disturbances without interfering with the anatomy and physiology of the turbinates.

These results indicate that the dramatic improvement in nasal airflow following complete resection of the inferior turbinates is accompanied by clinically significant loss of humidification and warming of the inspired air, efficiency of mucociliary transport activity, and reduced secretory IgA defense activities. Thus, even if turbinectomy has excellent results in relieving nasal obstruction it is associated with more pain, crusting, long-term dryness, and increased infection rate.

The follow-up of 4 years is long enough to evidence the normalization of physiological parameters when submucosal resection with or without lateral displacing is performed. During the same period of time no significant improvements are observed for non-conservative surgical procedures such as turbinectomy.

In our opinion a longer follow-up could only confirm our results: in fact the increased airflow and macroturbulence throughout the nasal cavities following turbinectomy represent the pathophysiological basis of nasal drying and crusting.

As a consequence the nasal physiological impairment must be considered permanent having as substratum irreversible anatomical alterations (21,22).

Without doubt elevation of a mucoperiosteal flap is technically more difficult than full thickness excision. This may be one of the reason because, many surgeons prefer total or partial turbinectomy to submucosal resection in spite of the better nasal physiology with the latter procedure.

We recommend submucosal resection combined with lateral displacement as first choice operation in case of nasal obstruction due to hypertrophy of inferior turbinates.

From the *Annals of Otology, Rhinology & Laryngology*, 2000 (June); 108:569–575. Reprinted with full permission.

References

1. Watkins ABK. Middle turbinate headache. Med J Aust 1970; 1:382–384.
2. Peynegre R, Bossard B, Koskas G, Borsik M, Bovaziz A, Gilain L. La chirurgie endoscopique des cornets: etude préliminaire. Ann Oto-Laryng (Paris) 1989; 106:537–540.
3. Moore GF, Bicknell PG. A comparison of cryotherapy and submucous diathermy in vasomotor rhinitis. J Laryngol Otol 1980; 94:1411–1431.
4. Motta G, Pucci V, Villari G, Motta G Jr, Salzano FA. Cryosurgery in the treatment of hypertrophic chronic rhinitis. In: Passàli D, ed. Around the Nose. Firenze, Italy: Conti Tipocolor, 1988.
5. Principato J. Chronic vasomotor rhinitis: cryogenic and other modes of treatment. Laryngoscope 1979; 89:616.
6. Fukutake T, Yamashita T, Tomoda K, Kumazawa T. Laser surgery for allergic rhinitis. Arch Otolaryngol Head Neck Surg 1986; 112:1280–1282.
7. Lenz H. Acht Jahre laserchirurgie an den unteren nasenmuscheln bei rhinopathia vasomotoria in form der laserstrichkarbonisation. HNO 1985; 33:422–425.
8. House HP. Submucous resection of the inferior turbinate. Laryngoscope 1951; 61:637–648.
9. Lizarraga VM, Arellano AM. Reseccion submucosa del cornete inferior oseo. Acta Otorrinolaringol Esp 1989; 40(5):363–364.
10. Mabry RL. Inferior turbinoplasty: patient selection technique and long-term consequences. Otolaryngol Head Neck Surg 1988; 98:60–66.
11. Elwany S, Harrison R. Inferior turbinectomy: comparison of four techniques. J Laryngol Otol 1990; 104:206–209.
12. Goode RL. Surgery of the turbinates. J Otolaryngol 1978; 7:262–268.
13. Ophir D, Schindel D, Halperin D, Marhak G. Long term follow-up of the effectiveness and safety of inferior turbinectomy. Plastic Reconstr Surg 1992; 90:980–984.

14. Clement PAR. Committee report on standardization of rhinomanometry. Rhinology 1984; 22:151–155.
15. Passàli D, Bellussi L, Bianchini-Ciampoli M, De Seta E. Our experiences in nasal mucociliary transport time determination. Acta Otolaryngol (Stockh) 1984; 97:319–323.
16. Pàssali D. L'Unità Rino-Faringo-Tubarica, ed. Milano: CRS Amplifon, 1985.
17. O'Flynn PE, Milford CA, Mackay IS. Short communication. Multiple submucosal out-fractures of inferior turbinates. J Laryngol Otol 1990; 104:239–240.
18. Dawes PJD. Inferior turbinectomy: is the risk of haemorrhage overstressed? J Laryngol Otol 1988; 102:590–591.
19. Cook JA, McCombe AW, Jones AS. Laser treatment of rhinitis-1 year follow-up. Clin Otolaryngol 1993; 18:209–211.
20. Salam MA, Wengraf C. Concho-antropexy or total inferior turbinotomy for hypertrophy of the inferior turbinates? A prospective randomized study. J Laryngol Otol 1993; 107:1125–1128.
21. Martinez SA, Nissen AJ, Stock CR, Tesmer T. Nasal turbinate resection for relief of nasal obstruction. Laryngoscope 1983; 93(7):871–875.
22. Moore GF, Freeman TJ, Orgen FP, Yonkers AJ. Extended follow-up of total inferior turbinate resection for relief of chronic nasal obstruction. Laryngoscope 1985; 95:1095–1099.

36

Long-Term Results of Endoscopic Sinus Surgery in Cystic Fibrosis

PETER A. R. CLEMENT and PIERRE BRIHAYE

Free University of Brussels,
Brussels, Belgium

Cystic fibrosis is the most common substantially lethal hereditary disease among young Caucasians (1). That infectious and polypoid degeneration of the nasal mucosa is part of this condition had not been recognized by the otolaryngologist until 1959 (2). The frequency of nasal polyposis in children is extremely low, about 0.1% (3). Schwachmann et al. (1962) (4) found nasal polyposis in 6.7%, Cepero et al. (1987) (5) in 10%, Neely et al. (1972) (6) in 24% and Stern et al. (1982) (7) in 26% of the patients with cystic fibrosis. Settipane (8) stated that any child of 16 years or younger with nasal polyps should be evaluated for cystic fibrosis. He found in cystic fibrosis the prevalence of nasal polyps to be 20%. Later the prevalence was estimated to be 32% in children and 40–48% in adults with cystic fibrosis (9), but at the same time these authors state that the detection of nasal polyps may be limited by the ability of the young child to tolerate nasal examination.

With the introduction of modern examination techniques [nasal endoscopy and computed tomography (CT) scanning], it was to be expected that the prevalence of nasal polyposis in cystic fibrosis was higher than estimated ever before. Brihaye et al. (10) found in a prospective clinical study of 84 patients during careful endoscopic examination after decongestion, topical anaesthesia and aspiration of the secretions, the presence of inflammatory polyps coming out of the middle meatus in 45% of the cases (mean age 15 years: range 5–34 years). The same authors performed a CT scan in 28 patients with cystic fibrosis and found in all cases a partial or complete opacification of the anterior complex (anterior ethmoid, maxillary sinus and when developed frontal sinus). In 42% of the patients the posterior complex was free of disease (posterior ethmoid, and—when developed—sphenoid sinus).

Initially, radical surgery for nasal polyposis in cystic fibrosis was estimated to be necessary and it was advised to remove the polyps as they appeared (2). When nasal obstruction occurred polypectomy was the rule (4). Regrowth, however, was sometimes observed within 3 weeks and many patients had multiple polypectomies going from 1 up to 12 procedures per child (4,7,11). Crockett et al. (1987) (12) was the first to stress the importance of a long-term follow-up (average 5 years) and showed that when intranasal ethmoidectomy and Caldwell-Luc procedures are combined with polypectomy, fewer recurrences and longer symptom-free intervals result. Cepero et al. (5) also advocated Caldwell-Luc procedure in conjunction with polypectomy. Unfortunately as a sublabial antrostomy is contra-indicated in children <10 years (13) a Caldwell-Luc procedure can only be performed in older children and adults.

Since the introduction of endoscopic sinus surgery (14–16), a sublabial antrostomy is not needed any longer to achieve radical surgery. With endoscopic sinus surgery (ESS), because of the optic control, not only more radical surgery can be achieved, but also the morbidity has decreased and the safety increased, all major advantages in pediatric surgery. The first results of this technique in children were reported by Lusk et al. (17). Duplechin et al. (18) reported for the first time the result of this kind of surgery in cystic fibrosis children and afterwards this type of surgery was used more or less successfully by many other authors (18–31). Many of these articles dealing with cystic fibrosis show one or more flaws, such as: no follow-up time mentioned (18,19,21), mixed patient population [cystic fibrosis, isolated polyposis, Woakes syndrome: Triglia et al. (27) cystic fibrosis patient with lung transplantation and sinonasal disease or only sinonasal disease], long term follow-up which is not long term for this disease [3 years (20,25,29); 2 years (24,26); 9 months (23)], inadequate follow-up [by phone (22); by questionnaire (25)], retrospective studies (24), majority of patients not children (21,24,26) or different surgical procedures had been performed [mostly endoscopic antrostomy with or without irrigation catheters, frontal trephination, transantral ethmoidectomy (24)] and the number of patients and average age not mentioned (29).

The aim of this study was to evaluate (subjective and objective evaluation done by one single ENT specialist) in a prospective way the long-term results (average follow-up time 8 years) of extensive sinus procedures from sinonasal polyposis in a pediatric population of cystic fibrosis patients suffering from sinonasal polyposis.

I. Material and Methods

A. Patients

All patients were seen before surgery and followed after surgery by one staff member of the ENT department who did not perform the surgery himself, but assisted all the surgical procedures. In all children a careful ENT history was taken as well as an endoscopic nasal examination and a CT scan before surgery. Thirty-five endoscopic ethmoidectomies were performed in 21 patients (mainly children). The average age was 8.7 years (3 months to 27 years) at the time of the first surgery.

All patients belong to a population of ± 100 cystic fibrosis patients who are followed continuously by the pneumologist in the pediatric department (life-time follow-up). The diagnoses of cystic fibrosis were confirmed in all cases by a positive sweat test. In all children endoscopic total sphenoidectomy was performed under general hypotensive anaesthesia. All operations were performed by one experienced ESS surgeon.

The number of recurrences was determined by history and nasal endoscopy. This prospective study was started in 1977 and ended in 1995.

B. Indications for Surgery

Indications for surgery were based mainly on history (referred to the ENT department by the paediatricians, because of medical therapy-resistant complaints, signs and symptoms), ENT examination and CT scan of the sinuses. All patients showed a satisfactory respiratory and nutritional status. An extensive nasal endoscopy was performed with a rigid 2.8 or 4 mm Panoview Wolf endoscope just prior to surgery, while the patient was already under general anaesthesia.

C. Postoperative Care

The postoperative care consisted in frequent cleansing of the nasal cavity after surgery, nasal lavage and antibiotic therapy. All the postoperative care was carried out again by the staff member, who did not perform the surgery.

II. Results

A. Complaints Before Surgery

The most common complaints ($n = 21$) at first consultation and ranked according to the frequency of occurrence were: nasal obstruction (94%), recurrent spells of acute rhinosinusitis (85%), rhinorrhea (75%), headache (69%) and poor quality of sleep (62%). The youngest patient was referred at the age of 3 months because of a failure to thrive caused by poor nutrition due to complete nasal obstruction which was not present at birth but occurred later, and at the time of surgery was accompanied by stridor.

In the older children it was the discomfort caused by the aforementioned complaints that resulted in chronic fatigue, decreased ability to concentrate and poor school results.

B. Signs and Symptoms Before Surgery

Again ranked according to frequency of occurrence, the sign that was always present was mouth breathing (100%), broadened nasal dorsum (72%), high arched palate and hypertrophy of the gum (22%).

During endoscopy nasal obstruction after decongestion was still present in 86%. The nasal obstruction was due to massive polyposis in 72% of the cases and to medialisation of the nasal lateral wall of the remaining 28% of the cases. Purulent secretions were seen in 67% and concomitant septal deviation in 44%. One case showed the presence of a unilateral antrochoanal polyp.

Main indications for surgery: recurrent spells of rhinosinusitis, rhinorrhea and sleep disturbances due to nasal obstructions.

In two older patients the indications for surgery had been headache caused by localised recurrence of polyps due to compartmentalisation of the frontal recess region and in one child surgery was necessary because of acute dacrycystitis due to a huge ethmoidal pyocoele, compressing the nasolacrimal duct on one side.

C. Associated Procedures

Apart from the complete spheno-ethmoidectomy, three septoplasties were performed because of severe septal deviation, obstructing one nasal cavity. Because of severe polypous degeneration of the middle turbinate three partial medial conchotomies, and eight nearly complete medical turbinectomies were performed. (If this septal deviation was not corrected it would continue to impair nasal breathing and it would make postoperative care on that side impossible.)

D. Results of the Surgery

Three to six months after surgery there was a 100% decrease of the nasal obstruction (main preoperative complaint). The quality of sleep and the daytime somnolence was also improved in 60%. The complaints of headache had mostly disappeared in 80% but some patients still complained of partial or total anosmia (20%), rhinorrhea (40%) and recurrent spells of rhinosinusitis (65%). Rhinoscopy showed persistent purulent secretions in practically all children. Two patients did not show any recurrence of polyps during that period, 12 showed limited recurrence. In three cases a massive recurrence was seen at 6 months after surgery, again resulting in severe nasal obstruction.

E.   Long-Term Follow-Up (Table 36.1)

The average follow-up was 7 years (9 months to 10 years). In that period surgery was performed 35 times in 21 children. Massive recurrence justifying repeated surgery was seen in 42% of the cases. Therefore, the number of operations for each child averaged 1.6 (one to four operations). Twelve patients (58%) were completely free of recurrence and needed no further surgery. Six children (29%) all younger than 10 years at the time of the first surgery showed recurrent massive polyposis. Three of these (14%) had more than one recurrence. The duration between the first and the second surgery (average 1.5 years, 6 months to 4 years) was always shorter than between the second and third surgery (average 4 years, in three cases only), or between the third and the fourth

Table 36.1   Long-Term Follow-Up of ESS in Cystic Fibrosis

Age at first surgery	Age at second surgery	Age at third surgery	Age at fourth surgery	Average follow-up time (years)
0	3			6
2				4
4				4
4	4			10
4	4	10		7
4	5	10		10
4	8	10	14	8
5	7	11		12
6	10			10
6				8
6				5
7				2
10				2
10				6
11				5
13				3
14				12
15				5
15				8
27				5
			Mean	6.6

surgery (4 years, in one case). Two older patients (10%) aged 12 and 15 years, respectively, at the time of the first surgery, showed localised recurrence in the frontal recess as mentioned before three and seven years after the initial surgery.

III. Discussion

Stern et al. (7) claimed that in 31% of the patients with massive polyposis in cystic fibrosis spontaneous and permanent disappearance of polyps occurs. In view of this statement one can wonder if surgery in these children is necessary at all, as spontaneous and permanent disappearance seems to be the natural evolution of the disease. This statement highlights the necessity to know more about the natural history of massive polyposis in cystic fibrosis children. Brihaye et al. (10) endoscopically studied a population of 84 cystic fibrosis patients. They found medial bulging of lateral nasal wall in 10 children (12%, six males and four females, mean age 5 years, range: 3 months to 8 years), inflammatory polyps coming out of the middle meatus in 30 patients (45%, 28 males and 10 females, mean age 15 years, range 5–34 years). These observations on the prevalence of the disease related to the age tell something about the natural history of the disease. It seems that the disease starts at early age (0–10 years) with a medialisation of the lateral nasal wall due to a mucopyosinusitis of the maxillary sinus, followed by nasal polyposis at later age (5–20 years), protruding from the middle meatus (mean age 15 years). The authors had seen CT evidence that at later age some patients show a kind of spontaneous ethmoidectomy with limited polyposis. So it seems that Stern et al. (7) are right in their statement on spontaneous improvement of the nasal polyposis in adult age (spontaneous and permanent disappearance however was not observed by the authors). Therefore, the remark of Marks (30) on the article of Nishioka et al. (25) that asymptomatic and minimally symptomatic patients with cystic fibrosis should not undergo sinus surgery and that extreme caution should be used before electing to operate on symptomatic patients with cystic fibrosis, looks meaningful. On the other hand in children with complete nasal obstruction resulting in facial deformation of the nasal dorsum and formation of a high arched palate and in a poor quality of life, or in the infant with respiratory distress and feeding disturbance, even the most conservative ENT surgeon or paediatrician will agree that surgery is the only alternative. One can of course argue that maybe a simple polypectomy is sufficient and complete sphenoidectomy is not necessary (4).

One sees, however, a very high recurrence rate of the polyposis in the series of patients treated only with polypectomy [61% Cepero et al. (5), 72% Schwachmann et al. 1962 (4), 87% Reilly et al. (11)]. When combining intranasal ethmoidectomy with Caldwell-Luc the recurrence rate dropped dramatically [12% Cepero et al. (5), 35% Crockett et al. (12)].

With the introduction of endoscopic sinus surgery, surgery became even more radical because of a better visualisation of the disease, and the morbidity decreased in such a way that the surgery can also be performed in children and young infants. The youngest patient ever operated upon in the literature (28) was a 13-month-old girl. She was operated upon because of nasal obstruction caused by medial displacement of the lateral nasal wall. The same condition was seen by the authors of this article in a 3-month-old boy, resulting in total nasal obstruction and stridor. Tunkel et al. (28) called this condition maxillary sinus mucocoeles. It is our opinion, however, that this condition is not caused by mucocoeles, but by mucopyosinusitis. The mucosa of the maxillary sinus shows already polypous degeneration (not found in mucocoeles) and the lumen is filled with the typical puttylike purulent secretions. Because of ostial dysfunction the pressure in the maxillary sinus increases and the nasal lateral wall is displaced medially. Parson (29) stated that the extent of intranasal surgery of polyposis was found to be inversely proportional to the recurrence rate. Even with a total sphenoidectomy, the recurrence rate will still be high if the follow-up time is long enough. Those articles that deal with long-term results (average of 2–3 years) showed recurrence rates of $\pm 50\%$ (25,26,29). The authors confirmed that the longer the follow-up is the higher the recurrence rate will be. In our series, the patients with no recurrence had an average follow-up of 5 years, those with one recurrence 8 years, two recurrences 9 years and the only one with three recurrences had a 12-year follow-up period. Also important, however, for the recurrence rate is the age at which the first surgery took place. The average age of the 12 patients with no recurrence was 11 years, with one recurrence 8 years, with two recurrences 5 years, and the one with three recurrences was also 5 years of age at the time of the first surgery.

So, the younger the child is at the first surgery, the higher the odds are to have a recurrence. Two factors may be responsible for this observation. First, it may be that an early nasal manifestation of cystic fibrosis represents a more aggressive type of the disease and/or second, it may also be that the after care in these young children (average 5 years of age) is very difficult and not adequate to prevent early recurrence (several general anesthesias are required for an adequate cleansing of the nasal cavity after surgery). The exception, however, confirms the rule. Some children were operated on at a very young age for nasal polyposis and they remained free of recurrence during a long follow-up time (one child was operated on for the first time at age 4 and was followed-up for 10 years).

Also in the authors' experience endoscopic sinus surgery for nasal polyposis in children with cystic fibrosis proved to be a safe technique. Two cases showed postoperative temperature that disappeared the day after surgery when the packing was removed. One case had an easy-to-control postoperative bleeding and another case showed a benign heart arrhythmia during the first postoperative day. Finally one patient showed a temporary ozaena for 6 months.

Due to the lower morbidity and better visualisation of the pathology during surgery, ESS is definitely a better (more radical and safer) technique than the headlight intranasal ethmoidectomy. Combined with hypotensive anaesthesia the safety is even higher (less bleeding results and better visualisation) and the blood loss can be limited on average to 130 mL (20–200 mL).

In conclusion, one can state that in consideration of the good clinical results (major improvement of the quality of life) and the absence of major complications (in the hands of an experienced surgeon) ESS in children with cystic fibrosis seems to be a better option than repeated polypectomies and/or headlight intranasal ethmoidectomy with or without Caldwell-Luc.

References

1. Vaughan VC, McKay RJ. Cystic fibrosis. The digestive system. In: Vaughan VC, McKay RJ, eds. Nelso WE, coed. Nelson Textboook of Pediatrics. Vol. 11. Philadelphia, PA: WB Saunders Company, 1975:906.
2. Lurie MH. Cystic fibrosis of the pancreas and nasal mucosa. Ann Otorhinolaryngol 1959; 478–486.
3. Lanoff G, Daddeno A, Johnson E. Nasal polyps in children: a ten-year study. Ann Allergy 1973; 31:551–554.
4. Schwachman H, Kulczycki LL, Mueller HL, Flake CG. Nasal polyposis in patients with cystic fibrosis. Pediatrics 1962; 389–401.
5. Cepero R, Smith RJH, Catlin FI, Bressler KL, Furruta GT, Shandeera KC. Cystic fibrosis: an otolaryngologic perspective. Otolaryngol Head Neck Surg 1987; 97(4):356–360.
6. Neely JG, Harrison GM, Jerger JF, Greenberg SD, Presberg H. The otolaryngologic aspects of cystic fibrosis. Trans Am Acad Ophthalmol Otol 1975; 76:313–324.
7. Stern RC, Boat TF, Wood RE, Matthews LW, Doershuk CF. Treatment and prognosis of nasal polyps in cystic fibrosis. Am J Dis Child 1982; 136:1067–1070.
8. Settipane GA. Nasal polyps. In: Settipane GA, ed. Rhinitis. Vol. 12. The New England and Regional Allergy Proceedings, Providence, RI, 1984:133–140.
9. Deane PMG, Schwartz RH. Nasal polyps in cystic fibrosis. In: Settipane GA, Lund VJ, Bernstein JM, Tos M, eds. Nasal Polyps: Epidemiology, Pathogenesis and Treatment. Vol. 17. Providence, RI, Oceanside Publications Inc., 1997:137–146.
10. Brihaye P, Clement PAR, Dab I, Desprechin B. Pathological changes of the lateral nasal wall in patients with cystic fibrosis (mucoviscidosis). Pediatr Otorhinolaryngol 1994; 28:141–147.
11. Reilly JS, Kenna MA, Stool SE, Bluestone CD. Nasal surgery in children with cystic fibrosis: complications and risk management. Laryngoscope 1985; 95:1491–1493.
12. Crockett DM, McGill TJ, Healy GB, Friedman EM, Salkeld LJ. Nasal and paranasal sinus surgery in children with cystic fibrosis. Ann Otorhinolaryngol 1987; 96:367–372.
13. Shurin PA. Inflammatory diseases of the nose and paranasal sinuses. In: Bluestone CD, Stool SE, Arjona, eds. Peditric Otolaryngology. Vol. 32. Philadelphia, PA: WB Saunders Company, 1983:781–790.
14. Kennedy DW. Functional endoscopic sinus surgery: technique. Arch Otolaryngol 1985; 111:643–649.

15. Stammberger H. Endoscopic endonasal surgery: concept in treatment of recurring rhinosinusitis—surgical technique. Otolaryngol Head Neck Surg 1986; 14:147–156.
16. Wigand ME. Transnasal ethmoidectomy under endoscopical control. Rhinology 1981; 19:7–15.
17. Lusk RP, Muntz HR. Endoscopic sinus surgery in children with chronic sinusitis: a pilot study. Laryngoscope 1990; 100:654–658.
18. Duplechain JK, White JA. Pediatric sinusitis. The role of endoscopic sinus surgery in cystic fibrosis and other forms of sinonasal disease. Arch Otolaryngol Head Neck Surg 1991; 117:422–426.
19. Cuyler JP, Monaghan AJ. Cystic fibrosis and sinusitis. J Otolaryngol 1989; 18(4):173–175.
20. Cuyler JP. Follow-up of endoscopic sinus surgery on children with cystic fibrosis. Arch Otolaryngol Head Neck Surg 1992; 118:505–506.
21. Davidson TM, Murphy C, Mitchell M, Smith C, Light M. Management of chronic sinusitis in cystic fibrosis. Laryngoscope 1995; 105:354–358.
22. Jones JW, Parsons DS, Cuyler JP. The results of functional endoscopic sinus (FESS) surgery on symptoms of patients with cystic fibrosis. Int J Pediatr Otorhinolaryngol 1993; 28:25–32.
23. Mark SC, Kissner DG. Management of sinusitis in adult cystic fibrosis. Am J Rhino 1997; 11:11–14.
24. Moss RB, King VV. Management of sinusitis in cystic fibrosis by endoscopic surgery and serial antimicrobial lavage. Arch Otolaryngol Head Neck Surg 1995; 121:566–571.
25. Nishioka GJ, Barbero GJ, König P, Parsons DS, Cook PR, Davis WE. Symptom outcome after functional endoscopic sinus surgery in patients with cystic fibrosis: a prospective study. Otolaryngol Head Neck Surg 1995; 113:440–445.
26. Rowe-Jones JM, MacKay IS. Endoscopic sinus surgery in the treatment of cystic fibrosis with nasal polyposis. Laryngoscope 1996; 106:1540–1544.
27. Triglia JM, Dessi P, Cannoni M, Peck A. Intranasal ethmoidectomy in nasal polyposis in children: indications and results. Int J Pediatr Otorhinolaryngol 1993; 23:125–131.
28. Tunkel DE, Naclerio RM, Baroody FM, Rosenstein BJ. Bilateral maxillary sinus mucoceles in an infant with cystic fibrosis. Head Neck Surg 1994; 111:116–120.
29. Parsons DS. Sinusitis and cystic fibrosis. In: Lusk RP, ed. Pediatric Sinusitis. Vol. 8. New York: Raven Press, 1992:65–70.
30. Marks S. Endoscopic sinus surgery in patients with cystic fibrosis. Otolaryngol Head Neck Surg 1996; 114:840–841.
31. Lusk RP. Pediatric endoscopic ethmoidectomy. In: Bluestone CD, Stool SE, eds. Atlas of Pediatric Otolaryngology. Vol. 13. Philadelphia, PA: WB Saunders Company, 1995:310–332.

Index